Eating Disorders in Women and Children

Prevention, Stress Management, and Treatment

Second Edition

Eating Disorders in Women and Children

Prevention, Stress Management, and Treatment

Second Edition

Edited by
Kristin L. Goodheart, James R. Clopton
Jacalyn J. Robert-McComb

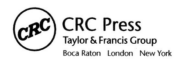

CRC Press
Taylor & Francis Group
Boca Raton   London   New York

CRC Press is an imprint of the
Taylor & Francis Group, an **informa** business

CRC Press
Taylor & Francis Group
6000 Broken Sound Parkway NW, Suite 300
Boca Raton, FL 33487-2742

© 2012 by Taylor & Francis Group, LLC
CRC Press is an imprint of Taylor & Francis Group, an Informa business

No claim to original U.S. Government works

Printed in the United States of America on acid-free paper
Version Date: 2011912

International Standard Book Number: 978-1-4398-2481-8 (Hardback)

Library of Congress Cataloging-in-Publication Data

Eating disorders in women and children : prevention, stress management, and treatment, second edition / editors, Kristin L. Goodheart, James R. Clopton, Jacalyn J. Robert-McComb. -- 2nd ed.
    p. cm.
  Includes bibliographical references and index.
  ISBN 978-1-4398-2481-8 (hardback)
  1. Eating disorders. 2. Eating disorders in children. 3. Women--Mental health. 4. Child mental health. 5. Stress management. I. Goodheart, Kristin L. II. Clopton, James R. III. Robert-McComb, Jacalyn J.

RC552.E18E2835 2011
618.92'8526--dc23
                                                  2011035863

Visit the Taylor & Francis Web site at
http://www.taylorandfrancis.com

and the CRC Press Web site at
http://www.crcpress.com

For the brave women working to overcome their eating problems, and for the friends and family members who support them, just as my friends and family supported me.

Kristin L. Goodheart

To Jane L. Winer and Kristin L. Goodheart, two remarkable individuals who made this book possible, each in her own special way. My collaboration on research and writing projects with Jacalyn Robert-McComb began when Jane introduced us and suggested that we work together. As Dean of Arts and Sciences at Texas Tech, she was exceptionally encouraging of faculty and skillful in bringing together people with similar interests.

Kristin's involvement with this book began over two years ago when she was asked to co-author one of the chapters. Due to her diligent and steady work, her impressive knowledge of eating disorders, and her maturity and good judgment, she became a co-editor for the book. Kristin's involvement in the editing and the writing of this book was indispensible. I am so grateful for the many ways in which she is devoted to providing hope to those individuals who have eating disorders.

Jim Clopton

To the two most important men in my life, my father, Vernon Robert, who died of cancer on August 8, 2010, while I was working on this book, and my faithful and loving husband, Robert McComb. I would also like to dedicate this book to women who have suffered the loss of someone they love.

Jacalyn Robert-McComb

In Memory of John Rohwer

John was truly devoted to children's health. He wrote two chapters for the first edition of this book, revised those chapters for this edition, and was a dependable and conscientious colleague throughout the work on these books. John died on December 25, 2010, of injuries from an accidental fall from his roof on Christmas Eve while shoveling snow. The editors join his family, friends, and other colleagues in honoring his life.

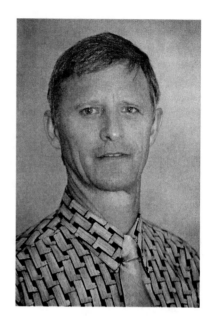

Contents*

PART I: Identifying and Understanding Eating Disorders

PART II: The Characteristics of Stress

PART III: Society and Eating Disorders

---

* The CD that accompanies this book contains a PowerPoint® presentation for each chapter.

PART VI: Therapeutic Approaches to the Treatment of Eating Disorders

Foreword

When I was a young woman being treated for an eating disorder, certain assumptions were made. If you had an eating disorder, you would be a white adolescent girl from a family with a controlling mother and an absent father. You would display a passive personality and low self-esteem. You would in all likelihood have signs of depression; whether you did or not, you would probably be treated for it. Your treatment team would see and treat you as childish and immature, and hold a variety of vague and often unfounded opinions about who you were, where you'd been, and what kind of chances of recovery you had. Those chances were considered, almost across the board, very low indeed.

I was treated for eating disorders in the 1980s and 1990s. The medical and therapeutic understanding of the etiology, nature, and treatment of disordered eating and body image had not changed markedly since the early days of eating disorder research 20 years before. Likewise, the limited understanding of the demographics of eating disordered populations ensured that thousands would go undiagnosed and untreated. While the eating disordered population exploded, research and treatment providers held fast to their notions of what they were dealing with and how they should proceed. Their abysmal success rates bewildered them; they attributed these low rates of recovery to the intractable, probably incurable nature of the diseases.

This second edition of *Eating Disorders in Women and Children: Prevention, Stress Management, and Treatment* is being released into a therapeutic community that has changed in many critical ways, and I believe the community will see further change as a result of the research done here. At the heart of this research is an assumption that was not always made, which must be made if treatment is to have the impact that it can and should have. This book sees the people who struggle with eating disorders as people—as individuals, with individual histories and reasons for developing their disease, and as individuals living in a society that is deeply stressful, and profoundly hospitable to the flourishing of eating disorders in more communities every day.

This book recognizes the multifaceted, multifactorial nature of these diseases, addresses the wide—and widening—demographic range of people who have them, and, importantly, delves into the deeper issues behind their development. This critically insightful perspective has enormous implications for advances in treatment. By exploring in detail the role of stress in eating disordered people's lives, and the use of eating disorders as a means of managing and easing that stress, this edition identifies etiological risk factors, physiological implications, and a range of treatment modalities that help patients create alternative methods of coping in their lives. The practical application of this information suggests enormous hope for an improvement in treatment and real help for the people who so painfully struggle with eating disorders every day.

By also stressing the importance of early identification and prevention—areas far too often overlooked in eating disorder literature—this book not only explores specific ways in which at-risk individuals can be helped but also explores critical measures that can be taken to help the larger population understand and work to prevent eating disorders in their communities. This emphasis goes to the heart of what our society must do if we hope to change our cultural perspective on how these disorders develop, and therefore our understanding of how to prevent their ongoing spread.

This book notes that "dissatisfaction with one's body appears to be ubiquitous for women." What sets this book apart from many others is its emphasis on the critically important factor of the social continuum on which eating disorders exist. Until we truly recognize and acknowledge the fact that body dissatisfaction and disordered eating have pervaded nearly every corner of our society, we will not understand clinical eating disorders. And until we understand the society in which people with eating disorders are developing their illnesses, we will remain unable to treat them effectively.

Eating Disorders in Women and Children: Prevention, Stress Management, and Treatment does—and goes beyond—what new eating disorder literature needs to do. It clearly explicates the nature of the disorders, explores a range of treatment modalities, and identifies critical risk factors; the research on the influence of stress in eating disordered populations published here represents enormously important new insights into the disorders, their treatment, and the people who have them.

In recognizing and exploring the individuality of people with eating disorders, and identifying the disorders' multifaceted social aspects, this book makes a significant contribution to the research currently informing treatment of these diseases. Departing from the tired, and increasingly inaccurate, notions that have so long governed eating disorder research and therapeutic models, this book moves into new territory, and does so with insight that will be of enormous benefit to its readers.

The work contained here has the potential to directly and dramatically improve the lives and recovery processes of real people. Eating disorders are not theoretical fields of research; they are devastating, too-often deadly illnesses, the treatment of which has a long way to go. This book is an enormous and important step in that direction, and it will be critical reading for anyone who hopes to understand, and help, people with eating disorders.

Marya Hornbacher, the author of *Wasted*

Editors

Kristin L. Goodheart, MS, completed her undergraduate and master's degrees at Fort Hays State University in Kansas. Her master's thesis research was on body image in late adolescence, and she has presented the results of that research at several national conferences. Currently, she is completing her PhD in clinical psychology at Texas Tech University and is conducting research about the relationships among shame, perfectionism, and symptoms of eating disorders. Kristin's interest in eating disorders emerged after overcoming a personal struggle with an eating disorder. Her positive experience of working with a psychologist inspired her current career goals. Kristin's commitment to serving others is reflected in her extensive public speaking, her volunteer work at the Southwest Cancer Center in Lubbock, Texas, and her service as co-president of the Clinical Psychology Graduate Student Council at Texas Tech University. Eventually, Kristin wants to have a private practice and work with a variety of people, especially people who are affected by dysfunctional relationships with food.

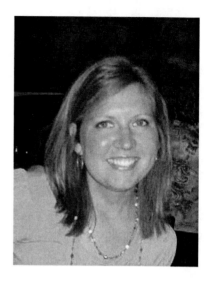

James R. Clopton, PhD, is a professor in clinical psychology at Texas Tech University. He is a licensed psychologist with over 20 years experience doing psychotherapy and psychological assessment with children, adolescents, and adults. After earning his PhD, he worked for 2 years in full-time clinical practice, mostly with children. During this time, he regularly received referrals from pediatricians to work with overweight children and their parents. That work led to an opportunity to work with a young woman with anorexia. The success of that courageous teenager was pivotal in encouraging his early interest in eating disorders. Over the years since then, a series of graduate students, beginning with Jan Kent, have asked Dr. Clopton to supervise their research on eating disorders. He is grateful for the opportunity to collaborate with Dr. McComb during the past 10 years, which led to the privilege of working on this book.

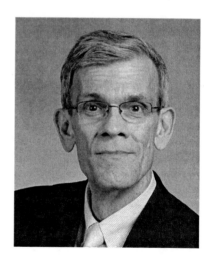

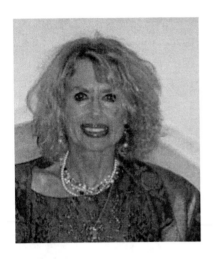

Jacalyn J. Robert-McComb, PhD, FACSM, is a professor of exercise physiology at Texas Tech University. She is certified by the American College of Sports Medicine as a Clinical Program Director (PD) and Clinical Exercise Specialist (CES). Her research interest is in teaching others to cope with the stressors in their daily lives through mindfulness-based exercise programs. She understands all too well the plight that young girls and women are going through in their struggle to find self-acceptance. As a young girl, she struggled with an eating disorder. Very little was known about the cause or the treatment of this disorder in her small hometown. It was through prayer and meditation, healthy exercise, and continual self-acceptance and renewal that she found the strength to change the behaviors associated with eating disorders. She became a professional athlete in spite of her struggles. However, this feat could never be accomplished alone; it took loving and caring parents, siblings, and friends, professional counselors, and others to share their stories through educational outlets. Hence, the inspiration for this book.

Contributors

Marcia M. Abbott, PhD
Private Practice
Lubbock, Texas

Barbara A. Barton, MPH, RN, CHES
Department of Health Studies
Texas Woman's University
Denton, Texas

Vanessa Bayer, MA
Department of Psychology
Texas Tech University
Lubbock, Texas

Julie Campbell-Ruggaard, PhD, RN, LPCC
Private Practice
Oxford, Ohio

James R. Clopton, PhD
Department of Psychology
Texas Tech University
Lubbock, Texas

Vanessa A. Coca-Lyle, BS
Department of Psychology
Texas Tech University
Lubbock, Texas

Angela Coker, PhD
Division of Counseling and Family
   Therapy
University of Missouri—St. Louis
St. Louis, Missouri

Stephen W. Cook, PhD
Department of Psychology
Texas Tech University
Lubbock, Texas

Brigitte Curtis, MD
Private Practice
Lubbock, Texas

Amanda J. Danielson, BA
Food Science and Human Nutrition
University of Wyoming
Laramie, Wyoming

Sheila Garos, PhD
Department of Psychology
Texas Tech University
Lubbock, Texas

Annette Gary, RN, PhD
Lubbock Regional MHMR Center
Lubbock, Texas

Heather L. Gibson, PhD
Private Practice
Ventura, California

Mandy Golman, PhD
Department of Health Studies
Texas Woman's University
Denton, Texas

Kristin L. Goodheart, MS
Department of Psychology
Texas Tech University
Lubbock, Texas

Stephanie L. Harter, PhD
Department of Psychology
Texas Tech University
Lubbock, Texas

Marta L. Hoes, BA
School of Law and School of Medicine
Texas Tech University
Lubbock, Texas

Deidre J. Holland, MPH, CHES
Department of Health Studies
Texas Woman's University
Denton, Texas

Hsin-hsin Huang, PhD
Social Work Department
Southern Illinois University—Edwardsville
Edwardsville, Illinois

Lucy Johnson, MEd
Auburn University
Auburn, Alabama

Susan Kashubeck-West, PhD
Division of Counseling and Family Therapy
University of Missouri—St. Louis
St. Louis, Missouri

Jan Snider Kent, PhD
Herndon Snider & Associates
Joplin, Missouri

Annette S. Kluck, PhD
Counseling Psychology
Auburn University
Auburn, Alabama

**Marilyn Massey-Stokes, EdD, CHES,
    FASHA, IC®**
Department of Health Studies
Texas Woman's University
Denton, Texas

Brittany McCullough, MS
Physical Medicine & Rehabilitation
University Medical Center
Lubbock, Texas

Jacalyn J. Robert-McComb, PhD, FACSM
Department of Health, Exercise, and Sport
    Sciences
Texas Tech University
Lubbock, Texas

John L. Rohwer, EdD†
Health and Human Performance Department
University of St. Thomas
St. Paul, Minnesota

Stephanie Rushing, MS, RD, LD, CEDRD
Private Practice
Dallas, Texas

Kendra Saunders, PhD
Millersville University
Millersville, Pennsylvania

Sean B. Stokes, PhD, LPC, LMFT
Texas Wesleyan University
Ft. Worth, Texas

Anna M. Tacón, PhD
Department of Health, Exercise, and Sport
    Sciences
Texas Tech University
Lubbock, Texas

Ann A. Thompson, PhD, RD, LD
Private Practice
Lubbock, Texas

Cathy L. Thompson, PhD
Federal Bureau of Prisons
Annapolis Junction, Maryland

Lindsay Wilson-Barlow, BA
Department of Psychology
Texas Tech University
Lubbock, Texas

Brett Owen Young, MS
Lifestyle Centre (Wellheart)
Covenant Health System
Lubbock, Texas

---

† Deceased

Part I

Identifying and Understanding Eating Disorders

1 An Overview of Eating Disorders

Jacalyn J. Robert-McComb, Lindsay Wilson-Barlow, and Kristin L. Goodheart

CONTENTS

1.1 LEARNING OBJECTIVES

After reading this chapter you should be able to

- Discuss the significance of an eating disorder
- Describe the varying types of eating disorders
- Identify the risk factors that contribute to the development of an eating disorder
- Identify differentiating and similar signs and symptoms of each disorder
- Explain how the SCOFF questionnaire is used to identify eating disorders

1.2   BACKGROUND AND SIGNIFICANCE

Eating disorders (EDs) are psychological disorders that are characterized by abnormal eating, dys-functional relationships with food, and a preoccupation with one's weight and shape. EDs affect daily functioning and often result in physical complications and psychological distress (American Psychiatric Association [APA] 2000). The current *Diagnostic and Statistical Manual of Mental Disorders* (*DSM-IV-TR*, APA 2000) recognizes two specific EDs: anorexia nervosa (AN) and bulimia nervosa (BN). There are two subtypes associated with each specific ED: anorexia nervosa, restricting type (AN-R); anorexia nervosa, binge/purge type (AN-BP); bulimia nervosa, purging type (BN-P); and bulimia nervosa, nonpurging type (BN-N). A third category, eating disorder not otherwise specified (EDNOS), is included for EDs of clinical significance that do not meet criteria for AN or BN. Within this broad category, there are currently three subdivisions: (1) binge eating disorder (BED), which is currently under review and has been recommended to be included in the *DSM-V* as a specific clinical ED (Wilfley et al. 2007); (2) subthreshold AN or BN (i.e., disorders very similar in symptoms or presentation to either AN or BN but not fully meeting the criteria for a diagnosis of either disorder); and (3) disorders with symptoms of both AN and BN but again not meeting the criteria for either disorder (Fairburn et al. 2007). Additionally, it has been recom-mended that purging disorder (PD) be included in the *DSM-V* under the EDNOS classification for further review so that the appropriateness of including PD as a full-threshold ED can be determined (Keel 2007).

It is difficult to estimate the true prevalence of EDs due to underreporting (Herpertz-Dahlmann 2008; Hoek 2006). Even with considerable underreporting, the incidence of EDs has increased over the past 50 years. Increase in the prevalence of EDs might be due to improved understanding of the symptomatology and risk factors, as well as changes in diagnostic criteria, referral practices, and accessibility to help (Hoek 2006).

Generally, the incidence of EDs decreases with age. Many young people suffer from some form of disordered eating, whereas the incidence of EDs in women ranges from 0.5% to 3% (Pearson et al. 2002; van Hoeken et al. 2003). Even though these numbers might seem low, this incidence rate is problematic as EDs are commonly listed in the top 10 causes of disability and mental ill-ness in young women (Stice et al. 2007; Striegel-Moore and Bulik 2007). Frequently, the onset age for AN and BN is between 15 and 19 (Bulik et al. 2005; Pearson et al. 2002; Stice et al. 2006, 2007). Although EDs and body dissatisfaction are typical for young women, they can occur in older women. In a randomly selected nonclinical sample of 1,000 women aged 60–70 years, more than 80% used strategies to control their weights and over 60% reported body dissatisfaction. Eighteen women (3.8%) met the criteria for an ED (Mangweth-Matzek et al. 2006). Because EDs can develop when people experience life transitions, are independent, and have an ample amount of privacy (Treasure 2008), one possible reason that some older women have EDs is because they have lost their spouses, are living alone, and are at a time of transition in their lives.

As one ages, there is also a slight change in the expression of EDs. Adolescents and young women are more likely to show signs and symptoms related to AN and BN, whereas older adults may exhibit signs and symptoms more closely aligned to BED (Stice et al. 2006, Striegel-Moore and Bulik 2007). These differences may exist because young people are more likely than older people to internalize cognitive distortions about body image and pressure from society to be thin (Hoek 2006).

At any age, EDs are complex, serious, maladaptive, and result in adverse health consequences (APA 2000; Herpertz-Dahlmann 2008; O'Brien and Vincent 2003). Eating disturbances that do not meet full criteria for a clinical ED are associated with elevated risk of depression, anxiety disorders, substance abuse, or health complications (Shaw et al. 2008). EDs typically last several years and tend to have high relapse rates (Shaw et al. 2008; Stice et al. 2007; Treasure 2008). Specifically, the average duration of BN is 8.3 years, and the average duration of BED and subthreshold levels of BED is 8.1 years and 7.2 years, respectively (Hudson et al. 2007). By the fifth year of the ED, the symptoms, pathology, and the clinical track of the ED will likely stabilize (Tozzi et al. 2005). Unfortunately, the chronicity of EDs can ultimately result in diminished health, decreased psychosocial functioning, and compromised interpersonal interactions (Herpertz-Dahlmann 2008; Shaw et al. 2008; Stice et al. 2007; Striegel-Moore et al. 2003).

Several characteristics that affect health outcomes are represented across EDs. Some of these characteristics include: (1) demographic characteristics, (2) experiences in adolescence, (3) low self-esteem and negative ideations, (4) medical and psychological comorbidity, and (5) issues with weight, shape, and the stereotype of beauty (Berkman et al. 2007). The majority of people with EDs experience other psychological disorders as well. Factors such as swiftness of weight loss, current weight, and chronicity of the ED are related to the intensity of the comorbid illness (Herpertz-Dahlmann 2008). One study found that 56.2% of individuals with AN, 94.5% with BN, 78.9% with BED, and 63.3% with subthreshold BED met the criteria for another mental disorder, most often mood disorders, anxiety disorders, impulse control disorders, or substance use disorders (Hudson et al. 2007). Additionally, some form of personality disorder affects between 27% and 93% of ED patients (Cassin and von Ranson 2005; Vitousek and Manke 1994).

Early identification of an ED is associated with shorter duration and fewer medical complications (Uyeda et al. 2002). Unfortunately, recent estimates show that only about 33% of AN patients and 6% of BN patients are receiving proper treatment for their illnesses (Hoek 2006). Comorbidity plays an important role in the treatment of EDs, as people are more likely to seek treatment for their non-ED mental health problems than for the ED itself (Hudson et al. 2007). In clinical settings, women and girls are ten times more likely than men and boys to receive treatment (Herpertz-Dahlmann 2008; Stice et al. 2007; Treasure 2008), but this ratio might not accurately represent the number of men and boys compared to women and girls who actually have EDs (Treasure 2008). Thus, increased understanding of EDs is imperative so that treatment for people with EDs is more accessible and more effective.

1.3 CURRENT FINDINGS

1.3.1 ANOREXIA NERVOSA

Anorexia nervosa (AN) is a drastic reduction in eating resulting in very low body weight (Treasure 2007). Although patients with AN consume food, they eat with extreme limitations. Strict calorie and food restriction, as well as obsessive exercise, can produce an unhealthy level of weight loss in AN patients (Herpertz-Dahlmann 2008; Treasure 2007). AN, particularly the restricting type (AN-R), is the most rare form of ED.

It is unclear if the prevalence rate for AN is increasing or has stabilized at this time (Bulik et al. 2006; Hoek 2006; Hudson et al. 2007). Prevalence rates for AN in westernized countries have been reported to range from 0.3% to 1.5%, and the prevalence of subthreshold AN is slightly higher, ranging from 0.37% to 3.0% (Berkman et al. 2007; Bulik et al. 2005, 2006; Bulik, Slof-Op't Landt et al. 2007; Gowers and Bryant-Waugh 2004;, Hudson et al. 2007; Steinhausen 2002; Stice et al. 2006; Treasure 2008). Up to 40% of all individuals with AN are young women between the ages 15 and 19 (Gowers and Bryant-Waugh 2004; van Hoeken et al. 2003), and the discrepancies traditionally seen in prevalence rates of AN in westernized versus developing countries and Caucasians versus ethnic minorities seem to be dissipating (Hoek 2006).

Chronicity of EDs has long been identified as a problem. Personality traits like obsessive-compulsiveness and maladaptive behaviors like self-induced vomiting, cycles of binge eating and purging, and the misuse of laxatives and substances that can induce purging have all been linked to the chronicity of EDs (Steinhausen 2002). AN patients experience varied courses of the illness. For some, the duration of the illness is shorter, whereas for others, the experience is chronic and fluctuates between temporary periods of remission and relapse (Bulik et al. 2005). Patients with AN typically deny the existence of the ED and present their condition to medical personnel as a physical problem or a different type of psychological problem in order to mask the ED (Currin et al. 2007; Herpertz-Dahlmann 2008; Treasure 2008). Many AN patients lack the willingness to change, even if they recognize the dangers of their ED. Unfortunately, resistance to intervention makes it difficult to treat these patients and can increase chronicity of the illness (Herpertz-Dahlmann 2008; Treasure 2008).

Crossover from one form of ED to another is fairly common. It has been estimated that between 8% and 62% of patients with AN eventually crossover to BN (Bulik et al. 2005; Tozzi et al. 2005). The highest percentage of crossover occurs when restricting AN patients crossover to the binge/purge subtype of AN (AN-BP) or to BN (Herpertz-Dahlmann 2008; Tozzi et al. 2005). Additionally, BN can crossover to BED (Fichter et al. 2005; Striegel-Moore and Bulik 2007). Crossover from one ED to another typically occurs during the first five years of the illness; after 10 years, the rate of crossover is substantially reduced (Bulik et al. 2005; Herpertz-Dahlmann 2008). Furthermore, certain personality traits in AN patients, such as novelty seeking and low self-directedness, have been associated with higher crossover probability compared to other AN patients without these traits (Wonderlich et al. 2005).

A combination of genetics, environmental factors, and specific personality traits likely contributes to the development and maintenance of AN (Karwautz et al. 2001). Research suggests that personality disorders most commonly associated with AN-R include avoidant, dependant, obsessive-compulsive, and borderline personality disorders (Bornstein 2001; Cassin and von Ranson 2005). Additionally, anxiety and mood disorders affect about 25% of people with AN (Steinhausen 2002), and comorbid conditions like depression, anxiety, phobias, and personality disorders might contribute to worse outcomes for AN patients (Steinhausen 2002).

1.3.1.1 Diagnostic Criteria for Anorexia Nervosa

DSM-IV-TR (APA 2000) includes specific diagnostic criteria for AN. Initially, the individual must be at a weight that is 85% or less of her expected weight, based on her height and her age. Additionally, individuals who have started menstruating will develop amenorrhea. For those girls who have not reached menarche, they will typically fail to begin menstruating at the expected time. Psychological criteria include extreme disturbance in self-perception of the body and an overwhelming fear of fatness. AN patients can be further subdivided into two subtypes: restricting subtype (AN-R) and binge/purge subtype (AN-BP). The AN-R subtype describes those individuals who severely restrict their food intake and do not use compensatory behaviors, like self-induced vomiting, to compensate for calories consumed. The AN-BP subtype is diagnosed when periods of restriction are accompanied by periods of overeating and extreme compensatory purging behaviors, like self-induced vomiting.

Some question the validity of the diagnostic criteria for AN that are included in the *DSM-IV-TR*. The strongest debate has risen regarding the inclusion of amenorrhea. Some suggest that the differences between AN patients who do and do not menstruate are very limited (Cachelin and Maher 1998; Garfinkel et al. 1996; Striegel-Moore and Marcus 1995). Additionally, a large number of females use birth control or other substances that affect hormones, so it can be difficult to determine if a woman would develop amenorrhea if she were not using these substances (Herpertz-Dahlmann 2008). Although some argue that fear of weight is a classic feature of AN, this fear may not be present in all individuals with AN (Wonderlich et al. 2007). Furthermore, the subtypes associated with AN have been questioned. The AN-R and AN-BP subtypes were originally differentiated because women in these two subgroups were thought to be different in terms of comorbidity and recovery cycles, but recent evidence suggests that the current separation might not be needed (Wonderlich et al. 2007). Still, others have pushed to eliminate the AN-BP subtype all together and limit AN to only those individuals who severely restrict their food intake, and to include AN-BP with BN and include a low-weight specifier (Gordon et al. 2007).

Another commonly used classification system for EDs and other illnesses is the 10th edition of the *International Classification of Diseases* (ICD-10). The ICD-10 specifies that patients with AN have a body mass index (BMI) equal to or below 17.5, which is well below the healthy range (18.5–24.9; World Health Organization 1992). Other ICD-10 criteria for AN include amenorrhea, weight loss that is self-induced and purposeful, a fear of fatness, and a perception of being fat. Unlike the *DSM-IV-TR* classification, the ICD-10 specifies that binge eating is an exclusionary criteria for AN. The ICD-10 criteria are based on behavioral symptoms and methods of weight loss, in contrast to the *DSM-IV-TR* that emphasizes psychological distortions and disturbances (Bulik et al. 2005; WHO 1992). Table 1.1 presents a comparison of the DSM and ICD-10 diagnostic criteria for AN.

Some research suggests that AN patients have lower levels of novelty seeking and higher levels of harm avoidance, and both factors can prevent a person from developing binge eating and purging behaviors (Cassin and von Ranson 2005; Fassino et al. 2004). However, AN-BP patients do develop binge eating and purging behaviors, and these behaviors are intermingled with periods of fasting, excessive exercise, and other compensatory behaviors (Herpertz-Dahlmann 2008).

1.3.1.2 Risk Factors for Anorexia Nervosa

It is difficult for researchers to design well-controlled studies for EDs, particularly studies that will distinguish the causes and early signs of EDs. There are multiple reasons for this difficulty. For instance, it is often difficult to accumulate a large enough sample of people with EDs, and AN and BN often consist of similar or overlapping characteristics (Bulik et al. 2005; Karwautz et al. 2001; Pearson et al. 2002). Risk factors for AN can be extrinsic and intrinsic, and these factors can act as a catalyst for AN or help to sustain the illness for a longer duration of time (Karwautz et al. 2001). Thus, it can be difficult to successfully and accurately determine distinct risk factors for each ED.

Female sex is recognized as the greatest risk factor for developing an ED (Striegel-Moore and Bulik 2007). Some argue that girls and women are more susceptible to and more influenced by the thin cultural ideal than boys and men and, therefore, develop EDs more frequently (Polivy and Herman 2002). In fact, the female-to-male ratio is 10:1 (Bulik, Slof-Op't Landt et al. 2007; Kaye et al. 2008; Pearson et al. 2002). Although an increase in the number of males with EDs has been reported, there is debate about whether this change is a rise in the incidence rate or whether mental health professionals are simply more aware of the disorder in men (Pearson et al. 2002). Researchers have recently been surprised by the discrepancy between the high number of men in the community who have AN or BN and the low number that are reported in treatment settings (Hudson et al. 2007).

Past negative life events, including abuse, teasing, or trauma, have been linked to AN (Bulik, Slof-Op't Landt et al. 2007). AN that develops during adolescence is often precipitated by stressful events, such as major life changes, academic pressures, and family conflict (McKnight Investigators 2003; Pike et al. 2006). Harmful and negative comments by loved ones and influential persons (e.g., friends, educators, family, and coaches) about weight and eating may result in binge eating and other eating-related pathology (Bachner-Melman et al. 2009; Karwautz et al. 2001).

Weight concerns, fear of fatness, social influence, distorted body shape, eating concerns, yearning for thinness, and body dissatisfaction are consistently found to be predictors of EDs and lie at the core of AN (Bulik, Slof-Op't Landt et al. 2007; Jansen et al. 2006; Lilenfeld et al. 2006; McKnight Investigators 2003; Shaw et al. 2008). Often, the AN patient is totally preoccupied by thoughts of shape and weight, including obsession about weight gain and the perceived largeness of her body, and she often sees herself as being overweight regardless of how much weight she loses (Bulik et al. 2005; Herpertz-Dahlmann 2008; McKnight Investigators 2003; Stice et al. 2006). Losing weight can be thrilling and challenging for those with AN, and they often have an unparalleled determination to diet and exercise. The endless drive to be thin results in severe caloric restriction and in an abnormally low BMI (Stice et al. 2006). Low past and current BMI are risk factors for AN. Recent studies show that lifetime AN is associated with a current low BMI, with many patients having a current BMI less than 18.5 (Hudson et al. 2007). Parallel to this finding, lightweight girls seem to be at the highest risk of developing AN (Karwautz et al. 2001).

TABLE 1.1

Comparison of *DSM-IV-TR* and ICD-10 Diagnostic Criteria for Anorexia Nervosa

	DSM-IV	ICD-10
Code	307.1	F50.0
Weight	Refusal to maintain body weight at or above minimal normal weight for age and height (e.g., weight loss leading to maintenance of body weight < 85% of expected weight) OR Failure to make expected weight gain during growth period, leading to weight < 85% of expected normal body weight	Body weight is maintained at least 15% below that expected (either lost or never achieved) Quetelets's body mass index is 17.5 kg/m2 or less OR Prepubertal patients may show failure to make the expected weight gain during the period of growth
Phobia/Associated behaviors	Intense fear of gaining weight or becoming fat, even though underweight *DSM-IV* behaviorally differentiates between types: Restricting = not engaging in binge eating or purging behavior Binge eating/purging = regularly engaging in binging or purging behavior	Weight loss self-induced by avoidance of "fattening foods" AND One or more of the following: self-induced vomiting, self-induced purging, excessive exercise, use of appetite suppressants and/or diuretics
Body perception	Disturbance in the way in which one's body weight and shape are experienced Undue influence of body weight or shape on self-evaluation OR Denial of the seriousness of the current low body weight	Body image distortion in the form of a specific psychopathology whereby a dread of fatness persists as an intrusive, overvalued idea AND Patient imposes a low weight threshold on himself or herself
Amenorrhea/Hormonal fluctuations	In postmenarcheal females, amenorrhea, that is, the absence of at least three consecutive menstrual cycles (amenorrhea exists if periods occur only via hormone induction)	In women, amenorrhea, and in men, loss of sexual interest and potency (an apparent exception is the persistence of vaginal bleeds in anorexic women who are receiving replacement hormonal therapy, most commonly taken as a contraceptive pill) There may also be elevated levels of growth hormone, raised levels of cortisol, changes in the peripheral metabolism of the thyroid hormone, and abnormalities of insulin secretion
Pubertal development	Not specified	With prepubertal onset, the sequence of pubertal events is delayed or even arrested (growth ceases; in girls, the breasts do not develop and there is a primary amenorrhea; in boys, the genitals remain juvenile). With recovery, puberty is often completed normally, but the menarche is late

Source: Data from Bulik, C. M., L. Reba, A. M. Siega-Riz, and T. Reichborn-Kjennerud. 2005. Anorexia nervosa: Definition, epidemiology, and cycle of risk. *Int J Eat Disord* 37: s2–s9. Reprinted with permission of John Wiley & Sons, Inc.

Social feedback and cultural ideals of what constitutes beauty may play a more complicated role in body image and perception than previously thought. In a study by Jansen and colleagues (2006), ED patients rated themselves on attractiveness. Similarly, a panel of judges also rated the women on attractiveness. Interestingly, the two groups rated specific body parts equally unattractive indicating that social feedback is especially important to those who develop EDs and that ideas about beauty are socially cultivated. Although the idea that cultural standards push women to achieve exaggerated thinness is commonly accepted, the results of the Jansen et al. study (2006) did not fully support this theory, as the ED patients were not rated as "the most attractive" women.

Perfectionistic behaviors, such as outstanding performance in academics or athletics, often precede the onset of AN (Bachner-Melman et al. 2009; Bulik, Slof-Op't Landt et al. 2007; Cassin and von Ranson 2005; Kaye et al. 2008). Evidence shows that low self-esteem coupled with body dissatisfaction and perfectionistic tendencies seem to be the greatest predictors for eating pathology (Stice et al. 2006; Vohs et al. 1999). Neurotic perfectionism (i.e., excessive worry about forgetting something or making a mistake) is found more often in AN patients than non-ED women (Ashby et al. 1998; Cassin and von Ranson 2005). Moreover, perfectionism has been found consistently in recovered AN patients, suggesting that it is a stable personality trait for AN patients (Karwautz et al. 2001; Ward et al. 1998).

High levels of self-discipline and persistence are also characteristic of AN patients, and patients with these characteristics are often resistant to treatment (Cassin and von Ranson 2005; Fassino et al. 2004; Stice et al. 2006). One risk factor for relapse is the continued experience of excessive weight preoccupation and body dissatisfaction after treatment (Fairburn et al. 1993; Jansen et al. 2006).

1.3.1.3 Signs and Symptoms of Anorexia Nervosa

The most obvious physical sign of AN is the emaciation resulting from starvation, making AN the most discernible ED (Bulik et al. 2005). AN patients often wear more clothing than others to hide their thinness and to keep warm (Lemberg and Cohn 1999; Uyeda et al. 2002). Thin, fuzzy hair called lanugo can develop over various parts of the body, and skin may appear thin and discolored and may become very pale, dry, and scaly (Lemberg and Cohn 1999; Strumia et al. 2001; Treasure 2008;Uyeda et al. 2002). Additionally, hair and nails are often brittle and easily damaged, and some AN patients lose a lot of hair without new hair growth (Lemberg and Cohn 1999; Uyeda et al. 2002). However, many of these symptoms clear up with the return of healthy eating behaviors (Strumia et al. 2001).

Aside from the physical effects of AN, behavioral changes can also be observed in AN patients. Behavioral clues include eating privately, taking unusually small bites, chewing food excessively, and attempting to conceal food on their plates to make it appear as though they ate it (Lemberg and Cohn 1999). Some AN patients develop a strong interest in collecting recipes and preparing and cooking food, but they rarely eat the food that they prepare. AN patients might also become fixated on nutritional values, caloric expenditure, and exercising frequently (Lemberg and Cohn 1999).

Many times, AN will begin as a diet, and the person might skip meals or greatly reduce portions to achieve weight loss. Eventually, many foods become forbidden to the AN patient until her food options are strictly limited (Herpertz-Dahlmann 2008). For example, she might forbid herself from consuming foods containing carbohydrates, fat, or sugar. Despite these restrictions, patients with AN do not lose their appetites. Instead, they become obsessed with food. Food restriction, however, might serve as a method of gaining control over some aspect of life.

There are different theories that attempt to explain the onset and continuation of AN. For example, denying food can be satisfying and gratifying, and can also serve as a distraction for unpleasant emotions for the AN patient (Polivy and Herman 2002). It has been suggested that AN patients have lower reward sensitivity than other individuals (Treasure 2007). For example, it might be easier for them to skip food because the food is not as pleasing for them as it is for people without AN. Similarly, there are theories attempting to explain why the crossover from AN to EDs with bingeing behavior occurs frequently. Several animal and historical studies have shown that restricted eating will result in binge eating later; therefore, many believe that the restricting behavior directly causes a person to begin binge eating (Treasure 2007).

Depression has been shown to correlate highly with EDs, including AN (Bulik et al. 2005; Bulik, Slof-Op't Landt et al. 2007; Klump et al. 2009; O'Brien and Vincent 2003). Recent studies have shown that depression, negative affect, and neurotisicm play a role in the development of AN (Bulik et al. 2006; Bulik, Hebebrand et al. 2007; Cassin and von Ranson 2005; Finzi-Dottan and Zubery 2009). Positive affect appears to be inversely related to EDs (Casper et al. 1992; Cassin and von Ranson 2005). Specific to AN, depression can be comorbid with AN and often dissipates when the AN patient recovers (Berkman et al. 2007; Halvorsen et al. 2004). Although some researchers suggest that depression is directly linked to the physical starvation associated with AN, other researchers suggest that depression precedes the onset of AN and can continue after one recovers (Herpertz-Dahlmann 2008; O'Brien and Vincent 2003).

Anxiety disorders are also highly correlated with AN (Bulik, Slof-Op't Landt et al. 2007; Cassin and von Ranson 2005; Herpertz-Dahlmann 2008). AN patients often have greater social functioning deficits than BN patients due to high levels of social anxiety, trouble feeling empathy for others, and extreme competitiveness (Hinrichsen et al. 2003; Kucharska-Pietura et al. 2004; Stice et al. 2006).

There is a large amount of research on obsessive-compulsive tendencies in relation to AN (Bulik, Slof-O'pt Landt et al. 2007; Cassin and von Ranson 2005; Kaye et al. 2008; Klump et al. 2009; Lilenfeld et al. 2006; O'Brien and Vincent 2003). Obsessive-compulsive tendencies may exist in childhood and manifest themselves as early as 5 years before the development of eating pathology (Cassin and von Ranson 2005; Herpertz-Dahlmann 2008; Lilenfeld et al. 2006; O'Brien and Vincent 2003; Treasure 2007), and some research suggests that more prominent obsessive-compulsive traits increase a person's chances of developing AN (Cassin and von Ranson 2005). Obsessive-compulsive tendencies can be associated with food, such as chewing food a certain number of times before swallowing or eating food at the exact same time every day, but can also occur in other ways, such as weighing oneself several times each day, running for exactly 1 h every single day, or even organizing all the clothes in one's closet by size and color (Herpertz-Dahlmann 2008; Polivy and Herman 2002; Treasure 2007). One research study suggested that up to 20% of AN patients do not have the desire to get rid of their obsessive thoughts, suggesting that AN patients might obsess to avoid other issues (Polivy and Herman 2002; Sunday et al. 1995). For example, obsessive-compulsive behavior might reduce the impulses and depression associated with AN (Finzi-Dottan and Zubery 2009). Although semi-starvation will induce mood disturbance as well as extreme obsessive-compulsive behaviors, obsessive-compulsive tendencies can also continue after normal eating patterns have been restored, which provides support for the idea that obsessive-compulsive tendencies are stable traits (Berkman et al. 2007; Cassin and von Ranson 2005; Karwautz et al. 2001; O'Brien and Vincent 2003; Stice et al. 2006; Treasure 2007). Additionally, there is some evidence suggesting that detailed tasks or tasks that require methodical and analytic thinking may be easier for AN patients because of their obsessive-compulsive tendencies, but that these individuals might have difficult shifting between tasks due to rigidity in thinking (Bulik et al. 2006; Treasure 2007).

Adolescents with AN differ somewhat from older people with AN. Some experts argue that prevention programs should be targeted towards girls before they reach sixth grade and should aim to reduce future weight preoccupation, body dissatisfaction, and social pressure to be thin (McKnight Investigators 2003). Additionally, the focal goal should be to decrease or eliminate obsessions and distortions about body weight (APA 2000). For young AN patients, positive outcomes seem to be correlated with few negative life events, short length of illness, high social status, and younger age at presentation (Gowers and Bryant-Waugh 2004; Treasure and Schmidt 2002). Vomiting, extreme weight loss, low self-esteem, personality disturbance, prior obesity, and the AN-R subtype seem to be associated with poorer outcomes in young AN patients (Gowers and Bryant-Waugh 2004). For adults, the features that have been found to correlate with a positive prognosis include short duration of illness, absence of a mood disorder, and higher average body weight at intake (Berkman et al. 2007; Herzog et al. 1999; Strober et al. 1996). Psychological pathology, low BMI, and social problems are related to worse long-term outcomes (Berkman et al. 2007; Lowe et al. 2001).

Although AN and BN are separate disorders, there are several traits commonly found in both AN and BN patients. Specifically, high neuroticism, perfectionism, obsessiveness, and low self-directedness are characteristic of both AN and BN patients and may increase the chance of crossover from AN to BN (Tozzi et al. 2005). Commonalities between AN and BN patients may be attributed to the symptom overlap between the two disorders or may help account for the high crossover rate from AN to BN (Bulik et al. 2005; Tozzi et al. 2005). Other traits associated with the crossover from AN to BN include prior anxiety, childhood sexual abuse, negative affect, and improvement in the AN condition (Karwautz et al. 2001; Tozzi et al. 2005).

AN is recognized as having the highest mortality rate of any psychiatric condition in young females (Bulik, Slof-Op't et al. 2007; Kaye et al. 2008; Klump et al. 2009; Stice et al. 2006, 2007; Striegel-Moore and Bulik 2007), and estimates of premature deaths in AN patients range from 5% to 6% (Herpertz-Dahlmann 2008; Steinhausen 2002). Causes of death in women with EDs include starvation, suicide, and electrolyte imbalance (Berkman et al. 2007; Birmingham et al. 2005; Hoek 2006; Steinhausen 2002). Several factors may be predictors of mortality, including having a body weight that is less than 77 pounds, repeated inpatient admissions, and severe alcohol and substance use disorders (Berkman et al. 2007; Patton 1988). Adults with AN also have a high mortality rate (Gowers and Bryant-Waugh 2004; Neilson et al. 1998). AN is also associated with elevated levels of suicide ideation and high rates of suicide (Birmingham et al. 2005; Herzog et al. 2000; Stice et al. 2006).

Patients with AN can experience hypotension, hypothermia, dehydration, bradycardia, and retardation of growth and pubertal development (APA 2000; Uyeda et al. 2002). Dehydration may produce lightheadedness, exhaustion, or muscle cramping (Lemberg and Cohn 1999). Additionally, AN patients often complain about constipation, abdominal pain, lethargy, exhaustion, inhibition, and weakness (APA 2000; Herpertz-Dahlmann 2008; Uyeda et al. 2002). There are other physical symptoms of AN, and most are due to malnutrition and starvation (Herpertz-Dahlmann 2008; Lemberg and Cohn 1999; Pearson et al. 2002). (For more information about the physical consequences of AN, refer to Chapter 3 of this book.)

1.3.2 Bulimia Nervosa

Prevalence rates of bulimia nervosa (BN) range from 1% to 4%, making BN approximately three times more common than AN (Berkman et al. 2007; Herpertz-Dahlmann 2008; Hoek 2006; Steinhausen 2002, Stice et al. 2006). Subthreshold rates of BN are thought to be even greater, between 2% and 5.4% (Berkman et al. 2007; Lewinsohn et al. 2000; Stice et al. 2006). Some reports show the rate of BN is increasing, but conflicting reports suggest that rates have remained stable or have decreased (Hoek 2006; Hudson et al. 2007). The onset of BN typically occurs in later adolescence and before the age of 21 (Gowers and Bryant-Waugh 2004, Striegel-Moore et al. 2007). Additionally, some evidence suggests that white women are diagnosed with BN more often than black women (Striegel-Moore et al. 2007).

The course of BN can be chronic, and patients with BN often go through cycles of improvement followed by relapse (Fairburn et al. 2000; Stice et al. 2006). Low self-directedness has been linked with poor outcomes for those with BN, but some evidence shows that cognitive behavior therapy can be used to boost self-directedness (Tozzi et al. 2005).

1.3.2.1 Diagnostic Criteria for Bulimia Nervosa

According to the *DSM-IV-TR*, BN is characterized by compulsive, extreme binge eating followed by a compensatory method like self-induced vomiting, misuse of diuretics or laxatives, or excessive exercise to make up for the excessive amount of calories consumed. Diagnostic criteria state that this type of cyclic behavior must occur for at least 3 months, and binge eating and purging episodes are to occur at least two times per week. The main psychological factor in BN is loss of control during episodes of binge eating. Additionally, the BN patient places high importance on body weight and physical appearance. There are two subtypes of BN: The purging subtype (BN-P) includes those people who make themselves vomit or use laxative or diuretics to compensate for a binge, and the nonpurging subtype (BN-N) includes those people who use other forms of compensatory behavior, such as excessive exercise or fasting (APA 2000).

The symptoms associated with AN-BP and both subtypes of BN overlap. A person's weight distinguishes those with BN from those with AN-BP. People with BN typically have a weight that is in the normal range, and some are overweight (Polivy and Herman 2002). Similar to AN, some diagnostic criteria for BN are controversial. For example, individuals who binge eat and purge once each week rather than twice each week experience similar levels of eating-related pathology, and the definition of a binge (i.e., "an amount of food that is larger than most people would eat") is not objective or easily measurable (Herpertz-Dahlmann 2008).

The ICD-10 criteria for BN are similar to the *DSM-IV-TR* criteria. The ICD-10 criteria for BN include having an adverse relationship or preoccupation with food, engaging in binge eating and purging behaviors, and attempting to keep body weight below a level that would optimize health (WHO 1992). Table 1.2 provides a comparison of the DSM and ICD-10 diagnostic criteria for BN.

1.3.2.2   Risk Factors for Bulimia Nervosa

Like those with AN, BN patients are highly concerned about the size and shape of their bodies, and they have distorted views of the ideal female body size. It is well-documented that the "perfect" female body size and weight have decreased over the past 70 years. Westernized society is bombarded by images of thin men and women, so people often receive the message that they must be thin in order to be happy (Bachner-Melman et al. 2009). Fear of fatness has been associated with BN pathology (Bulik, Hebebrand et al. 2007; Herpertz-Dahlmann 2008), and that fear likely develops from cultural messages telling young girls to fear becoming fat. BN patients and other people with EDs may internalize these cultural values of beauty more than other people, resulting

---

TABLE 1.2

Comparison of *DSM-IV-TR* and ICD-10 Diagnostic Criteria for Bulimia Nervosa

	DSM-IV-TR	ICD-10
Code	307.51	F 50.2
Relationship with food	binge/purge cycle must occur for at least 3 months, at a rate of two times per week, on average	continued obsession with food strong cravings fear of weight gain
Binge eating	eating, in 2 h or less, a portion of food that is substantially larger than most others would eat loss of control when consuming this food	period of overeating when are a great deal of food is eaten quickly
Purging tendencies	recurrent methods of compensation (vomiting, diuretics, other medications, fasting or exercise)	methods to compensate for the binge vomiting, restriction of food intake, drug use may include appetite suppressants, thyroid treatments or diuretics
Beauty ideal	weight and shape are a major influence in defining the identity of a BN patient	strives to achieve a weight that is well standard weight or weight expected for a particular person

Source: Data from Bulik, C. M., L. Reba, A. M. Siega-Riz, and T. Reichborn-Kjennerud. 2005. Anorexia nervosa: Definition, epidemiology, and cycle of risk. *Int J Eat Disord* 37: s2–s9. Adapted with permission of John Wiley & Sons, Inc.

in dysfunctional relationships with food and other eating problems (Bachner-Melman et al. 2009; Polivy and Herman 1985; Stice et al. 2006).

The sociocultural model of EDs includes contact with and acceptance of the thin ideal and a subsequent disparity between the ideal self and the current self (Striegel-Moore and Bulik 2007). Factors such as weight teasing may also increase the perceived discrepancy between a BN patient's actual weight and her perceived ideal body shape (Stice et al. 2006). The thin ideal is often referred to as a westernized value (Striegel-Moore and Bulik 2007); however, it appears that globalization of the thin beauty ideal has contributed to an increased number of EDs worldwide. Based on this conceptualization of BN, addressing the patient's internalization of the cultural body ideal seems necessary to reduce her body dissatisfaction and other symptoms of BN (Stice et al. 2006).

Dieting and calorie restriction can contribute to eating pathology, particularly episodes of binge eating and subsequent compensatory behaviors (McKnight Investigators 2003; Shaw et al. 2008). Oftentimes, BN patients will attempt to restrict their calorie consumption. However, when they are unable to stick to a plan to eat a small amount of food, they might binge eat because consuming a large amount of food and water will make it easier to vomit later (Uyeda et al. 2002). Studies have shown that up to 82% of women attribute binge eating to food cravings (Fassino et al. 2004; Gendall et al. 1997). Additionally, research has shown that stressors will increase eating in women who diet but might decrease eating in women who do not diet, and that dieting women are more likely to blame their distress on food and overeating (Polivy and Herman 2002). There is also evidence that eating patterns during childhood contribute to the development and maintenance of an ED. For example, ED patients often report that during childhood, they consumed more fast food and snack foods and lacked regular eating schedules (Treasure et al. 2008).

Negative affect has been associated with EDs and has been shown to predict the onset of BN (Lilenfeld et al. 2006; Stice and Agras 1998; Stice et al. 2006). Research has shown that a person can experience negative affect before, during, and after an episode of binge eating (Stein et al. 2007), and several theories have been developed to try to explain how negative affect relates to episodes of binge eating. The trade-off theory and the emotional regulation theory both suggest that negative emotions are replaced by less negative emotions that follow a binge, so it may be less painful for the BN patient to binge and feel guilty than it is to not binge and experience negative affect (Burton et al. 2007; Finzi-Dottan and Zubery 2009; Stein et al. 2007).

Several personality variables have been linked to BN. For example, neuroticism may be a factor in predicting the onset of BN and other EDs (Lilenfeld et al. 2006, Stice et al. 2006), and patients with BN often have problems responding to negative emotions (Klump et al. 2009; Rosval et al. 2006). Another personality trait associated with BN is impulsivity (Finzi-Dottan and Zubery 2009). In a meta-analysis, individuals with EDs who were characterized by binge eating and purging were also high in novelty seeking and low in self-directedness, and had an intolerance of routine (Cassin and von Ranson 2005; Fassino et al. 2004; Rossier et al. 1993). Substance abuse, sexual promiscuity, stealing, and suicide attempts are behaviors often observed in BN (Polivy and Herman 2002; Stice et al. 2006). Because of these risky and impulsive characteristics that can accompany BN, some researchers have proposed a "multi-impulsive disorder" that can include all of these risky behaviors (Herpertz-Dahlmann 2008; O'Brien and Vincent 2003; Wiseman et al. 1999). Several studies have found mixed results regarding the role of impulsivity in EDs (Stice et al. 2006). Impulsivity may result from unpredictable eating and extreme affect, rather than being a stable personality trait (Cassin and von Ranson 2005), and impulsivity may help explain why many patients with AN eventually develop BN (Polivy and Herman 2002; Stice et al. 2006).

Axis I and Axis II psychopathology is highly comorbid with BN (Cassin and von Ranson 2005; Fassino et al. 2004; O'Brien and Vincent 2003). It has been estimated that 56% of BN patients have at least one personality disorder (Fassino et al. 2004; Mulder et al. 1999). Furthermore, women with personality disorders are more likely to have EDs than people with other psychopathology (O'Brien and Vincent 2003). The personality disorders that are most commonly comorbid with BN are dependant, avoidant, and borderline personality disorders (Bornstein 2001; Cassin and von

Ranson 2005; Fassino et al. 2004; Mulder et al. 1999; O'Brien and Vincent 2003). Personality traits that are related to BN, such as unstable affect and an inability to regulate emotions, are also related to some personality disorders, such as borderline personality disorder (BPD; Finzi-Dottan and Zubery 2009; Westen and Hamden-Fischer 2001). Although BN symptoms frequently dissipate following treatment, BPD symptoms often remain (O'Brien and Vincent 2003). Because BPD and BN symptoms are so closely related, it may be difficult to determine where one disorder ends and the other one begins (O'Brien and Vincent 2003). Finally, some research suggests that prior sexual abuse is a risk factor for BN and may be indirectly associated with BN and BPD (O'Brien and Vincent 2003; Polivy and Herman 2002).

In summary, body dissatisfaction and issues related to body weight and shape can be considered the basis of ED behaviors; however, the exact influence that sociocultural factors have on the development of EDs is not clear (Polivy and Herman 2002). Evidence from studies shows that internalizing the thin beauty ideal, in combination with body dissatisfaction and higher than ideal body weight, predict the onset of BN and are also associated with a worse prognosis (Berkman et al. 2007; Gowers and Bryant-Waugh 2004; Stice et al. 2007). Additionally, people in occupations that place high value on attractiveness, body weight, and body shape (e.g., dancers, actresses, models, gymnasts, figure skaters) are at an increased risk for developing EDs (Uyeda et al. 2002). Evidence also shows that jobs involving travel, rotating shifts, or food handling may interfere with normal, healthy eating behaviors and can lead to ED symptoms (Uyeda et al. 2002). Interventions and programs aimed at reducing internalization of the thin ideal, addressing body and weight concerns, and improving negative mood have been successful at reducing some eating psychopathology (Burton et al. 2007; Stice et al. 2007).

1.3.2.3 Signs and Symptoms of Bulimia Nervosa

Binge eating is a defining feature of BN, and a typical binge episode is defined as eating a large amount of food that a person typically considers "off-limits" in everyday settings, particularly foods that are high in fat, sugar, and calories (Herpertz-Dahlmann 2008; Stice et al. 2006). During an episode of binge eating, BN patients typically eat whatever is readily available, regardless of hunger cues or satiation, and approximately 80% to 90% of BN patients engage in purging behaviors following the binge, including self-induced vomiting and misuse of laxatives (APA 2000). Those who do not purge use other methods to attempt to compensate for binge eating, such as fasting or excessive exercise. Binge eating and purging are done almost exclusively in private (Herpertz-Dahlmann 2008; Latner and Clyne 2008). Initially, the beginning phases of binge eating are often stress induced, but the illness becomes ritualized with time (Herpertz-Dahlmann 2008).

People with BN can use various methods to compensate for binge eating, and some people use a combination of compensatory behaviors. Typical methods of compensation include self-induced vomiting, excessive exercise, and fasting, but compensatory behaviors may also include the use of diuretics, laxatives, suppositories, or herbal remedies (Uyeda et al. 2002). Medications such as diet pills and thyroid stimulants can also be abused to induce weight loss (Uyeda et al. 2002). Although BN patients typically yearn to stop binge eating, they often want to continue engaging in compensatory behaviors, which makes it very difficult to break the maladaptive cycle of binge eating and purging (Treasure 2008).

Anxiety plays a central role in BN pathology and often causes major distress for the BN patient (Herpertz-Dahlmann 2008; Stice et al. 2006). A specific type of anxiety, social phobia, is often found in BN patients (Herpertz-Dahlmann 2008; Swinbourne and Touyz 2007). Shame is also an important contributor to BN. In fact, BN patients often choose to seek treatment because they find the cycle of binge eating and purging to be very disturbing and shameful (Stice et al. 2006), and this motivation to decrease distress is thought to aid in the treatment process (Polivy and Herman 2002; Stice et al. 2006).

As is true with AN, depression and other affective disorders are highly correlated with BN (Cassin and von Ranson 2005; Klump et al. 2009). It is estimated that 36% of women with BN also have depression (Dansky et al. 1998; O'Brien and Vincent 2003), and a meta-analysis reported a positive relationship between depression and body dissatisfaction (Berkman et al. 2007). Various stressors such as personal losses, interpersonal problems, and threats to one's safety have been catalysts for the onset of BN (O'Brien and Vincent 2003). BN has also been shown to precede the onset of depression, anxiety, and various health problems (Johnson et al. 2002; Stice et al. 2006). A less favorable prognosis has been associated with the presence of depression, substance use, and low impulse control (Berkman et al. 2007; Keel et al. 2000). Given the relation between ED symptoms and affective disorders, cognitive behavioral therapy (CBT) is often used in the treatment of BN, with specific emphasis on mending irregular eating patterns and identifying distorted cognitions that are contributing to eating disturbances and negative affect (Fairburn and Harrison 2003; Gowers and Bryant-Waugh 2004).

Physical signs of BN can occur in a variety of forms. Vomiting can cause erosion of enamel, damaged teeth, aching and raw throats, sores in the mouth, or dry and cracked lips (APA 2000; Gowers and Bryant-Waugh 2004; Lemberg and Cohn 1999). Induced vomiting may also cause scars to develop on the back of the hand. BN patients using laxatives may suffer from stomach pain, nausea, irregular bowels, bloating, or constipation (Lemberg and Cohn 1999). Additionally, lack of appropriate fluids in the body or kidney dysfunction may result from diuretic abuse (Lemberg and Cohn 1999). (For more information about the physical consequences of BN, refer to Chapter 4 of this book.)

1.3.3 Eating Disorder Not Otherwise Specified

The Eating Disorder Not Otherwise Specified (EDNOS) diagnosis was established as a residual category for troublesome eating behavior that does not meet criteria for a full-syndrome disorder, as defined by the *DSM-IV-TR* (Herpertz-Dahlmann 2008). Many believe that EDNOS are significant because they may develop into specific EDs, like AN or BN (Ackard et al. 2007; Schmidt et al. 2008). Demographic traits, longevity of illness, and food-related pathology are similar among many BN patients and EDNOS patients (Schmidt et al. 2008).

Some mental health professionals are beginning to question the diagnostic criteria for EDs because the majority of ED patients fall into the residual category of EDNOS (Herpertz-Dahlmann 2008; Rockert et al. 2007). Furthermore, the number of individuals with EDNOS in clinical treatment or research studies is probably much lower than their actual prevalence (Machado et al. 2007). The majority of ED patients can be included in the EDNOS category; however, this category includes so many different patterns of symptoms that it is difficult to tell what percentage of the EDNOS group is subclinically AN, BN, or BED (APA 2000; Herpertz-Dahlmann 2008; Striegel-Moore and Franko 2008).

EDNOS accounts for approximately 60% of ED cases, whereas AN and BN account for only 14.5% and 25.5% of ED patients, respectively (Fairburn and Bohn 2005; Hoek 2006; Machado et al. 2007). One study found that approximately 3% of girls in a community sample had disordered eating and 77% of these girls had symptoms that fell in the EDNOS diagnostic category (Machado et al. 2007). Even though EDNOS holds the majority of ED cases (Keel et al. 2005; Schmidt et al. 2008), it is the least studied ED, so relatively little is known about EDNOS (Hoek 2006; Machado et al. 2007; Rockert et al. 2007).

1.3.3.1 Diagnostic Criteria for Eating Disorder Not Otherwise Specified

The EDNOS group includes individuals with disordered eating behaviors that do not fully meet the diagnostic criteria for AN or BN. For example, if a young woman met all of the other diagnostic criteria for AN but did not have amenorrhea, then her diagnosis would be EDNOS. Other criteria that could qualify an individual for an EDNOS diagnosis include weight falling within normal limits despite highly erratic eating, and binge eating and compensatory behaviors occurring less frequently than the diagnostic criteria specify (APA 2000).

Most people in the EDNOS category are people of normal weight who severely restrict their food intake, people who engage in purging without binge eating, or people who engage in binge eating and purging behaviors less than two times per week (Rockert et al. 2007). Thus, many individuals who are classified as EDNOS can be considered to have less severe cases of AN and BN (Turner and Bryant-Waugh 2004). Yet, the psychological distress that people with EDNOS experience is similar to those with specific EDs (Turner and Bryant-Waugh 2004). Comorbidity of psychological disorders in EDNOS is also similar to AN and BN (Klump et al. 2009). Table 1.3 presents a comparison of the DSM and ICD-10 diagnostic criteria for EDNOS.

1.3.3.2   Risk Factors for EDNOS

The signs and risk factors for EDNOS are highly similar to those for AN and BN. All of these EDs demonstrate high levels of harm avoidance, anxiety, perfectionism, and obsessive-compulsive traits, as well as low levels of self-directedness and cooperativeness (Cassin and von Ranson 2005). This substantial overlap supports the idea that these traits are a fundamental core of ED risk factors. However, there are some important differences between the disorders. For instance, AN-R patients show more restraint and diligence than patients with BN, BED, or AN-BP (Cassin and von Ranson 2005). Impulsivity, novelty seeking, and sensation seeking are traits often found in EDs with binge-purge behaviors, including BN and AN-BP (Cassin and von Ranson 2005). These differences are important in identifying high-risk individuals and predicting treatment response and prognosis (Cassin and von Ranson 2005).

Body image distortion and compensatory methods, such as vomiting, laxative abuse, or excessive exercise, are frequent among adolescents, even those without diagnosed EDs (Ackard et al. 2007). Adolescents are more frequently diagnosed with EDNOS than AN or BN. This may be due

TABLE 1.3
Comparison of the *DSM-IV-TR* and ICD-10 Diagnostic Criteria for Eating Disorder Not Otherwise Specified

	DSM-IV-TR	ICD-10
Code	307.50	F50.1, F50.3, F50.5
Subthreshold AN	An individual will be diagnosed EDNOS if they meet criterion for AN except amenorrhea or established weight cutoffs	An individual will be diagnosed with atypical AN when significant weight loss occurs but not all criterion are met for a full-threshold diagnosis. Other physical and medical disorders must be ruled out
Subthreshold BN	An individual will be diagnosed as EDNOS if they meet criterion for BN except that binging and purging occur too infrequently or the b/p cycle has not met the time criteria of 2 months	An individual will be diagnosed with atypical BN when the individual binges and purges but does not meet criteria for a full-threshold diagnosis
Compensatory behaviors	An individual may be diagnosed with EDNOS if she engages in compensatory behaviors after eating only a small amount of food or if she chews but does not swallow food	An individual will be diagnosed with "vomiting associated with other psychological disturbances" if there is another psychological disorder diagnosis combined with repeated vomiting (with emotional factors playing a role)

Sources: Adapted with permission from the American Psychiatric Association. 2000. *Diagnostic and statistical manual of mental disorders: Fourth Edition, Text Revision.* Washington DC: American Psychiatric Association. Adapted with permission from the World Health Organization. 1992. *International statistical classification of diseases and related health problems.* 10th ed. Geneva, Switzerland: World Health Organization.

to the fact that adolescents usually begin treatment early in their illness, so they may not have had enough time to develop full-syndrome disorders (Fisher et al. 2001; Gowers and Bryant-Waugh 2004). Adolescents with EDNOS often display eating irregularities as well as exaggerated interest in food, weight, and shape (Gowers and Bryant-Waugh 2004). For adolescents, a few specific risk factors have been identified, including negative mood, low thoughtfulness, low introspective reflection, neuroticism, and perfectionistic tendencies, and these risk factors can also contribute to the maintenance of EDs (Leon et al. 1999; Wonderlich et al. 2005).

1.3.3.3 Signs and Symptoms of EDNOS

Signs and symptoms of EDNOS are very similar or the same as those for full-syndrome AN and BN (Turner and Bryant-Waugh 2004). In one study, BN patients were more fixated on food and calories, and they considered weight and shape more important than patients in the EDNOS group (Turner and Bryant-Waugh 2004). Often, individuals with EDNOS experience psychological distress that is similar to those with full-syndrome disorders even though the behavioral symptoms or physical signs of EDNOS are slightly different than for other EDs (Turner and Bryant-Waugh 2004). For example, one study showed that 35% of patients were diagnosed as EDNOS instead of AN because their weight was not under 85% of the expected level or because they continued menstruating. Likewise, 37% of EDNOS were classified as such because their binge eating and compensatory behaviors were not frequent enough for a BN diagnosis (Turner and Bryant-Waugh 2004). Still, these physical differences do not result in psychological differences in distress, so the seriousness and persistence of subthreshold disorders is a central reason why people believe that the diagnostic criteria for full-syndrome disorders should be reconsidered (Herpertz-Dahlmann 2008; Turner and Bryant-Waugh 2004).

1.3.4 BINGE EATING DISORDER

Binge Eating Disorder (BED) is behaviorally similar to BN, without the compensatory behaviors. Many mental health professionals seek to discern a more distinct line between BED and the BN-N subtype, and the revised criteria for BN in the *DSM-V* might reflect the desire to distinguish the two disorders (Cooper and Fairburn 2003; Mathes et al. 2009; Striegel-Moore and Franko 2008). The most prominent characteristic of BED is binge eating, which involves eating an excessively large portion of food rapidly over a short period of time (Latner and Clyne 2008; Mathes et al. 2009; Striegel-Moore and Franko 2008). Additionally, people with BED eat much faster during episodes of binge eating than during periods of regular eating (Latner and Clyne 2008). BED has been shown to be as chronic and long-lasting as AN or BN (Hudson et al. 2007). However, binge eating is reported less often in adolescents than adults and young adults, so the onset of BED is generally later than the onset for other EDs (Fisher et al. 2001). Table 1.4 presents information about the circumstances when binge eating occurs.

Binge eating is a public health concern, as research shows BED to be more prevalent than any of the other EDs (Hudson et al. 2007; Striegel-Moore and Franko 2008). Up to 5% of people will develop BED sometime during their lives, and even more people will develop subthreshold levels of BED (Mathes et al. 2009; Treasure 2008). Additionally, obesity is linked with BED, and studies suggest that 5% to 50% of obese individuals have BED (Berkman et al. 2007; Bruce and Agras 1992; Hudson et al. 2007; Latner and Clyne 2008).

BED can remit at a high rate, and relapse and crossover rates are low (Striegel-Moore and Franko 2008). However, BED can also be chronic before treatment and recovery (Striegel-Moore and Franko 2008). The longevity of BED can be significantly detrimental to health, contributing to increased blood pressure, blood sugar, heart rate, and cholesterol levels (Striegel-Moore and Franko 2008). Few patients seek treatment for BED, even though many BED patients report impaired daily functioning (Striegel-Moore and Franko 2008). For those who seek treatment, however, psychotherapy has been shown to be effective in treating BED (Stice et al. 2006).

TABLE 1.4
Topography of Binge Eating: Where and with Whom Does It Occur

Circumstances	Frequency
Where	
Kitchen	30.7%
Bedroom	7.2%
Dining Room	3.8%
Car	10.2%
Restaurant	1.9%
Living Room	31.1%
Work	10.2%
Other	4.9%
With Whom	
No One	58.3%
Partner	17.4%
Friend	1.1%
Other Family	14.8%
Coworker	5.3%
Other	3.0%

Source: Data from Stein, R. I., J. Kenardy, C. V. Wiseman, J. Z. Dounchis, B. A. Arnow, and D. E. Wilfley. 2007. What's driving the binge in binge eating disorder? A prospective examination of precursors and consequences. *Int J Eat Disord* 40: 195–203. Reprinted with permission from John Wiley & Sons, Inc.

1.3.4.1 Diagnostic Criteria for Binge Eating Disorder

In the *DSM-IV-TR*, BED is classified under the EDNOS category (APA 2000), but many have suggested that BED should be a distinct ED. However, there are problems with the current diagnostic criteria for BED. For instance, the definition of a binge, according to *DSM-IV-TR*, includes consuming a large amount of food within a short period of time and experiencing a perceived loss of control (APA 2000; Latner and Clyne 2008; Striegel-Moore and Franko 2008). The lack of clarity for those diagnostic criteria makes it difficult for a researcher or clinician to determine whether a person engages in rapid eating, to differentiate an unusually large amount of food from a normal amount of food, and to determine what constitutes a discrete amount of time (Cooper and Fairburn 2003; Mathes et al. 2009; Polivy and Herman 2002; Striegel-Moore and Franko 2008). However, some evidence shows that self-reported "binges" are not always noticeably large (Latner and Clyne 2008; Rosen et al. 1986). Furthermore, the subjectivity of measuring loss of control while eating is very difficult, even for the BED patient (Cooper and Fairburn 2003; Mathes et al. 2009; Polivy and Herman 2002; Striegel-Moore and Franko 2008). Additionally, the criterion that requires binge eating to occur at least twice per week was set arbitrarily, as there are only small differences between patients that meet this criterion and those who do not (Latner and Clyne 2008, Striegel-Moore and Franko 2008).

According to *DSM-IV-TR* criteria, the BED patient must experience a loss of control during the binge, and loss of control has been associated with negative mood (Mathes et al. 2009; Stein et al. 2007). Given the subjective nature of the characteristic, "lack of control" must be decided by the individual with BED (Latner and Clyne 2008). Latner and Clyne (2008) showed that loss of control was used to classify binges by 82% of women, but loss of control, as reported by individuals with BED, may depend upon their frame of mind. When asked what caused the loss of control during a binge, 27% of women reported that they were trying to change their mood. However, in this same study, 8% of BED patients reported no loss of control. Thus, solid diagnostic criteria for BED still need to be determined. A comparison of the *DSM-IV-TR* and ICD-10 diagnostic criteria for BED is presented in Table 1.5.

1.3.4.2   Risk Factors Contributing to Binge Eating Disorder

Risk factors for BED vary from person to person and are related to personality traits and individual experiences (Striegel-Moore et al. 2007). Stress is a significant factor in other EDs and likely plays a role in BED as well. In one study, higher perceived levels of stress predicted binge eating in some BED patients (Striegel-Moore et al. 2007). In a different study, BED women reported a larger number of stressful life events, especially during the year preceding the onset of BED, and the rate of risk found in the BED patients with the most life-event stressors was six times higher than others (Pike et al. 2006). Even individuals not suffering from BED show that the combination of dieting and stress are predictors of binge eating (Mathes et al. 2009). Stressors found to affect BED patients often include weight-related criticism, physical abuse, interpersonal problems, worries about physical safety, and work and school stress (Pike et al. 2006). Furthermore, any stress that is paired with weight criticism is a predictor of BED onset (Pike et al. 2006).

Men seem to experience much higher levels of BED than other EDs, making female sex less of a predictor of BED (Hudson et al. 2007; Striegel-Moore and Bulik 2007). However, men experiencing BED may be less psychologically affected than women, as they report lower levels of participation in weight-control behaviors, such as compensatory methods (Hay 1998; Striegel-Moore and Bulik 2007). Recent literature has demonstrated no significant ethnicity differences in BED (Striegel-Moore and Bulik 2007; Striegel-Moore and Franko 2008). However, BED seems to be more prevalent in highly developed countries. Many BED patients show onset after 21 years of age and are comparatively older than other ED patients; however, longevity of the disease may play a role in the higher age of BED patients (Striegel-Moore et al. 2007; Striegel-Moore and Franko 2008).

Severe dieting causes extreme hunger, and BED patients rate their hunger as being very strong prior to a binge (Stein et al. 2007). Not surprisingly, abstaining from eating throughout the day is associated with binge eating (Stein et al. 2007). Evidence supports the theory that binge eating may produce neurochemical pathways in the brain that are similar to the pathways seen in those with

---

TABLE 1.5

Comparison of the *DSM-IV-TR* and ICD-10 Diagnostic Criteria for Binge Eating Disorder

	DSM-IV	**ICD-10**
Code	**Proposed Disorder**	**F50.4**
Duration of binge	2 h	
Food intake	Consummation of food is larger than others might consume in equitable situations	Overeating
Psychological factors	Binge eaters must experience lack of control binging	Stressful events (bereavement, anxiety, life changes)

Sources: Adapted with permission from the American Psychiatric Association. 2000. *Diagnostic and statistical manual of mental disorders: Fourth Edition, Text Revision.* Washington DC: American Psychiatric Association. Adapted with permission from the World Health Organization. 1992. *International statistical classification of diseases and related health problems.* 10th ed. Geneva, Switzerland: World Health Organization.

addictive behaviors (Mathes et al. 2009). Eating appetizing food also releases dopamine, which is highly rewarding and encourages continued eating.

The restraint theory has been proposed to account for BED, hypothesizing that drive for thinness promotes food restriction that will result in binge eating to replenish the body with energy (Howard and Porzelius 1999; Stein et al. 2007). Similar to the restraint theory, the abstinence violation effect claims that severe black-and-white thinking may trigger a binge after a strict dietary rule is broken (Stein et al. 2007). Additionally, "binge priming" is sometimes used to describe how dieting is associated with binge eating (Treasure et al. 2008). In studies with animals, researchers often try to elicit the circumstances that precipitate binge eating in humans, such as inducing stress or restraint, and research has shown that denying animals food for only 2 h can lead to increased food intake later (Mathes et al. 2009). Thus, there may be a correlation between dieting and the onset of binge eating (Hagan et al. 2002).

Stress plays an important role in BED. Evidence suggests that BED patients may not be able to read physiological hunger cues like other people do, which results in eating due to stress, not hunger (Stein et al. 2007). To date, many theories of binge eating involve stress and other factors such as dieting, emotional eating, female sex, obesity, disinhibition, and factors related to stress (Crowther et al. 2001; Mathes et al. 2009). Consistent evidence has shown that BED patients will interpret stressful situations as more stressful than those without BED (Harrington et al. 2006). Specifically, Crowther et al. (2001) found that the level of stressors experienced by people who engaged in episodes of binge eating was comparable to the comparison group; however, those who binged perceived stressors as being more stressful and consumed more calories on high-stress days than low-stress days (Crowther et al. 2001). Thus, binge eating may be used as a coping strategy to handle the stressors (Harrington et al. 2006).

In addition to stress, negative affect may be related to BED (Mathes et al. 2009). Negative mood may trigger binge eating, and eating might alleviate the negative mood temporarily (Mathes et al. 2009; Stein et al. 2007). Over the long term, however, affect will worsen and stress related to binge eating will increase (Latner and Clyne 2008). As a person continues to use food in an attempt to improve mood, the negative affect cycle is perpetuated because mood decreases after eating too much food (Hagan et al. 2002). Although negative mood is more likely than hunger to be attributed as the cause of a binge, when hunger is added to negative affect, the likelihood of a binge rises (Stein et al. 2007).

1.3.4.3 Signs and Symptoms of Binge Eating Disorder

Compared to other EDs, BED seems to be associated with less severe psychopathology. For example, BN patients reported less inhibition, greater fear of fatness, higher avoidance of foods, more purging behaviors, and more restrained eating than BED patients (Deaver et al. 2003; Latner and Clyne 2008). These characteristics may contribute to the elevated psychopathology experienced by BN patients, including higher levels of depression, anxiety, and personality disorders (Latner and Clyne 2008; Raymond et al. 1995). However, BED patients report more secretive eating than BN patients (Latner and Clyne 2008), and some research suggests that the binge eating for those with BN is very different from the binge eating of those with BED, including the types of foods used to binge, the number of calories ingested, and the level of self-control exercised (Striegel-Moore and Franko 2008). Despite these differences, there are also important similarities between BED and other EDs. Specifically, evidence shows that BED and BN patients experience similar levels of body dissatisfaction and concerns about shape and weight (Latner and Clyne 2008). Yet, not all overeaters display weight and shape concerns, and those who do not display weight and shape concerns have reported less psychological distress, suggesting that weight and shape concerns may be specifically related to ED psychopathology (Striegel-Moore and Franko 2008). Disorders found in BED patients that may be linked to binge eating include mood disorders, anxiety disorders, and substance abuse disorders as well as health problems like obesity (Latner and Clyne 2008; Pike et al. 2006). Thus, it seems that binge eating is strongly associated with psychological comorbidity, low self-esteem, and interpersonal problems (Latner and Clyne 2008).

Research has consistently shown that BED patients tend to have higher weights and BMIs than people who do not binge (Pike et al. 2006), but not all overweight or obese patients have BED and not all patients with BED are overweight or obese. Weight, however, is particularly important for people with BED, because BED patients often identify obesity and weight gain as their greatest personal concern (Hagan et al. 2002). Additionally, research has shown that being overweight or obese can complicate BED. For example, gastric capacity is greater in obese patients with BED compared to obese patients without BED and is likely due to binge eating behaviors (Latner and Clyne 2008). Also, research has shown that obese patients with BED are significantly more impaired than obese people who do not binge, and specific areas of impairment can include employment, sexual functioning, self-esteem, and general quality of life (Latner and Clyne 2008; Reiger et al. 2005).

Some studies have produced valuable information about the binge characteristics of those with BED. Specifically, BED patients reported eating other people's food, stockpiling or hiding food items, and looking through the garbage for food that has been thrown away (Hagan et al. 1999, 2002). Research has also suggested that chaotic binge eating characteristics include overeating to the point of being painfully full, eating in private, and experiencing negative feelings after eating, such as remorse and shame (Hagan et al. 2002). Additionally, people with BED typically binge eat at night, usually between 6 PM and 1 AM, and binge eating usually occurs in one's own home and is unlikely to occur in public places, such as work settings (Stein et al. 2007). BED patients also described their food consumptions during episodes of binge eating as "large" or "unusually large," and those classifications are linked to more stress and less control (Stein et al. 2007). Intentionality was also shown to be related to binge eating, and binges that were considered "large" by BED patients were rated as more intentional but were also associated with much higher loss of control (Stein et al. 2007).

BED is associated with a variety of psychological and physical health problems, many of which are related to obesity (APA 2000; Hudson et al. 2007; Latner and Clyne 2008; Mathes et al. 2009; Stice et al. 2006; Striegel-Moore and Franko 2008; Treasure 2008). It is estimated that 5% to 50% of people who have BED are also obese (Berkman et al. 2007; Bruce and Agras 1992; Hudson et al. 2007; Latner and Clyne 2008).

Because individuals with BED are often overweight or obese, it is likely that people seek treatment primarily for weight problems rather than for BED. Depression, poor adjustment, psychiatric disturbance, impaired functioning, eating pathology, body dissatisfaction, weight and shape concerns, and shame and guilt are commonly found in individuals with obesity and BED who seek treatment (Latner and Clyne 2008, Stice et al. 2006; Striegel-Moore and Franko 2008). Research has also shown that BED patients visit their physicians more frequently and report more health problems than people without BED (Striegel-Moore and Franko 2008). Clearly, BED has negative personal and social consequences, so recognizing and treating BED are as important as recognizing other types of EDs (Mathes et al. 2009; Striegel-Moore and Franko 2008).

1.4 CONCLUDING REMARKS AND NEW INSIGHTS

1.4.1 New Insights

Because of the overlapping symptoms among EDs, diagnosing specific EDs can be challenging, especially if the ED is comorbid with other illnesses. Commonly, the patient will seek treatment for non-ED symptoms and may deny the existence of an ED (Berkman et al. 2007). Often, the ED patient is young or is unable to understand the consequences of her eating behavior (Berkman et al. 2007). However, clinicians need to look for signs and symptoms of EDs in all people, including young women, young men, adolescents, ethnic minorities, and overweight people (Berkman et al. 2007; Currin et al. 2007; Gowers and Bryant-Waugh 2004).

In the past, EDs, particularly AN, have been viewed as disorders that only occurred in affluent White women, perhaps because these women are able to seek treatment and are also more likely to be involved in research studies (Pearson et al. 2002; Striegel-Moore and Bulik 2007). As understanding of EDs has increased, researchers and clinicians have become increasingly aware that EDs can be a problem for people of any age, race, or gender. However, some research has suggested lower prevalence of EDs for some groups. For example, it has been reported that African-American girls display fewer behavioral eating problems and have greater contentment with their bodies than Caucasian or Hispanic girls (McKnight Investigators 2003). One challenge, however, is that minority women in the United States might be less likely to seek mental health care, even if they have EDs, so prevalence rates of EDs in minority groups could be higher (Striegel-Moore and Bulik 2007; Striegel-Moore et al. 2007). Conversely, healthcare providers may not consider EDs in the initial consultation with ethnic minority women in the same way that they do with Caucasian women (Striegel-Moore et al. 2007). Although some evidence suggests that higher socioeconomic status might be a bigger risk factor for developing an ED than ethnicity, results in these studies are mixed, and the evidence may be due to differences in having the means to seek treatment and be involved in research studies (Sobal and Stunkard 1989; Striegel-Moore and Bulik 2007).

Purging disorder (PD) has sparked research interest and is characterized by recurring purging episodes in the absence of binge eating (Keel et al. 2005). In research thus far, PD patients have demonstrated similar levels of ED severity, psychopathology, dietary restraint, and distorted body image to patients with BN (Keel et al. 2001, 2005; Rockert et al. 2007). Much research is still needed to understand PD, but one possible reason that PD patients do not engage in binge eating is that they report much lower levels of hunger and disinhibition around food than BN patients (Keel et al. 2005). It has been recommended that PD be included in the *DSM-V* as a specific type of EDNOS that needs to be researched more thoroughly before accurate diagnostic criteria are determined (Keel 2007).

1.4.2 THE IMPORTANCE OF EARLY DETECTION AND SCREENING

Early diagnosis of an ED is related to a better prognosis because the patient is more receptive to treatment. Earlier diagnosis is an important first step for many patients and allows for intervention before the adverse eating patterns are ingrained due to repetition (Gowers and Bryant-Waugh 2004). Vigilant friends and family can notice signs and symptoms of the ED and attempt to seek proper help. If an ED is suspected, one of the most practical screening tools to use in the primary care setting is the SCOFF questionnaire (Morgan et al. 1999; see Appendix 1.A). Because of its 12.5% false-positive rate, this test is not sufficiently accurate for diagnosing EDs, but it is an appropriate screening tool that physicians can use as a first step in identifying and treating the ED. (For more information about other screening measures for EDs, refer to Chapter 5 of this book.) Although a substantial amount of progress has been made in the field of ED research and treatment, there are still many questions without answers. By reading this book, you will see where we are on the journey towards better understanding and treating EDs.

APPENDIX 1.A   THE SCOFF QUESTIONNAIRE

SCOFF QUESTIONS

Do you make yourself **S**ick (induce vomiting) because you feel uncomfortably full?
Do you worry that you have lost **C**ontrol over how much you eat?
Have you recently lost more than **O**ne stone (14 lb [6.4 kg]) in a 3-month period?
Do you think you are too **F**at, even though others say you are too thin?
Would you say that **F**ood dominates your life?

One point for every yes answer; a score ≥ 2 indicates a likely case of anorexia nervosa or bulimia nervosa (sensitivity: 100%; specificity: 87.5%).

Source: Morgan J. F., F. Reid, and J. H. Lacey. 1999. The SCOFF questionnaire: Assessment of a new screening tool for eating disorders. *BMJ* 319: 1467–8. Reprinted with permission.

REFERENCES

Ackard, D. M., J. A. Fulkerson, and D. Neumark-Sztainer. 2007. Prevalence and utility of DSM IV eating disorder diagnostic criteria among youth. *Int J Eat Disord* 40: 409–417.

American Psychiatric Association. 2000. *Diagnostic and statistical manual of mental disorders: Fourth Edition, Text Revision.* Washington DC: American Psychiatric Association.

Ashby, J. S., T. Kottman, and E. Schoen. 1998. Perfectionism and eating disorders reconsidered. *J Ment Health Couns* 20: 261–271.

Bachner-Melman, R., A. H. Zohar, Y. Elizur, I. Kremer, M. Golan, and R. Ebstein. 2009. Protective self-presentation style: Association with disordered eating and anorexia nervosa mediated by sociocultural attitudes towards appearance. *Eat Weight Disord* 14: 1–12.

Berkman, N. D., K. N. Lohr, and C. M. Bulik. 2007. Outcomes of eating disorders: A systematic review of the literature. *Int J Eat Disord* 40: 293–309.

Birmingham, L. C., J. Su, J. A. Hlynsky, E. M. Goldner, and M. Gao. 2005. Mortality rates from anorexia nervosa. *Int J Eat Disord* 38: 143–146.

Bornstein, R. F. 2001. A meta-analysis of the dependency-eating-disorders relationship: Strength, specificity, and temporal stability. *J Psychopathol Behav Assess* 23: 151–162.

Bruce, B., and W. S. Agras. 1992. Binge eating in females: A population-based investigation. *Int J Eat Disord* 12: 365–373.

Bulik, C. M., J. Hebebrand, A. Keski-Rahkonen, K. L. Klump, T. Reichborn-Kjennerud, S. E. Mazzeo, and T. D. Wade. 2007. Genetic epidemiology, endophenotypes and eating disorder classification. *Int J Eat Disord* 40: s52–s60.

Bulik, C. M., L. Reba, A. M. Siega-Riz, and T. Reichborn-Kjennerud. 2005. Anorexia nervosa: Definition, epidemiology, and cycle of risk. *Int J Eat Disord* 37: s2–s9.

Bulik, C. M., M. C. Slof-Op't Landt, E. F. van Furth, and P. F. Sullivan. 2007. The genetics of Anorexia Nervosa. *Annu Rev Nutrition,* 27: 263–275.

Bulik, C. M., P. F. Sullivan, F. Tozzi, H. Furberg, P. Lichtenstein, and N. L. Pederson. 2006. Prevalence, heritability and prospective risk factors for anorexia nervosa. *Arch Gen Psychiatry* 63: 305–313.

Burton, E., E. Stice, S. K. Bearman, and P. Rohde. 2007. Experimental test of the affect-regulation theory of bulimic symptoms and substance use: A randomized trial. *Int J Eat Disord* 40: 27–36.

Cachelin, F., and B. Maher. 1998. Is amenorrhea a critical criterion for anorexia nervosa? *J Psychosom Res* 44: 435–440.

Casper, R. C., D. Hedeker, and J. F. McClough. 1992. Personality dimensions in eating disorders and their relevance for subtyping. *J Am Acad Child Adol Psychiatry* 31: 830–840.

Cassin, S. E., and K. M. von Ranson. 2005. Personality and eating disorders: A decade in review. *Clin Psychol Rev* 25: 895–916.

Cooper, Z., and C. G. Fairburn. 2003. Refining the definition of binge eating disorder and nonpurging bulimia nervosa. *Int J Eat Disord* 34: s89–s95.

Crowther, J. H., J. Sanftner, D. Z. Bonifazi, and K. L. Shepherd. 2001. The role of daily hassles in binge eating. *Int J Eat Disord* 29: 449–454.

Currin, L., U. Schmidt, and G. Waller. 2007. Variables that influence diagnosis and treatment of the eating disorders within primary care settings: A vignette study. *Int J Eat Disord* 40: 257–262.

Dansky, B. S., T. D. Brewerton, D. G. Kilpatrick, P. M. O'Neil, H. S. Resnick, C. L. Best, and B. E. Saunders. 1998. The nature and prevalence of binge eating disorder in a national sample of women. In *DSM-IV sourcebook,* ed. T. A. Widiger, A. J. Frances. H. A. Pincus, R. Ross, M. B. First, W. F. Davis and M. Kline, 515–531. Washington: American Psychiatric Association Press.

Deaver, C. M., R. G. Miltenberger, I. Smyth, A. Meidinger, and R. Crosby. 2003. An evaluation of affect and binge eating. *Behav Modif* 27: 578–599.

Fairburn, C. G., and K. Bohn. 2005. Eating disorder NOS (EDNOS): An example of the troublesome "not otherwise specified" (NOS) category in DSM-IV. *Behav Res Ther* 43: 691–701.

Fairburn, C. G., Z. Cooper, and K. Bohn. 2007. The severity and status of eating disorder NOS: Implications for DSM-V. *Behav Res Ther* 45: 1705–1715.

Fairburn, C.G., Z. Cooper, H. A. Doll, P. A. Norman, and M. E. O'Connor. 2000. The natural course of bulimia nervosa and binge eating disorder in young women. *Arch Gen Psychiatry* 57: 659–665.

Fairburn, C. G., and P. J. Harrison. 2003. Eating disorders. *The Lancet* 361: 407–416.

Fairburn, C. G., R. C. Peveler, R. Jones, R. A. Hope, and H. A. Doll. 1993. Predictors of twelve-month outcome in bulimia nervosa and the influence of attitudes to shape and weight. *J Consult Clin Psychol* 61: 696–698.

Fassino, S., F. Amianto, C. Gramaglia, F. Facchini, and G. Abbate Daga. 2004. Temperament and character in eating disorders: Ten years of studies. *Eat Weight Disord* 9: 81–90.

Fichter, M. M., N. Quadflieg, and S. Hedlund. 2005. Twelve-year course and outcome predictors of anorexia nervosa. *Int J Eat Disord* 39: 310–322.

Finzi-Dottan, R., and E. Zubery. 2009. The role of depression and anxiety in impulsive and obsessive-compulsive behaviors among anorexic and bulimic patients. *Eat Disord* 17: 162–182.

Fisher, M., M. Schneider, J. Burns, H. Symons, and F. S. Mandel. 2001. Differences between adolescents and young adults at presentation to an eating disorders program. *J Adolesc Health* 28: 222–227.

Garfinkel, P., E. Lin, P. Goering, and C. Spegg. 1996. Should amenorrhea be necessary for the diagnosis of anorexia nervosa? Evidence from a Canadian community sample. *Brit J Psychiatry* 168: 500–506.

Gendall, K. A., P. F. Sullivan, P. R. Joyce, J. L. Fear, and C. M. Bulik. 1997. Psychopathology and personality of young women who experience food cravings. *Addict Behav* 22: 545–555.

Gordon, K., J. Holm-Denoma, A. Smith, E. Fink, and T. Joiner. 2007. Taxometric analysis: Introduction and overview. *Int J Eat Disord* 40: S35–S39.

Gowers, S., and R. Bryant-Waugh. 2004. Management of child and adolescent eating disorders: The current evidence base and future directions. *J Child Psychol Psychiatry* 45: 63–83.

Hagan, M. M., E. S. Shuman, K. D. Oswald, K. J. Corcoran, J. H. Profitt, K. Blackburn, M. W. Schwieber, P. C. Chandler, and M. C. Birbaum. 2002. Incidence of chaotic eating behaviors in binge eating disorder: Contributing factors. *Behav Med* 28: 99–105.

Hagan, M. M., R. H. Whitworth, and D. E. Moss. 1999. Semistarvation-associated eating behaviors among college binge eaters: A preliminary description and assessment scale. *Behav Med* 25: 125–133.

Halvorsen, I., A. Andersen, and S. Heyerdahl. 2004. Good outcome of adolescent onset anorexia nervosa after systematic treatment: Intermediate to long-term follow-up of a representative country-sample. *Eur Child Adolesc Psychiatry* 13: 295–306.

Harrington, E. F., J. H. Crowther, H. C. Payne Hendrickson, and K. D. Mickelson. 2006. The relationship among trauma, stress, ethnicity and binge eating. *Cultur Divers Ethnic Minor Psychol* 12: 212–229.

Hay, P. 1998. The epidemiology of eating disorder behaviors: An Australian community-based survey. *Int J Eat Disord* 23: 371–382.

Herpertz-Dahlmann, B. 2008. Adolescent eating disorders: Definitions, symptomatology, epidemiology and comorbidity. *Child Adolesc Psychiatr Clin N Am* 18: 31–47.

Herzog, D. B., D. J. Dorer, P. K. Keel, S. E. Selwyn, E. R. Ekeblad, A. T. Flores, D. N. Greenwood, R. A. Burwell, and M. B. Keller. 1999. Recovery and relapse in anorexia and bulimia nervosa: A 7.5-year follow-up study. *J Am Acad Child Adolesc Psychiatry* 38: 829–837.

Herzog, D. B., D. N. Greenwood, D. J. Dorer, A. T. Flores, and E. R. Richards. 2000. Mortality in eating disorders: A descriptive study. *Int J Eat Disord* 28: 20–26.

Hinrichsen, H., F. Wright, and C. Meyer. 2003. Social anxiety and coping strategies in the eating disorders. *Eat Behav* 4: 117–126.

Hoek, H. W. 2006. Incidence, prevalence and mortality of anorexia nervosa and other eating disorders. *Curr Opin Psychiatry* 19: 389–394.

Howard, C. E., and L. K. Porzelius. 1999. The role of dieting in binge eating disorder: Etiology and treatment implications. *Clin Psychol Rev* 19: 25–44.

Hudson, J. I., Hiripi, E., Pope, H. G., and R. C. Kessler. 2007. The prevalence and correlates of eating disorders in the national comorbidity survey replication. *Biol Psychiatry* 61: 348–358.

Jansen, A., T. Smeets, C. Martijn, and C. Nederkoorn. 2006. I see what you see: The lack of a self-serving body-image bias in eating disorders. *B J Clin Psychol* 45: 123–135.

Johnson, J. G., P. Cohen, S. Kasen, and J. S. Brook. 2002. Eating disorders during adolescence and the risk for physical and mental disorders during early adulthood. *Arch Gen Psychiatry* 59: 545–552.

Karwautz, A., S. Rabe-Hesketh, X. Hu, J. Zhao, P. Sham, D. A. Collier, and J. L. Treasure. 2001. Individual-specific risk factors for anorexia-nervosa: A pilot study using a discordant sister-pair design. *Psychol Med* 31: 317–329.

Kaye, W. H., C. M. Bulik, K. Plotnicov, L. Thornton, B. Devlin, M. M. Fichter, J. Treasure, et al. 2008. The genetics of anorexia nervosa collaborative study: Methods and sample description. *Int J Eat Disord* 41: 289–300.

Keel, P. K. 2007. Purging disorder: Subthreshold variant or full-threshold eating disorder? *Int J Eat Disord* 40: S89–S94.

Keel, P. K., A. Haedt, and C. Edler. 2005. Purging disorder: An ominous variant of bulimia nervosa? *Int J Eat Disord* 38: 191–199.

Keel, P. K., S. A. Mayer, and J. H. Harnden-Fischer. 2001. Importance of size in defining binge eating episodes in bulimia nervosa. *Int J Eat Disord* 29: 294–301.

Keel, P. K., J. C. Mitchell, K. B. Miller, T. L. Davis, and S. J. Crow. 2000. Predictive validity of bulimia nervosa as a diagnostic category. *Am J Psychiatry* 157: 136–138.

Klump, K. L., C. M. Bulik, W. H. Kaye, J. Treasure, and E. Tyson. 2009. Academy for Eating Disorders position paper: Eating disorders are serious mental illnesses. *Int J Eat Disord* 42: 97–103.

Kucharska-Pietura, K., V. Nikolaou, M. Masiak, and J. Treasure. 2004. The recognition of emotion in the faces and voice of anorexia nervosa. *Int J Eat Disord* 12: 377–384.

Latner, J. D., and C. Clyne. 2008. The diagnostic validity of the criteria for binge eating disorder. *Int J Eat Disord* 41: 1–14.

Lemberg, R., and L. Cohn. 1999. *Eating disorders: A reference sourcebook.* Phoenix, Arizona: Oryx Press.

Leon, G. R., J. A. Fulkerson, C. L. Perry, P. K. Keel, and K. L. Klump. 1999. Three to four year prospective evaluation of personality and behavioral risk factors for later disordered eating in adolescent girls and boys. *J Youth Adolesc* 28: 181–196.

Lewinsohn, P. M., R. H. Striegel-Moore, and J. R. Seeley. 2000. Epidemiology and natural course of eating disorders in young women from adolescence to young adulthood. *J Abnormal Psych* 39: 1284–1292.

Lilenfeld, L. R. R., S. Wonderlich, R. P. Lawrence, R. Crosby, and J. Mitchell. 2006. Eating disorders and personality: A methodological and empirical review. *Clin Psychol Rev* 26: 299–320.

Lowe, B., S. Zipfel, C. Buchholz, Y. Dupont, D. L. Reas, and W. Herzog. 2001. Long-term outcome of anorexia nervosa in a prospective 21-year follow-up study. *Psychol Med* 31: 881–890.

Machado, P. P. P., B. C. Machado, S. Goncalves, and H. W. Hoek. 2007. The prevalence of eating disorder not otherwise specified. *Int J Eat Disord* 40: 212–217.

Mangweth-Matzek B., C. I. Rupp, A. Hausmann, K. Assmayr, E. Mariacher, G. Kemmler, A. B. Whitworth, and W. Biebl. 2006. Never too old for eating disorders or body dissatisfaction: A community study of elderly women. *Int J Eat Disord* 39: 583–587.

Mathes, W. F., K. M. Brownley, X. Mo, and C. M. Bulik. 2009. The biology of binge eating. *Appetite* 52: 545–553.

McKnight Investigators. 2003. Risk factors for the onset of eating disorders in adolescent girls: Results of the McKnight longitudinal risk factor study. *Am J Psychiatry* 160: 248–254.

Morgan J. F., F. Reid, and J. H. Lacey. 1999. The SCOFF questionnaire: Assessment of a new screening tool for eating disorders. *BMJ* 319: 1467–1468.

Mulder, R. T., P. R. Joyce, P. F. Sullivan, C. M. Bulik, and F. A. Carter. 1999. The relationship among three models of personality psychopathology: DSM-III-R personality disorder, TCI scores and DSQ defenses. *Psychol Med* 29: 943–951.

Nielsen, S., S. Moller-Madsen, T. Isager, J. Jorgensen, K. Pagsberg, S. Theander. 1998. Standardized mortality in eating disorders: A quantitative summary of previously published and new evidence. *J Psychosom Res* 44: 412–434.

O'Brien, K. M., and N. K. Vincent. 2003. Psychiatric comorbidity in anorexia and bulimia nervosa: Nature, prevalence and causal relationships. *Clin Psychol Rev* 23: 57–74.

Patton, G. C. 1988. Mortality in eating disorders. *Psychol Med* 18: 947–951.

Pearson, J., D. Goldklang, and R. H. Striegel-Moore. 2002. Prevention of eating disorders: Challenges and opportunities. *Int J Eat Disord* 31: 233–239.

Pike, K. M., D. Wilfley, A. Hilbert, C. G. Fairburn, F. A. Dohm, and R. H. Striegel-Moore. 2006. Antecedent life events of binge-eating. *Psychiatry Res* 142: 19–29.

Polivy J., and C. P. Herman. 1985. Dieting and binge eating: A causal analysis. *Am Psychol* 40: 193–204.

Polivy, J., and C. P. Herman. 2002. Causes of eating disorders. *Annu Rev Psychol* 53: 187–213.

Raymond, N. C., M. P. Mussell, J. E. Mitchell, M. de Zwann, and R. D. Crosby. 1995. An age matched comparison of subjects with binge eating disorder and bulimia nervosa. *Int J Eat Disord* 18: 135–143.

Rieger, E., D. E. Wilfley, R. I. Stein, V. Marino, and S. J. Crow. 2005. A comparison of quality of life in obese individuals with and without binge eating disorder. *Int J Eat Disord* 37: 234–240.

Rockert, W., A. S. Kaplan, and M. P. Olmsted. 2007. Eating disorder not otherwise specified: The view from a tertiary care treatment center. *Int J Eat Disord* 40: s99–s103.

Rosen, J. C., H. Leitenberg, C. Fisher, and C. Khazam. 1986. Binge eating episodes in bulimia nervosa: The amount and type of food consumed. *Int J Eat Disord* 5: 255–267.

Rossier, E. M., W. S. Agras, C. F. Telch and J. A. Schneider. 1993. Cluster B personality disorder characteristics predict outcome in the treatment of bulimia nervosa. *Int J Eat Disord* 13: 349–357.

Rosval, L., H. Steiger, K. R. Bruce, M. Israel, J. Richardson, and M. Aubut. 2006. Impulsivity in women with eating disorders: Problem of response inhibition, planning, or attention? *Int J Eat Disord* 39: 590–593.

Schmidt, U., S. Lee, S. Perkins, I. Eisler, J. Treasure, J. Beecham, M. Berelowitz, et al. 2008. Do adolescents with eating disorder not otherwise specified or full-syndrome bulimia nervosa differ in the clinical severity, comorbidity, risk factors, treatment outcome or cost? *Int J Eat Disord* 41: 498–504.

Shaw, H., E. Stice, and C. B. Becker. 2008. Preventing eating disorders. *Child Adolesc Psychiatr Clin N Am* 18: 199–207.

Sobal, J., and A.J. Stunkard. 1989. Socioeconomic status and obesity: A review of the literature. *Psychol Bull* 105: 260–275.

Stein, R. I., J. Kenardy, C. V. Wiseman, J. Z. Dounchis, B. A. Arnow, and D. E. Wilfley. 2007. What's driving the binge in binge eating disorder?: A prospective examination of precursors and consequences. *Int J Eat Disord* 40: 195–203.

Steinhausen, H. C. 2002. The outcome of anorexia nervosa in the 20th century. *Am J Psychiatry* 159: 1284–1293.

Stice, E. and W. S. Agras. 1998. Predicting onset and cessation of bulimic behaviors during adolescence: A longitudinal grouping analysis. *Behav Ther* 29: 257–276.

Stice, E., H. Shaw, and C. N. Marti. 2007. A meta-analytic review of eating disorder prevention programs: Encouraging findings. *Annu Rev Clin Psychol* 3: 207–231.

Stice, E., S. Wonderlich, and E. Wade. 2006. Chapter 20, Eating disorders. In *Comprehensive Handbook of Personality and Psychopathology,* ed. M. Hersen, J.C. Thomas and R.T. Ammerman, 330–347. Hoboken, NJ: John Wiley.

Striegel-Moore, R. H., and C. M. Bulik. 2007. Risk factors for eating disorders. *Am Psychol* 62: 181–198.

Striegel-Moore, R. H., F. A. Dohm, H. C. Kraemer, C. B. Taylor, S. Daniels, P. B. Crawford, and G. B. Schreiber. 2003. Eating disorders in white and black women. *Am J Psychiatry* 160: 1326–1331.

Striegel-Moore, R. H., F. A. Dohm, H. C. Kraemer, G. B. Schreiber, C. B. Taylor, and S. R. Daniels. 2007. Risk factors for binge-eating disorders: An exploratory study. *Int J Eat Disord* 40: 81–487.

Striegel-Moore, R. H., and D. L. Franko. 2008. Should binge eating disorder be included in the DSM-V? A critical review of the state of the evidence. *Annu Rev Clin Psychol* 4: 305–323.

Striegel-Moore, R. H., and M. D. Marcus. 1995. Eating disorders in women: Current issues and debates. In *The psychology of women's health: Progress and challenges in research and application,* ed. A. L. Stanton and S. J. Gallant, 445–487. Washington, DC: American Psychological Association.

Strober, M., R. Freeman, S. Bower, and J. Rigali. 1996. Binge eating in anorexia nervosa predicts later onset of substance use disorder: A ten-year prospective, longitudinal follow-up of 95 adolescents. *J Youth Adolesc* 25: 519–532.

Strumia, R., E. Varotti, E. Manzato, and M. Gualandi. 2001. Skin signs in anorexia nervosa. *Dermatology* 203: 314–317.

Sunday, S. R., K. A. Halmi, and A. Einhorn. 1995. The Yale-Brown-Cornell eating disorder scale: A new scale to assess eating disorder symptomatology. *Int J Eat Disord* 18: 237–245.

Swinbourne, J. M. and S. W. Touyz. 2007. The co-morbidity of eating disorders and anxiety disorders: A review. *Eur Eat Disord Rev* 15: 253–274.

Tozzi, F., L. M. Thornton, K. L. Klump, M. M. Fichter, K. A. Halmi, A. S. Kaplan, M. Strober et al. 2005. Symptom fluctuation in eating disorders: Correlates of diagnostic crossover. *Am J Psychiatry* 162: 732–740.

Treasure, J. L. 2007. Getting beneath the phenotype of anorexia nervosa: The search for viable endophenotypes and genotypes. *Can J Psychiatry* 52: 212–219.

Treasure, J. 2008. Eating disorders. *Medicine* 36: 430–435.

Treasure, J., and U. Schmidt. 2002. Anorexia nervosa. *Clin Evid* 7: 824–833.

Treasure, J. L., E. R. Wack, and M. E. Roberts. 2008. Models as a high-risk group: The health implications of a size zero culture. *Br J Psychiatry* 192: 243–244.

Turner, H., and R. Bryant-Waugh. 2004. Eating disorder not otherwise specified (EDNOS): Profiles of clients presenting at a community eating disorder service. *Eur Eat Disord Rev* 12: 18–26.

Uyeda, L., I. Tyler, J. Pinzon, and C. L. Birmingham. 2002. Identification of patients with eating disorders. The signs and symptoms of anorexia nervosa and bulimia nervosa. *Eat Weight Disord* 7: 116–123.

van Hoeken, D., J. Seidell and H. Hoek. 2003. Epidemiology. In *Handbook of eating disorders,* ed. J. Treasure, U. Schmidt, and E. van Furth, 11–34. Chichester: Wiley.

Vitousek, K., and F. Manke. 1994. Personality variables and disorders in anorexia nervosa and bulimia nervosa. *J Abnorm Psychol* 103: 137–147.

Vohs, K. D., A. M. Bardone, T. E. Joiner, L. Y. Abramson, and T. F. Heatherton. 1999. Perfectionism, perceived weight status, and self-esteem interact to predict bulimic symptoms: A model of bulimic symptom development. *J Abnorm Psychol* 108: 695–700.

Ward, A., N. Brown, S. Lightman, I. C. Campbell, and J. Treasure. 1998. Neuroendocrine, appetitive and behavioural responses to d-fenfluramine in women recovered from anorexia nervosa. *Br J Psychiatry* 172: 351–358.

Westen, D., and J. Hamden-Fischer. 2001. Personality profiles in eating disorders: Rethinking the distinction between axis I and axis II. *Am J Psychiatry* 158: 547–562.

Wilfley, D. E., M. E. Bishop, G. T. Wilson, and W. S. Agras. 2007. Classification of eating disorders: Toward DSM-V. *Int J Eat Disord* 40: S123–S129.

Wiseman, C. V., S. R. Sunday, P. Halligan, S. Korn, C. Brown, and K. A. Halmi. 1999. Substance dependence and eating disorders: Impact of sequence on comorbidity. *Compr Psychiatry* 40: 332–336.

Wonderlich, S. A., T. E. Joiner Jr., P. K. Keel, D. A. Williamson, and R. D. Crosby. 2007. Eating disorder diagnoses. *Am Psychol* 62: 167–180.

Wonderlich, S. A., L. A. Lilenfeld, L. P. Riso, S. Engel, and J. E. Mitchell. 2005. Personality and anorexia nervosa. *Int J Eat Disord* 37: s68–s71.

World Health Organization. 1992. *International statistical classification of diseases and related health problems.* 10th ed. Geneva, Switzerland: World Health Organization.

2 The Psychology of Eating Disorders

Kristin L. Goodheart, Heather L. Gibson, and James R. Clopton

CONTENTS

2.1 LEARNING OBJECTIVES

After completing this chapter, you should be able to

- Identify aspects of adolescence that contribute to the development of eating disorders
- Explain why certain people are more susceptible to developing eating disorders than others
- Identify psychological characteristics, including aspects of personality and emotional experiences, that are often associated with eating disorders, and understand how those characteristics might precipitate or perpetuate the disorder
- Use your knowledge of psychological characteristics typically associated with eating disorders to devise the most appropriate treatment plan for eating disordered women
- Identify reasons why ignoring comorbid psychological characteristics in the treatment of eating disorders might lead to relapse or failure to recover

2.2 RESEARCH BACKGROUND, SIGNIFICANCE, AND CURRENT FINDINGS

Eating disorders are psychological disorders marked by irregular eating patterns, distress related to food consumption, and an overwhelming desire for thinness. They interfere with a person's ability to function and often result in physical complications such as infertility, decreased heart rate, and lowered bone density (APA 2000). The term "eating disorder" might give the misperception that the problems associated with dysfunctional eating patterns are fairly simple to define and easy to understand. When describing eating disorders, the focus is often on the behavioral or observable symptoms associated with eating disorders. For example, anorexia nervosa may be conceptualized as severe food restriction leading to emaciation. Bulimia nervosa may be conceptualized as engaging in episodes of binge eating and purging behaviors, like self-induced vomiting. The internal experience of a person struggling with an eating disorder may not be considered. However, "eating disorders are not just about eating or about food, but about the use of the body-self as a unique vehicle of communication" (Freedman and Lavender 2002, 183). So, questions that explore what drives a person to the point of self-induced starvation or uncontrollable cycles of binge eating and purging need to be raised. Additionally, a person's feelings about herself, the disorder, and the world in general must not be overlooked.

Eating disorders are complex, and the associated symptoms are intense. A person's life often revolves around the eating disorder, as days can be spent consciously avoiding food consumption, bingeing and purging in secrecy, and exercising compulsively while attempting to seem normal, healthy, and flawless to friends and family (Hornbacher 1999). The complicated, consuming nature of eating disorders combined with the physiological need for food makes it difficult for people to understand why a friend or family member might develop an eating disorder. It is also difficult for the person struggling with the disorder to understand the problems surrounding the dysfunction and the reasons for the problem. In fact, some people with eating disorders are unaware that they have a problem at all. Others may be aware that something is "not quite right" but are unsure how to ask for help, and some are in denial about the severity of the problem.

One reason that eating disorders and associated symptoms are not always detected is because people receive mixed messages about healthy and unhealthy behaviors and attitudes about food, weight, diet, and exercise. Body dissatisfaction and suggestions about diet and exercise are omnipresent in American society and other Western cultures, so it can be difficult to determine when a person has a problem that merits clinical attention. For example, distress associated with body image is so common among women of all ages that it is considered normal (Garner et al. 1980; Kjaerbye-Thygesen et al. 2004; Ohring et al. 2002; Peat et al. 2008). Additionally, dieting is a very common practice among individuals within our society (McCreary and Sasse 2000). Therefore, it is not always obvious when a diet becomes too restrictive or when dissatisfaction with one's appearance becomes such a problem that some type of intervention is necessary.

Because people within our culture have conflicting opinions about what constitutes healthy and unhealthy behaviors, people can be positively reinforced for engaging in unhealthy behaviors. For example, there is not a universal agreement about an amount of exercise that would classify a person as engaging in an excessive amount of exercise, nor is there an amount of calories that suggests a diet is too restrictive. As a result, people may be praised for potentially dangerous behaviors. Severely restricting one's diet might be viewed by some people as exercising an incredible amount of willpower, a coveted trait by some standards. Similarly, an individual might be praised for the amount of time she spends exercising, even if the amount of exercise she is doing is hazardous to her health. Additionally, weight loss often accompanies behaviors like restrictive dieting and excessive exercise, so people are often praised for their weight loss because of the value commonly associated with thinness. Receiving compliments that are specific to appearance, such as losing weight, can feel really good, so the behaviors that contributed to the weight loss, which are often framed as "controlled diet" and "commitment to exercise," persist. For some people, weight loss continues to a deadly level, as is seen in women who develop anorexia nervosa. For other individuals, steady weight loss eventually plateaus to a weight that may be considered healthy, but more destructive behaviors, such as binge eating or purging, are developed to attempt to maintain or resume the weight loss. Eventually, the preoccupation with weight, food, exercise, and physical appearance become more important than anything else, so other areas of life, including family, friends, and school, are neglected. Even if a person recognizes her severely unbalanced lifestyle, the thoughts and behaviors that she has developed become so ingrained in her mind and in her daily routine that abandoning these behaviors may seem terrifying, undesirable, or even impossible. In fact, many people with them do not receive treatment (Hoek and Hoeken 2003), and symptoms often persist throughout their lives (Fichter and Quadflieg 2007). Sometimes, eating disorders can result in death from suicide, starvation, or an electrolyte imbalance (Birmingham et al. 2005). In fact, mortality rates for people with eating disorders, especially those with anorexia nervosa, are among the highest of any mental disorder (APA 2000).

2.2.1 PREVALENCE OF EATING DISORDERS

Despite the overwhelming presence of factors associated with eating disorders, such as dieting and body dissatisfaction, specific eating disorders are rare. The estimated prevalence rates for all women with anorexia nervosa and bulimia nervosa are 0.3% and 1%, respectively (Hoek and Hoeken 2003). More often, women experience symptoms of eating disorders that do not meet full criteria for a diagnosis of anorexia nervosa or bulimia nervosa (Dalle Grave and Calugi 2007; Fairburn and Bohn 2005), but the distress associated with unspecified eating disorders is often as severe as the distress experienced in individuals with anorexia nervosa or bulimia nervosa (Fairburn et al. 2007; Striegel-Moore and Marcus 1995). The estimated prevalence rate for unspecified eating disorders is 5%, and approximately 60 to 75% of all eating disorder cases fall into the unspecified eating disorder category (Fairburn et al. 2003; Machado et al. 2007).

Although specific eating disorders are rare among the general population, adolescent to college-aged women living in advanced countries like the United States are particularly susceptible to developing eating disorders like anorexia nervosa and bulimia nervosa (Alexander 1998; Hoek and Hoeken 2003). Regarding specific symptoms associated with eating disorders, estimated prevalence rates for binge eating, fasting, and purging in the general population are 3.2%, 1.6%, and .8%, respectively (Hay and Fairburn 1998). However, these rates were found to be much higher for college women: 19%, 12.4%, and 2.7% (Heatherton et al. 1995). Other research suggests that between 25 and 40% of college women endorse moderate problems associated with eating disorders, such as concern about body image, weight management, and lack of control when eating (Schwitzer et al. 2001).

Due to the high incidence of eating disorders and associated symptoms in adolescent girls and college-aged women, much of the current understanding about eating disorders has been gained through research with these populations. However, children, young men, older women, and people from other ethnic backgrounds are not immune from developing or experiencing eating disorders or associated symptoms (Muise et al. 2003; Peat et al. 2008; Soh et al. 2006). Therefore, a common criticism is that our currently available knowledge about eating disorders may not be true for these other individuals.

There is growing evidence, however, to suggest that much of the current understanding about eating disorders can be applied to adolescent males (McCabe and Vincent 2003). For example, both male and female adolescents can be dissatisfied with their bodies and feel pressure to lose weight, especially when they perceive themselves as being overweight (Halliwell and Harvey 2006). Additionally, some research suggests that boys experience similar risk factors as girls for developing eating disorders, including perfectionism, anxiety, and low self-esteem (McCabe and Vincent 2003). Other factors, such as involvement in athletics and having a same-sex or bisexual orientation, may increase a young man's susceptibility to developing an eating disorder (Muise et al. 2003). Although girls are more likely than boys to diet to lose weight (McCreary and Sasse 2000), binge eating and compensatory behaviors may occur as frequently in boys as in girls (McCabe and Vincent 2003). Furthermore, some young men experience dysfunctional eating problems that are as severe as, and similar in presentation to, young women (McCabe and Vincent 2003). Therefore, even though prevalence rates for males with eating disorders are considerably lower than the prevalence rates for females, it is equally important to recognize dysfunctional eating patterns in young men as it is to recognize these patterns in young women.

Another criticism is that the current understanding of eating disorders may not be applicable to younger children (Nicholls et al. 2000). This is problematic because symptoms of eating disorders are now being detected earlier in life. Obviously, there are clear biological, cognitive, and emotional differences that distinguish children and young adolescents from adults, and these developmental differences complicate the consequences of dysfunctional eating pathology for younger people (Sokol et al. 2005). Specifically, physical complications can occur more quickly during childhood and early adolescence. Additionally, these physical complications can be more detrimental, since children and younger adolescents are not fully developed like adults, and can result in developmental delays or permanent problems (Sokol et al. 2005). Despite the need to understand and to address issues associated with this vulnerable phase of life, eating disorders that develop during childhood have been researched less and therefore are less well understood.

Eating disorders in older adults have also been researched less, yet women can experience body dissatisfaction at any age (Peat et al. 2008). However, it is rare for an older woman to develop an eating disorder or symptoms associated with eating disorders. Instead, problems associated with food, eating, weight, and physical appearance likely persisted into adulthood. Older women might be less susceptible to developing eating disorders because they typically place less value on physical appearance than children, adolescents, and younger women (Peat et al. 2008). In fact, having more life experience might aid in developing healthier views about one's body, and therefore protect older women against symptoms associated with eating disorders (Peat et al. 2008). Yet, life experience does not protect all older women from developing eating disorders or experiencing associated symptoms, so an eating disorder diagnosis may be appropriate for a woman of any age.

Although earlier researchers suggested that young women living in countries where thinness is valued, such as the United States, were most susceptible to developing eating disorders, more recent research suggests that people from other cultural backgrounds are not immune from developing eating disorders or experiencing associated symptoms, especially if they are highly acculturated (Soh et al. 2006). Still, symptoms of eating disorders are most common during adolescence, particularly for adolescent females, and typically decrease in frequency following the adolescent stage of development (Steinhausen et al. 1997). Therefore, a more thorough discussion of adolescent vulnerability to developing eating disorders and associated symptoms follows.

2.2.2 EATING DISORDERS IN ADOLESCENTS

The period between childhood and adulthood is often a difficult but vital phase of a person's development. During adolescence, many dramatic and significant transitions occur that physically change a person and influence his or her sense of self-worth (Kearney-Cooke 1999). New social pressures, rapid physical changes, and heightened emotional experiences accompany this developmental phase. For example, adolescents are quickly expected to begin acting more like adults. Many people begin driving, earning money, attending college, and living independently during this time. Increased self-consciousness, desire for independence, and a greater awareness of, and a desire to interact with, potential sexual partners are also associated with this developmental period (Furman et al. 1999).

Because society demands that adolescents quickly learn to behave and think like adults rather than like children, young people may not be adequately prepared to cope with the physical and emotional changes that accompany adolescence. As a consequence, young people are highly vulnerable to engaging in risky behaviors, such as extreme dieting or drug use (Banister and Schreiber 2001). Adolescence is also a prime time for body dissatisfaction to surface (Hill 2002), which could be attributed to unwelcome biological and physical changes in the body (McCabe and Ricciardelli 2004) or an increased awareness of or exposure to sociocultural factors, such as the media, peer influence, and societal ideals (Clay et al. 2005; Guerzina 1998; Pinhas et al. 1999; Taylor et al. 1998; Wiseman et al. 2005).

Additionally, young people are susceptible to developing dysfunctional eating patterns. It is estimated that between 3 and 4% of children and adolescents struggle with eating disorders (Sancho et al. 2007), and nearly 3% of adolescents with eating disorders die (Steinhausen et al. 2003). An even greater number of individuals suffer from subclinical eating disorders or experience some, but not all, of the symptoms associated with clinical eating disorders, like anorexia nervosa or bulimia nervosa (Chamay-Weber et al. 2005). In fact, it is suggested that about 12% of adolescent boys and 14% of adolescent girls endorse subclinical eating problems (Sancho et al. 2007). For example, it is estimated that nearly half of all adolescent females are dieting to lose weight (McCreary and Sasse 2002), which is often a precursor to developing an eating disorder (Garrow et al. 2000). Common experiences, such as body dissatisfaction and involvement in romantic relationships, increase the likelihood of dieting in young people (Halpern et al. 2005). Unfortunately, unhealthy behaviors and beliefs that are established in adolescence, such as dieting and body dissatisfaction, often persist into adulthood (Ohring et al. 2002; Peat et al. 2008).

Clinical eating disorders that develop during adolescence may be chronic, and if untreated, the distress and symptoms associated with eating disorders often become increasingly severe (Sancho et al. 2007; Steinhousen et al. 2003). It is estimated that 30% of adolescent girls with anorexia nervosa will continue to have this disorder throughout their lifespan. Approximately half of the persistent cases will require a second hospitalization, and one quarter will require a third hospitalization (Steinhausen et al. 2003). However, dysfunctional eating patterns that are diagnosed during early adolescence are associated with more favorable outcomes. Therefore, detecting disordered eating patterns in young people may prevent some of them from developing a clinical eating disorder, like anorexia nervosa or bulimia nervosa (Steinhausen et al. 2003).

Perhaps the most prominent characteristic of adolescence is the rapid biological and hormonal changes that occur during this time period (Rembeck and Gunnarsson 2004). During adolescence, young girls experience substantial physiological and biochemical changes, during which their bodies alter from those of children to those of young women in a relatively short amount of time (De Castro and Goldstein 1995). As a result, young girls may place more emphasis on the appearance of the body. Although some adolescents welcome these changes and like their adult-like bodies, others may find it difficult to cope with the physical changes that their bodies are experiencing and attempt to control these changes through destructive behaviors like fasting or purging. Therefore, some of the physical changes that occur during adolescence may contribute to the onset of eating disturbances and eventually eating disorders.

Social pressure during this developmental period also contributes to adolescent girls' vulnerability to body dissatisfaction associated with the physical changes that they experience. For example, adolescents are highly influenced by their peers (Taylor et al. 1998), and physical appearance is often scrutinized. Unfortunately, younger people, compared to any other age group, are more critical of one another and are less accepting of others whose bodies differ from what is considered physically normal (Rand and Wright 2000). Therefore, an adolescent's physical appearance is particularly vulnerable to peer criticism (Taylor et al. 1998). As a result, an adolescent girl could develop extreme dissatisfaction for her physical appearance and engage in unhealthy behaviors, like food restriction or purging, to attempt to alleviate her dissatisfaction and avoid further scrutiny.

Beyond the occurrence of puberty, some research suggests that the timing of the onset of puberty is critical in the development of symptoms of eating disorders, like body dissatisfaction (Siegel et al. 1999). Specifically, girls who develop earlier than their peers may be more susceptible to symptoms associated with eating disorders than girls who develop at the same time or later than most of their peers. For example, a young girl who begins to develop into a woman at an earlier age than her peers may feel uncomfortable because she is larger (i.e., taller, heavier) than her friends. Her peers or family members might tease her about her growing body. If she begins to develop at an unusually early age, she may endure this ridicule for several years before her peers catch up with her physical development. Additionally, the rate of her cognitive and emotional development may not match that of her physical development, and thus she might have difficulty understanding the changes that she is experiencing and the reasons for the physical differences between herself and her peers. As a result, she may develop unhealthy eating patterns, such as binge eating, to attempt to cope with the uncomfortable emotion that she experiences. She may also resort to unhealthy practices like food restriction, excessive exercise, or self-induced vomiting to attempt to regain her childlike body or prevent further growth.

Although early development might contribute to dysfunctional eating patterns or associated symptoms, not all girls who develop earlier than their peers experience problems associated with food, eating, and body image. Furthermore, girls whose physical development occurs at about the same time or later than most of their peers can develop eating disorders or associated symptoms (Lieberman et al. 2001). Even if a young girl is not the recipient of criticism, she can be sensitive to or influenced by teasing. For example, she might observe her older sister being teased by other family members because of her changing appearance. In order to avoid a similar experience, a young girl might attempt to avoid or delay physical development by restricting her food intake, increasing her physical activity, or engaging in purging behaviors, like self-induced vomiting. Therefore, factors beyond age and physical characteristics, like body weight and menstrual functioning, must be considered when attempting to understand the development and persistence of disordered eating.

In addition to social pressures and the physical changes experienced during adolescence, various psychological factors can contribute to the development of eating disorders. Table 2.1 provides a list of psychological factors related to eating disorders that are well-supported by research. Although it is encouraging that general knowledge about eating disorders and associated factors is increasing, there is not one clear trajectory or group of risk factors that determines the development of an eating disorder. Therefore, attempting to address every psychological factor that has been associated with the development or maintenance of eating disorders is beyond the scope of a single chapter. In the following section, aspects of personality and emotional experiences will be addressed. Although these variables are not unique to adolescents, the changing demands that are associated with adolescence may amplify some of the psychological risk factors addressed in the following sections.

TABLE 2.1

Psychological Characteristics Related to Eating Disorders

Avoidance[a,b]	Body Dissatisfaction[a,c]	Dieting[a]
Exposure to mass media[d]	Exposure to disturbed eating[c]	History of teasing[a]
Impulsivity[b,e]	Low self-esteem[a]	Maladaptive coping[a,b]
Negative affect[c]	Perceived pressure to be thin[c]	Perceived stress[b]
Perfectionism[a,c,e]	Predisposition to anxiety[f]	Stressful life events[b]
Substance use[c]	Thin ideal[a,c]	

Notes: References below provide research support for these characteristics.

[a] Ghaderi, A. 2001. Review of risk factors for eating disorders: Implications for primary prevention and cognitive behavioural therapy. *Scand J Behav Ther* 30: 57–74.

[b] Ball, K., and C. Lee. 2000. Relationship between psychological stress, coping and disordered eating: A review. *Psychol Health* 14: 1007–1035.

[c] Stice, E. 2002. Risk and maintenance factors for eating pathology: A meta-analytic review. *Psychol B* 128: 825–848.

[d] Levine, M. P., and S. K. Murnen. 2009. "Everybody knows that mass media are/are not [pick one] a cause of eating disorders": A critical review of evidence for a causal link between media, negative body image, and disordered eating in females. *J Soc Clin Psychol* 28: 9–42.

[e] Cassin, S. E., and K. M. von Ranson. 2005. Personality and eating disorders: A decade in review. *Clin Psychol Rev* 25: 895–916.

[f] Swinbourne, J. M., and S. W. Touyz. 2007. The co-morbidity of eating disorders and anxiety disorders: A review. *Eur Eat Disord Rev* 15: 253–274.

2.2.3 Psychological Factors Contributing to the Development and Maintenance of Eating Disorders

Because of the physical consequences associated with eating disorders, it can be argued that eating disorders are medical disorders that merit medical attention. As a consequence, psychological aspects contributing to the development and maintenance of these disorders may get overlooked. However, psychological variables, such as aspects of personality and emotional experiences are important when considering eating disorders. Research suggests that a variety of psychological factors may be related to eating pathology. Consistent relationships between eating disorders and internal factors, such as low self-esteem and high body dissatisfaction, have been found (Kearney-Cook 1999; Hill 2002). Additionally, relationships between eating disorders and symptoms of other psychological dysfunction, such as anxiety and depression, have been well documented (Swinbourne and Touynz 2007; Santos et al. 2007). Aspects of one's personality, such as perfectionism and impulsivity, have also been strongly connected to eating disorders (Cassin and von Ranson 2005). Relationships with peers and family members are also related to eating disorders (Lieberman et al. 2001). A person's cognitions, or the way a person thinks, may contribute to the development or maintenance of an eating disorder (Fairburn et al. 2003). These variables are only a few examples of factors that might contribute to the eating pathology.

Various aspects of personality can be related to eating disorders. Specifically, features like perfectionism, neuroticism, obsessiveness, harm avoidance, low self-directedness, low cooperativeness, and general avoidance are often present in individuals who are diagnosed with eating disorders (see Cassin and von Ranson 2005; Vitousek and Manke 1994 for reviews). Additionally, some personality factors, such as persistence and need for control, are especially seen in individuals who restrict their diets (Cassin and von Ranson 2005; Vitousek and Manke 1994). Other personality factors, such as impulsivity and a desire for spontaneity and new experiences, are more common in individuals who binge and purge (Cassin and von Ranson 2005; Vitousek and Manke 1994). Personality disorders, such as borderline personality disorder, dependent personality disorder, avoidant personality disorder, and obsessive-compulsive personality disorder, are often seen in individuals with eating disorders (Cassin and von Ranson 2005). Although several aspects of personality and other psychological factors have been linked to eating disorders, this chapter will focus specifically on perfectionism, obsessiveness and need for control, shame, and depression in individuals with eating disorders.

2.2.3.1 Perfectionism

One area of eating disorder research that has received much attention is perfectionism. Presenting oneself as being perfect is common among individuals with symptoms of eating disorders. Because of their desire to be flawless, perfectionists are at increased risk of developing symptoms of an eating disorder, and they may go to great lengths to conceal their imperfections (McGee et al. 2005). In fact, some research suggests that perfectionism is a greater risk factor for dysfunctional eating patterns and behaviors than body dissatisfaction (Kiemle et al. 1987). Additionally, perfectionism often contributes to the development of clinical eating disorders like anorexia nervosa and bulimia nervosa (Cassin and von Ranson 2005; Fairburn et al. 1997, 1999; Tyrka et al. 2002) or accounts for the persistence of eating disorder pathology (Fairburn et al. 2003; Santonastaso et al. 1999).

Perfectionists often set unreasonable standards for themselves, such as striving to wear a size 0 when a more realistic expectation might be wearing a size 6. Furthermore, they cannot accept failure. Therefore, when their personal standards are not met, perfectionists may experience shame associated with their bodies and their perceived failures. The shame they experience can contribute to the maintenance of the dysfunctional relationship with food and is likely complicated by their perfectionistic attitudes and beliefs. As the experience of both perfectionism and shame persists, the dysfunction can become more severe and affect a person's self-esteem and overall welfare. Eventually, a person may develop an eating disorder or associated symptoms while attempting to cope with these negative emotions.

Women with eating disorders often think in absolute terms, meaning that they view the world as being either black or white, either good or bad. For example, if a perfectionistic woman believes that weighing more than 99 pounds is unacceptable, she will view herself as a bad person if she exceeds that weight, even if by only one pound, despite her other positive attributes. Additionally, perfectionists have high standards for themselves and constantly compare themselves to other people. Therefore, they are highly prone to criticism. These maladaptive ways of thinking combined with unreasonable expectations often put these women at great risk for developing psychological dysfunctions like eating disorders (Riebel 1985).

When personal standards are not met, perfectionists feel dissatisfied and unhappy with themselves. They may feel unwanted, unattractive, undesirable, stupid, or incompetent. As a consequence, perfectionists may resort to extreme measures, like binge eating or self-induced vomiting, to alleviate these negative feelings and escape from the self-ridicule (Joiner et al. 1997). However, rather than alleviating the negative feelings that prompted the maladaptive behaviors, engaging in these behaviors may elicit additional negative emotions, like shame, in the perfectionist.

Some perfectionistic women who develop eating pathology are motivated to avoid feeling inferior to other people (Bellew et al. 2006). Therefore, it is possible that the way in which women view competition in their environments and among their social groups may influence the development of eating disorders. This is particularly important in societies in which appearance is salient. For example, one way that perfectionistic women living in an appearance-focused society can attempt to avoid feelings of inferiority is to focus on their physical appearance, specifically being thinner and therefore more attractive than other women. Unfortunately, this may cause some women to resort to unhealthy practices to meet their own high standards and avoid feeling inferior to others.

Perfectionism may be linked to specific aspects of eating disorders. For example, research has shown that perfectionism is associated with dieting, fasting, and bulimic symptoms like purging (Downey and Chang 2007; Forbush et al. 2007) and cognitive symptoms of eating disorders, such as feeling fat and unattractive (Pollock-BarZiv and Davis 2005). Other research has investigated specific aspects of perfectionism that are related to general eating pathology. For example, concern about mistakes, a component of negative or unhealthy perfectionism, has been shown to strongly predict disordered eating behavior in college women (Humphreys et al. 2007). Additionally, high parental expectations, a component of perfectionism, have been shown to predict lower bulimic symptoms in college women (Young et al. 2004), suggesting that some components of perfectionism may actually be beneficial.

Healthy perfectionism is an aspect of one's personality that can help a person be successful. In highly competitive environments, such as athletics, business, medicine, and academia, some perfectionistic tendencies may be necessary. A person's expectations and attitudes when these perfectionistic expectations are not met can differentiate healthy and unhealthy perfectionists (Franco-Paredes et al. 2005; Terry-Short et al. 1995). More specifically, healthy or adaptive perfectionists set high but reasonable standards and enjoy working diligently to achieve their goals. Additionally, healthy perfectionists are able to relax their personal expectations when necessary. In contrast, unhealthy perfectionists have unrealistic and inflexible expectations for themselves. Therefore, they rarely meet these expectations, yet they are unable to alter their personal standards (Hamachek 1978). For example, a healthy perfectionist who loses five pounds in 2 months instead of ten as she originally intended can be proud of herself for losing some weight. She may not have met the goal that she originally set, but she can still view her weight loss as an achievement and can continue working toward her goal. For an unhealthy perfectionist, the weight loss goal might be unrealistic, such as losing ten pounds in 1 week, and losing five pounds instead of the expected ten would be considered a failure because the original goal was not achieved. She would view her five-pound loss as unacceptable and may even resort to inappropriate and unhealthy behaviors, such as purging or excessive exercise, in an attempt to achieve her goal.

Motivation also distinguishes healthy and unhealthy perfectionists. Fear of failure motivates unhealthy perfectionists, whereas desire for personal improvement or achievement motivates healthy perfectionists (Hamachek 1978; Terry-Short et al. 1995). For example, an unhealthy perfectionist might diet because she is afraid of looking unattractive in her bathing suit and wants to avoid the ridicule of others. Conversely, a healthy perfectionist might diet to improve her overall health and feeling of wellness.

Different dimensions of perfectionism can affect our mood and functioning in beneficial or damaging ways. Specifically, unhealthy perfectionism has been linked to both anxiety disorders and depressive disorders (Bieling et al. 2004; Kawamura et al. 2001; Rice et al. 1998). Obviously, potentially negative experiences such as depression, shame, guilt, shyness, procrastination, and self-depreciation can accompany the experience of unhealthy perfectionism (Hamachek 1978). Because unhealthy perfectionists use unrealistic, maladaptive strategies to cope with stress (Burns and Fedewa 2005), it is not surprising that unhealthy perfectionism has also been linked to disordered eating (Ashby et al. 1998; Campbell 2003; Haase et al. 1999; Pearson and Gleaves 2006). Using bingeing and purging to cope with negative emotions is obviously maladaptive. Additionally, unhealthy perfectionism may predict symptom severity and affect a woman's ability to recover from an eating disorder, as recent research has shown that unhealthy perfectionism may be a risk factor for relapse in those with eating disorders (Soenens et al. 2007).

Although it might seem that "healthy" perfectionism might protect a person from psychological dysfunction, research studies have also linked healthy perfectionism to psychological dysfunction, such as eating disorders (Davis 1997; Haase et al. 2002; Terry-Short et al. 1995). For example, in a study comparing depressed women, elite women athletes, women with eating disorders, and a nonclinical comparison group of women, those in the elite athlete group and those in the eating disorder group reported higher levels of healthy perfectionism than the other groups (Terry-Short et al. 1995). Furthermore, athletes who reported high levels of healthy perfectionism also reported low levels of unhealthy perfectionism, and those with eating disorders who reported high levels of healthy perfectionism also reported high levels of unhealthy perfectionism. Therefore, both healthy and unhealthy perfectionism may be important when attempting to understand the relationship between perfectionism and eating disorders.

Recognizing the relationships between various component of perfectionism and eating disorder symptoms will be advantageous in the therapeutic context. Some research suggests that decreases in perfectionism are correlated with decreases in eating disorder symptoms (Campbell 2003). Yet, other research suggests that general levels of healthy and unhealthy perfectionism rarely change despite recovery from an eating disorder (Bardone-Cone et al. 2007). Perhaps this reflects the tendency to address the physically obvious symptoms, such as weight restoration and discontinuing bingeing and purging behaviors, rather than addressing psychological issues that accompany eating disorders. Additionally, it is possible that the wrong aspects of perfectionism are being addressed in therapy. For example, some research suggests that working with people with eating disorders to lower personal standards (i.e., reducing extreme levels of healthy perfectionism) may be less important than working with them to decrease concern about mistakes and anxiety about performance (i.e., reducing unhealthy perfectionism) (Ashby et al. 1998).

Clearly, there is a relationship between perfectionism and eating disorders. Furthermore, some research suggests that perfectionism might help to explain the relationships between eating disorders and other types of pathology. For example, perfectionism may be problematic for people with eating disorders because of the obsessive thoughts that often accompany eating disorders (Humphreys et al. 2007). However, the specific relationships among components of perfectionism and various eating disorder symptoms are less obvious. Despite extensive research on perfectionism and eating disorders, much research still needs to be conducted to investigate unique relationships to eating disorder symptoms. Increased knowledge of these relationships will contribute to the overall understanding and treatment of eating disorders. Therefore, perfectionism may be increasingly important when considering future diagnostic criteria for eating disorders (Herzog and Delinsky 2001).

2.2.3.2 Obsessiveness and Desire for Control

In addition to perfectionism, other aspects of personality are often observed in women with eating disorders. Obsessiveness is a common trait among women with eating disorders and may be a predisposing factor for developing an eating disorder (Lilenfeld et al. 2006). Obsessiveness is characterized by persistent and obtrusive thoughts or ideas (APA 2000). For example, a woman with an eating disorder might be plagued with persistent thoughts that she is overweight or that eating certain foods will result in weight gain. Furthermore, some women with eating disorders are actually diagnosed with obsessive-compulsive disorder or obsessive-compulsive personality disorder (Lilenfeld et al. 2006; Swinbourne and Touyz 2007). Thus, a person who obsessively counted her books or arranged her dolls as a child may find that ruminating about caloric consumption or body weight is appropriate, feels natural, and accommodates her need for control.

Like obsessiveness, an individual's need for control is also a common feature in people with eating disorders (Polivy and Herman 2002). More specifically, eating disorders can originate from concerns about personal control, particularly in those who feel out of control in some way and have a strong desire to regain control over their lives (Surgenor et al. 2002). For example, if a young woman feels as though she is not in control of her life because she has demanding, overly critical parents or because she is not performing as well in school as she would like, she might attempt to compensate for the lack of control by overcontrolling a different area of her life, such as her food intake. Rather than addressing the problem directly, she focuses all of her attention on controlling her diet. Dietary restriction might seem like an effective strategy to a young woman because she can physically see evidence that she is "in control" by staying within a specific weight range, gradually losing weight over time, or restricting herself to a low range of calories each day (Fairburn et al. 1998). Therefore, a young woman could feel compelled to remain in control of her weight or to regain control of her weight as quickly as possible when she sensed that she had lost control of her weight or eating habits.

This pattern and extreme need for control can be observed in women who restrict as well as women who binge and purge. For example, a woman who severely restricts her caloric intake shows her strong need for control by strictly monitoring the amount of food she eats. She may view this restriction as a great accomplishment because she is able to exercise a level of will power around food that others do not have (Peters et al. 1992). A woman who binges and purges also shows a high need for control. Although she likely loses control during an episode of binge eating, she attempts to regain control by engaging in inappropriate compensatory behavior, such as self-induced vomiting, laxative misuse, or excessive exercise.

Recognizing the degree to which an obsessive style perpetuates the course of an eating disorder and addressing the need for control in people with eating disorders are essential when treating the eating disorder, because both factors can strongly influence the effectiveness of therapy. For example, a woman who is obsessed with counting calories may not benefit from keeping a food journal because it reinforces her obsession. Rather, she may be directed to avoid such obsessions or to use her obsessive thinking in healthier ways. Additionally, women with eating disorders can become quite fearful when they sense that control is lost or forfeited. Therefore, following a dietary plan as advised by a licensed nutritionist or not purging after binge eating can be overwhelming and terrifying experiences for a person with an eating disorder. Therapists should work to make clients aware that, even though they might believe that behaviors like restriction and purging help maintain a level of control over their lives, these behaviors actually reflect an extreme loss of control because the obsession with weight and food eventually dominates every aspect of their lives.

2.2.3.3 Shame

Various emotional experiences are salient when considering psychological factors associated with eating disorders. One especially salient emotion is the experience of shame, which can affect a person's self-esteem and body image and can contribute to the development and maintenance of dysfunctional relationships with food (Burney and Irwin 2000; Skarderud 2007). When shame is associated with psychological dysfunction, one can experience alienation, loneliness, and inferiority, and an eating disorder may be an attempt to deal with or regulate these negative emotions (Kaufman 1989; Skarderud 2007). This shame may be related to a person's body, to herself as a person, or to her inability to control her "chaotic" life (Pettersen et al. 2008).

Some behaviors associated with the experience of shame, such as avoidance and secrecy, are common among those with eating disorders (Gilbert 1998). In fact, eating disorders have been described as "disorders of shame" (Kaufman 1989). Additionally, the frequent experience of shame may distinguish those with clinical eating disorders from those with other types of psychological dysfunction (Frank 1991). Indeed, research has shown that those women who experience shame are more likely to binge and then compensate for the binge in an inappropriate way (Denious 2004). Shame is also important in predicting the severity of specific eating disorder symptoms. For example, higher reported levels of shame are related to higher reported levels of bulimic symptoms for college women, women with subclinical symptoms of bulimia nervosa, and women with bulimia nervosa (Hayaki et al. 2002). Therefore, even if a woman is not diagnosed with an eating disorder but experiences some bulimic symptoms, the experience of shame is likely.

Research has shown that feelings of shame fluctuate during the binge–purge cycle, and fluctuations are most evident in people who binge eat (Sanftner and Crowther 1998). Specifically, research has shown that shame increases following episodes of binge eating and that this increased shame persists even after purging (Corstophine et al. 2006). Similarly, strong feelings of shame, guilt, and anxiety prior to vomiting have been shown to increase the urge to vomit (Hinrichsen et al. 2007), suggesting that shame might play a role in triggering self-induced vomiting and may cause the individual to actually vomit. Therefore, a woman may experience shame after bingeing, and this shame may motivate her to purge. Although she may experience relief, she might also feel ashamed of the purging behavior as well as the hypothesized shame that motivated the purge.

Part of the difficulty in recognizing and treated eating disorders is the secrecy associated with some symptoms of eating disorder, and the experience of shame can drive women to attempt to conceal the shame they experience. For example, women who binge and purge often describe internal experiences that differ from their social experiences. Specifically, women who engage in bulimic behaviors are often outgoing and engaged in personal relationships. Because they associate bulimic behaviors, such as binge eating and purging, with shame and a fear of stigmatization, extreme efforts may be made to conceal their behavior to avoid public shame. However, even when bulimic behavior is successfully concealed, they often feel ashamed for engaging in these behaviors and for concealing these behaviors. As a result, they might plan, at least to some degree, episodes of bingeing and purging to help protect themselves from the experience of shame and public scrutiny (Pettersen et al. 2008).

Although shame plays an obvious role in the persistence of eating disorder symptoms, shame may prevent people from seeking help. For many people with eating disorders, actually discussing their eating disorder symptoms could result in perceived negative evaluations from others and lead to greater shame. Some people may seek treatment for other psychological dysfunction, such as depression or obsessive-compulsive disorder, but not report symptoms of an eating disorder (Striegel-Moore and Marcus 1995). Some women who are in treatment for an eating disorder stop reporting symptoms prematurely to avoid the experience of shame. As a consequence, these women could be inaccurately diagnosed as being in remission. Therefore, reducing shame may be one of the most important components of treatment for these individuals (Pettersen et al. 2008).

In addition to general feelings of shame, a specific type of shame, body shame, has also been linked to eating disorders (Brock 2000; Chervinko 2005; Denious 2004; Skarderud 2007; Troop et al. 2006; Tyla and Hill 2004). Body shame is the perception that others find one's physical appearance unattractive, which could result in rejection (Skarderud 2007). The experience of body shame is likely when there is a discrepancy between the way a person actually views herself and the way she would like to look. The greater the discrepancy, the more body shame she experiences (Kellett and Gilbert 2001), and research suggests that body shame might develop in girls as early as age

11 (Grabe et al. 2007). Additionally, the experience of body shame might distinguish people with eating disorders from those who experience normal body dissatisfaction (Brock 2000). Beyond a simple association with eating disorders, the experience of body shame has also been shown to predict specific eating disorder symptoms, including fasting, bingeing, and purging (Chervinko 2005; Denious 2004). Additionally, women who experience body shame might suppress their hunger, satiety, and emotional cues in an attempt to decrease body shame (Tyla and Hill 2004). Even the expectation of experiencing body shame has been linked to dysfunctional eating patterns (Troop et al. 2006). Therefore, increasing understanding of body shame will enhance psychological conceptualizations of eating disorders.

Much of the current research on body shame explains the experience, development, and maintenance of body shame through Objectification Theory (Fredrickson and Roberts 1997). Specifically, Fredrickson and Roberts (1997) propose that women in Western society are "treated as bodies ... that exist for the use and pleasure of others" (p. 175). Therefore, women view their own bodies as objects that they readily evaluate and criticize. Women learn in our culture to engage in self-objectification—to consider how attractive they are to others instead of focusing on whether they feel well and are engaged in behavior to promote good health. Since the standard for physical attractiveness imposed on women in Western society is unattainable for most, women are predisposed to criticize themselves. This repeated evaluation and surveillance of one's body, together with exposure to idealized images, can lead to negative consequences, such as body shame (Monro and Huon 2005). These constant experiences of objectification, self-criticism, and shame can result in psychological dysfunction, such as disordered eating or depression. Further, those who are more tempted to adopt impossible goals regarding their bodies (e.g., perfectionists) have more opportunities to experience body shame (Fredrickson and Roberts 1997).

2.2.3.4 Depression

Depression or symptoms of depression are often seen in people with eating disorders (Chamay-Weber et al. 2005; Santos et al. 2007; Zerbe et al. 1991). Symptoms associated with eating disorders, such as dieting and body dissatisfaction, are often accompanied by depressive symptoms and decreased self-esteem (McCreary and Sasse 2002). However, it is unclear if depression is present prior to the onset of eating disturbance, serving as a risk factor for disordered eating patterns, or if depression is the result of disturbed eating patterns (Fava et al. 1997). Regardless of the relationship between eating disorders and depression, it is clear that depression is a significant problem for many people with eating disorders and merits attention throughout the course of treatment, as the co-occurrence of both eating and depressive symptoms is linked with greater levels of distress and poorer treatment outcomes (Graber and Brooks-Gunn 2001).

Although it might seem that depressive symptoms in people with eating disorders would be linked exclusively to difficulties surrounding food, weight, and body image, in actuality, negative thoughts and feelings can be much more pervasive. As described in the first edition of this book (Haas and Clopton 2001), women with eating disorders frequently report feeling generally sad and hopeless about life. Additionally, they often show other characteristics of depression, such as withdrawing from others or experiencing less pleasure in activities that were once enjoyable. As a result, they may have a weak social support system and limited range of enjoyable activities, both of which may be obstacles in therapeutic endeavors.

The coexistence of depressive symptoms and disturbed eating patterns has significant implications for the diagnosis and treatment of these dysfunctions. Treating the depressive symptoms with psychotropic medication, psychotherapy, or both may help to alleviate the eating disorder symptoms (Fava et al. 1997). However, if the depressive symptoms are not addressed, these symptoms can persist even after eating disorder symptoms dissipate (Haas and Clopton 2001). Therefore, it is imperative to help people prepare to cope with future depressive symptoms in order to prevent relapses.

2.2.4 SUMMARY

Eating disorders are a relatively new phenomenon. Although much research is being conducted to enhance understanding of these disorders, many questions remain regarding risk factors for development and maintenance of these disorders. Because each individual is unique, it is impossible to identify one specific combination of risk factors that lead to the development and maintenance of eating disorders. Yet, understanding the psychological risk factors that might contribute to the development and maintenance of eating pathology is imperative in treating individuals with eating disorders.

Long-term follow-up studies have shown that 30% of eating disordered women relapse, and up to 40% still show symptoms of disturbed eating thoughts and behaviors even after improvement in treatment (Steinhausen et al. 2003; Zerbe et al. 1991). A therapist, teacher, or parent could spend hours lecturing a young woman on the life-threatening physical consequences of self-starvation or purging, but never get through to her because of a failure to understand and incorporate the deep-seated needs of the young woman to be attractive and accepted. Exploring other psychological characteristics, such as perfectionism, obsessiveness, need for control, shame, and depression, may be essential to truly helping women with eating disorders recover. With additional understanding of these issues, a therapist or other influential person may be able to help a person with an eating disorder find other ways to feel attractive or help her become less reliant on the need for approval from others. A greater understanding of the issues associated with eating disorders may greatly benefit people in the struggle to treat and prevent eating disorders.

2.3 RESEARCH APPLICATION

The application of the information presented in this chapter is in the conceptualization and treatment of eating disorders. The importance of assessing related characteristics among women with eating disorders should now be clear. Clinicians have found that dealing with characteristics that coexist with eating disorders greatly complicates the treatment of the disorders but, at the same time, can greatly improve the quality of these women's lives and reduce the likelihood that eating disorders will recur (Steinhausen et al. 2003). Several instruments have been developed to assess for various psychological characteristics associated with eating disorders. The use of such assessments can greatly enhance clinicians' abilities to determine the most important psychological characteristics exhibited by young women and, in addition, can help them to develop the most effective treatment plans.

Several measures can assist with the assessment of comorbid psychological characteristics. For example, the Beck Depression Inventory (BDI-II) is a 21-item forced-choice measure of the cognitive, motivational, and physiological symptoms of depression (Beck et al. 1996). The Revised Almost Perfect Scale (Slaney et al. 2001) is a 23-item measure that assesses overall perfectionism, as well as positive and negative components of perfectionism. The Body Shame Scale (Troop et al. 2006) is an 11-item measure that contains three subscales: current body shame, anticipated body shame, and perceived unattractiveness of being overweight.

REFERENCES

Aime, A., W. M. Craig, D. Pepler, D. Jiang, and J. Connolly. 2008. Developmental pathways of eating problems in adolescents. *Int J Eat Disord* 41: 686–696.

Alexander, L. 1998. The prevalence of eating disorders and eating disordered behavior in sororities. *Coll Student J* 32: 66–75.

American Psychiatric Association. 2000. *Diagnostic and statistical manual of mental disorders*. 4th ed text revision. Washington, DC: American Psychiatric Association.

Ashby, J. S., T. Kottman, and E. Schoen. 1998. Perfectionism and eating disorders reconsidered. *J Ment Health Couns* 20: 261–271.

Ashby, J. S., K. G. Rice, and J. L. Martin. 2006. Perfectionism, shame, and depressive symptoms. *J Couns Dev* 84: 148–156.

Ball, K., and C. Lee. 2000. Relationship between psychological stress, coping and disordered eating: A review. *Psychol Health* 14: 1007–1035.

Banister, E., and R. Schreiber. 2001. Young women's health concerns: Revealing paradox. *Health Care Women Int* 22: 633–647.

Bardone-Cone, A. M., S. A. Wonderlich, R. O. Frost, C. M. Bulik, J. E. Mitchell, S. Uppala, and H. Simonich. 2007. Perfectionism and eating disorders: Current status and future directions. *Clin Psychol Rev* 27: 384–405.

Beck A. T., R. A. Steer, and G. K. Brown. 1996. *Manual for the Beck Depression Inventory-II.* San Antonio, TX: Psychological Corporation.

Bellew, R., P. Gilbert, A. Mills, K. McEwan, and C. Gale. 2006. Eating attitudes and striving to avoid inferiority. *Eat Disord* 14: 313–322.

Bieling, P. J., A. L., Israeli, and M. M. Antony. 2004. Is perfectionism good, bad, or both? Examining models of the perfectionism construct. *Pers Individ Dif* 36: 1373–1385.

Birmingham, C., J. Su, J. Hlynsky, E. Goldner, and M. Gao. 2005. The mortality rate from anorexia nervosa. *Int J Eat Disord* 38: 143–146.

Brock, K. J. 2000. Exploring evidence for a continuum of eating disturbances: Self-objectification, parental attachment, and sociotrophy-autonomy in college women. *Diss Abstr* 60: 6354.

Burney, J., and H. Irwin. 2000. Shame and guilt in women with eating-disorder symptomatology. *J Clin Psychol* 56: 51–61.

Burns, L., and B. Fedewa. 2005. Cognitive styles: Links with perfectionistic thinking. *Pers Individ Dif* 38: 103–113.

Campbell, L. A. 2003. Dimensions of perfectionism in eating disorders: Diagnostic specificity and prognostic significance. *Diss Abstr* 64: 2909.

Cassin, S. E., and K. M. von Ranson. 2005. Personality and eating disorders: A decade in review. *Clin Psychol Rev* 25: 895–916.

Chamay-Weber, C., F. Narring, and P. Michaud. 2005. Partial eating disorders among adolescents: A review. *J Adolesc Health* 37: 417–427.

Chervinko, S. 2005. Potential moderators of the relationship between dietary restraint and binge eating: Affect intensity, body shame, and coping styles. *Diss Abstr* 65: 4821.

Clay, D., V. L. Vignoles, and H. Dittmar. 2005. Body image and self-esteem among adolescent girls: Testing the influence of sociocultural factors. *J Res Adolesc* 15: 451–477.

Corstophine, E., G. Waller, V. Ohanian, and M. Baker. 2006. Changes in internal states across the binge-vomit cycle in bulimia nervosa. *J Nerv Ment Dis* 194: 446–449.

Dalle Grave, R., and S. Calugi. 2007. Eating disorder not otherwise specified in an inpatient unit: The impact of altering the DSM-IV criteria for anorexia nervosa and bulimia nervosa. *Eur Eat Disord Rev* 15: 340–349.

Davis, C. 1997. Normal and neurotic perfectionism in eating disorders: An interactive model. *Int J Eat Disord* 22: 421–426.

Denious, J. E. 2004. Understanding the relationship of shame to eating-disordered symptomology. *Diss Abstr Int* 65: 1071.

Downey, C. A., and E. C. Chang. 2007. Perfectionism and symptoms of eating disturbances in female college students: Considering the role of negative affect and body dissatisfaction. *Eat Behav* 8: 497–503.

Fairburn, C. G., and K. Bohn. 2005. Eating disorder NOS (EDNOS): An example of troublesome 'not otherwise specified' (NOS) category in DSM-IV. *Behav Res Ther* 43: 691–701.

Fairburn, C. G., Z. Cooper, and K. Bohn. 2007. The severity and status of eating disorder NOS: Implications for DSM-V. *Behav Res Ther* 45: 1705–1715.

Fairburn, C. G., Z. Cooper, H. A. Doll, and S. L. Welch. 1999. Risk factors for anorexia nervosa: Three integrated case-control comparisons. *Gen Psychiatry* 56: 468–476.

Fairburn, C. G., Z. Cooper, and R. Shafran. 2003. CBT for eating disorders: A transdiagnostic theory and treatment. *Behav Res Ther* 41: 509–517.

Fairburn, C. G., S. L. Welch, H. A. Doll, B. A. Davies, and M. E. Connor. 1997. Risk factors for bulimia nervosa: A community-based case-control study. *Gen Psychiatry* 54: 509–517.

Fava, M., M. Abraham, K. Clancy-Colecchi, J. A. Pava, J. Matthews, and J. Rosenbaum. 1997. Eating disorders symptomatology in major depression, *J Nerv Ment Dis* 185: 140–144.

Fichter, M. M., and N. Quadflieg. 2007. Long-term stability of eating disorder diagnoses. *Int J Eat Disord* 40: 561–566.

Forbush, K., T. F. Heatherton, and P. K. Keel. 2007. Relationships between perfectionism and specific disorder eating behaviors. *Int J Eat Disord* 40: 37–41.

Franco-Paredes, K., J. M. Mancilla-Diaz, R. Vazquez-Arevalo, X. Lopez-Aguilar, and G. Alvarez-Rayon. 2005. Perfectionism and eating disorders: A review of the literature. *Eur Eat Disord Rev* 13: 61–70.

Frank, E. S. 1991. Shame and guilt in eating disorders. *Am J Orthopsychiatry* 61: 303–306.

Fredrickson, B. L., and T. A. Roberts. 1997. Objectification theory: Toward understanding women's lived experiences and mental health risks. *Psychol Women Q* 21: 173–206.

Freedman, N., and J. Lavender. 2002. On desymbolization: The concept and observations on anorexia and bulimia. *Psychoanalysis and Contemporary Thought* 25: 165–199.

Furman, W., B. B. Brown, and C. Feiring. 1999. *The development of romantic relationships in adolescence.* New York: Cambridge Univ. Press.

Garner, D. M., P. E. Garfinkel, D. Schwartz, and M. Thompson. 1980. Cultural expectations of thinness in women. *Psychol Rep* 47: 483–491.

Garrow, J. S., James, W. P. T., and A. Ralph. 2000. *Human nutrition and dietetics.* London: Harcourt.

Ghaderi, A. 2001. Review of risk factors for eating disorders: Implications for primary prevention and cognitive behavioural therapy. *Scand J Behav Ther* 30: 57–74.

Gilbert, P. 1998. What is shame? Some core issues and controversies. In *Shame: interpersonal behavior, psychopathology, and culture,* ed. P. Gilbert and B. Andrews, 3–38. New York: Oxford Univ. Press.

Grabe, S., J. Shibley, and S. M. Lindberg. 2007. Body objectification and depression in adolescents: The role of gender, shame, and rumination. *Psychol Women Q* 31: 164–175.

Graber, J. A., and J. Brooks-Gunn. 2001. Co-occurring eating and depressive symptoms: An 8-year study of adolescent girls. *Int J Eat Disord* 30: 37–47.

Haas, H. L., and J. R. Clopton. 2001. Psychology of an eating disorder. In *Eating disorders in women and children: Prevention, stress management, and treatment,* ed. J. J. Robert-McComb, 39–48. Boca Raton, FL: CRC Press.

Haase, A. M., H. Prapavessis, and R. G. Owens. 1999. Perfectionism and eating attitudes in competitive rowers: Moderating effects of body mass, weight classification and gender. *Psychol Health* 14: 643–657.

Halliwell, E., and M. Harvey. 2006. Examination of a sociocultural model of disordered eating among male and female adolescents. *Brit J Health Psychol* 11: 235–248.

Hamachek, D. E. (1978). Psychodynamics of normal and neurotic perfectionism. *Psychol: J Human Behav* 15: 27–33.

Hay, P., and C. Fairburn. 1998. The validity of the DSM-IV scheme for classifying bulimic eating disorders. *Int J Eat Disord* 23: 7–15.

Hayaki, J., M. A. Friedman, and K. D. Brownell. 2002. Shame and severity of bulimic symptoms. *Eat Behav* 3: 73–83.

Heatherton, T. F., P. Nichols, F. Mahamedi, and P. Keel. 1995. Body weight, dieting, and eating disorder symptoms among college students, 1982–1992. *Am J Psychiatry* 152: 1623–1629.

Herzog, D. B., and S. S. Delinsky. 2001. Classification of eating disorders. In *Eating disorders: Innovative directions in research and practice,* ed. R. H. Striegel-Moore and L. Smolak, 31–50. Washington, DC: American Psychological Association.

Hill, A. J. 2002. Developmental issues in attitudes to food and diet. *Proceed Nutr Soc* 61: 259–266.

Hinrichsen, H., T. Morrison, G. Waller, and U. Schmidt. 2007. Triggers of self-induced vomiting in bulimic disorders: The roles of core beliefs and imagery. *J Cogn Psychotherapy* 21: 261–272.

Hoek, H., and D. Hoeken. 2003. Review of the prevalence and incidence of eating disorders. *Int J Eat Disord* 34: 383–396.

Hornbacher, M. 1999. *Wasted: A memoir of anorexia nervosa and bulimia nervosa.* New York: Harper Collins.

Humphreys, J. D., J. R. Clopton, and D. A. Reich. 2007. Disordered eating behavior and obsessive compulsive symptoms in college students: Cognitive and affective similarities. *Eat Disord* 15: 247–259.

Joiner, T. E., T. F. Heatherton, M. D. Rudd, and Schmidt, N. B. (1997). Perfectionism, perceived weight status, and bulimic symptoms: Two studies testing a diathesis-stress model. *J Ab Psychol* 106: 145–153.

Kansi, J., L. Wichstrom, and L. R. Bergman. 2005. Eating problems and their risk factors: A 7-year longitudinal study of a population sample of Norwegian adolescent girls. *J Youth Adolesc* 34: 521–531.

Kaufman, G. 1989. *The psychology of shame.* New York: Springer.

Kawamura, K., S. Hunt, R. Frost, and P. DiBartolo. 2001. Perfectionism, anxiety, and depression: Are the relationships independent? *Cogn Ther Res* 25: 291–301.

Kearney-Cooke, A. 1999. Gender differences and self-esteem. *J Gen Spec Med* 2: 46–52.

Kellett, S., and P. Gilbert. 2001. Acne: A biopsychosocial and evolutionary perspective with a focus on shame. *Brit J Health Psychol* 6: 1–24.

Kiemle, G., P. D. Slade, and M. E. Dewey. 1987. Factors associated with abnormal eating attitudes and behaviors: Screening individuals at risk of developing an eating disorder. *Int J Eat Disord* 6: 713–724.

Kjaerbye-Thygesen, A., C. Munk, B. Ottesen, and S. Kjaer. 2004. Why do slim women consider themselves too heavy? A characterization of adult women considering their body weight as too heavy. *Int J Eat Disord* 35, 275–285.

Levine, M. P., and S. K. Murnen. 2009. "Everybody knows that mass media are/are not [pick one] a cause of eating disorders": A critical review of evidence for a causal link between media, negative body image, and disordered eating in females. *J Soc Clin Psychol* 28: 9–42.

Lieberman, M., L. Gauvin, W. Bukowski, and D. White. 2001. Interpersonal influence and disordered eating behaviors in adolescent girls: The role of peer modeling, social reinforcement, and body-related teasing. *Eat Behav* 2: 215–236.

Lilenfeld, L. R. R., S. Wonderlich, L. P. Riso, R. Crosby, and J. Mitchell. 2006. Eating disorders and personality: A methodological and empirical review. *Clin Psychol Rev* 26: 299–320.

Machado, P. P., B. C. Machado, S. Goncalves, and H. W. Hoek. 2007. The prevalence of eating disorders not otherwise specified. *Int J Eat Disord* 40: 212–217.

McCabe, M. P., and L. A. Ricciardelli. 2004. A longitudinal study of pubertal timing and extreme body change behaviors among adolescent boys and girls. *Adolesc* 39: 145–166.

McCabe, M. P., and M. A. Vicent. 2003. The role of biodevelopmental and psychological factors in disordered eating among adolescent males and females. *Eur Eat Disord Rev* 11: 315–328.

McCreary, D. R., and D. K. Sasse. 2002. Gender differences in high school students' dieting behavior and their correlates. *Int J Men's Health* 1: 195–213.

McGee, B. J., P. L. Hewitt, S. B. Sherry, M. Parkin, and G. L. Flett. 2005. Perfectionistic self-presentation, body image, and eating disorder symptoms. *Body Image* 2: 29–40.

Monro, F., and G. Huon. 2005. Media-portrayed idealized images, body shame, and appearance anxiety. *Int J Eat Disord* 38: 85–90.

Muise, A. M., D. G. Stein, and G. Arbess. 2003. Eating disorders in adolescent boys: A review of the adolescent and young adult literature. *J Adolesc Health* 33: 427–435.

Nicholls, D., R. Chater, and B. Lask. 2000. Children into DSM don't go: A comparison of classification systems for eating disorders in childhood and early adolescence. *Int J Eat Disord* 28: 317–324.

Ohring, R., J. A. Graber, and J. Brooks-Gunn. 2002. Girls recurrent and concurrent body dissatisfaction: Correlates and consequences over 8 years. *Int J Eat Disord* 31: 404–415.

Pearson, C. A., and D. H. Gleaves. 2006. The multiple dimensions of perfectionism and their relation with eating disorder features. *Pers Individ Dif* 41: 225–235.

Peat, C. M., N. L. Peyerl, and J. J. Muehlenkamp. 2008. Body image and eating disorders in older adults: A review. *J Gen Psychol* 135: 343–358.

Peters, C., C. S. Swassing, P. Butterfield, and G. McKay. 1984. Assessment and treatment of anorexia nervosa and bulimia in school age children. *Sch Psychol Rev* 13: 183–191.

Pettersen, G., J. H. Rosenvinge, and B. Ytterhus. 2008. The "double life" of bulimia patients' experiences of daily life interactions. *Eat Disord* 16: 204–211.

Polivy, J., and C. P. Herman. 2002. Causes of eating disorders. *Annu Rev Psychol* 53: 187–213.

Pollock-BarZiv, S. M., and C. Davis. 2005. Personality factors and disordered eating in young women with Type I Diabetes Mellitus. *Psychosom: J Consult Liaison Psychiatry* 46: 11–18.

Rand, C. S. W., and B. A. Wright. 2000. Continuity and change in the evaluation of ideal and acceptable body sizes across a wide age span. *Int J Eat Disord* 28: 90–100.

Rembeck, G. I., and R. K. Gunnarsson. 2004. Improving pre- and postmenarcheal 12-year old girls' attitudes towards menstruation. *Health Care Women Int* 25: 680–698.

Rice, K. G., J. S. Ashby, and R. B. Slaney. 1998. Self-esteem as a mediator between perfectionism and depression: A structural equations analysis. *J Couns Psychol* 45: 304–314.

Riebel, L. 1985. Eating disorders and personal constructs. *Transactional Anal J* 15: 42–47.

Sancho, C., M. V. Arija, O. Asorey, and J. Canals. 2007. Epidemiology of eating disorders: A two year follow up in an early adolescent school population. *Eur Child Adolesc Psychiatry* 16: 495–504.

Sanftner, J. L., and J. H. Crowther. 1998. Variability in self-esteem, moods, shame, and guilt in women who binge. *Int J Eat Disord* 23: 391–397.

Santonastaso, P., S. Friederici, and A. Favaro. 1999. Full and partial syndromes in eating disorders: A 1-year prospective study of risk factors among female students. *Psychopathol* 32: 50–56.

Santos, M., C. S. Richards, and M. K. Bleckley. 2007. Comorbidity between depression and disordered eating in adolescents. *Eat Behav* 8: 440–449.

Schwitzer, A. M., L. E. Rodriguez, C. Thomas, and L. Salimi. 2001. The eating disorder NOS diagnostic profile among college women. *J Am Coll Health* 49: 157–166.

Siegel, J. M., A. K. Yancey, C. S. Aneshensel, and R. Schuler. 1999. Body image, perceived pubertal timing, and adolescent mental health. *J Adolesc Health* 25: 155–165.

Skarderud, F. 2007. Shame and pride in anorexia nervosa: A qualitative description. *Eur Eat Disord Rev* 15: 81–97.

Slaney, R. B., K. G. Rice, M. Mobley, J. Trippi, and J. S. Ashby. 2001. The revised almost perfect scale. *Meas Eval Couns Dev* 34: 130–145.

Soenens, B., W. Nevelsteen, and W. Vandereycken. 2007. The significance of perfectionism in eating disorders: A comparative study. *J Psychiatry* 49: 709–718.

Soh, N. L., S. W. Touyz, and L. J. Surgenor. 2006. Eating and body image disturbances across cultures: A review. *Eur Eat Disord Rev* 14: 54–65.

Sokol, M. S., T. K. Jackson, and C. T. Selser. 2005. Review of clinical research in child and adolescent eating disorders. *Prim Psychiatry* 12: 52–58.

Steinhausen, H. C., S. Boyadjieva, M. Griogoroiu-Serbanescu, and K. J. Neumärker. 2003. The outcome of adolescent eating disorders: Findings from an international collaborative study. *Eur Child Adolesc Psychiatry* 12: i91–i98.

Steinhausen, H. C., C. Winkler, and M. Meier. 1997. Eating disorders in adolescence in a Swiss epidemiological study. *Int J Eat Disord* 22: 147–151.

Stice, E. 2002. Risk and maintenance factors for *eating* pathology: A meta-analytic *review. Psychol B* 128: 825–848.

Striegel-Moore, R. H., D. L. Franko, D. Thompson, B. Barton, G. B. Schreiber, and S. R. Daniels. 2005. An empirical study of the typology of bulimia nervosa and its spectrum variants. *Psychol Med* 35: 1563–1572.

Striegel-Moore, R. H., and M. D. Marcus. 1995. Eating disorders in women: Current issues and debates. In *The psychology of women's health: Progress and challenges in research and application,* ed. A. L. Stanton and S. J. Gallant, 445–487. Washington, DC: American Psychological Association.

Surgenor, L. J., J. Horn, E. W. Plumridge, and S. M. Hudson. 2002. Anorexia nervosa and psychological control: A reexamination of selected theoretical accounts. *Eur Eat Disord Rev* 10: 85–101.

Swinbourne, J. M., and S. W. Touyz. 2007. The co-morbidity of eating disorders and anxiety disorders: A review. *Eur Eat Disord Rev* 15: 253–274.

Tangney, J. P. 2002. Perfectionism and the self-conscious emotions: Shame, guilt, embarrassment, and pride. In *Perfectionism: Theory, research, and treatment,* ed. G. L. Flett and P. L. Hewitt, 199–215. Washington, DC: American Psychological Association.

Taylor, C., T. Sharpe, C. Shisslak, S. Bryson, L. Estes, N. Gray, K. McKnight, M. Crago, H. Kraemer, and J. Killen. 1998. Factors associated with weight concern in adolescent girls. *Int J Eat Disord* 24: 31–42.

Terry-Short, L., R. G. Owens, P. Slade, and M. Dewey. 1995. Positive and negative perfectionism. *Pers Individ Dif* 18: 663–668.

Troop, N. A., S. Sotrilli, and L. Serpell. 2006. Establishing a useful distinction between current and anticipated bodily shame in eating disorders. *Eat Weight Disord* 11: 83–90.

Tylka, T. L., and M. S. Hill. 2004. Objectification theory as it relates to disordered eating among college women. *Sex Roles* 51: 719–730.

Tyrka, A. R., I. Waldron, J. A. Grader, and J. Brooks-Gunn. 2002. Prospective predictors of the onset of anorexic and bulimic syndromes. *Int J Eat Disord* 32: 282–290.

Vitousek, K., and F. Manke. 1994. Personality variables and disorders in anorexia nervosa and bulimia nervosa. *J Ab Psychol* 103: 137–147.

Wiseman, C. V., S. R. Sunday, and A. E. Becker. 2005. Impact of the media on adolescent body image. *Child Adolesc Psychiatr Clin North Am* 14: 453–471.

Young, E. A., J. R. Clopton, and M. K. Bleckley. 2004. Perfectionism, low self-esteem, and family factors as predictors of bulimic behavior. *Eat Behav* 5: 273–283.

Zerbe, K. J., S. R. Marsh, and C. Lolafay. 1991. Comorbidity in an inpatient eating disordered population: clinical characteristics and treatment implications. *Psychiatr Hosp* 24: 3–8.

3 The Physiology of Anorexia Nervosa

Annette Gary, Julie Campbell-Ruggaard, Kristin L. Goodheart, and James R. Clopton

CONTENTS

3.1   LEARNING OBJECTIVES

After reading this chapter, you should be able to

- Describe the physiological signs and symptoms of anorexia nervosa
- Discuss the physiological changes that occur in anorexia nervosa, such as the electrocardiograph (EKG), blood pressure, body fat percentage, heart rate, and metabolic rate
- Identify abnormal laboratory values associated with anorexia nervosa
- Describe the potential long-term physiological consequences of anorexia nervosa

3.2   INTRODUCTION

Eating disorders, such as anorexia nervosa, typically begin as plans to lose some weight through diet and sometimes exercise. What begins as a seemingly benign diet, however, can eventually consume a person's life, and the person becomes more restrictive with her caloric intake, more obsessed with weight loss and the shape of her body, and more disconnected from other aspects of life that were once important to her. Because of the strong emphasis on weight loss and physical appearance, people with anorexia nervosa often overlook or ignore physical consequences associated with being malnourished and severely underweight. Although anorexia nervosa is classified as a psychological disorder, the physical consequences associated with starvation and emaciation are severe and potentially life-threatening. For this reason, medical professionals are vital in treating people with anorexia nervosa.

Diagnostic criteria for anorexia nervosa include several criteria that reflect the physical manifestation of the disorder. Specifically, the current *Diagnostic and Statistical Manual of Mental Disorders* (*DSM-IV-TR;* American Psychiatric Association 2000) indicates that women with anorexia nervosa are severely underweight (i.e., 85% or less of the weight that would be expected based on age and height) and experience amenorrhea (i.e., absence of menstruation for at least 3 months). Individuals with this disorder also engage in behaviors that contribute to the physical signs and symptoms of anorexia nervosa. These behaviors, such as excessive exercise, self-induced vomiting, and laxative abuse, complicate the physical consequences of starvation (Fairburn 1995). Physical complications from anorexia nervosa may also increase a person's sense of vulnerability or personal inadequacy and can lead to an increase in psychological symptoms, such as increased anxiety or a depressed mood. (For more information on the psychological consequences of eating disorders, see Chapter 2 of this book.)

"Eating is such a fundamental biological process necessary to life that families and friends are left perplexed when a young girl starves herself. The irony is that she most often does not intend to starve herself or want to die, but to the contrary, she wants to become a better, more noble, and more attractive person" (Lucas 2004, x). The starvation of a young woman with anorexia causes biological changes that have profound effects on her physical development and functioning, her emotions, her thinking, and her interaction with family members. There is a danger in observing those effects of anorexia and assuming that they are causes (Lucas 2004, 5).

This chapter will discuss the physical signs and symptoms of anorexia nervosa. Since behaviors, such as calorie restriction and frequency of purging occur at varying degrees, the information presented in this chapter is most closely linked to the physical consequences of semi-starvation. Although purging behaviors, such as vomiting and laxative abuse, are problematic for many with anorexia nervosa (Fairburn 1995), the primary focus of this chapter will be on the physical consequences of starvation. Although this chapter contains some information about binge eating and purging, refer to Chapter 4 of this book for additional information on the physical consequences of binge eating and purging.

3.3   RESEARCH BACKGROUND AND SIGNIFICANCE

"Although patients with anorexia nervosa look and behave very much alike once their starvation is well advanced, there is no single cause" (Lucas 2004, 33). There are no laboratory tests or distinctive biological markers for anorexia. Its diagnosis depends on abnormally low weight and on interviewing the girl or woman about her history and present condition. "Anorexia nervosa arises in ordinary families … . It does not require extraordinary circumstances. … Blaming parents for causing the disease is unjustified" (Lucas 2004, 11).

Cases of self-starvation have been traced back as far as the Middle Ages, but the disorder was not familiar to American society until the 1970s (Bruch 1978). However, physicians, psychologists, and other professionals encountered individuals with anorexia nervosa long before the 1970s. Lucas and his colleagues (1991, 1999) reviewed the medical records of people in Rochester, Minnesota, for a 55-year time period, and they specifically identified individuals who either definitely had anorexia nervosa or who may have had it. Among those individuals, the youngest person was a 10-year-old girl, and the oldest was a 59-year-old woman who developed anorexia at that age for the first time. Most people with anorexia were young women between the ages of 15 and 24, and 90% of those identified were women. Although there was no statistically significant increase in anorexia over time for the entire sample, among young women (ages 15–24), there was a significant increase from 1935 to 1989. Among older teenage girls, the prevalence of anorexia was about

1 in 200 (Lucas et al. 1999), and that 0.5% rate is nearly the same as the prevalence rate found in three other studies (Crisp et al. 1976; Kent and Clopton 1992; Råstam et al. 1989).

Although few studied anorexia nervosa prior to the 1970s, early research that examined the effects of semi-starvation can be applied to people with anorexia nervosa. In 1950, Ancel Keys, a nutritionist who established "K" rations for World War II soldiers, conducted the Minnesota Starvation Experiment. He and his colleagues conducted this research to gain insight into the physical and psychological effects associated with semi-starvation and to explore problems with re-feeding. A small sample of healthy men was subjected to semi-starvation. Most of these men lost more than 25% of their original body weight, and many experienced anemia, fatigue, apathy, irritability, extreme weakness, neurological deficits, and lower extremity edema. It is noteworthy that all of these symptoms can occur in people with anorexia nervosa. Additionally, they experienced many of the same cognitive, social, and emotional changes that are observed in clients with eating disorders. Specifically, these men were preoccupied by thoughts of food, they showed great interest in recipes and cooking, and they spent most of their waking time thinking about eating and how to eat their allowable amount of food. One man compulsively looked through garbage cans for food, and many men increased their intake of non-nutritive substances, such as coffee, tea, and gum. In fact, one man reportedly chewed forty packs of gum each day.

With regard to the emotional effects of semi-starvation, the men in the Minnesota Starvation Experiment were reportedly tearful, angry, depressed, and anxious, and sometimes these emotional consequences interfered with their abilities to function and perform daily routines. For a few, the emotional consequences of semi-starvation were so severe that they resorted to extreme measures. For example, one man chopped off three fingers in response to his distress. Cognitive changes were also observed. The men were irritable, less alert, experienced difficulty concentrating, and reported feeling "foggy" in their thinking. Additionally, they reported loss of interest in romantic partners and friendships.

By the end of the 6-month period, participants experienced a 40% reduction, on average, in metabolic functioning, so their bodies compensated for the restrictive eating by burning fewer calories. During the re-feeding period, men who ate larger amounts of food increased metabolic functioning more than men who ate only slightly increased portions. Medical complications were also observed, including cardiac problems, mood fluctuations, hormonal changes, fertility problems, decreased bone density, neurological problems, and blood disorders.

The findings from the Minnesota Starvation Experiment are significant because symptoms that were once thought to be purely psychiatric were linked to the effects of physical starvation (e.g., fatigue, isolation, changes in mood and concentration, preoccupation with food and eating, increased consumption of non-nutritive substances). Additionally, results of this study confirmed that prolonged semi-starvation produces significant increases in depression, hysteria, and hypochondrias, as measured using the Minnesota Multiphasic Personality Inventory (MMPI; Greene 1980). Thus, the findings from this study contributed to current understanding of the physical and psychological consequences associated with anorexia nervosa.

The remainder of this chapter will focus on specific physical consequences of anorexia nervosa and will include information summarizing earlier research studies as well as more current research findings.

3.4 SUMMARY OF RESEARCH AND CURRENT FINDINGS

Numerous physiological signs and symptoms are associated with anorexia nervosa, and many of these physical symptoms are life-threatening. In fact, mortality rates for people with anorexia nervosa are among the highest of all mental disorders with reported rates as high as 18% (Steinhausen 2002). In addition to severe weight changes, individuals with anorexia nervosa may experience fluid and electrolyte disturbances, as well as cardiovascular problems, gastrointestinal abnormalities, endocrine problems, central nervous system abnormalities, and other abnormalities. A summary of some of the physical consequences of anorexia nervosa is provided in Table 3.1.

TABLE 3.1
Physical Consequences of Anorexia Nervosa

Cardiovascular	Gastrointestinal
Bradycardia	Abdominal discomfort
Tachycardia	Bloating/feeling of fullness
Arrhythmias	Constipation
Hypotension	Delayed gastric emptying
Fainting	Decreased gastric and intestinal motility
Dizziness	Pancreatitis
Endocrine	**Integumentary**
Amenorrhea	Dry, flaky/scaly, yellowish orange skin
Oligomenorrhea	Decreased body fat
Anovulation	Lanugo (fine facial and body hair)
Cold sensitivity	Thinning hair
	Brittle nails
Hematologic	**Central Nervous System**
Anemia	Poor problem-solving skills and memory
Leukopenia	Decreased concentration and attention
Thrombocytopenia	Depressed mood
Pancytopenia	Peripheral neuropathy
Hypercortisolism	Seizures
Skeletal	**Fluids and Electrolytes**
Osteopenia	Electrolyte imbalance
Osteoperosis	Dehydration
Bone fractures	Rebound peripheral edema
Stunted growth	Renal failure
	Metabolic acidosis

3.4.1 WEIGHT CHANGES

Individuals who are diagnosed with anorexia nervosa have an intense preoccupation with body weight and body shape. The individual may practice numerous behaviors focused on weight control, such as calorie restriction, excessive exercise, and purging behaviors, such as vomiting and laxative abuse. Unfortunately, a young woman who is concerned about being fat and loses a significant amount of weight because she has been restricting her food intake might make the mistake of regarding her loose skin as a sign that she is flabby or fat (Lucas 2004, 9).

The body weight of the individual with anorexia nervosa generally reflects the degree of calorie restriction, the severity of purging behaviors (if present), and the amount of exercise engaged in by the individual. Adults who are diagnosed with anorexia nervosa generally show extreme weight loss and may be described as thin or emaciated. Children and adolescents may not lose an extreme amount of weight, because weight loss goes against the body's natural tendency to grow larger. Rather, children and adolescents might lose smaller amounts of weight (e.g., 5 to 10 pounds) or might not grow to a weight that would be expected for them based on their height, age, and developmental level. The *DSM-IV* (APA 2000) diagnostic criterion that the body weight of a person with anorexia nervosa is 85% or less of what would be expected, based on her age and height, is equivalent to a body mass index (BMI) of less than 18 (a BMI that falls between 18.5 and 24.9 is considered to be in the healthy weight range).

In contrast to the *intentional* weight loss in anorexia due to fear of becoming fat or a desire to be thinner or healthier, there are other illnesses that can produce *unintentional* weight loss in girls and young women. In some of these, the individual consumes an adequate amount of food, but her body cannot absorb or metabolize it in a normal way, as in malabsorption disorders, inflammatory bowel disease, diabetes mellitus, and hyperthyroidism. In contrast, when a girl or young woman has cancer, her body may require such an increased amount of food that she rapidly loses weight when she eats what would normally be an adequate amount of food (Lucas 2004, 8).

In addition to the conditions just described, depression may lead to a lack of appetite and unintentional weight loss, although the amount of weight lost is usually much less than in anorexia (Lucas 2004, 8). Although depression often occurs for young women who have anorexia for a while, the two conditions are often quite distinctive. Individuals with anorexia have increased activity and exercise, whereas depression often leads to reduced activity and a lack of exercise due to fatigue. The main difference, however, is that individuals who are depressed have a "true loss of appetite" and lose interest in food, but do not intend to lose weight (Lucas 2004, 79). Similarly, adolescents with inflammatory bowel disease or endocrine disorders may lose significant amounts of weight, but interviewing will often demonstrate that they have no intention to lose weight, no fear of being fat, and no distortion in body image (Lucas 2004, 79–81).

3.4.2 Fluid and Electrolyte Abnormalities

Individuals with anorexia nervosa can develop imbalances in body fluid and electrolyte levels due to prolonged malnutrition and dehydration. These imbalances can reduce fluid and mineral levels and produce a condition known as *electrolyte imbalance*. Electrolytes, such as calcium and potassium, are critical for maintaining the electric currents necessary for a normal heartbeat. These imbalances can be very serious and can even be life-threatening unless fluids and minerals are replaced.

Fluid and electrolyte imbalances can become more serious when an individual also engages in purging behaviors, such as vomiting and laxative abuse. Dehydration may result from inadequate fluid intake or excessive fluid loss during purging or exercise. Dehydration leads to increased blood levels of urea, urate, and creatinine, and dehydration may result in decreased urine volume and renal failure. A *rebound peripheral edema* (i.e., swelling of body tissue due to excessive fluid retention) may also occur and can contribute to a dramatic increase in body weight (approximately 10 to 45 pounds). *Metabolic acidosis*, a condition when the body produces too much acid or the kidneys do not remove enough acid, may result from vomiting and loss of stomach acid and sodium bicarbonate. If the individual also engages in laxative abuse, the loss of alkaline bowel fluids may result in metabolic acidosis (Mitchell et al. 1986), and individuals who abuse laxatives are four times more likely to suffer serious medical complications than non-laxative abusers (Mitchell et al. 1987).

Heart problems are also a particular risk when anorexia nervosa is compounded with purging behaviors. Irregular heartbeat, slow heartbeat (i.e., a rate under 50 beats or even fewer per minute instead of the normal resting rate of 70 to 80 beats per minute; Lucas 2004, 82), reduced blood flow, and lower blood pressure have all been linked to electrolyte imbalance. More information on cardiovascular abnormalities associated with anorexia nervosa is included in the next section of the chapter.

3.4.3 Cardiovascular Abnormalities

Some of the most serious and life-threatening complications of anorexia nervosa result from impairment of the cardiovascular system. Individuals with anorexia nervosa can develop a number of serious cardiac abnormalities. For example, people with anorexia nervosa might complain of heart palpitations, dizziness, fainting, shortness of breath, and chest discomfort. If these cardiovascular abnormalities are not recognized and treated, they could result in death.

Heart disease is the most common medical cause of death in people with anorexia nervosa, and a primary danger to the heart is from abnormalities in the balance of minerals, such as potassium, calcium, magnesium, and phosphate. Prolonged starvation leads to decreased sympathetic tone in the heart and blood vessels. The heart's ability to pump and the vessels' ability to transport blood may be altered, which could result in *bradycardia* (i.e., heart beats too slowly), *tachycardia* (i.e., heart beats too quickly), or extremely low blood pressure (Carney and Andersen 1996). Tachycardia can occur when the circulating fluid volume decreases as a result of dehydration, and the heart is forced to pump faster to compensate for the decrease. Bradycardia may occur due to a starvation-induced metabolic decrease controlled by circulating *catecholamines* (i.e., "fight or flight" hormones released in response to stress) and a change in thyroid hormone levels (Hall et al. 1989). The reduction in blood pressure may lead to light-headedness or dizziness, and the individual with anorexia may experience orthostatic hypotension (light-headedness when standing up or getting out of bed; Lucas 2004, 83). Episodes of fainting may occur because of abnormally low blood pressure. Studies have shown that 91% of individuals with anorexia nervosa have pulse rates less than 60 beats per minute (Fohlin 1977), and up to 85% of patients with anorexia nervosa also have hypotension, with blood pressures below 90/60 (Warren and van de Wiele 1973). Individuals with anorexia nervosa have been found to have higher incidences of mitral valve abnormalities and left ventricular dysfunction than individuals who do not have eating disorders (De Simone et al. 1994). All of these factors contribute to a significant risk of sudden death due to cardiovascular problems in this population (Hall and Beresford 1989; Schocken et al. 1989).

Cardiovascular abnormalities also contribute to the coldness that people with anorexia nervosa experience. Because the blood circulates more slowly, a person's hands and feet turn cold and also appear blue because red blood cells have been depleted of oxygen (Lucas 2004, 82). However, another reason that individuals with anorexia feel cold is the loss of the insulation normally provided by a thin layer fat all over the body (Lucas 2004, 85).

3.4.4 ENDOCRINE ABNORMALITIES

Anorexia nervosa affects the endocrine system by producing numerous alterations in neuroendocrine mechanisms. Changes in the hypothalamic-pituitary-adrenal axis (HPA axis) result in hypercortisolemia and increased cerebrospinal fluid (CSF) levels of corticotropin-releasing hormones. Since the hypothalamus controls the pituitary gland, pituitary function is also inhibited, resulting in alterations in the normal circulating levels of gonadotropins, cortisol, growth hormone, and thyroid hormones. As a result, prepubertal patients may have altered sexual maturation and arrested physical development and growth patterns (American Psychiatric Association 1993).

Starvation and weight loss are known to create hypothalamic abnormalities that profoundly affect other organs within the endocrine system. A chain of interrelated events begins when the hypothalamus fails to signal the release of gonadotropin-releasing hormones from the pituitary. The absence of this signal causes a decrease in luteinizing hormone (LH) and follicular-stimulating hormone (FSH) levels and inhibits the positive feedback mechanism to the ovaries. Consequently, the ovaries do not release estrogen or progesterone in normal amounts, which further inhibits the pituitary gland. Ovarian volume and uterine volume are decreased, and the vaginal mucosa becomes atrophic (Carney and Andersen 1996).

Normal functioning of the thyroid gland is also disrupted in individuals who have eating disorders. Individuals with anorexia nervosa frequently demonstrate thyroid abnormalities as a result of decreased calorie intake and starvation. Free thyroxine (free T4) decreases to low normal levels, whereas triiodothyronine (T3) levels decrease to abnormally low levels in proportion to the degree of weight loss (Carney and Andersen 1996), but thyroid-stimulating hormone (TSH) levels are usually within normal range (Schwabe et al. 1981).

Hormonal problems are one of the most serious effects of anorexia nervosa. People with anorexia nervosa have decreased levels of reproductive hormones, including estrogen and dehydroepiandrosterone (DHEA). Estrogen is important for heart health and bone health. DHEA, a weak male hormone, is also important for bone health. Additionally, compared to healthy people, thyroid hormones and growth hormones are lower in people with anorexia nervosa, and stress hormones are higher in those with anorexia nervosa. Consequently, children and adolescents with anorexia nervosa may experience retarded growth. For women, these hormonal abnormalities may result in menstrual cycle disruptions, including anovulation (lack of regular ovulation), oligomenorrhea (infrequent menstruation), and amenorrhea (absent menstruation; Fairburn 1995; Stewart et al. 1990), and these abnormalities can occur even *before* a person has lost a significant amount of weight. Estrogen levels are usually restored and menses usually resume after a person has been treated and her weight has increased. However, in some cases, menstruation may never return, resulting in infertility.

3.4.5 EFFECTS ON PREGNANCY

Research suggests that most pregnant women with a history of eating disorders have healthy pregnancies (Ekeus et al. 2006). However, some research suggests that women who have had eating disorders may face higher risks for a number of complications, including cesarean sections, postpartum depression, miscarriages, complicated deliveries, and premature birth (Lucas 2004; Russell et al. 1998). In one of the few studies that investigated pregnancy outcomes for women who had a previous diagnosis of anorexia nervosa, a large sample of women who were discharged from the hospital with a diagnosis of anorexia nervosa during 1973 to 1996 and who gave birth during 1983 to 2002 were compared with a large sample of healthy women who gave birth during the same years. The researchers collected information about preeclampsia (i.e., pregnancy-induced hypertension), instrumental delivery, prematurity, small for gestational age, birth weight, Apgar score, and perinatal mortality. Results showed that the main birth outcome measures in women with a history of anorexia nervosa were very similar to those without a history of anorexia nervosa. The only observed difference was a slightly lower mean birth weight for babies whose mothers had a history of anorexia nervosa (Ekeus et al. 2006). This research suggests that women who have a history of anorexia nervosa and who have been treated for the disorder are often able to become pregnant and have healthy pregnancies.

3.4.6 GASTROINTESTINAL ABNORMALITIES

Individuals with anorexia nervosa frequently describe mealtime as an uncomfortable experience associated with symptoms of anxiety, such as sweating and increased pulse and respiratory rates. Occasionally, when the patient is required to eat more than a small amount, bloating occurs primarily due to delayed gastric emptying (Treasure and Szmulker 1995). As poor nutrition and caloric restriction continue, individuals develop gastrointestinal motility disturbances, hypothermia, and other evidence of hypometabolism. Complaints of chronic constipation and abdominal pain are common in individuals who are evaluated for anorexia nervosa (Rock and Zerbe 1995).

When a person eats little food, a series of adverse consequences affect normal digestion. Food is held for longer periods in the stomach and intestines, which can produce bloating and a feeling of being full, stomachache, and constipation. Food normally passes through the stomach in about an hour, but when the consumption of food is restricted, food may stay in the stomach for 4 or 5 hours (Lucas 2004, 84). So, it may be difficult for a young woman with anorexia to resume a normal pattern of eating. After eating a normal amount of food for lunch, she may still feel full when it is time for supper.

Due to malnutrition (Rock and Zerbe 1995) and repeated episodes of binge eating (Gavish et al. 1987), pancreatitis is a common occurrence in patients with eating disorders. Patients with pancreatitis may complain of steady and intense upper abdominal pain that may diffuse to the back, chest, or lower abdomen. Numerous mechanisms have the potential to cause pancreatitis, including a sudden increase in calorie intake after malnutrition or the ingestion of various medications including the laxatives and diuretics used in purging (McClain et al. 1993).

3.4.7 Central Nervous System Abnormalities

During periods of severe food restriction, the brain and the central nervous system undergo structural changes and operate abnormally. The nerve damage that results from anorexia nervosa affects the brain and other parts of the body. Seizures, disordered thinking, and *peripheral neuropathy* (i.e., numbness or odd nerve sensations in the hands or feet) have all been reported in people with anorexia nervosa. Additionally, severe starvation has been linked to depressed mood, decreased concentration and attention, and poor problem-solving skills and memory. These problems may contribute to poor judgment about the severity of the illness and, therefore, hamper the individual's recognition of the need for treatment (Treasure and Szmulker 1995).

Disruptions in neuroendocrine and neurotransmitter systems are prevalent in people with anorexia nervosa. Structural changes in the brain have also been shown in people with anorexia nervosa, including widening of the sulcal spaces and cerebroventricular enlargement (Palazidou et al. 1990) and reductions in the size of the pituitary (Husain et al. 1992). People with anorexia nervosa also demonstrate increased metabolism in the cortex and caudate nucleus (Kreig et al. 1991).

3.4.8 Hematologic and Immunologic Abnormalities

Hematologic and immunologic abnormalities are often found in patients with anorexia nervosa. Poor nutrition with severe weight loss often results in dramatic decreases in red blood cells, white blood cells, and blood platelets. Anemia is a common result of anorexia and starvation. One particularly serious blood problem is pernicious anemia, which can be caused by severely low levels of vitamin B12. In some severe cases of anorexia nervosa, the bone marrow dramatically reduces its production of blood cells, a life-threatening condition called *pancytopenia*. Impairment of the immune system is also common and is believed to be a consequence of *hypercortisolism* (i.e., excessive amounts of the hormone cortisol). These effects can be corrected with nutritional improvement and weight restoration.

3.4.9 Integumentary Abnormalities

Patients with anorexia nervosa often experience changes in skin and tissues that are likely related to malnutrition, loss of body fat, and dehydration. Frequently, the skin is dry, scaly, and covered with *lanugo*, a fine, downy hair resembling that of newborn babies. Fingernails and hair are often brittle, and hair loss may occur in patches or uniformly over the scalp and other body areas (Schwartz and Thompson 1981). A yellowish or orangish discoloration of the skin occurs in approximately 80% of patients with anorexia nervosa (Sharp and Freeman 1993). This unusual skin color, which is "most noticeable on the palms of the hands, the soles of the feet, and the creases inside the elbows," is due to faulty metabolism of β-carotene in the liver leading an excessive level of β-carotene circulating in the blood, some of which is deposited under the skin (Lucas 2004, 85).

3.4.10 Skeletal Problems

Bone loss and decreased bone density are common problems for people with anorexia nervosa. Approximately 90% of women with anorexia experience osteopenia (decrease in bone mass) and some have osteoporosis (brittle and fragile bones; Grinspoon et al. 2000). In a study assessing decreased bone density and bone loss in women with anorexia nervosa, nearly half of the women had osteopenia at the hip, and 16% had osteoporosis at the hip. More than half had osteopenia at the spine, and almost 25% had osteoporosis at the spine. Over 90% of women had abnormally low bone density at one or more sites in the skeleton. Additionally, weight was the factor most related to bone loss. The less a woman weighed, the more likely it was that she would have substantial bone loss (Grinspoon et al. 2000).

The bone loss that women with anorexia nervosa experience is largely due to low estrogen levels that occur with anorexia nervosa. Other factors contributing to bone loss include high levels of stress hormones (which impair bone growth) and low levels of calcium, certain growth factors, and DHEA. Unfortunately, weight gain does not completely restore bone loss, but achieving regular menstruation as soon as possible can protect against permanent bone loss. The longer the eating disorder persists the more likely the bone loss will be permanent.

Although long-term complications of anorexia nervosa can involve any of the body's systems, the bones are significantly affected. Since puberty is a critical time for skeletal development, developing anorexia nervosa during this period can interfere with the development of peak bone mass and, therefore, produce permanent long-term skeletal effects (Treasure and Szmukler 1995). When a young child is severely underweight, there is a danger that the child's growth will be limited. However, if anorexia nervosa starts after puberty begins and ends before the growth plates in her bones have closed, then a young woman's growth in height will not be stunted (Pfeiffer et al. 1986).

Decreased bone density is known to be particularly prevalent in individuals with anorexia nervosa who have been severely emaciated for a prolonged period of time (Biller et al. 1989; Hay et al. 1992; Kiriike et al. 1992). Fractures of the long bones, vertebrae, and sternum have been reported in individuals with anorexia nervosa who have had amenorrhea for as short a period as 1 year (Mitchell 1983). In a long-term study of 103 patients with anorexia nervosa, osteoporosis with multiple fractures and terminal renal deficiency accounted for the most severe disabilities experienced by the patients (Herzog et al. 1992).

Bone loss, osteopenia, and associated stress fractures have been linked to endocrine disturbances that alter normal hormonal mechanisms and lead to oligomenorrhea and amenorrhea (Rigotti et al. 1991). Dietary deficiency, low circulating estrogen levels, hypercortisolism, laxative misuse, and disturbed acid–base balance also contribute to adverse physical consequences (Garner 1993). Skeletal problems can be minimized or prevented by early recognition and intervention, but long-term complications can be expected to occur and progress as long as an individual continues to exercise without proper nutritional intake (Katz 1995).

3.5 APPLICATION OF THE RESEARCH

"The treatment of patients with anorexia nervosa is both a science and an art. The science deals with the physical aspects that resulted from under-nutrition, and the art deals with the person in whom the disorder exists" (Lucas 2004, 102). Specific information regarding treatment of people with eating disorders can be found in Chapters 19, 20, and 21 of this book. However, the information in these chapters was not written for people with anorexia nervosa, specifically. Therefore, this section of the chapter will briefly describe specific strategies for treating women with anorexia nervosa.

Individuals with anorexia nervosa frequently lack insight into their problems and often deny the existence of problems related to eating. They are often reluctant to seek help from friends, family members, or health professionals, because the eating disorder becomes a lifestyle and they fear changing their habits and gaining weight. When they do seek help on their own, it may be due to severe distress over physical or psychological problems that occur as a result of the eating disorder or in conjunction with the eating disorder. In an attempt to conceal their disorder from health professionals, individuals with anorexia nervosa may try to hide signs of this disorder or might provide inaccurate information to the clinician. For example, an individual with anorexia nervosa might drink a lot of water prior to being weighed by a professional or might hide weights in her clothing to increase the number on the scale.

"Because there is such variation among patients, with a wide spectrum of severity, the same treatment does not fit all. … Since there is so much variability among patients and among their family circumstances, treatment must be tailored to fit each individual patient's uniqueness. … Inflexible treatment protocols and rigid programs that treat all patients alike should be viewed with suspicion" (Lucas 2004, 109). Effective treatment of individuals with anorexia nervosa should include weight restoration and restoring healthy eating habits. However, successful treatment of anorexia nervosa requires more than a focus on eating and weight gain. Focus on emotional issues that are related to the disorder and family conflicts that contribute to the disorder are also needed (Lucas 2004, 113).

Successful treatment depends on the individual with anorexia nervosa gaining weight and maintaining a normal weight and adequate nutrition. Initially in treatment, the focus is on supporting the individual with anorexia nervosa and building a cooperative relationship with her while she gains weight. Because of the cognitive impairments resulting from semi-starvation, it will be difficult to deal with emotional and interpersonal problems until the individual's weight returns to the normal range (Lucas 2004, 112). Sometimes, however, the focus on weight gain may be too narrow, so that the person gains weight during treatment, but has not accepted that weight gain or changed her attitudes and perceptions related to weight and eating. Many patients with anorexia gain weight in treatment but then lose it soon after leaving treatment. Also, some treatment programs focus on rapid weight gain, which will be difficult for the individual with anorexia both psychologically and physically, and may expose the individual to some serious health risks, such as heart failure (Lucas 2004, 46–47, 111). Weight restoration must be done gradually and patiently. Additionally, returning the individual with anorexia nervosa to a normal pattern of eating can be either easily accomplished or extremely difficult, depending on how long the disorder has persisted. Therefore, enlisting the help of a dietitian can assist in educating the person about her nutritional needs. However, including too many professionals into the treatment might pose problems for the person being treated for anorexia nervosa, so an ideal approach might be for the therapist to work closely with the nutritionist (Lucas 2004, 124).

It would be great if anorexia nervosa could be prevented from occurring (primary prevention), but that goal seems unattainable based on the research on past prevention programs. (For a review of prevention programs, see Chapter 13 of this book.) Efforts to prevent eating disorders have produced temporary results, a change in knowledge but no change in attitudes or behavior, or an increase in symptoms of eating disorders (Carter et al. 1997; Killen et al. 1993; Mann et al. 1997). Unfortunately, prevention efforts can lead girls and young women to focus even more than they had before on their bodies and on dieting, and may promote unhealthy behaviors among especially vulnerable girls (Lucas 2004, 155). Another reason that primary prevention is so difficult is that any prevention programs are unlikely to have as much of an effect on girls and young women as the influence of their peers and of media messages. "Effective prevention would require a wholesale change in the priorities and values expressed in our society" (Lucas 2004, 157). Therefore, the best type of prevention for anorexia nervosa may be secondary prevention—identifying the early signs of trouble and starting treatment as soon as possible.

Health professionals must be educated about the dangers and warning signs of anorexia nervosa and other eating disorders to promote early recognition, evaluation, and treatment. Parents, teachers, and coaches who recognize common signs of anorexia nervosa in girls or young women should express their concerns to these individuals and their parents and should also encourage them to seek further evaluation. Because individuals often develop an eating disorder in the aftermath of a diet, overweight individuals should be encouraged to lose weight through nutritionally balanced meals and exercise rather than by strict dieting that can trigger binge eating and purging cycles (Rock and Zerbe 1995). Health professionals must develop realistic attitudes about body weight and shape in order to communicate information effectively and to promote appropriate preventive efforts.

3.6 SUMMARY

The key feature of anorexia nervosa is the refusal of the girl or woman to eat an adequate amount of food. All of the physiological changes that occur in anorexia nervosa are caused by malnutrition or "semi-starvation" (Lucas 2004, 82). Those changes are the adaptive responses of the body to survive despite inadequate intake of food: conservation of energy, shifts in electrolyte balances, attempts to use fat and spare the body's glucose and protein, and changes in the functioning of the hypothalamus and the pituitary gland.

The initial evaluation of an individual with an eating disorder must include a comprehensive physical exam and health history to rule out existing physiological pathology. Several lab tests, including a complete blood count (i.e., full blood chemistry, electrolyte profile, liver and function tests, and urinalysis) should also be performed. An EKG is essential to evaluate the cardiovascular system and to rule out potentially life-threatening arrhythmias, and a chest X-ray may be performed to evaluate heart size and placement (Garner 1993).

Although numerous physical abnormalities may be found in people with anorexia nervosa, research findings indicate that laboratory results may be normal even in the presence of profound malnutrition (Sharp and Freeman 1993). Over 60% of patients with anorexia nervosa have leuko-penia (a reduction in the number of leukocytes in the blood), and this abnormality may be related to bone marrow hypoplasia and decreased neutrophil (a granular leukocyte having a nucleus of three to five lobes) lifespan (Sharp and Freeman 1993). Leukopenia accompanied by a relative lym-phocytosis has also been reported (Mitchell 1983). Normochromic anemia, normocytic anemia, and thrombocytopenia have been found in approximately one-third of patients with anorexia ner-vosa. Hypoglycemia, hypercortisolemia, hypercholesterolemia, low serum zinc levels, and various other electrolyte disturbances, such as decreased levels of potassium, chloride, and magnesium may be found, depending upon the degree of dehydration. Thyroid function tests reveal low T3 levels in proportion to weight loss, low normal T4 levels, and decreased metabolic rates (Carney and Andersen 1996).

A number of long-term complications may result from the prolonged and severe malnutrition that often accompanies anorexia nervosa. Medical complications can be expected to progress as long as the individual continues to exercise without proper nutritional intake (Katz 1995). Without early, aggressive intervention, anorexia nervosa will most likely last for several years, and it may persist or reoccur throughout the individual's life (Lucas 2004, 42). Long-term follow-up studies reveal a mortality rate as high as 18%, with the majority of deaths related to medical complications of the disorder (Steinhausen 2002).

When a girl or young woman has anorexia nervosa and is severely emaciated, restoring her health must often be a gradual process. She may rebel against a 2000- to 3000-calorie diet because she will feel as though she is being overfed and may therefore also stop cooperating with other aspects of treatment. There are also physical reasons that she will be unable to resume a normal diet immediately. Attempting rapid weight gain in a person who has been starving may lead to exces-sive fluid retention with a risk of heart failure. In addition, any nourishment may be difficult for her because of her empty and shrunken stomach. So, eating may trigger nausea and vomiting, and these physical responses must be carefully distinguished from common psychological variables, such as revulsion at food and self-induced vomiting (Lucas 2004, 46–47, 111).

Although malnutrition is common to all eating disorders, it is particularly prominent for those with anorexia nervosa. Inadequate nutritional intake and poor absorption of nutrients result in physi-cal consequences, including extreme weight loss, electrolyte imbalances, cardiac abnormalities, hor-monal changes, central nervous system abnormalities, bone loss, and muscle wasting. Unfortunately, these physical consequences can result in death; therefore, adequate nutritional intake and weight restoration are vital in the treatment of anorexia nervosa.

REFERENCES

American Psychiatric Association. 2000. *Diagnostic and statistical manual of mental disorders.* 4th ed text revi-
     sion. Washington, DC: American Psychiatric Association.
American Psychiatric Association. 1993. Practice guidelines for eating disorders. *Am J Psychiatry* 150:
     212–218.

Biller, B. M. K, V. Saxe, D. B. Herzog, D. I. Rosenthal, S. Holzman, and A. Klibanski. 1989. Mechanisms of osteoporosis in adult and adolescent women with anorexia nervosa. *J Clin Endocrinol Metab* 68: 548–554.

Bruch, H. 1978. *The golden cage: The enigma of anorexia nervosa*. Cambridge, MA: Harvard Univ. Press.

Carney, C. P., and A. E. Andersen. 1996. Eating disorders: Guide to medical evaluation and complications. *Psychiatr Clin North Am* 19: 657–679.

Carter, J. C., D. A. Stewart, V. J. Dunn, and C. G. Fairburn. 1997. Primary prevention of eating disorders: Might it do more harm than good? *Int J Eat Disord* 22: 167–172.

Crisp, A. H., R. L. Palmer, and R. S. Kalucy. How common is anorexia nervosa? A prevalence study. *Brit J Psychiatry* 128: 549–554.

De Simone, G., L. Scalfi, M. Galderisi, A. Celentano, G. Di Biase, P. Tammaro, M. Garofalo, G. F. Mureddu, O. De Divitiis, and F. Contaldo. 1994. Cardiac abnormalities in young women with anorexia nervosa. *Brit Heart J* 71: 278–292.

Ekeus, C., L. Lindberg, F. Lindblad, and A. Hjern. 2006. Birth outcomes and pregnancy complications in women with a history of anorexia nervosa. *BJOG* 113: 925–929.

Fairburn, C. G. 1995. Physiology of anorexia nervosa. In *Eating disorders and obesity: A comprehensive handbook,* ed. K. D. Brownell and C. G. Fairburn, 251–254 (Ch 44). New York: Guilford.

Fohlin, L. 1977. Body composition, cardiovascular and renal function in adolescent patients with anorexia nervosa. *Acta Paediatr Scand Suppl* 268: 1–20.

Garner, D. M. 1993. Pathogenesis of anorexia nervosa. *Lancet* 341: 1631–1635.

Gavish, D., S. Eisenerg, E. M. Berry, Y. Kleinman, E. Witztum, J. Norman, and E. Leitersdorf. 1987. Bulimia: An underlying behavioral disorder in hyperlipidemic pancreatitis: A prospective multidisciplinary approach. *Arch Intern Med* 147: 705–708.

Greene, R. L. 1980. *The MMPI: An interpretive manual.* New York: Grune and Stratton.

Grinspoon, S., E. Thomas, S. Pitts, E. Gross, D. Mickley, K. Miller, D. Herzog, and A. Klibanski. 2000. Prevalence and predictive factors for regional osteopenia in women with anorexia nervosa. *Ann Intern Med* 133: 828–830.

Hall, R. C. W., and T. P. Beresford. 1989. Medical complications of anorexia and bulimia. *Psychiatr Med* 7: 165–192.

Hall, R. C., R. S. Hoffman, T. P. Beresford, B. Wooley, A. K. Hall, and L. Kubasak. 1989. Physical illness encountered in patients with eating disorders. *Psychosomatics* 30: 174–191.

Hay, P. J., J. W. Delahunt, A. Hall, A. W. Mitchell, G. Harper, and C. Salmond. 1992. Predictors of osteopenia in premenopausal women with anorexia nervosa. *Calcif Tissue Int* 50: 498–501.

Herzog, W., H. C. Deter, D. Schellberg, S. Seilkopf, E. Sarembe, F. Kroger, H. Minne, H. Mayer, and S. Petzold. 1992. Somatic findings at 12-year follow-up of 103 anorexia nervosa patients: Results of the Heidelberg-Mannheim follow-up. In *The comprehensive medical text,* ed. W. Herzog, H. C. Deter, and W. Vandereycken, 85–107. Berlin: Springer-Verlag.

Husain, M. M., K. J. Black, P. M. Doraiswamy, S. A. Shah, W. J. K. Rockwell, E. H. Ellinwood, and K. R. Krishnan. 1992. Subcortical brain anatomy in anorexia and bulimia. *Biol Psychiatry* 31: 735–738.

Katz, J. L. 1995. Eating disorders. In *Women and exercise: Physiology and sports medicine,* 2nd edn, ed. M. Shangold and G. Mirkin, 292–312. Philadelphia: F. A. Davis.

Kent, J. S., and J. R. Clopton. 1992. Bulimic women's perceptions of their family relationships. *J Clin Psychol* 48: 281–292.

Keys, A., J. Brošek, A. Henschel, O. Mickelson, and H. L. Tayor. (1950). *The biology of human starvation.* Minneapolis, MN: Univ. of Minnesota Press.

Killen, J. D., C. B. Taylor, L. D. Hammer, I. Litt, D. M. Wilson, T. Rich, C. Hayward, B. Simmonds, H. Kraemer, and A. Varady. 1993. An attempt to modify unhealthful eating attitudes and weight regulation practices of young adolescent girls. *Int J Eat Disord* 13: 369–384.

Kiriike, N., T. Iketani, S. Nakanishi, T. Nagata, K. Inoue, M. Okuno, H. Ochi, and K. Kawakita. 1992. Reduced bone density and major hormones regulating calcium metabolism in anorexia nervosa. *Acta Psychiatr Scand* 86: 358–363.

Kreig, J. C., V. Holthoff, W. Schreiber, K. M. Pirke, and K. Herholz. 1991. Glucose metabolism in the caudate nuclei of patients with eating disorders, measured by PET. *European Archives of Psychiatry and Clinical Neuroscience* 240: 331–333.

Lucas, A. R. 2004. *Demystifying anorexia nervosa: An optimistic guide to understanding and healing.* New York: Oxford Univ. Press.

Lucas, A. R., C. M. Beard, W. M. O'Fallon, and L. T. Kurland. 1991. 50-year trends in the incidence of anorexia nervosa in Rochester, Minnesota: A population-based study. *Am J Psychiatry* 148: 917–922.

Lucas, A. R., C. S. Crowson, W. M. O'Fallon, and L. J. Melton III. 1999. The ups and downs of anorexia nervosa. *Int J Eat Disord* 26: 397–405.

Mann,T., S. Nolen-Hoeksema, K. Huang, D. Burgard, A. Wright, and K. Hanson. 1997. Are two interventions worse than none? *Health Psychol* 16: 215–225.

McClain, C. J., L. L. Humphries, K. K. Hill, and N. J. Nicki. 1993. Gastrointestinal and nutritional aspects of eating disorders. *JACN* 12: 466–474.

Mitchell, J. E. 1983. Medical complications of anorexia nervosa and bulimia. *Psychiatr Med* 1: 229–255.

Mitchell, J. E., L. I. Boutacoff, D. Hatsukami, R. L. Pyle, and E. D. Eckert. 1986. Laxative abuse as a variant of bulimia. *J Nerv Ment Dis* 174: 174–176.

Mitchell, J. E., D. Hatsukami, R. L. Pyle, E. D. Ekert, and L. I. Boutacoff, 1987. Metabolic acidosis as a marker for laxative abuse in patients with bulimia. *Int J Eat Disord* 6: 557–560.

Palazidou, E., P. Robinson, and W. A. Lishman. 1990. Neuroradiological and neuropsychological assessment in anorexia nervosa. *Psychol Med* 20: 521–527.

Pfeiffer, R. J., A. R. Lucas, and D. M. Ilstrup. 1986. Effect of anorexia nervosa on linear growth. *Clin Pediatr* 25: 7–12.

Råstam, M., C. Gillberg, and M. Garton. 1989. Anorexia nervosa in a Swedish urban region: A population-based study. *Br J Psychiatry* 155: 642–646.

Rigotti, N. A., R. M. Neer, S. J. Skates, D. B. Herzog, and S. R. Nussbaum. 1991. The clinical course of osteoporosis in anorexia nervosa: A longitudinal study of cortical bone mass. *JAMA* 265: 1133–1138.

Rock, C. L. and K. J. Zerbe. 1995. Keeping eating disorders at bay. *Patient Care* 11: 78–86.

Russell, G. F., J. Treasure, and I. Eisler. 1998. Mothers with anorexia nervosa who underfeed their children: Their recognition and management. *Psychol Med* 28: 93–108.

Schocken, D. D., J. D. Holloway, and P. S. Powers. 1989. Weight loss and the heart: Effects of anorexia nervosa and starvation. *Arch Intern Med* 149: 877–881.

Schwabe, A. D., B. M. Lippe, R. J. Chang, M. A. Pops, and J. Yager. 1981. Anorexia nervosa. *Ann Intern Med* 94: 371–381.

Schwartz, D. M., and M. G. Thompson. 1981. Do anorexics get well? Current research and future needs. *Am J Psychiatry* 138: 319–323.

Sharp, C. W., and C. P. L. Freeman. 1993. Medical complications of anorexia nervosa. *Brit J Psychiatry* 162: 452–462.

Steinhausen, H. C. 2002. The outcome of anorexia nervosa in the 20th century. *Am J Psychiatry* 159: 1284–1293.

Stewart, D. E., E. Robinson, D. S. Goldbloom, and C. Wright. 1990. Infertility and eating disorders. *Am J Obstet Gynecol* 163: 1196–1199.

Treasure, J., and G. Szmukler. 1995. Medical complications of chronic anorexia nervosa. In *Handbook of eating disorders: Theory, treatment and research*, ed. G. Szmukler, C. Dare, and J. Treasure, 197–220. New York: Wiley.

Warren, M. P., and R. L. van de Wiele. 1973. Clinical and metabolic features of anorexia nervosa, *Am J Obstet Gynecol* 117: 435–449.

4 The Physiology of Bulimia Nervosa

Jacalyn J. Robert-McComb and Brittany McCullough

CONTENTS

4.1 LEARNING OBJECTIVES

After completing this chapter, you should be able to

- State the prevalence rate for bulimia nervosa
- Describe the risk factors and health consequence of bulimia nervosa
- Describe the *DSM-IV-TR* criteria for bulimia nervosa
- Explain the importance of genetics, neurotransmitters, and key hormones in bulimia nervosa

4.2 INTRODUCTION

4.2.1 PREVALENCE RATES FOR BULIMIA NERVOSA

Alarmingly, more than 4 million individuals are believed to experience some type of an eating disorder (ED) in the United States (Hudson et al. 2007). Even though this book is about women and children with EDs, maladaptive eating patterns also occur in men, particularly men who participate in sports with either a weight requirement (e.g., wrestling, horse racing) or a low body fat requirement (e.g., bodybuilding; Ackard et al. 2007). The lifetime prevalence of bulimia nervosa (BN) is reported to range from 0.5 to 3% (Garfinkel et al. 1995; Kendler et al. 1991; Klein and Walsh 2004) in the United States and as high as 4% in other countries (Resch et al. 2004). Internationally, EDs are believed to be more common in industrialized countries; however, appropriate epidemiologic studies have not been conducted in developing countries.

4.2.2 RISK FACTORS FOR BULIMIA NERVOSA

Risk factors for BN are multifactorial; there is no single cause for BN. Some of the many contributing risk factors for BN are the following: (1) major life changes; (2) poor body image; (3) low self-esteem; (4) a history of trauma or abuse; (5) appearance-oriented professions or activities; (6) cultural and parental pressure to be thin; (7) biological and hormonal disturbances in the digestive and central nervous system; (8) birth after 1960; (9) low parental care; (10) a history of wide weight fluctuation, dieting, or frequent exercise; (11) and external locus of control; (12) high levels of neuroticism; and (13) specific genetic factors (Kendler et al. 1991; Klein and Walsh 2004; Sim et al. 2004).

EDs in general are more common in women than in men. Thirty-two percent of girls and twenty percent of boys reported using compensatory factors and binge eating to control weight, within this subset, 11% of girls and approximately 3% of boys engaged in binge eating in a manner that felt out of control (Ackard et al. 2007). This would indicate that being female is a risk factor for the development of BN. Age is also a risk factor for BN because EDs tend to begin during late adolescence or early adulthood (Klein and Walsh 2004). The development of BN symptoms at an even earlier age may be associated with a more severe disorder. Among individuals with either anorexia nervosa (AN) or BN, age at onset has decreased significantly through the generations, so that members of younger generations develop these disorders at younger ages than members of older generations did (Favaro et al. 2009). Differences have been found between AN and BN for peak age of onset; AN has a peak age of onset in early to mid-adolescence, whereas BN has a peak age of onset during or after late adolescence (Kohn and Golden 2001).

Common threads in the risk factors for BN are environmental (cultural and parental pressure to be thin) and emotional (low self-esteem) sources of *distress*. Most individuals with BN have trouble managing their emotions in a healthy way. Eating can be an emotional release so it is not surprising that people engage in binge eating and purging when feeling angry, depressed, stressed, or anxious.

A study by Buckholdt (2010) found that individuals who engaged in binge eating and compensatory behavior, and who also showed a lack of emotional control, were extremely likely to have parents who had difficulty regulating their own emotions. Therefore, the behavior of an adolescent girl's parents may contribute to the development of disordered eating behaviors (Morris et al. 2007). Difficulty in regulating emotional behavior is a major aspect of individuals with BN (Markey and Vander Wal 2007; Sim and Zeman 2004), and emotional dysregulation may be a key mechanism through which parents' responses to emotions influence disordered eating behaviors in their daughters.

Family influences play a *major* role in triggering and perpetuating EDs. Interestingly, even families that are trying to teach their children good eating habits may trigger a reverse reaction. For example, families who are vegetarians may be putting their children at increased risk for binge eating with loss of control and increased risk for extreme unhealthful weight-control behaviors (Robinson-O'Brien et al. 2009).

4.2.3 *DSM-IV* CRITERIA FOR BULIMIA NERVOSA

BN is a complex disorder characterized by recurrent binge eating, compensatory behaviors to avoid weight gain, and related behavioral and physiological symptoms. The diagnostic criteria for BN include several criteria that reflect the physical manifestation of the disorder. Specifically, the current *Diagnostic and Statistical Manual for Mental Disorder (DSM-IV-TR)* indicates that all women with BN have recurrent episodes of binge eating (American Psychiatric Association [APA] 2000).

An episode of binge eating is characterized by both of the following: (1) eating within any 2-h period an amount of food that is definitely larger than most people would eat; and (2) a sense of lack of control over eating, or a feeling that one cannot stop eating or control what or how much is being consumed. To compensate for the large amount of food that has been consumed during the eating binge, the individual engages in behaviors to prevent weight gain, such as (1) self-induced vomiting; (2) misuse of laxatives, diuretics, enemas, or other medications; (3) fasting; or (4) excessive exercise. To be diagnosed with BN using the current DSM criteria, the binge eating and compensatory behaviors must occur, on average, at least twice a week for 3 months. Another diagnostic criterion for BN is that self-evaluation is unduly influenced by body shape and weight (Klein and Walsh 2004).

According to the *DSM-IV-TR,* there are two types of BN—the purging type and the nonpurging type (APA 2000). An individual with the purging type regularly engages in self-induced vomiting or the misuse of laxatives, diuretics, or enemas. An individual with the nonpurging type compensates for her large food intake through fasting or excessive exercise, but engage in self-induced vomiting, and she does not misuse laxatives, diuretics, or enemas.

4.3 BACKGROUND AND SIGNIFICANCE

4.3.1 SHORT-TERM ADVERSE HEALTH EFFECTS OF BULIMIA NERVOSA

Behaviors associated with BN may have few adverse consequences for individuals who briefly engage in self-induced vomiting, purging, or fasting (Roberts and Tylenda 1989). However, when those behaviors are recurrent and persistent enough to lead to a diagnosis for BN, individuals are likely to have these physiological consequences: (1) erosion of the teeth, (2) enlargement of the parotid salivary glands, and (3) acidic stomachs leading to regurgitation of acidic stomach and heartburn (Barlett et al. 1996; Roberts and Tylenda 1989). Signs and symptoms related to BN are listed in Table 4.1. This table is not all inclusive but lists some of the more common pathologies in BN.

Excessive vomiting causes erosion on the enamel and dentin on teeth, increasing the susceptibility to cavities and gum disease (Barlett et al. 1996; Roberts and Tylenda 1989). It can also cause acid from the stomach to rise up to the esophagus, which leads to infections, gastro-esophageal reflux disease, and may eventually cause a ruptured esophagus (Barlett et al. 1996). Other short-term complications resulting from BN include impaired satiety, decreased resting metabolic rate, and abnormal neuroendocrine responses. These symptoms increase in severity with continued disordered

---

TABLE 4.1

Signs and Symptoms of Bulimia Nervosa

• Anovulation	• Hypotension
• Calluses on back of hand and fingers	• Integumentary
• Cardiomyopathy	• System
• Cheilosis	• Disorders
• Constipation	• Metabolic
• Dental abscesses	• Acidosis
• Dental caries	• Alkalosis
• Diarrhea	• Mitral valve prolapse
• Dry, flaky skin	• Muscle cramps
• Dyspepsia	• Musculoskeletal weakness
• Endocrine disorders	• Palpitations
• Esophagitis	• Pancreatitis
• Heart failure	• Pruitis
• Hematemesis	• Sore throat
	• Tetany

eating (Birketvedt et al. 2006). These complications should be thought of as occurring on a continuum, and in some cases, the symptoms are reversible.

4.3.2 Long-Term Adverse Health Effects of Bulimia Nervosa

Gynecological problems are one of the most frequent long-term complications of EDs (Crow et al. 2002; Resch and Szendei 2004). The unsatisfactory nutrition in BN results in hormonal dysfunction, menstrual disturbances, and infertility (Freizinger et al. 2010). These symptoms may be reversible with early treatment of the ED (Crow et al. 2002; Resch and Szendei 2004). Menstrual irregularities as a result of BN may be caused by weight fluctuations, nutritional deficiency, and prolonged stress (Yager 1988). This same menstrual irregularity or oligomenorrhea can lead to polycystic ovary syndrome in individuals who are bulimic, especially if they are also obese (Seidenfeld et al. 2001; Yager 1988).

Gonadal steroids are among the many factors that influence food intake and body weight in mammals (Butera 2009). A key role of estradiol is related to food intake and energy balance. The actions of estradiol may have a gender-specific effect on the regulations of eating, which could explain why BN is more common in women than men (Sodersten and Bergh 2003). During the estrogen-releasing cycle, the amount of food being consumed fluctuates in response to ovarian rhythms in bulimic women (Butera 2009; Dalvit-McPhillips 1983).

Disturbances in hormonal regulation in BN can lead to severe mood changes and aggressive behavior patterns. Researchers have found that individuals with BN have a decrease in plasma levels of prolactin and estradiol, and an increase in cortisol and testosterone (Cotrufo et al. 2000; Naessén et al. 2006). There is a positive correlation between testosterone plasma levels (Monteleone, Luisi et al. 2003) and aggressiveness in individuals with BN that is not seen in other individuals (Cotrufo et al. 2000; Naessén et al. 2006). Individuals with BN tend to have a higher score when rating depressive symptoms and aggressiveness on eating-related psychopathology assessments, which suggests that BN plays a role in the modulation of aggressiveness (Cotrufo et al. 2000).

Hypercholesteremia (the presence of high levels of cholesterol in the blood) is another cardiovascular risk factor associated with BN. Pauporte and Walsh (2000) found that the mean serum cholesterol levels of patients with BN were significantly higher than the cholesterol levels of individuals in a comparison group (patients: 194 +/− 36 mg/dL; comparison group: 176 +/− 34 mg/dL; $t = 2.77$; $df = 159$; $p = .006$). Hypercholesterolemia is not a disease but an abnormal metabolic state that can be secondary to many diseases and can also contribute to many forms of disease, most notably cardiovascular disease (Matzkin et al. 2006). Additionally, individuals who binge or overeat, or who are obese, are also at high risk for developing hypertension, which is another pathway to long-term cardiovascular disease.

Mira et al. (1985) found that individuals with BN and other EDs not only had higher levels of cholesterol, but they also had lower levels of electrolytes, such as, potassium, chloride, and phosphate in the plasma. The misuse of laxatives and weight loss supplements over time can cause these electrolyte imbalances and gastrointestinal abnormalities. Individuals who engage in binge eating also commonly engage in the excessive use of weight loss supplements. According to Reba-Harrelson et al. (2008), women with BN are more likely to use diet pills if they have a higher BMI, higher novelty seeking, anxiety disorders, alcohol abuse, or borderline personality disorder. Many of these characteristics are commonly found to co-occur with BN.

Cardiac autonomic regulation and stress reactivity may also be altered in BN patients due to energy restriction. Altered eating patterns in BN can result in metabolic and cardiovascular abnormalities (Vögele et al. 2009). Messerli- Bürgy et al. (2010) found that heart rate stress reactivity was highest in BN patients when looking at biological stress responses. During the stress recovery stage of the laboratory stressor, heart rate variability (HRV) decreased in the participants with BN compared to a group of other women. A decrease in HRV is associated with coronary artery disease and congestive heart failure (Casolo et al. 1989; Gordon et al. 1988; Kienzle et al. 1992; Mortara et al. 1994; Nolan et al. 1992). A similar study investigated cardiac autonomic regulation and stress reactivity in relation to biochemical markers of dietary restriction in women diagnosed with BN. These investigators found that women with BN who were fasting (compared to women who had BN but were not fasting or women who did not have BN) showed increased vagal dominance and decreased sympathetic modulation during both resting and recovery periods. These results support the notion of cardiac sympathetic inhibition and vagal dominance during dietary restriction, and suggest the specificity of starvation related to biochemical changes for cardiac autonomic control (Tanaka et al. 2006). Vögele et al. (2009) also found that individuals with BN have higher resting cardiac vagal tone than controls. Based on the findings from their studies, Murialdo et al. (2007) hypothesized that BN patients have sympathetic failure, prevalent vagal activity, and impaired sympathetic activation. These findings indicate a relationship between energy restriction and vagal dominance.

Elevated homocysteine levels (an amino acid in the blood) are associated with cognitive decline in dementia and healthy elderly people and are also associated with a high risk of cardiovascular diseases, stroke, and peripheral vascular disease (Bostom et al. 1997; Frieling et al. 2005). While elevated homocysteine levels are more common in AN than BN patients, BN patients also exhibit signs of elevated homocysteine levels (Frieling et al. 2005; Wilhelm et al. 2005). This condition can be caused by several conditions, such as malnutrition, starvation, alcohol abuse, or genetic predisposition (Geisel et al. 2003). Deficiencies of three vitamins—folic acid (B_9), pyridoxine (B_6), or cyanocobalamin (B_{12})—can also lead to high homocysteine levels. Wilhem et al. (2010) found a small decrease in levels of homocysteine following a 12-week treatment period for individuals with ED; however, the change was small and statistically nonsignificant. Nonetheless, their conclusion was that during effective treatment that concomitantly increased BMI, hyperhomocysteinemia was partially reversible. In light of the findings from Frieling et al. (2005), decreasing homocysteine levels may not improve memory in an ED population. Interestingly, in a mixed group of patients (14 with AN and 12 with BN), elevated homocysteine levels were associated with normal short- and long-term verbal memory, and normal plasma homocysteine levels were associated with poorer memory performance. These results indicate that, under the special circumstances of ED, elevated homocysteine levels improve memory signaling, possibly by facilitating long-term potentiation.

Individuals with BN may also have a comprised immune system. Several studies have reported changes in immune cells and natural killer cells important for immunity in patients with AN and BN (e.g., Vaz- Leal et al. 2010). With a decrease in lymphocyte number, individuals with BN are more vulnerable to disease.

4.3.3 Comorbidities and Mortality Rates for Bulimia Nervosa

BN is a long-term disorder with a waxing and waning course. Comorbid medical and psychiatric conditions associated with BN include: (1) irritable bowel syndrome; (2) fibromyalgia; (3) mood disorders, such as major depression; (4) anxiety disorders, such as generalized anxiety disorder, panic disorder, and phobias; (5) alcoholism and substance abuse, (6) personality disorders, and (7) aggressive behavior and poor impulse control (Kendler et al. 1991). These comorbid conditions are similar for BN and AN (Kendler et al. 1991).

Recent data suggest that mortality rates for BN are around 3.9% (Crow et al. 2009). Mortality rates are slightly higher (5.2%) for Eating Disorders Not Otherwise Specified (EDNOS), a disorder in which an individual's behavior may meet some but not all of the diagnostic criteria for BN (Crow et al. 2009).

4.4 CURRENT FINDINGS

4.4.1 Genetic Variables and Bulimia Nervosa

An area of increasing research activity is the role that genetics plays in EDs. Genetic research is attempting to explicate the behavioral, neurobiological, and temperamental variables that represent the core features of the bulimic phenotype. However, there is shared variance between genetic variables and other risk factors, such as an individual's environment or her attempts at dieting and losing weight. The behavior components of BN, such as, self-induced vomiting, have also been found to be inheritable (Bulik et al. 2003). Some have suggested that overeating or behaviors consistent with BN are related to genetically determined, dysfunctional neurotransmitter systems (Kaye et al. 2000). However, an inherent limitation in the research methodology is the difficulty in linking the symptoms of BN to one single variable, such as genetics.

The role of genetics in the etiology of EDs has long been postulated to be a risk factor based on information about the relatives and siblings of individuals with EDs. For example, individuals are more susceptible to developing an ED if a close relative also has an ED (Klump et al. 2001), and twins have a tendency to share specific patterns of ED symptoms, such as obesity, AN, or BN (Bulik et al. 2010). The importance of genetic predisposition in BN is shown by the difference in concordance rates for monozygotic and dizygotic twins. The concordance rate for BN is 23% for monozygotic twins and 9% for dizygotic twins (Bulik et al. 2010; Kendler 1992). In other words, when one member of a twin pair has BN, the other twin is more likely to also have BN if the twins are identical genetically than if their genetic similarity is that of any other pair of siblings. The fact that the concordance rates for BN found in twin studies are nowhere near 100% demonstrates clearly that many factors other than genetic predisposition contribute to BN.

The role of shared environmental influences must be considered in studies of twins and other siblings, given our knowledge of the importance of environment in the development of an ED. Evidence supports a strong association between genetically determined factors, such serotonin (5-hydroxytryptamine [5-HT]) and dopamine (DOP) levels, and environmental risk factors, suggesting that environmental risk factors play a large role in the expression of behaviors that are also genetically determined (Hollander 1998). However, others investigators have noted that only a small overlap between genetically determined and environmental risk factors. Thus, their conclusion was that there is considerable independence between these two types of risk factors in the development of BN (Bulik et al. 2000, 2007; Fairburn and Harrison 2003; Gorwood et al. 2003; Tracey et al. 2009).

4.4.2 NEUROTRANSMITTERS AND NEUROPEPTIDES

The ingestion of food produces chemical changes in the brain that cause a variety of neurochemical responses throughout the body. Specific hormones are released to create instructional pathways for neural communication. Tryptophan is an essential amino acid that is found in many common foods, such as nuts, meats, and dairy products, and it is a precursor for serotonin (5-HT). Dietary deficiency of tryptophan may lead to low levels of 5-HT. Low levels of tryptophan and 5-HT are commonly seen in individuals with psychological disorders, such as depression and BN (Bruce et al. 2009). A decrease in 5-HT can contribute to the abnormal eating patterns seen in individuals with BN by interfering with the homeostatic regulation of eating by the hypothalamus (Jimerson et al. 1997).

Serotonin is a monoamine neurotransmitter that helps the body regulate appetite, sleep patterns, and mood. As stated previously, serotonin (5-HT) is biochemically derived from tryptophan and is primarily found in the gastrointestinal tract, platelets, and central nervous system of humans and animals. Serotonin is synthesized extensively in the human gastrointestinal tract (about 90%), and the major storage place is platelets in the bloodstream.

Serotonin is likely involved in the etiology of BN by modulating physiological and behavioral functions including anxiety, perception, and appetite (Hammer et al. 2009). Regulation of serotonin is important in the pathophysiology of an ED (Bailer et al. 2010; Wurtman and Wurtman 1995). Serotonin is responsible for regulation or involvement in some of the main functions of the central nervous system, such as control of mood, appetite, sleep, muscle contraction, pain sensitivity, blood pressure, and some cognitive functions including memory and learning (Berger et al. 2009; Hildebrandt et al. 2010).

The neural signaling that occurs in response to food consumption is a link in the feedback mechanisms that normally keep carbohydrate and protein intake more or less constant (Wurtman 1988). Carbohydrate consumption causes insulin secretion, which also increases 5-HT release, whereas the consumption of protein lacks this effect on insulin. The consumption of carbohydrates causes the secretion of insulin from the pancreas into the blood, reducing plasma levels of glucose and allowing the uptake of tryptophan in the brain. Tryptophan enhances 5-HT release and also increases the saturation of tryptophan hydroxlase (Wurtman 1988; Wurtman and Wurtman 1995). Hydroxlase is the enzyme responsible for 5-HT synthesis. When BN patients are given a pharmacological stimulus for the production of 5-HT (serotonin-stimulated prolactin secretion), the number of their eating binges decreases (Jimerson et al. 1997).

Other investigators have suggested that protein should be added to the diet of BN patients in order to reduce binge eating (Latner and Wilson 2004). Individuals whose eating binges consist of primarily protein have fewer eating binges than those whose eating binges consist primarily of carbohydrates (Wurtman and Wurtman 1995). In that study, individuals with BN reported less hunger and greater fullness, and consumed less food at test meals, after protein intake than after carbohydrate intake (673 vs. 856 kcal). This discrepancy between protein and carbohydrate consumption during eating binges deserves attention in future research.

The pharmacology of 5-HT is extremely complex, with its actions being mediated by a large and diverse range of 5-HT receptors. At least seven different receptor subtypes (5-HT1–7) are known to exist, each located in different parts of the body and triggering different responses. Associations between a functional variant in the 5-HT transporter gene have been found with other psychiatric symptoms such as depression, alcoholism, and suicidal behavior (Gorwood et al. 2000). By conferring the allele-specific transcriptional activity on the 5-HT transporter gene promoter in humans, it has been found that the 5-HT transporter gene-linked polymorphic region (5-HTTLPR-a serotonin-transporter-linked promoter region) influences a constellation of personality traits related to anxiety and increases the risk for neurodevelopmental, neurodegenerative, and psychiatric disorders (Lesch et al. 1997). (Alleles are different forms of the DNA sequence of a particular gene.)

The S, G, and A alleles have been implicated in the transmission of an ED from mother to child (Mikolajczyk et al. 2009). It has been hypothesized that alterations in the S-allele contributes to the pathophysiology of binge eating (Steiger et al. 2005). A study by Akkermann (2010) investigated the association between the 5-HTTLPR (serotonin-transporter-linked promoter region) and binge eating to determine if the 5-HTTLPR genotype influenced the severity of binge eating. Women prone to binge eating and carrying the S-allele showed significantly higher levels of BN scores. Among these women, the women with s/s genotype also had higher levels of state anxiety and a tendency for higher impulsivity (Akkermann et al. 2010).

Not all researchers are in agreement about the relationship of the S-allele and the pathophysiology of BN. Lee (2009) found that overall EDs were significantly associated with the S-allele and genotype, but a meta-analysis led to the conclusion that while AN was associated with the S-allele and the S carrier genotype, BN was not associated with this allele (Lee 2009). Racine et al. (2009) found that the T-allele and the S-allele gene were associated with higher levels of impulsivity, but there were no main effects for the 5-HT genotypes on any binge-eating measure, and interaction between genotypes, impulsivity, and dietary restraint were nonsignificant (Racine et al. 2009).

Another important neurotransmitter (neural messenger) that merits discussion in the pathophysiology of BN is dopamine (DOP). DOP is classified as a catecholamine (a class of molecules that serve as neurotransmitters and hormones). DOP is a precursor (forerunner) of adrenaline and another closely related molecule, noradrenaline. Central DOP mechanisms are involved in the reward and motivational aspects of eating and food choices, and they play a role in the compulsive feeding patterns observed in BN and purging disorders (Bello and Hajnal 2010). DOP has been hypothesized that deficiencies in DOP may promote reward-seeking behaviors that result in instant gratification such as carbohydrate eating binges (Baptista et al. 1999; Erlanson-Albertsson 2005; Noble 2003). Foods high in fats and sugars are likely to promote DOP stimulation (Avena et al. 2006).

Although not classified as a neurotransmitter, catechol-O-methyltransferase (COMT) is an important protein in the degradation of DOP and other catecholamines in the brain, so it deserves attention in the discussion of BN. It is one of several enzymes that degrade catecholamines, such as DOP, epinephrine, and norepinephrine. Dysregulation of DOP has been implicated in many genetic studies related to BN (Avena et al. 2006; Bello and Hajnal 2010).

The COMT gene lies in a chromosomal region that is of interest in investigations of psychosis and mood disorders (Mikolajczyk et al. 2009). In particular, regions on chromosome10 have been linked to BN and obesity (Scherag et al. 2010). However, despite a considerable research effort, a clear relationship between the genetic variation in specific chromosomes and the psychiatric phenotype has not been substantiated (Craddock et al. 2006).

4.4.3 Peptides and Proteins

Individuals with BN are less sensitive to the satiating effects of food; after eating, they report lower subjective ratings of fullness than other individuals (Zimmerli et al. 2010). Ample evidence supports the notion that individuals with BN have a disturbance in satiation, which helps to explain the consumption of very large amounts of food that is recorded during binge meals in laboratory settings (Guss et al. 1994; Keel et al. 2007; Kissileff et al. 1986; LaChaussee et al. 1992; Walsh et al.1989). There are several specific physiological mechanisms that help to explain the deficit in the normal development of satiation when individuals with BN consume food.

Abnormal levels of leptin, ghrelin (the satiety peptide), cholecystokinin (CCK), and androgens have all been implicated as playing a role in satiety signaling and binge-eating behavior (Bailer and Kaye 2003). Leptin is a protein hormone that plays a key role in regulating energy intake and energy expenditure, including appetite and metabolism. It is one of the most important adipose-derived hormones (Brennan and Mantzoros 2006). Some studies have found that individuals with BN have low levels of serum leptin (Jimerson et al. 2009; Murialdo et al. 2007; Tanaka et al. 2006; Wolfe et al. 2004), but one study found that leptin concentrations were significantly higher in patients with BN than they were for individuals in a comparison group (Gáti et al. 2007). There is also no consensus among researchers examining ED patients about whether plasma levels of leptin are significantly related with patients' body weight or BMI (Ferron et al. 1997; Hebebrand et al. 1997; Mantzoros and Moschos 1998; Mantzoros et al. 1997; Mathiak et al. 1999; Monteleone et al. 2000).

Ghrelin is a hormone that stimulates hunger that is produced mainly by P/D1 cells lining the fundus of the human stomach and by the epsilon cells of the pancreas. Ghrelin levels increase before meals and decrease after meals. It is considered the counterpart to the hormone leptin, produced by adipose tissue, which induces satiation when present at higher levels. Both acute and chronic fasting increase ghrelin levels (Xi et al. 2008). Weight loss brought about by dieting causes ghrelin levels to rise as body weight and body fat decline. Ghrelin may blunt the appetite-reducing effect of leptin (Monteleone, Martiadis et al. 2003). Individuals with BN have high ghrelin levels (Kojima et al. 2005), but those elevated ghrelin levels have all been found to decrease significantly after treatment, despite similar BMI, percent body fat, and leptin levels (Tanaka et al. 2006). When ghrelin levels return to normal for an individual with an ED, abnormal eating behavior and depressive symptoms both improve (Tanaka et al. 2006).

Supporting the hypothesis that individuals with BN have high ghrelin levels, Kojima et al. (2005) found that patients with BN exhibit elevated ghrelin levels before meals and reduced ghrelin suppression after eating. They found that postprandial ghrelin suppression was significantly attenuated in patients with BN compared to individuals who did not have BN. Monteleone, Monteleone et al. (2003) also found that the ghrelin levels of individuals with BN did not decrease as much as would be expected after a meal. In healthy women, circulating ghrelin showed a drastic decrease after food intake, whereas this response was significantly blunted for individuals with BN. The blunted ghrelin response to food ingestion for individuals with BN may explain the impaired suppression of the drive to eat following a meal, which can lead to binge eating (Monteleone, Martiadis et al. 2003).

CCK is a peptide hormone of the gastrointestinal system responsible for stimulating the digestion of fat and protein. It also acts as a hunger suppressant and contributes to the feeling of satiation (Helm et al. 2003). Individuals with BN have a reduced level of postprandial CCK compared to individuals who do not have EDs (Devlin et al. 1997; Geliebter et al. 1992; Geracioti Jr. and Liddle 1988; Keel et al. 2007, 2010; Pirke et al. 1994).

The development of CCK and satiety has been greatly explored in BN, including gastric capacity, gastric emptying, gastric relaxation reflex, and the postprandial release of CCK (Klein and Walsh 2004). It has been found that there is a significant enlarged gastric capacity in women with BN compared to non-BN women (Geliebter and Hashim 2000). This suggests that a larger amount of food must be consumed before the development of gastric signals. Along with this gastrointestinal abnormality, gastric emptying has found to be delayed in women with BN (Cuellar et al. 1988; Devlin et al. 1997; Kiss et al. 1990; Shih et al. 1987). As a result of this irregularity, there may be a delay in the development of satiety cues that result from the presence of food in the intestine. Finally, another gastrointestinal problem that arises in BN is that there is a reduced gastric relaxation occurring following food ingestion (Walsh et al. 2003).

Lastly, certain proteins, such as brain-derived neurotrophic factor (BDNF), have been implicated in the etiology of an ED. This protein may influence an individual's vulnerability to AN and BN (Scherag et al. 2010). Specifically, the genetic contribution of the BDNF-specific receptor neurotrophic tyrosine kinase receptor type 2 (NTRK2) is implicated in the susceptibility of developing an ED (Ribases et al. 2005).

4.5 CONCLUSIONS

BN is an ED that involves binge eating and the use of inappropriate methods to avoid weight gain. Both genetics and environmental factors (culture and family) play large roles in the behavioral, neurobiological, and temperamental variables that represent the core features of BN. The family environment is especially important in the development of BN, since adolescence is a particularly vulnerable age for females. Although BN is more common in females, if can occur for males, especially those who are concerned about their weight for specific sports and activities (Ackard et al. 2007).

The psychological and physiological aspects of BN are often tightly linked (Sim and Zeman 2004). Biomarkers associated with BN include, but are not limited to the dysregulation of hormones that contribute to irregular dieting behaviors, possibly through serotonergic mechanisms (Klein and Walsh 2004). Alterations in 5-HT and DOP can result in the dysregulation of mood, satiety, appetite, sleep, muscle contraction, and some cognitive functions including memory and learning (Berger et al. 2009; Hildebrandt et al. 2010).

With fluctuating eating patterns, individuals with BN are at risk for developing cardiovascular health problems (Vögele et al. 2009), such as coronary artery disease, hypertension, and congestive heart failure (Casolo et al. 1989; Gordon et al. 1988; Kiensle et al. 1992; Mortara et al. 1994; Nolan et al. 1992). Many other adverse health conditions are associated with the disorder such as alcoholism, panic disorder, generalized anxiety disorder, phobia, and major depression (Kendler et al. 1991). Two of the most prevalent co-occurring conditions for individuals with BN are anxiety and depression (Kaye 2004).

There are many effective treatment options for individuals with BN, such as pharmacology (most commonly antidepressant medications; Zhu and Walsh 2002), psychological treatment, therapeutic exercise such as yoga, and behavioral modification. Short-term multidisciplinary therapy is effective in reducing the symptoms of BN and binge-eating disorder (Cariner et al. 2008). However, even though improvement over a short-term period is commonly found in the research literature, treatment may have a more limited effect over the longer term (Keel and Mitchell 1997). Vigilance is needed in helping girls and women to have healthy eating patterns and to avoid BN and other EDs in a culture that places so much emphasis on physical appearance and has such unrealistic ideals regarding the weight and shape of the human body.

REFERENCES

Ackard, D. M., J. A. Fulkerson, and D. Neumark-Sztainer. 2007. Prevalence and utility of DSM-IV eating disorder diagnostic criteria among youth. *Int J Eat Disord* 40: 409–417.

Akkermann, K., N. Nordquist, L. Oreland, and J. Harro, 2010. Serotonin transporter gene promoter polymorphism affects the severity of binge eating in general population. *Prog Neuropsychopharmacol Biol Psychiatry* 34: 111–114.

American Psychiatric Association. 2000. *Diagnostic and Statistical Manual of Mental Disorders, Fourth Edition*. Washington, DC: American Psychiatric Association Press.

Avena, N. M., P., Rada, N. Moise, and B. G. Hoebel. 2006. Sucrose sham feeding on a binge schedule accumbens dopamine repeatedly and eliminated the acetylcholine satiety response. *Neuroscience* 139 813–820.

Bailer, U. F., C. S. Bloss, G. K. Frank, J. C. Price, C. C. Meltzer, C. A. Mathis, M. A. Geyer, A. Wagner, C. R. Becker, and W. H. Kaye. 2010. 5-HT (1A) receptor binding is increased after recovery from bulimia nervosa compared to control women and is associated with behavioral inhibition in both groups. *Int J Eat Disord* 85 (In press).

Bailer, U. F., and W. H. Kaye. 2003. A review of neuropeptide and neuroendocrine dysregulation in anorexia and bulimia nervosa. *Curr Drug Targets CNS Neurol Disord* 2: 53–59.

Baptista, T., D. Reyes, and L. Hernandez. 1999. Antipsychotic drugs and reproductive hormones: Relationship to body weight regulation. *Pharmacol Biochem Behav* 62: 409–417.

Bartlett, D. W., D. F. Evans, and B. G. Smith. 1996. The relationship between gastro-oesophageal reflux disease and dental erosion. *J Oral Rehabil* 23: 287–297.

Bello, N., and A. Hajnal. 2010. Dopamine and binge eating behaviors. *Pharmacol Biochem Behav* 97: 25–33.

Berger, M., J. A. Gray, and B. L. Roth, 2009. The expanded biology of serotonin. *Annu Rev Med* 60: 355–366.

Birketvedt, G. S., E. Drivenes, I. Agledahl, J. Sundsfjord, R. Olstad, and J. R. Florholmen. 2006. Bulimia nervosa—A primary defect in the hypothalamic-pituitary-adrenal axis? *Appetite* 46: 164–167.

Bostom A. G., D. Shemin, P. Verhoef, M. R. Nadeau, P. F. Jacques, J. Selhub, L. Dworkin, I. H. Rosenberg. 1997. Elevated fasting total plasma homocysteine levels and cardiovascular disease outcomes in maintenance dialysis patients: A prospective study. *Arterioscler Thromb Vasc Biol.* 17: 2554–2558.

Brennan, A. M., and C. S. Mantzoros. 2006. Drug Insight: the role of leptin in human physiology and pathophysiology—Emerging clinical applications. *Nat Clin Pract Endocrinol Metab* 2: 318–327.

Bruce, K. R. H., S. N. Steiger, N. Young, M. K. N. Y., Kin, M. Israël, and M. Lévesque. 2009. Impact of acute tryptophan depletion on mood and eating-related urges in bulimic and nonbulimic women. *J Psychiatry Neurosci* 34: 376–382.

Buckholdt, K. E., G. R. Para, and L. Jobe-Shields. 2010. Emotion dysregulation as a mechanism through which parental magnification of sadness increase risk for binge eating and limited control of eating behaviors. *Eat Behav* 11: 122–126.

Bulik, C. M., B. Devlin, and S. A. Bacanu. 2003. Significant linkage on chromosome 10p families with bulimia nervosa. *Am J of Hum Genet* 72: 200–7.

Bulik, C. M., M. C. Slof-Op't Landt, E. F. van Furth, and P. F. Sullivan. 2007. The genetics of anorexia nervosa. *Annu Rev Nutr* 27: 263–275.

Bulik, C. M., P. F. Sullivan, T. D. Wade, and K. S. Kendler. 2000. Twin studies of eating disorders: A review. *Int J Eat Disord* 27: 1–20.

Bulik, C. M., L. M. Thorton, T. L. Root, E. M. Pisetsky, P. Lichtenstein, and N. L. Pedersen. 2010. Understanding the relation between anorexia nervosa and bulimia nervosa in a Swedish national twin sample. *Biol Psychiatry* 67: 71–77.

Butera, P. C. 2009. Estradiol and the control of food intake. *Physiol Behav* 99: 175–180.

Casolo, G., E. Balli, T. Taddei, J. Amuhasi, and C. Gori. 1989. Decreased spontaneous heart rate variability on congestive heart failure. *Am J Cardiol* 64: 1162–1167.

Contrufo, P., P. Monteleone, M. D'Istria, A. Fuschino, I. Serino, and M. Maj. 2000. Aggressive behavioral characteristics and endogenous hormones in women with bulimia nervosa. *Neuropsychobiology* 42: 58–61.

Craddock, N., M. J. Owen, and M. C. O'Donovan. 2006. The catechol-*O*-methyl transferase (*COMT*) gene as a candidate for psychiatric phenotypes: evidence and lessons. *Mol Psychiatry* 11: 446–458.

Crow, S. J., C. B. Peterson, S. A. Swanson, N. C. Raymond, S. Specker, E. D. Eckert, and J. E. Mitchell. 2009. Increased mortality in bulimia nervosa and other eating disorders. *Am J Psychiatry* 166: 1342–1346.

Crow, S. J., P. Thuras, P. K. Keel, and J. E. Mitchell. 2002. Long-term menstrual and reproductive function in patients with bulimia nervosa. *Am J Psychiatry* 159: 1048–1050.

Cuellar, R. E., W. H. Kaye, L. K. Hsu, and D. H. VanThiel. 1988. Upper gastrointestinal tract dysfunction in bulimia. *Dig Dis Sci* 33: 1549–1553.

Dalvit-McPhillips, S. 1983. The effect of the human menstrual cycle on nutrient intake. *Physiol Behav* 31: 209–212.

Devlin, M. J., B. T. Walsh, J. L. Guss, H. R. Kissileff, R. A. Liddle, and E. Petkova. 1997. Postprandial cholecystokinin release and gastric emptying in patients with bulimia nervosa. *Am J Clin Nutr* 65: 114–120.

Erlanson-Albertsson, C. 2005. How palatable food disrupts appetite regulation. *Basic Clin Pharmacol Toxicol* 97: 61–73.

Fairburn, C. G., and P. J. Harrison. 2003. Eating Disorders. *Eat Disord* 361:407–416.

Favaro, A., L. Caregaro, E. Tenconi, R. Bosello, and P. Santonastaso. 2009. Time trends in age at onset of anorexia and bulimia nervosa. *J Clin Psychiatry* 70: 1715–1721.

Ferron, F., R. V. Considine, R. Peino, I. G. Lado, C. Dieguez, and F. F. Casanueva. 1997. Serum leptin concentrations in patients with anorexia nervosa, bulimia nervosa and non-specific eating disorders correlate with the body mass index but are independent of the respective disease. *Clin Endocrinol* 46: 289–293.

Freizinger, M., D. L. Franko, M. Dacey, B. Okun, and A. D. Domar. 2010. The prevalence of eating disorders in infertile women. *Fertil Steril* 93: 72–78.

Frieling, H., K. D. Romer, B. Sabine, T. Hillemacher, J. Wilhelm, G. E. Jacoby, M. de Zwaan, J. Kornhuber, and S. Bliech. 2006. Depressive symptoms may explain elevated plasma levels of homocysteine in females with eating disorders. *J Psychiatr Res* 42:83–86.

Frieling, H., B. Röschke, J. Kornhuber, J. Wilhelm, K. D. Römer, B. Gruss, D. Bönsch, T. Hillemacher, M. de Zwaan, G. E. Jacoby, and S. Bleich. 2005. Cognitive impairment and its association with homocysteine plasma levels in females with eating disorders—Findings from the HEaD-study. *J Neural Trans* 112: 1591–1598.

Garfinkel, P. E., E. Lin, P. Goering, C. Spegg, D. S. Goldbloom, S. Kennedy, A. S. Kaplan, and D. B. Woodside. 1995. Bulimia nervosa in a Canadian community sample: Prevalence and comparison of subgroups. *Am J Psychiatry* 152: 1052–1058.

Gáti, A., B. Pászthy, I. Wittman, I. Abrahám, S. Jeges, and F. Túry. 2007. Leptin and glucose metabolism in eating disorders. *Psychiatr Hung* 22: 163–169.

Geisel, J., U. Hubner, M. Bodis, H. Schorr, J. P. Knapp, R. Obeid, and W. Herrman. 2003. The role of genetic factors in the development of hyperhomocysteinemia. *Clin Chem Lab Med* 41: 1427–1434.

Geliebter, A., and S. A. Hashim. 2000. Gastric capacity in normal, obese, and bulimic women. *Physiol. Behav* 74: 743–746.

Geliebter, A, P. M. Melton, R. S. McCray, D. R. Gallagher, D. Gage, and S. A. Hashim. 1992. Gastric capacity, gastric emptying, and test-meal intake in normal and bulimic women. *Am J Clin Nutr* 56: 656–661.

Geracioti, Jr.,T. D, and R. A. Liddle. 1988. Impaired cholecystokinin secretion in bulimia nervosa. *N Engl J Med* 319: 683–688.

Gordon, D., V. L. Herrera, L. McAlpine, R. J., Cohen, S. Akselrod, P. Lang, and W. I. Norwood. 1988. Heart rate spectral analysis: A noninvasive probe of cardiovascular regulation in critically ill children with heart disease. *Pediatr Cardiol* 9: 69–77.

Gorwood, P., P. Batel, J. Adèsb, M. Hamon, and C. Bonid. 2000. Serotonin transporter gene polymorphisms, alcoholism, and suicidal behavior. *Biol Psychiatry* 48: 259–64.

Gorwood, P., A. Kipman, and C. Foulon. 2003. The human genetics of anorexia nervosa. *J Eur Pharmacol* 480: 163–170.

Guss, J. L., H. R. Kissilef, B. T. Walsh, and M. J. Devlin. 1994. Binge eating behavior in patients with eating disorders. *Obes Res* 2: 355–363.

Hammer, C. 2009 Functional variants of the serotonin receptor type 3A and B gene are associated with eating disorders. *Pharmacogent Geonomics* 19: 790–799.

Hebebrand, J., W. F. Blum, N. Barth, H. Coners, P. Englaro, A. Juul, A. Ziegler, A. Warnke, W. Rascher, and H. Remschmidt.1997. Leptin levels in patients with anorexia nervosa are reduced in the acute stage and elevated upon short-term weight restoration. *Mol Psychiatry* 2: 330–334.

Helm, K. A., P. Rada, and B. G. Hoebel. 2003. Cholecystokinin combined with serotonin in the hypothalamus limits accumbens dopamine release while increasing acetylcholine: A possible satiation mechanism. *Brain Res* 963: 290–297.

Hollander, E. 1998. Treatment of obsessive-compulsive spectrum disorders with SSRIs. *Br J Psychiatry* 35: 7–12.

Hudson, J. I., E. Hiripi, H. G. Pope, and R. C. Kessler. 2007. The prevalence and correlates of eating disorders in the National Comorbidity Survey Replication. *Biol Psychiatry* 61: 348–358.

Jimerson, D. C., B. E. Wolfe, D. P. Carroll, and P. K. Keel. 2009. Psychobiology of purging disorder: Reduction in circulating leptin levels in purging disorder in comparison with controls. *Int J Eat Disord* 43: 584–588.

Jimerson, D. C., B. E. Wolfe, E. D. Metzger, D. M. Finkelstein, T. B. Cooper, and J. M. Levine. 1997. Decreased serotonin function in bulimia nervosa. *Arch Gen Psychiatry* 54: 529–534.

Kaye, W. H., B. M. Cynthia, L. Thornton, N. Barbarich, K. Masters, and the Price Foundation Collaborative Group. 2004. Comorbidity of anxiety disorders with anorexia and bulimia nervosa. *Am J Psychiatry* 161: 2215–2221.

Kaye, W. H., K. L. Klump, G. K. Frank, and M. Strober. 2000. Anorexia and bulimia nervosa. *Annu Rev Med* 51: 299–313.

Keel, P. K., and J. E. Mitchell. 1997. Outcome in bulimia nervosa. *Am J Psychiatry* 154: 313–321.

Keel, P. K., B. E. Wolfe, R. A. Liddle, K. P. De Young, and D. C. Jimerson. 2007. Clinical features and physiology response to a test meal in purging disorder and bulimia nervosa. *Arch Gen Psychiatry* 64: 1058–1066.

Kendler, K. S., C. MacLean, M. Neale, R. Kessler, A. Heath, and L. Eaves. 1991. The genetic epidemiology of bulimia nervosa. *Am J Psychiatry* 148: 1627–1637.

Kienzle, M. G., D. W. Ferguson, C. L. Birkett, G. A. Myers, W. J. Berg, and D. J. Mariano. 1992. Clinical hemodynamic and sympathetic neural correlates of heart rate variability in congestive heart failure. *Am J Cardiol* 69: 482–485.

Kiss, A., H. Bergmann, T. A. Abatzi, C. Schneider, S. Wiesnagrotzki, J. Höbart, G. Steiner-Mittelbach, G. Gaupmann, A. Kugi, and G. Stacher-Janotta. 1990. Oesophageal and gastric motor activity in patients with bulimia nervosa. *Gut* 31: 259–265.

Kissileff, H.R., B.T. Walsh, J.G. Kral, and S.M. Cassidy. 1986. Laboratory studies of eating behavior in women with bulimia. *Physiol Behav* 38: 563–570.

Klein, D. A., and T. B. Walsh. 2004. Eating disorders: Clinical features and pathophysiology. *Physiol Behav* 81: 359–374.

Klump, K. L., W. H. Kaye, and M. Strober. 2001. The evolving genetic foundations of eating disorders. *Psychiatr Clin North Am* 24: 215–225.

Kohn, M., and N. H. Golden. 2001. Eating disorders in children and adolescents: Epidemiology, diagnosis and treatment. *Paediatr Drugs* 3: 91–99.

Kojima, S., T. Nakahara, N. Nagai, T. Muranaga, M. Tanaka, D. Yasuhara, A. Masuda, Y. Date, H. Ueno, M. Nakazato, and T. Narou. 2005. Altered ghrelin and peptide YY responses to meals in bulimia nervosa. *Clin Endocrinol* 62: 74–78.

LaChaussee, J. L., H. R. Kissileff, B. T. Walsh, and C. M. Hadigan. 1992. The single-item meal as a measure of binge-eating behavior in patients with bulimia nervosa. *Physiol Behav* 51: 593–600.

Latner, J. D., and G. T. Wilson. 2004. Binge eating and satiety in bulimia nervosa and binge eating disorder: effects of macronutrients intake. *Int J Eat Disord* 36: 402–415.

Lee, Y. 2009. Association between serotonin transporter gene polymorphism and eating disorders: A meta analytic study. *Int J Eat Disord* 43: 498–504.

Lesch, K. P., J. Meyer, K. Glatz, G. Fliigge, A. Hinney, J. Hebebrand, S. M. Klauck, A. Poustka, F. Poustka, and D. Bengel. 1997. The 5-HT transporter gene-linked polymorphic region (5-HTTLER) in evolutionary perspective: alternative biallelic variation in rhesus monkeys. *J Neural Transm* 104: 1259–1266.

Mantzoros, C., J. S. Flier, M. D. Lesem, T. D. Brewerton, and D. C. Jimerson. 1997. Cerebrospinal fluid leptin in anorexia nervosa: Correlation with nutritional status and potential role in resistance to weight gain. *J Clin Endo Metab* 82: 1845–1851.

Mantzoros, C. S., and S. J. Moschos. 1998. Leptin: In search of roles in human physiology and pathophysiology. *Clin Endocrinol* 49: 551–567.

Markey, M. A., and J. S. Vander Wal. 2007. The role of emotional intelligence and negative affect in bulimia symptomatology. *Compr Psychiatry* 48: 458–464.

Mathiak, K., W. Gowin, J. Hebebrand, A. Ziegler, W. F. Blum, D. Felsenberg, H. Lubbert, and W. Kopp. 1999. Serum leptin levels, body fat deposition, and weight in females with anorexia or bulimia nervosa. *Hor Metabol Res* 31: 274–277.

Matzkin, V. B., C. Geissler, R. Coniglio, J. Selles, and M. Bello. 2006. Cholesterol concentrations in patients with Anorexia Nervosa and in healthy controls. *Int J Psychiatr Nurs Res* 11: 1283–1293.

Messerli-Bürgy, N., C.Engesser, E. Lemmenmeier, A. Steptoe, and K. Laederach-Hofmann. 2010. Cardiovascular stress reactivity and recovery in bulimia nervosa and binge eating disorder. *Int J Psychophysiol* 98: 229–234.

Mikolajczyk, E., A. Grzywacz, and J. Samochowiec. 2009. The association of the catechol-O-methyltransferase genotype with the phenotype of women with eating disorders. *Br Res* 1307: 142–148.

Mira, M., P. M. Stewart, and S. Abraham. 1985. Hormonal and biochemical abnormalities in women suffering from eating disorders. *Pediatrician* 12: 148–156.

Monteleone, P., A. D. Lieto, A. Tortorella, N. Longobardi, and M. Maj. 2000. Circulating leptin in patients with anorexia nervosa, bulimia nervosa or binge-eating disorder: Relationship to body weight, eating patterns, psychopathology and endocrine changes. *Psychiat Res* 94: 121–129.

Monteleone, P., M. Luisi, G. De Filippis, B. Colurcio, P. Monteleone, A. R. Genazzani, and M. Maj. 2003. Circulating levels of neuroactive steroids in patients with binge eating disorder: A comparison with non-obese health controls and non-binge eating obese subjects. *Int J Eat Disord* 34: 432–440.

Monteleone, P., V. Martiadis, M. Fabrazzo, C. Serritella, and M. Maj. 2003b. Ghrelin and leptin responses to food ingestion in bulimia nervosa: implications for binge-eating and compensatory behaviors. *Psychol Med* 33: 1387–1394.

Morris, A. S., J. S. Silk, L. Steinberg, S. S. Myers, and L. R. Robinson. 2007. The role of the family context and development of emotion regulation. *Soc Dev* 16: 361–388.

Mortara, A., M. T. La Rovere, M. G. Signorini, P. Pantaleo, G. Pinna, L. Martinelli, C. Ceconi, S. Cerutti, and L. Tavazzi. 1994. Can power spectral analysis of heart rate variability identify a high risk subgroup of congestive heart failure patients with excessive sympathetic activation? A pilot study before and after heart transplantation. *Br Heart J* 71: 422–430.

Murialdo, G., M. Casu, M. Falchero, A. Brugnolo, V. Patrone, P. F. Cerro, P. Ameri, G. Andraghetti, L. Briatore, F. Copello, R. Cordera, G. Rodriguez, and A. M. Ferro. 2007. Alterations in the autonomic control of heart rate variability in patients with anorexia or bulimia nervosa: Correlations between sympathovagal activity, clinical features, and leptin levels. *J Endocrinol Invest* 30: 356–362.

Naessén, S., K. Carlström, R. Glant, H. Jacobsson, and A. L. Hirschberg. 2006. Bone mineral density in bulimic women—Influence of endocrine factors and previous anorexia. *Eur J Endocrinol* 155: 245–251.

Noble, E. P. 2003. D2 dopamine receptor gene in psychiatric and neurologic disorders and its phenotypes. *Am J Med Genet B Neuropsychiatr Genet* 116: 103–125.

Nolan, J., A. D. Flapan, S. Capewell, T. M. MacDonald, J. M. M. Neilson, and D. J. Ewing. 1992. Decreased cardiac parasympathetic activity in chronic heart failure and its relation to left ventricular function. *Br Heart J* 69: 761–767.

Pauporte, J., and B. T. Walsh. 2000. Serum cholesterol in bulimia nervosa. *Int J Eat Disord* 30: 294–298.

Pirke, K. M., M. B. Kellner, E. Friess, J. C. Krieg, and M. M. Fichter. 1994. Satiety and cholecystokinin. *Int J Eat Disord* 15: 63–69.

Racine, S. E., K. M. Culbert, C. L. Larson, and K. L. Klump. 2009. The possible influence of impulsivity and dietary restraint on associations between serotonin genes and binge eating. *J Psychiatr Res* 43: 1278–1286.

Reba-Harrelson, L., A. Von Holle, L. M. Thronton, K. L. Klump, W. H. Berrettini, H. Brandt, S. Crawford, S. Crow, M. M. Fichter, D. Goldman, K. A. Halmi, C. Johnson, A. S. Kaplan, P. Keel, M. LaVia, J. Mitchell, K. Plotnicov, A. Rotondo, M. Strober, and J. Treasure. 2008. Features associated with diet pill used in individuals with eating disorders. *Eat Behav* 9: 73–81.

Resch, M., G. Szendei, and P. Haasz. 2004, Bulimia from a gynecological view: Hormonal changes. *J Obstet Gynaecol* 24: 907–910.

Ribases, M., M. Gratacos, A. Badia, L. Jimenez, R. Solano, J. Vallejo, F. Fernandez-Aranda, and X. Estivill. 2005. Contribution of NTRK2 to the genetic susceptibility to anorexia nervosa, harm avoidance and minimum body mass index. *Mol Psychiatry* 10: 851–860.

Roberts, M. W., and C. A. Tylenda. 1989. Dental aspects of anorexia and bulimia nervosa. *Pediatrician* 16: 178–184.

Robinson-O'Brien, R., C. L. Perry, M. M. Wall, M. Story, and D. Neumark-Sztainer. 2009. Adolescent and young adult vegetarianism: Better dietary intake and weight outcomes but increased risk of disordered eating behaviors. *J Am Diet Assoc* 109: 648–655.

Scherag, S., J. Heberbrand, and A. Hinney. 2010. Eating disorders: The current status of molecular genetic research. *Eur Child Adolesc Psychiatry* 19: 211–226.

Seidenfeld, M. E. K., and V. I. Rickert. 2001. Impact of anorexia, bulimia and obesity on the gynecologic health of adolescents. *Am Fam Physician* 64: 445–450.

Shih, W. J., L. Humphries, G. A. Digenis, F. X. Castellanos, P. A. Domstad, and F. H. DeLand. 1987. Tc-99 m labeled triethelene tetraamine polysterene gastric emptying studies in bulimia patients. *Eur J Nucl Med* 13: 192–196.

Sim, L., and J. Zeman. 2004. Emotion awareness and identification skills in adolescent girls with bulimia nervosa. *J Clin Child Adolesc Psychol* 33: 760–771.

Sodersten, P., and C. Bergh. 2003. Anorexia nervosa: towards a neurobiologically based therapy. *J Eur Pharm* 480: 67–74.

Steiger, H., R. Joober, M. Israel, S. N. Young, N. M. Ng Ying Kin, L. Gauvin, K. R. Bruce, J. Joncas, and A. Torkaman-Zehi. 2005. The 5HTTLPR polymorphism, psychopathologic symptoms, and platelet [3H-] paroxetine binding in bulimic syndromes. *Int J Eat Disord* 37: 57–60.

Tanaka, M., T. Nakahara, T. Muranaga, S. Kojima, D. Yasuhara, H. Ueno, M. Nakazato, and A. Inui. 2006. Ghrelin concentrations and cardiac vagal tone are decreased after pharmacologic and cognitive-behavioral treatment in patients with bulimia nervosa. *Horm Behav* 50: 261–265.

Tracey D., T. D. Wade, S. A. Treloar, A. C. Heath, and N. G. Martin. 2009. An examination of the overlap between genetic and environmental risk factors for intentional weight loss and overeating. *Int J Eat Disord* 42: 492–497.

Vaz-Leal, F. J., L. Rodriquez-Santos, J. M. Melero-Ruiz, I. M. Ramos-Fuentes, and A. M. Garcia-Herraiz. 2010. Psychopathology and lymphocyte subsets in patients with bulimia nervosa. *Nutri Neurosci* 13: 109–115.

Vögele, C., A. Hilbert, and B. Tushchen-Caffier. 2009. Dietary restriction, cardiac autonomic regulation and stress reactivity in bulimic women. *Physiol Behav* 98: 229–234.

Walsh, B. T., E. Zimmerli, M. J. Devlin, J. Guss, and H. R. Kissileff. 2003. A disturbance of gastric function in bulimia nervosa. *Biol Psychiatry* 54: 929–933.

Walsh, B. T., H. R. Kissileff, S. M. Cassidy, and S. Dantzic. 1989 Eating behavior of women with bulimia. *Arch Gen Psychiatry* 46: 54–58.

Wilhelm, J., E. Müller, M. de Zwaan, J. Fischer, T. Hillemacher, J. Kornhuber, S. Bleich, and H. Frieling. 2010. Elevation of homocysteine levels is only partially reversed after therapy in females with eating disorders. *J Neural Transm* 117: 521–527.

Wilhelm, J., K. D. Römer, B. Gruss, D. Bönsch, T. Hillemacher, M. de Zwaan, G. E. Jacoby, and S. Bleich. 2005. Cognitive impairment and its association with homocysteine plasma levels in females with eating disorders—Findings from the HEaD-study. *J Neural Trans* 112: 1591–1598.

Wolfe, B. E., D. C. Jimerson, C. Orlova, and C. S. Mantzoros. 2004. Effect of dieting on plasma leptin, soluble leptin receptor, adiponectin and resistin levels in healthy volunteers. *Clin Endocrinol* 61: 332–338.

Wurtman R. J., and Wurtman J. J. 1995. Brain serotonin, carbohydrate-craving, obesity and depression. *Obes Res* 3: 477S–480S.

Wurtman, J. J. 1988. Carbohydrate craving, mood changes, and obesity. *J Clin Psychiatry* 49: 37–39.

Xi, Q., J. T. Reed, G. Wang, S. Han, E. W. Englander, and G. H. Greeley. 2008. Gherlin secretion is not reduced by increase fat mass during diet-induced obesity. *Am J Physiol Regul Integr Comp* Physiol 295: R429–435.

Yager, J., J. Landsverk, C. K. Edelstein, and M. Jarvik. 1988. A 20-month follow-up study of 628 women with eating disorders: II course of associated symptoms and related clinical features. *Int J Eat Disord* 7: 503–513.

Zhu, A. J., and B. T. Walsh. 2002. Pharmacologic treatment of eating disorders. *Can J Psychiatry* 47: 227–234.

Zimmerli, E. J., M. J. Devlin, H. R. Kissileff, and T. B. Walsh. 2010. The development of satiation in bulimia nervosa. *J Phys Behav* 100: 346–349.

5 Measures of Eating Disorder Symptoms and Body Image Disturbance

Susan Kashubeck-West, Kendra Saunders, and Hsin-hsin Huang

CONTENTS

5.1 LEARNING OBJECTIVES

After reading this chapter you should be able to

- Identify the types of measures of eating-disordered behavior and body image that are available
- Describe the limitations of various methods for assessing disordered eating and body image
- Describe some widely used measures of disordered eating and body image
- Explain how to conduct an assessment of body image and eating disorder symptoms

5.2   RESEARCH BACKGROUND, SIGNIFICANCE, AND CURRENT FINDINGS

The purpose of this chapter is to review methods for assessing the behavioral and psychological characteristics of individuals with problems that are suggestive of eating disorders. Some of the most widely used instruments for assessing these disorders will be considered, including self-report inventories and structured interview methods. Psychometric data, including reliability and validity, will be discussed for each method. Reliability refers to the degree to which a test can be repeated with the same results in the same type of participants. In other words, reliability involves the consistency shown by a test with specific samples of participants. When tests demonstrate high reliability in a sample, it means the scores of participants in the sample are less susceptible to insignificant or random changes in the test taker or the testing environment. Reliability coefficients above .80 typically are considered satisfactory, and coefficients below .70 often are viewed as unacceptable. Validity refers to the degree to which a questionnaire measures what it is intended to measure in a given sample of participants. For example, does a measure of body dissatisfaction really assess a person's negative feelings toward her body, or does it capture some other phenomenon, such as depression or anxiety? The validity of an assessment procedure in a given sample will affect the appropriateness, meaningfulness, and usefulness of the test data. The greater the reliability and validity, the more confident one can be in the accuracy of the data gathered from a sample of participants.

5.2.1   Self-Report Inventories for Eating Disorder Symptoms

Numerous self-report instruments have been created to assess symptoms related to eating disorders. By self-report, we mean paper-and-pencil measures or online versions of these measures that the individual completes by herself. Self-report questionnaires offer several advantages. They are typically inexpensive and usually require less time to administer than an interview. Furthermore, administration of a self-report questionnaire is simple, and such a measure can often be administered and scored by nonprofessional staff, although professionals with knowledge about eating disorders should interpret the results. In addition, self-report measures can be given to groups of individuals, making it possible to collect data from large samples.

There are disadvantages to self-report inventories, however. They are vulnerable to various types of error and biases, including difficulty distinguishing between individuals who deny the existence of psychological problems and those who are psychologically healthy (Shedler et al. 1993). Sometimes, people may not be truthful in completing the questions, or respondents might circle more than one answer, leave an answer blank, or pick what they think is the right answer when they do not feel that they identify with the options presented (Pike et al. 1995). Questions asked by an interviewer can often determine nuances to people's answers that are not available when using a self-report measure. In addition, it may be difficult to accurately assess complex concepts with a paper-and-pencil measure, and many self-report measures are based on outdated diagnostic criteria for eating disorders (Mintz et al. 1997). Finally, most self-report questionnaires do not provide a diagnosis for eating disorders, but instead assess the symptoms of the eating problem. Individuals who score above certain cutoff scores on these measures need to be evaluated with a clinical interview to assess the presence of an eating disorder.

Because of their advantages, and despite their limitations, self-report instruments are widely used. Researchers often use them to get information from a large number of people so that relationships between eating disorder symptoms and other variables can be determined. Also, a clinician who suspects a client has symptoms associated with an eating disorder might ask her to fill out a self-report measure to get an initial assessment of the problem. Summaries of commonly used self-report inventories for the measurement of eating disorder symptoms are provided in the following sections of this chapter.

5.2.1.1   Eating Disorder Inventory-3 (EDI-3)

The EDI-3 is a popular, 91-item, self-report questionnaire that was constructed to measure the cognitive and behavioral traits found in individuals with eating disorders (Garner 2004). The original EDI (Garner 1983) was developed to address a wide range of psychological issues related to eating disorders and to aid in differentiating among individuals with eating disorders, those with subclinical levels of eating disorders, and those without eating disorder symptoms (Mintz and Kashubeck-West 2004). In 1991, Garner introduced the EDI-2, containing the original 64 EDI items and 27 additional items, and those 91 items were classified into 11 subscales. The primary purpose of the EDI-2 was to assess a client's symptoms and to aid in treatment planning. In 2004, Garner published the EDI-3; it contained the same 91 items as the EDI-2 but was reconfigured into 12 subscales to better reflect current knowledge about eating disorders. In addition to these subscales, the EDI-3 also offers three indicators of response style to assess inconsistency, impression management tendencies, and infrequent responses. This is an important addition, given the tendency of individuals with eating disorders to engage in denial and approval seeking, and their increased risk of cognitive impairment (Cumella 2006).

The EDI-3 has three subscales that are specific to eating disorders: (1) Drive for thinness measures a person's concern with thinness, weight, and dieting; (2) Bulimia measures the frequency of episodes of uncontrollable overeating (binge eating) and the urge to engage in self-induced vomiting (purging); and (3) Body Dissatisfaction assesses the belief that certain body parts that change at puberty (hips, thighs, stomach, buttocks) are too large. These three subscales make up the composite scale entitled Eating Disorder Risk Composite. The remaining nine subscales assess general psychological constructs that are thought to be related to eating disorders: Low Self-Esteem, Personal Alienation, Interpersonal Insecurity, Interpersonal Alienation, Interoceptive Deficits, Emotional Dysregulation, Perfectionism, Asceticism, and Maturity Fears.

One can use scores on the 12 subscales individually, one can total the scores on the subscales for an overall score, or one can calculate six composite scores. If respondents are suspected to have an eating disorder, they should be evaluated further. A companion measure, the Eating Disorder Inventory-3 Symptom Checklist, assesses the frequency of specific symptoms and can be used in conjunction with the EDI-3 to make a *DSM-IV-TR* diagnosis. The EDI-3 may be purchased through the publisher, Psychological Assessment Resources, Inc. (800–331-8378, www.parinc.com). Administration of the EDI-3 does not require a trained examiner, but the test interpreter should have a mental health background and some knowledge of the test and the intended variables of interest. The EDI-3 can be administered individually or in groups, is designed for ages 13–53, and requires approximately 20 minutes to complete.

The EDI was founded on the authors' clinical experience and research with anorexic and bulimic patients. In samples of European American women with and without eating disorders, the internal consistency reliability for all three versions of the EDI generally has been above .70 (Espelage et al. 2003; Garner et al. 1983; Schaefer et al. 1998). However, Limbert (2004) reported less than acceptable internal consistency estimates for 5 of the 8 original EDI subscales in a large sample of female university students.

Factor analytic results with the various versions of the EDI have been mixed, with some researchers (e.g., Welch et al. 1990) reporting an eight-factor solution that corresponded to the original eight subscales proposed by the EDI authors. However, other researchers suggest that many subscales of the EDI measure dimensions of general psychological disturbance and do not adequately differentiate individuals with eating disorders from individuals with other psychological disorders (Cooper et al. 1985). Furthermore, most support for the factorial integrity of the EDI has come from studies using clinical populations (Cooper et al. 1985; Hurley et al. 1990; Norring 1990; Schoemaker et al. 1997; Welch et al. 1990). Unfortunately, studies using nonpatients have revealed that the factorial integrity and validity of the EDI may not be adequate. For example, different studies with college women report different factor structures (Williamson et al. 1995). Such findings suggest that the individuals who have eating disorders interpret the EDI items differently than individuals without eating disorders (Mintz and Kashubeck-West 2004), and some authors have proposed that the EDI should not be used for screening purposes until its validity for this purpose has been better established (Klemchuk et al. 1990).

Espelage et al. (2003) used data from clinical and nonclinical participants in the U.S. to evaluate the construct validity of the EDI. Their results indicated partial support for the eight-factor structure and revealed that certain EDI items were better indicators of their hypothesized constructs than other items. Results of a confirmatory factor analysis suggested that the EDI assesses two distinct constructs: one related to eating and weight-related problems and the other related to personality variables. A similar conclusion was reached by Podar and Allik (2009), who aggregated data from 94 different studies that reported mean values for EDI subscales. The two-factor structure they found contained one factor that had the three subscales that are specific for eating disorders (Drive for Thinness, Bulimia, and Body Dissatisfaction), and a second factor comprised of three personality subscales (Interoceptive Deficits, Maturity Fears, and Impulse Regulation). Interestingly, Podar and Allik (2009) found that the same factor structure was present in both clinical and nonclinical samples and across Western and nonwestern samples.

Although the EDI has been used in a number of research studies with U.S. ethnic minority women (Franko et al. 2004), little research has investigated the psychometric qualities of the EDI with such samples (Kashubeck-West et al. 2001). Similarly, the EDI has been translated into numerous languages and used around the world, often without attention to establishing the psychometric properties of the new measure (Mintz and Kashubeck-West 2004).

Many authors have recommendations for potential uses of the EDI-3. For example, some have recommended using it as a tool for screening for eating disorders in nonclinical samples, since some data show that the EDI can discriminate between individuals with eating disorders and nonpsychiatric individuals in comparison groups (Crowther and Sherwood 1997; Garner 1991; Gross et al. 1986; Raciti and Norcross 1987). However, other authors disagree, citing data demonstrating that the EDI has low discriminate power (Bennett and Stevens 1997; Klemchuk et al. 1990). If the EDI-3 is used as a screening instrument, the administrator needs to remember that its ability to differentiate among types and subtypes of eating disorders is questionable. The EDI was reported to be useful for measuring change in therapy over time (Dare et al. 2000; Sunday et al. 1992) and Crowther and Sherwood (1997) suggested that EDI items could be used for developing a psychological profile to use in setting treatment goals for clients with eating disorders. Readers are cautioned, however, that these recommendations are only for white individuals, given the lack of psychometric data on the EDI-3 with members of ethnic minority groups.

5.2.1.2 Eating Attitudes Test (EAT)

The EAT (Garner and Garfinkel 1979) is one of the most widely used measures of eating-disordered behavior. The original EAT contains 40 self-rated items that assess behaviors and attitudes associated with anorexia nervosa. An abbreviated 26-item version of the EAT (EAT-26) is also available, and it is highly correlated with the EAT-40 (Garner et al. 1982). The EAT has been translated into many different languages, and psychometric evaluations of some of these translated versions have been carried out (e.g., Rivas, Bersabe, and Jimenez 2004). Unfortunately, no psychometric evaluation of the EAT appears to have been conducted with racial and ethnic minority individuals in the United States (Mintz and Kashubeck-West 2004). Both the EAT-40 and the EAT-26 (see Appendix 5.A) are available free of charge from the authors, and numerous websites have the EAT posted on them (e.g., http://psychcentral.com/quizzes/eat.htm). The EAT has a 5th-grade reading level. A children's version of the EAT (ChEAT; Maloney et al. 1988) has been developed and was found to be useful in identifying younger children (i.e., elementary-school aged children) at risk for eating disorders (Anderson et al. 2009).

Changes in the *Diagnostic and Statistical Manual of Mental Disorders* (*DSM*; American Psychiatric Association 2000) criteria have resulted in confusion over what eating disorder symptoms the EAT assesses. Mintz and Kashubeck-West (2004) noted that, although many of the items still seem to capture *DSM-IV* symptoms for anorexia nervosa, many of the items also reflect criteria for bulimia nervosa. In addition, some EAT items are likely to be endorsed by women who chronically diet or are preoccupied with their weight (Mintz and O'Halloran 2000). Therefore, many individuals who score high on the EAT are not formally diagnosed with an eating disorder but instead are identified as having abnormal eating patterns that interfere with daily functioning (Garner and Garfinkel 1979). Cutoff scores to identify individuals with eating-disordered behaviors and attitudes have been recommended by the authors of the EAT (30 for the EAT-40 and 20 for the EAT-26; Garner and Garfinkel 1979; Garner et al. 1982).

The EAT generally appears to discriminate between women who are diagnosed with either anorexia nervosa or bulimia nervosa and women without eating disorders (Williamson et al. 1993). However, there is no evidence that the EAT discriminates between women with anorexia nervosa and women with bulimia nervosa. Furthermore, the factor structure of the EAT has been shown to vary among different populations (Doninger et al. 2005; Ocker et al. 2007). The EAT has been found to have a high false-positive rate, as many individuals with high scores on the EAT do not qualify for full-syndrome anorexia or bulimia diagnoses (Garkinkle and Newman 2001; Mintz and O'Halloran 2000). Based on their review of the validity data available on the EAT and EAT-26, Mintz and O'Halloran (2000) recommended that, with nonclinical samples, the EAT be used for identifying individuals who might have symptoms of eating disorders, either in the clinical or the subclinical range, and who need to be assessed further. It does appear that women with higher scores on the EAT show more eating pathology (Mintz and O'Halloran 2000). The EAT appears to be sensitive to therapeutic changes in women with eating disorders. Thus, it has been used as an outcome measure in clinical groups to assess whether treatment has been effective (Mintz and Kashubeck-West 2004; Williamson et al. 1995).

5.2.1.3 Bulimia Test—Revised (BULIT-R)

The BULIT-R (Thelen et al. 1991) is a frequently used self-report questionnaire developed to measure behavioral, physiological, and cognitive aspects of bulimia nervosa. Respondents answer 36 items, and 28 of the items are scored using a five-choice format. Questions on the BULIT-R investigate binge eating, purging behavior, negative affect, and weight fluctuations, and the test is recommended to be used as a screening instrument (Thelen et al. 1991). An individual who scores at or above a cutoff score of 104 on the BULIT-R is considered to be at risk for being diagnosed with bulimia nervosa in a clinical interview. However, Thelen et al. (1991) suggested that researchers interested in identifying individuals with problematic eating behaviors use a lower cutoff of 85 points. The BULIT-R is available free of charge from Mark Thelen at 573-445-4689. It takes approximately 10 minutes to complete and has an 11th-grade reading level.

The BULIT-R has been shown to be a reliable and valid measure for identifying individuals who may suffer from bulimia nervosa in both clinical and nonclinical samples (Thelen et al. 1996). The internal consistency in these samples was very high, test–retest reliability over a 2-month interval was very stable, and the BULIT-R consistently differentiated bulimic individuals from normal controls (Thelen et al. 1991). Thelen et al. (1991) indicated that the BULIT-R, although originally based on *DSM-III-R* criteria for bulimia, also captures the *DSM-IV* criteria for bulimia. Recent research also suggests that the Spanish and Korean versions of the BULIT-R have sound psychometric properties in nonclinical samples and can be used to screen for bulimia nervosa (Berrios-Hernandez et al. 2007; Morejon et al. 2007). Generally, the BULIT-R is a useful self-report inventory for the assessment of bulimia nervosa, and it has achieved increased popularity (see Appendix 5.B).

5.2.1.4 Questionnaire for Eating Disorder Diagnoses (Q-EDD)

The Questionnaire for Eating Disorder Diagnoses (Mintz et al. 1997) was developed to assess the *DSM-IV* criteria for eating disorders in a self-report format. The Q-EDD differentiates (1) between women who have and do not have an eating disorder diagnosis; (2) between women with an anorexia diagnosis and women with a bulimia diagnosis; and (3) between women with eating disorders, those women who have symptoms of eating disorders but do not meet DSM criteria for eating disorders, and women with no symptoms of eating disorders. The Q-EDD contains 13 items, some of which have multiple questions (see Appendix 5.C) for a total of 43 questions. Scoring yields frequency data for behaviors related to disordered eating and labels that can be used to place individuals into categories, such as eating disordered or noneating disordered, symptomatic (some symptoms but no diagnosable disorder), anorexia nervosa, bulimia nervosa, and four types of Eating Disorder—Not Otherwise Specified. The items take approximately 5–10 minutes to complete, and scoring is conducted using a manual (available from Laurie Mintz at MintzL@missouri.edu) that contains simple flowchart decision rules.

Initial reliability and validity studies by Mintz et al. (1997) indicate that the Q-EDD had strong psychometric support in two samples of college women and a small sample of women with eating disorders. Test–retest reliabilities were in the expected range, and there were significant relationships between the results of the Q-EDD and scores on the BULIT-R and the EAT. Importantly, diagnoses based on the Q-EDD showed a high correspondence with diagnoses made through clinical interviews and clinician judgments. Finally, the Q-EDD was slightly better than the BULIT-R in differentiating women with bulimia from all other women (those with anorexia, those women with subclinical symptoms of eating disorders, and asymptomatic women). Psychometric evaluation of the Q-EDD with a sample of African-American women indicated that the measure had a very high accuracy rate for differentiating women with and without eating disorders and a high accuracy rate for distinguishing between those women with eating disorders, those with subclinical symptoms of eating disorders, and those with no symptoms (Mulholland and Mintz 2001). There was some evidence that eating disorder symptoms were underestimated in this sample. Both a French translation (Callahan et al. 2003) and a Spanish translation (Rivas et al. 2001) were found to be reliable and valid with samples of adolescents and adults.

Overall, the Q-EDD has demonstrated good predictive ability and accuracy for differentiating between women who have eating disorders and those who do not, and between women with eating disorders, women with symptoms of eating disorders (but not full-blown disorders) and women who are asymptomatic (Mintz and Kashubeck-West 2004). The Q-EDD can be used for screening individuals, for counseling intake sessions to gather frequency data on eating-disordered behavior, and for assessing change over the course of therapy in eating-disordered symptoms.

5.2.1.5 Eating Disorder Examination—Questionnaire (EDE-Q)

A popular interview measure for diagnosing eating disorders is the Eating Disorder Examination (Fairburn and Cooper 1993), described below in the interview section. A 36-item, self-report version of the EDE (EDE-Q; Fairburn and Beglin 1994) also has been developed and evaluated. Participants respond to the forced-choice items based on the past 28 days, and scores on each item range from 0 to 6. There are four subscales that assess both attitudes and behaviors (Restraint, Eating Concern, Weight Concern, and Shape Concern), and a global score can be calculated from the 22 items that address attitudes (Mond et al. 2008). Other items assess the frequency of eating disorder behaviors during the past 28 days.

Research on the psychometric adequacy of the EDE-Q has been quite promising. Internal consistency estimates have been high in a community sample of women with bulimia nervosa (Peterson et al. 2007), and test–retest reliability has been good for attitudinal items in a sample of adult women from the community (Mond et al. 2004a) and for objective bulimic episodes in a sample of women diagnosed with Binge Eating Disorder (Reas et al. 2005). Scores on the EDE-Q tend to be higher than scores obtained when the same individuals are evaluated with the EDE (Mond et al. 2004b). Thus, one should be aware that use of the EDE-Q could result in overestimation of eating disorders. Good convergent validity of the EDE-Q compared to the EDE has been reported in community samples (Mond et al. 2004b) and in adolescents diagnosed with eating disorders (Binford et al. 2005). Mond et al. (2008) reported that the EDE-Q detected individuals with eating disorders in a sample of young women from a primary care clinic. However, factor analytic studies (e.g., Hrabosky et al. 2008; Peterson et al. 2007) have not replicated the original subscales proposed by Fairburn and Beglin (1994), and more evaluation of the factor structure of the EDE-Q is needed. Finally, the EDE-Q has been translated and evaluated in both German (Hilbert et al. 2007) and Spanish (Elder and Grilo 2007) and was found to have acceptable reliability and validity. More psychometric investigation of the EDE-Q with racial and ethnic minority women in the United States is needed.

5.2.2 STRUCTURED INTERVIEW MEASURES FOR EATING DISORDER SYMPTOMS

Structured interviews offer a methodical way to gather information about eating-disordered behavior, thoughts, and attitudes that then can be used, along with other information, to make a diagnosis. A paramount advantage of structured interviews is the ability to gather an abundance of information that may not be accessible through self-report measures. However, structured interviews also require more time and effort from the assessor, and often the examiner must be well trained in the administration and scoring of the interview. In addition, individuals may lie to the examiner due to shame or concern about negative evaluation, or they may simply fail to give the examiner accurate and complete information. Two structured interviews for the assessment of eating disorders are described next.

5.2.2.1 Eating Disorders Examination (EDE)

The EDE is a 62-item, semistructured clinical interview developed to measure behavioral and cognitive features of eating disorders, including extreme concerns about weight and shape (Cooper and Fairburn 1987). The authors designed the EDE to correct for problems found in self-report measures, such as the lack of a commonly accepted definition of the word *binge* (Williamson et al. 1995). The four subscales, which assess pertinent aspects of eating disorders, are Eating Concern, Shape Concern, Dietary Restraint, and Weight Concern (Fairburn and Cooper 1993). For each topic, there is at least one mandatory question as well as several optional questions. In addition, the interviewer is encouraged to ask further questions to obtain additional information. Most responses are rated on a 7-point scale, with four defined anchor points. Other questions are scored by the frequency of occurrence of a particular behavior. The interview takes about 45 minutes to complete, and the examiner must know both the techniques of interviewing and the concepts governing the ratings of the EDE (Cooper and Fairburn 1987).

The EDE has been revised numerous times in order to increase its reliability and validity and is now in its 12th edition. Several studies have examined the validity and reliability of the EDE, and all have supported the interview as a sound psychometric measure in adults (Beglin 1990; Fairburn and Cooper 1993; Guest 2000; House et al. 2008; Rizvi et al. 2000; Wilson and Smith 1989). Indeed, it has been called the gold standard assessment of eating disorder psychopathology (Guest 2000; Wade et al. 2008). The EDE can discriminate between individuals with anorexia and individuals with bulimia, and between individuals with bulimia and individuals with restrained eating (Cooper et al. 1989; Wilson and Smith 1989). In a sample of female twins aged 12–15 years, Wade et al. (2008) reported that the EDE was able to discriminate between age groups (12 vs. 13 vs. 14 vs. 15–16) and between those who did and did not have an eating disorder. However, Wade et al. (2008) found the factor structure of the EDE to be unstable, as they were not able to replicate the intended four-subscale structure and could only derive one eight-item factor. Such findings are consistent with factor analyses on the EDE-Q, as noted in Section 5.2.1.5. Wade et al. (2008) reported that the EDE should perform well as a diagnostic and predictive tool with young adolescents. At the same time, House et al. (2008) found that the EDE was not effective in identifying 35% of the individuals with eating disorders (anorexia nervosa or EDNOS) in a sample of adolescents seen at an eating disorder clinic in London. House et al. (2008) suggested that adolescents may have more trouble being open about symptoms in a face-to-face interview, and that the EDE therefore may not be suitable for this population. Such findings are consistent with those of Couturier et al. (2007), who found that adolescents with anorexia nervosa scored much lower on the EDE than parents and clinicians scored when answering questions about the adolescents. The EDE has been recommended: (1) as a measure of treatment outcome, (2) as a measure of binge-eating and vomiting frequencies, (3) for use in research on the nature and course of eating disorders, and (4) for investigations into the effectiveness of treatment (Wilson and Smith 1989). However, the EDE is not intended to be used by itself to make an eating disorder diagnosis (Cooper and Fairburn 1987). A children's version of the EDE (ChEDE) was developed by Bryant-Waugh et al. (1996). Watkins et al. (2005) reported that the ChEDE showed good inter-rater reliability (agreement of different judges as to what the diagnosis should be) and internal consistency, and it was able to differentiate between children with anorexia nervosa and children with other symptoms of disordered eating.

5.2.2.2 Structured Clinical Interview for Axis I *DSM-IV* Disorders (SCID)

The Structured Clinical Interview for Axis I *DSM-IV* Disorders (SCID) for Module H (Eating Disorders) was designed to assess the *DSM-IV* criteria for eating disorders (First et al. 1994). Interviewers ask questions that are based on each criterion (Pike et al. 1995). Test–retest reliabilities of earlier versions of the SCID for eating disorders are good or excellent. For example, the coefficients ranged from .82 to .90 for the bulimia nervosa section based on *DSM-III-R* criteria (Pike et al. 1995). Using *DSM-IV* criteria, Zanarini et al. (2000) found the inter-rater reliability to be satisfactory and the test–retest reliability (7–10 days apart) to be acceptable. Validity studies of the SCID suggest that it provides "valid assessment of binge eating and purging relevant to the diagnosis of the eating disorders. ... [The SCID] provides the essential information for discriminating among the eating disorders, in particular" (Pike et al. 1995, 323). Basco et al. (2000) found that administering the SCID resulted in improved accuracy over what was found with routine diagnostic procedures in a sample of 200 patients from a community mental health center. To use the SCID, interviewers should have some clinical experience, be familiar with the *DSM-IV*, and be trained and supervised in conducting the interview appropriately. SCID materials, including a clinician version and a research version, are available from the SCID website (www.scid4.org).

5.2.3 Assessment of Body Image Disturbance

Many studies have shown a connection between body image disturbance and eating-disordered behavior (Cash and Deagle 1997; Stice and Hoffman 2004). Generally, body image disturbance has been conceptualized as a multidimensional phenomenon and has been assessed via three primary dimensions: (1) perceptual measures of body image distortion, which occurs when one over- or underestimates one's current body size; (2) body-size dissatisfaction, which is a function of the discrepancy between one's current body size and one's ideal body size; and (3) attitudinal measures, which investigate affective and cognitive components of body image. Individuals with eating disorders often overestimate their actual body sizes, manifest large discrepancies between their perceived body size and ideal body size, and experience significant emotional distress and cognitive distortions related to their body image.

Since the publication of the first edition of this book (Kashubeck-West and Saunders 2001), the number of assessments measuring different aspects of body image has increased dramatically. There are now over 50 measures of body image disturbance. For a comprehensive review of factors to consider when choosing an assessment strategy, please see Thompson (2004). The following sections describe commonly used or innovative assessment techniques for measuring different aspects of body image disturbance, including methods for assessing size-perception accuracy and body-size dissatisfaction, as well as measures that assess subjective feelings and thoughts about one's body.

5.2.3.1 Measures of Body Size Perception

5.2.3.1.1 *Contour Drawing Rating Scale (CDRS)*

Figural rating scales are frequently used in assessing body image. The Contour Drawing Rating Scale (Thompson and Gray 1995) is a measure of body-size dissatisfaction that determines an individual's perceived current and ideal body sizes. The discrepancy between these two measures is thought to indicate level of body dissatisfaction. The scale consists of nine male and nine female schematic figures that range from underweight to overweight (Thompson and Gray 1995). Unlike a number of other figural stimulus materials, the CDRS features precisely graduated increments from the smallest to largest figures (Thompson 1995). Using these stimuli, individuals choose the figure they think most accurately depicts their current body size and the figure that represents their ideal body size. The larger the discrepancy between these two figures, the greater the presumed body dissatisfaction. The CDRS has demonstrated moderate to high reliability and high validity in a sample of female undergraduate students (Thompson and Gray 1995) and in a large sample of 7th and 8th grade girls (Wertheim et al. 2004). However, Doll et al. (2003) found that the manner in which figures are presented to respondents (e.g., ordered from thin to obese, not ordered, or presented individually on separate cards) greatly influenced their ratings of their body image, suggesting that what is being measured by figural rating scales is not entirely clear. In addition, the figures used in these types of scales usually have European American characteristics, and their ability to assess body perception in racial and ethnic minority individuals typically is unknown (Gardner 2003). The scale is available in Thompson and Gray (1995).

5.2.3.1.2 *Body Morph Assessment Version 2.0 (BMA 2.0)*

Thompson et al. (2005) asserted that recent developments in body morphing techniques via use of computer technology have led to some of the most impressive advances in the assessment of body image. One recent example of the body morphing technique is the Body Morph Assessment 2.0 (BMA 2.0; Stewart et al. 2009). The BMA 2.0 uses a computer-generated "morph" technique to measure both size estimation and body dissatisfaction (the discrepancy between a respondent's current and ideal size). It uses a continuous response scale of 100 figures from thin to obese that increase in size in equal gradients. The BMA 2.0 can be used with Caucasian and African-American men and women, and it has exhibited both validity and reliability with these samples (Stewart et al. 2009). The BMA 2.0 is available from the Pennington Biomedical Research Center at (225) 763–2500.

5.2.3.2 Measures of Attitudes and Body Dissatisfaction

5.2.3.2.1 *Multidimensional Body-Self Relations Questionnaire (MBSRQ)*

The MBSRQ (Brown et al. 1990; Cash 2000) is one of the most widely used measures of body image attitudes and weight-related variables. The MBSRQ (see Appendix 5.D) consists of 69 items that comprise three subscales: The Body-Areas Satisfaction Scale, the Overweight Preoccupation Scale, and the Self-Classified Weight Scale (Cash 2000). The Body-Areas Satisfaction Scale assesses satisfaction with specific body features, while the Overweight Preoccupations Scale assesses anxiety about fat, dieting, eating restraint, and weight vigilance, and the Self-Classified Weight Scale asks respondents to rate their weight, ranging from underweight to overweight (Cash 2000). In addition, the MBSRQ includes seven factor subscales: Appearance Evaluation, Appearance Orientation, Fitness Evaluation, Fitness Orientation, Health Evaluation, Health Orientation, and Illness Orientation. In addition to the full 69-item measure, a 34-item Appearance Scales version (MBSRQ-AS) that consists of five subscales (Appearance Orientation, Appearance Evaluation, Self-Classified Weight, Overweight Preoccupation, and the BASS) is also available. Generally, research has indicated that the MBSRQ has excellent psychometric characteristics, demonstrating solid reliability and validity in a number of studies (Cash 2000). In addition, unlike other instruments, the MBSRQ assesses both affective components of body image and cognitive-behavioral or motivational aspects. Finally, the MBSRQ has been validated with many diverse samples (Thompson 2004). One caution is that a large-scale study (Rusticus and Hubley 2006) investigating the measurement invariance of the MBSRQ across men and women ranging in age from young adulthood to older adulthood found that body image was perceived differently across the groups. Thus, the MBSRQ should not be used to make comparisons across gender and age groups without first evaluating the measurement invariance in each sample. As Rusticus and Hubley (2006) noted, their findings call into question many of the correlational and cross-group mean difference findings reported in the past based on the MBSRQ. The MBSRQ and a users' manual are available from Thomas F. Cash at Old Dominion University or at http://www.body-images.com/assessments/mbsrq.html.

5.2.3.2.2 Body Dissatisfaction Subscale of the Eating Disorder Inventory–3

One of the most popular methods for assessing body image dissatisfaction is to administer the Body Dissatisfaction Subscale from the EDI-3 (Garner 2004). This scale consists of nine items that assess an individual's level of satisfaction with the shape and size of her hips, thighs, stomach, and buttocks. Higher scores represent greater dissatisfaction. The EDI-3 is described in Section 5.2.1.1.

5.2.3.2.3 Body Shape Questionnaire (BSQ)

The Body Shape Questionnaire (Cooper et al. 1987) is a frequently used 34-item, self-report questionnaire that assesses concern with body shape and size. Both the 34-item questionnaire and its shortened versions use a 6-point scale ranging from never (1) to always (6) and have exhibited sound psychometric properties (Evans and Dolan 1993; Warren et al. 2008). Specifically, high internal consistency, high test–retest reliability, and strong construct validity have been reported in samples of women from the community and women with eating disorders. In addition, the BSQ is available in multiple languages and is a widely used questionnaire of body image disturbance among Spanish speakers (Warren et al. 2008). The 34-item BSQ is available in the original article by Cooper et al. (1987). Warren et al. (2008) identified a 10-item version of the BSQ that appeared invariant across four samples of women from the United States and Spain, both English and Spanish speaking.

5.2.3.2.4 Body Image Disturbance Questionnaire (BIDQ)

The 7-item Body Image Disturbance Questionnaire (BIDQ; Cash et al. 2004) was derived from the Body Dysmorphic Disorder Questionnaire (Phillips 1996, as cited in Cash et al. 2004) and was created to comprehensively measure body image disturbance, not simply body image dissatisfaction. It uses a 5-point rating scale and measures concern about parts of the body, mental preoccupation with these concerns, emotional distress due to a perceived defect, impairment in functioning because of the perceived defect, such as interference with one's social life, school, job, or role functioning, and avoidance of things because of the perceived defect. The initial psychometric evaluation of the BIDQ was conducted using a relatively diverse college student population in terms of age and ethnicity. In this nonclinical sample, the BIDQ was shown to be both reliable and valid in measuring negative body image (Cash and Grasso 2005; Cash et al. 2004). Furthermore, scores on the BIDQ predicted psychosocial functioning above and beyond measures of body dissatisfaction. The BIDQ is published in Cash et al. (2004).

5.2.3.2.5 Body Appreciation Scale (BAS)

The Body Appreciation Scale (BAS; Avalos et al. 2005) was created in response to the assertion that body image assessment has primarily focused on individuals' negative orientations toward their bodies. The construct of body appreciation reflects unconditional approval and respect for the body, and the BAS items assess such aspects as favorable opinions of one's body, acceptance of one's body, and engagement in behaviors that are healthy for the body. The 13 items are rated on a 5-point scale ranging from *never* to *always*, and responses are averaged to obtain an overall body appreciation score. Higher scores indicate a more positive body image. In several samples of college women, the BAS demonstrated excellent psychometric properties. For additional information, please see the study by Avalos et al. (2005).

5.3 APPLICATION OF RESEARCH QUESTION

Given the variety of measures described in the previous sections of this chapter, which represents only a fraction of the many measures available for use, how does a clinician pick which measure to use with a client? We suggest the clinician consider a number of factors when deciding how to assess a client. First, the clinician needs to identify the purpose of the assessment. Is it to rule out the possibility of an eating disorder? Is it to make a diagnosis of an eating disorder that the clinician suspects the client has? If the clinician wants to rule out an eating disorder, he or she could administer several of the self-report screening measures described in this chapter. If the client scores in the normal range or does not score in the clinically significant range on the instruments, the clinician has evidence that the client does not have an eating disorder. However, clinicians must remember that these screening measures are not 100% accurate, and follow-up information obtained through interview questions or other sources is needed. If the clinician suspects that the client has an eating disorder and wants to make a diagnosis, then he or she ought to consider administering a self-report instrument such as the Q-EDD and a structured interview such as the EDE or the SCID. It is always important to gather information from as many sources as possible, so the clinician might interview the client's friends, family, and teachers to obtain their perspective on the client's eating behaviors and symptoms. In addition, the clinician ought to send the client for a full medical check-up from a physician due to the serious physical consequences of many eating disorder symptoms.

Second, clinicians need to keep in mind the psychometric properties of the assessment tools that they are using. As indicated earlier, the reliability and validity of measures vary, and none are perfectly reliable or valid. In addition, the reliability and validity of measures may vary depending on the client's race or ethnicity and on whether the client is from a nonclinical or a clinical population. It is very difficult to accurately measure some constructs, such as food intake, activity level, purging behavior, and obesity (Agras 1995). Third, clinicians need to keep in mind the limitations of the self-report measures and the interview tools that were mentioned previously. For example, few of these measures have been assessed for their psychometric utility with individuals who are not white and middle class. Finally, it is possible that the client might fail to provide accurate and complete information or might lie, given the secretive nature of eating disorders. Clinicians need to be prepared to handle such inaccurate responses in a manner that does not alienate the client yet also does not ignore the potential health risks to the client of continuing to engage in eating-disordered behaviors.

Crowther and Sherwood (1997) noted the importance of conducting eating disorder assessments in a multidimensional fashion. Clinicians need to establish a sense of trust and rapport with their clients prior to engaging in assessment. Thus, the assessment process may need to take place over several sessions with the client (Kashubeck-West et al. 2001). Assessment should not consist solely of administration of a self-report measure or a structured interview, but should be comprehensive so that the clinician is able to develop a well-rounded picture of the client (including her behaviors, thoughts, and feelings) that situates her in her social, environmental, and cultural context. By understanding the client in this fashion, clinicians improve their ability to develop a trusting relationship with the client and thereby increase their chances of being able to effectively help the client with eating-disordered behavior.

APPENDIX 5.A   EATING ATTITUDES TEST (EAT-26)

✓ **Please choose one response by marking a check to the right for each of the following statements:**

		Always	Usually	Often	Some-times	Rarely	Never	Score
1.	Am terrified about being overweight.	☐	☐	☐	☐	☐	☐	
2.	Avoid eating when I am hungry.	☐	☐	☐	☐	☐	☐	
3.	Find myself preoccupied with food.	☐	☐	☐	☐	☐	☐	
4.	Have gone on eating binges where I feel that I may not be able to stop.	☐	☐	☐	☐	☐	☐	
5.	Cut my food into small pieces.	☐	☐	☐	☐	☐	☐	
6.	Aware of the calorie content of foods that I eat.	☐	☐	☐	☐	☐	☐	
7.	Particularly avoid food with a high carbohydrate content (i.e. bread, rice, potatoes, etc.)	☐	☐	☐	☐	☐	☐	
8.	Feel that others would prefer if I ate more.	☐	☐	☐	☐	☐	☐	
9.	Vomit after I have eaten.	☐	☐	☐	☐	☐	☐	
10.	Feel extremely guilty after eating.	☐	☐	☐	☐	☐	☐	
11.	Am preoccupied with a desire to be thinner.	☐	☐	☐	☐	☐	☐	
12.	Think about burning up calories when I exercise.	☐	☐	☐	☐	☐	☐	
13.	Other people think that I am too thin.	☐	☐	☐	☐	☐	☐	
14.	Am preoccupied with the thought of having fat on my body.	☐	☐	☐	☐	☐	☐	
15.	Take longer than others to eat my meals.	☐	☐	☐	☐	☐	☐	
16.	Avoid foods with sugar in them.	☐	☐	☐	☐	☐	☐	
17.	Eat diet foods.	☐	☐	☐	☐	☐	☐	
18.	Feel that food controls my life.	☐	☐	☐	☐	☐	☐	
19.	Display self-control around food.	☐	☐	☐	☐	☐	☐	
20.	Feel that others pressure me to eat.	☐	☐	☐	☐	☐	☐	
21.	Give too much time and thought to food.	☐	☐	☐	☐	☐	☐	
22.	Feel uncomfortable after eating sweets.	☐	☐	☐	☐	☐	☐	
23.	Engage in dieting behavior.	☐	☐	☐	☐	☐	☐	
24.	Like my stomach to be empty.	☐	☐	☐	☐	☐	☐	
25.	Have the impulse to vomit after meals.	☐	☐	☐	☐	☐	☐	
26.	Enjoy trying new rich foods.	☐	☐	☐	☐	☐	☐	

APPENDIX 5.B   BULIMIA TEST—REVISED (BULIT-R)

Answer each question by circling the appropriate response. Please respond to each item as honestly as possible; remember all of the information you provide will be kept strictly confidential.

1. I am satisfied with my eating patterns.
   1. agree
   2. neutral
   3. disagree a little
   4. disagree
   +5. disagree strongly

2. Would you presently call yourself a "binge eater"?
   +1. yes, absolutely
   2. yes
   3. yes, probably
   4. yes, possibly
   5. no, probably not

3. Do you feel you have control over the amount of food you consume?
   1. most or all of the time
   2. a lot of the time
   3. occasionally
   4. rarely
   +5. never

4. I am satisfied with the shape and size of my body.
   1. frequently or always
   2. sometimes
   3. occasionally
   4. rarely
   +5. seldom or never

5. When I feel that my eating behavior is out of control, I try to take rather extreme measures to get back on course (strict dieting, fasting, laxatives, diuretics, self-induced vomiting, or vigorous exercise).
   +1. always
   2. almost always
   3. frequently
   4. sometimes
   5. never or my eating behavior is never out of control

6. X I use laxatives or suppositories to help control my weight.
   1. once a day or more
   2. 3–6 times a week
   3. once or twice a week
   4. 2–3 times a month
   5. once a month or less (or never)

7. I am obsessed about the size and shape of my body.
   +1. always
   2. almost always
   3. frequently
   4. sometimes
   5. seldom or never

8. There are times when I rapidly eat a very large amount of food.
   +1. more than twice a week
   2. twice a week
   3. once a week
   4. 2–3 times a month
   5. once a month or less (or never)

9. How long have you been binge eating (eating uncontrollably to the point of stuffing yourself)?
   1. not applicable; I don't binge eat
   2. less than 3 months
   3. 3 months–1 year
   4. 1–3 years
   +5. 3 or more years

10. Most people I know would be amazed if they knew how much food I can consume at one sitting.
   +1. without a doubt
   2. very probably
   3. probably
   4. possibly
   5. no

11. X I exercise in order to burn calories
   1. more than 2 h per day

    2. about 2 h per day

    3. more than 1 but less than 2 h per day

    4. 1 h or less per day

    5. I exercise but not to burn calories or I don't exercise

12. Compared with women your age, how preoccupied are you about your weight and body shape?

    +1. a great deal more than average   4. a little more than average

    2. much more than average   5. average or less than average

    3. more than average

13. I am afraid to eat anything for fear that I won't be able to stop.

    +1. always   4. sometimes

    2. almost always   5. seldom or never

    3. frequently

14. I feel tormented by the idea that I am fat or might gain weight.

    +1. always   4. sometimes

    2. almost always   5. seldom or never

    3. frequently

15. How often do you intentionally vomit after eating?

    +1. 2 or more times a week   4. once a month

    2. once a week   5. less than once a month or never

    3. 2–3 times a month

16. I eat a lot of food when I'm not even hungry.

    +1. very frequently   4. sometimes

    2. frequently   5. seldom or never

    3. occasionally

17. My eating patterns are different from the eating patterns of most people.

    +1. always   4. sometimes

    2. almost always   5. seldom or never

    3. frequently

18. After I binge eat, I turn to one of several strict methods to try to keep from gaining weight (vigorous exercise, strict dieting, fasting, self-induced vomiting, laxatives, or diuretics).

    1. never or I don't binge eat   4. a lot of the time

    2. rarely   +5. most or all of the time

    3. occasionally

19. X I have tried to lose weight by fasting or going on strict diets.

    1. not in the past year   4. 4–5 times in the past year

    2. once in the past year   5. more than 5 times in the past

    3. 2–3 times in the past year year

20. X I exercise vigorously and for long periods of time in order to burn calories.

    1. average or less than average   4. much more than average

    2. a little more than average   5. a great deal more than average

    3. more than average

21. When engaged in an eating binge, I tend to eat foods that are high in carbohydrates (sweets and starches).

    +1. always   4. sometimes

    2. almost always   5. seldom, I don't binge

    3. frequently

22. Compared to most people, my ability to control my eating behavior seems to be:

    1. greater than others' ability   4. much less

    2. about the same   +5. I have absolutely no control

    3. Less

23. I would presently label myself a 'compulsive eater,' (one who engages in episodes of uncontrolled eating).

    +1. absolutely   4. yes, possibly
    2. yes   5. no, probably not
    3. yes, probably

24. I hate the way my body looks after I eat too much.

    1. seldom or never   4. almost always
    2. sometimes   +5. always
    3. frequently

25. When I am trying to keep from gaining weight, I feel that I have to resort to vigorous exercise, strict dieting, fasting, self-induced vomiting, laxatives, or diuretics.

    1. never   4. a lot of the time
    2. rarely   +5. most or all of the time
    3. occasionally

26. Do you believe that it is easier for you to vomit than it is for most people?

    +1. yes, it's no problem at all for me   4. about the same
    2. yes, it's easier   5. no, it's less easy
    3. yes, it's a little easier

27. X I use diuretics (water pills) to help control my weight.

    1. never   4. frequently
    2. seldom   5. very frequently
    3. sometimes

28. I feel that food controls my life.

    +1. always   4. sometimes
    2. almost always   5. seldom or never
    3. frequently

29. X I try to control my weight by eating little or no food for a day or longer.

    1. never   4. frequently
    2. seldom   5. very frequently
    3. sometimes

30. When consuming a large quantity of food, at what rate of speed do you usually eat?

    +1. more rapidly than most people have ever eaten in their lives
    2. a lot more rapidly than most people
    3. a little more rapidly than most people
    4. about the same rate as most people
    5. more slowly than most people (or not applicable)

31. X I use laxatives or suppositories to help control my weight.

    1. never   4. frequently
    2. seldom   5. very frequently
    3. sometimes

32. Right after I binge eat I feel:

    +1. so fat and bloated I can't stand it
    2. extremely fat
    3. fat
    4. a little fat
    5. OK about how my body looks or I never binge eat

33. Compared to other people of my sex, my ability to always feel in control of how much I eat is:

    1. about the same or greater   4. much less
    2. a little less   +5. a great deal less
    3. less

34. In the last 3 months, on the average how often did you binge eat (eat uncontrollably to the point of stuffing yourself)?
    1. once a month or less (or never)
    2. 2–3 times a month
    3. once a week
    4. twice a week
    +5. more than twice a week
35. Most people I know would be surprised at how fat I look after I eat a lot of food.
    +1. yes, definitely   4. yes, possibly
    2. yes   5. no, probably not or I never eat a
    3. yes, probably   lot of food
36. X I use diuretics (water pills) to help control my weight.
    1. 3 times a week or more   4. once a month
    2. once or twice a week   5. never
    3. 2–3 times a month

Scoring: X denotes questions whose answers are not added to determine the total BULIT-R score; + denotes the most strongly symptomatic response, which receives a score of five points

Source: The BULIT-R may not be copied. All copies of this test must be obtained from Mark H. Thelen, PhD, 573-445-4689. With permission.

APPENDIX 5.C   QUESTIONNAIRE FOR EATING DISORDER DIAGNOSES (Q-EDD)

Please complete the following questions as honestly as possible. The questions refer to *current behaviors and beliefs*, meaning those that have occurred in the past 3 months.

Sex: (Please circle)   Male   Female

Age:

School/Occupational Status: (Please circle)
     Junior High or younger (*specify* grade: _____)
     High School Freshman
     High School Sophomore
     High School Junior
     High School Senior
     College Freshman
     College Sophomore
     College Junior
     College Senior
Not in School/Employed (specify: _____)
Race/Ethnicity: Caucasian/White
(Please circle)   African-American/Black
                 Hispanic /Latino/Mexican-American
                 American Indian
                 Asian-American/Pacific Islander
                 Other: _____ (specify)
Present height:_____ feet _____ inches
Present weight: _____ pounds
My body frame is: small   medium   large (Please circle)
I would like to weigh   _____ pounds.

1. Do you experience recurrent episodes of binge eating, meaning eating in a discrete period of time (e.g., within any 2-h period) an amount of food that is definitely larger than most people would eat during a similar time period?

   YES   NO

   If YES: Continue to answer the following questions.

   If NO*:*   Skip to Question #4 (on the next page)

2. Do you have a sense of lack of control during the binge-eating episodes (i.e., the feeling that you cannot stop eating or control what or how much you are eating)?

   YES NO

3. Circle the answers within the *two* sets of **[bold brackets]** below that best fit for you:

   On the average, I have had **[1, 2, 3, 4, 5, 6 or more]** binge-eating episodes a *WEEK* for at least

   [1 month, 2 months, 3 months, 4 months, 5 months, 6–12 months, more than one year]

4. Please circle the appropriate responses below concerning things you may do *currently to prevent weight gain*. If you circle yes to any question, please indicate how often on the average you do this and how long you have been doing this.

   a) **Do you make yourself vomit?** YES NO

   How often do you do this?

   Daily Twice/Week Once/Week Once/Month

   How long have you been doing this?

   1 month 2 months 3 months 4 months 5–11 months More than a year

   b) **Do you take laxatives?** YES NO

   How often do you do this?

   Daily Twice/Week Once/Week Once/Month

   How long have you been doing this?

   1 month 2 months 3 months 4 months 5–11 months More than a year

   c) **Do you take diuretics (water pills)?** YES NO

   How often do you do this?

   Daily Twice/Week Once/Week Once/Month

   How long have you been doing this?

   1 month 2 months 3 months 4 months 5–11 months More than a year

   d) **Do you fast (skip food for 24 h)?** YES NO

   How often do you do this?

   Daily Twice/Week Once/Week Once/Month

   How long have you been doing this?

   1 month 2 months 3 months 4 months 5–11 months More than a year

   e) **Do you chew food but spit it out?** YES NO

   How often do you do this?

   Daily Twice/Week Once/Week Once/Month

   How long have you been doing this?

   1 month 2 months 3 months 4 months 5–11 months More than a year

   f) **Do you give yourself an enema?** YES NO

   How often do you do this?

   Daily Twice/Week Once/Week Once/Month

   How long have you been doing this?

   1 month 2 months 3 months 4 months 5–11 months More than a year

   g) **Do you take appetite control pills?** YES NO

   How often do you do this?

   Daily Twice/Week Once/Week Once/Month

   How long have you been doing this?

   1 month 2 months 3 months 4 months 5–11 months More than a year

h) **Do you diet strictly?**   YES   NO
How often do you do this?
Daily   Twice/Week   Once/Week   Once/Month
How long have you been doing this?
1 month   2 months   3 months   4 months   5–11 months   More than a year

i) **Do you exercise a lot?**   YES   NO
How often do you do this?
Daily   Twice/Week   Once/Week   Once/Month
How long have you been doing this?
1 month   2 months   3 months   4 months   5–11 months   More than a year

5. If you answered YES to "exercise a lot," please answer questions #5a, 5b, 5c, and 5d. If you answered NO to "exercise a lot," skip to question #6.

5a. Fill in the blanks below:

I _____ (types of exercise, e.g., jog, swim) for an average of _____ hours at a time.

5b. My exercise sometimes significantly interferes with important activities.
    YES   NO

5c. I exercise despite injury and/or medical complications.
    YES   NO

5d. Is your primary reason for exercising to counteract the effects of binges or to prevent weight gain?
    YES   NO

For the following questions, circle the response that best reflects your answer:

6. Does your weight and/or body shape influence how you feel about yourself?

1	2	3	4	5
Not at all	A Little	A moderate amount	Very Much	Extremely or Completely

7. How afraid are you of becoming fat?

1	2	3	4	5
Not at all	A Little	A moderate amount	Very Much	Extremely or Completely

8. How afraid are you of gaining weight?

1	2	3	4	5
Not at all	A Little	A moderate amount	Very Much	Extremely or Completely

9. Do you consider yourself to be:

1	2	3	4	5	6
Grossly Obese	Moderately Obese	Overweight	Normal Weight	Low Weight	Severely Underweight

10. Certain parts of my body (e.g., my abdomen, buttocks, thighs) are too fat.
    YES   NO

11. I feel fat all over.
    YES   NO

12. I believe that how little I weigh is a serious problem.
    YES   NO

13. I have missed at least 3 consecutive menstrual cycles (not including those missed during a pregnancy).
    YES   NO

Source: The Q-EDD is available from Laurie Mintz, Ph.D. Please contact her at MintzL@missouri.edu. With permission.

APPENDIX 5.D   MULTIDIMENSIONAL BODY-SELF RELATIONS QUESTIONNAIRE (MBSRQ)

INSTRUCTIONS—PLEASE READ CAREFULLY

The following pages contain a series of statements about how people might think, feel, or behave. You are asked to indicate *the extent to which each statement pertains to you personally.* Your answers to the items in the questionnaire are anonymous, so please do not write your name on any of the materials. In order to complete the questionnaire, read each statement carefully and decide how much it pertains to you personally. Using a scale like the one below, indicate your answer by entering it to the left of the number of the statement.

EXAMPLE:

_____   I am usually in a good mood.

In the blank space, enter a **1** if you **definitely disagree** with the statement; enter a **2** if you **mostly disagree**; enter a **3** if you **neither agree nor disagree**; enter a **4** if you **mostly agree**; or enter a **5** if you **definitely agree** with the statement.

1	2	3	4	5
Definitely Disagree	Mostly Disagree	Neither Agree Nor Disagree	Mostly Agree	Definitely Agree

_____   1.   Before going out in public, I always notice how I look.
_____   2.   I am careful to buy clothes that will make me look my best.
_____   3.   I would pass most physical fitness tests.
_____   4.   It is important that I have superior physical strength.
_____   5.   My body is sexually appealing.
_____   6.   I am not involved in a regular exercise program.
_____   7.   I am in control of my health.
_____   8.   I know a lot about things that affect my physical health.
_____   9.   I have deliberately developed a healthy lifestyle.
_____   10.   I constantly worry about being or becoming fat.
_____   11.   I like my looks just the way they are.
_____   12.   I check my appearance in a mirror whenever I can.
_____   13.   Before going out, I usually spend a lot of time getting ready.
_____   14.   My physical endurance is good.
_____   15.   Participating in sports is unimportant to me.
_____   16.   I do not actively do things to keep physically fit.
_____   17.   My health is a matter of unexpected ups and downs.
_____   18.   Good health is one of the most important things in my life.
_____   19.   I don't do anything that I know might threaten my health.
_____   20.   I am very conscious of even small changes in my weight.
_____   21.   Most people would consider me good-looking.
_____   22.   It is important that I always look good.
_____   23.   I use very few grooming products.
_____   24.   I easily learn physical skills.
_____   25.   Being physically fit is not a strong priority in my life.
_____   26.   I do things to increase my physical strength.
_____   27.   I am seldom physically ill.
_____   28.   I take my health for granted.
_____   29.   I often read books and magazines that pertain to health.
_____   30.   I like the way I look without my clothes on.
_____   31.   I am self-conscious if my grooming isn't right.
_____   32.   I usually wear whatever is handy without caring how it looks.

_____ 33. I do poorly in physical sports or games.

_____ 34. I seldom think about my athletic skills.

_____ 35. I work to improve my physical stamina.

_____ 36. From day to day, I never know how my body will feel.

_____ 37. If I am sick, I don't pay much attention to my symptoms.

_____ 38. I make no special effort to eat a balanced and nutritious diet.

_____ 39. I like the way my clothes fit me.

_____ 40. I don't care what people think about my appearance.

_____ 41. I take special care with my hair grooming.

_____ 42. I dislike my physique.

_____ 43. I don't care to improve my abilities in physical activities.

_____ 44. I try to be physically active.

_____ 45. I often feel vulnerable to sickness.

_____ 46. I pay close attention to my body for any signs of illness.

_____ 47. If I'm coming down with a cold or flu, I just ignore it and go on as usual.

_____ 48. I am physically unattractive.

_____ 49. I never think about my appearance.

_____ 50. I am always trying to improve my physical appearance.

_____ 51. I am very well coordinated.

_____ 52. I know a lot about physical fitness.

_____ 53. I play a sport regularly throughout the year.

_____ 54. I am a physically healthy person.

_____ 55. I am very aware of small changes in my physical health.

_____ 56. At the first sign of illness, I seek medical advice.

_____ 57. I am on a weight loss diet.

For the remainder of the items use the response scale given with the item, and enter your answer in the space beside the item.

_____ 58. I have tried to lose weight by fasting or going on crash diets.

     1. Never

     2. Rarely

     3. Sometimes

     4. Often

     5. Very Often

_____ 59. I think I am:

     1. Very Underweight

     2. Somewhat Underweight

     3. Normal Weight

     4. Somewhat Overweight

     5. Very Overweight

_____ 60. From looking at me, most other people would think I am:

     1. Very Underweight

     2. Somewhat Underweight

     3. Normal Weight

     4. Somewhat Overweight

     5. Very Overweight

61–69. Use this 1 to 5 scale to indicate how dissatisfied or satisfied you are with each of the following areas or aspects of your body:

1	2	3	4	5
Very Dissatisfied	Mostly Dissatisfied	Neither Satisfied Nor Dissatisfied	Mostly Satisfied	Very Satisfied

_____ 61. Face (facial features, complexion)
_____ 62. Hair (color, thickness, texture)
_____ 63. Lower torso (buttocks, hips, thighs, legs)
_____ 64. Mid torso (waist, stomach)
_____ 65. Upper torso (chest or breasts, shoulders, arms)
_____ 66. Muscle tone
_____ 67. Weight
_____ 68. Height
_____ 69. Overall appearance

Source: The MBSRQ is a copyright protected assessment by Thomas F. Cash, PhD and is reprinted here with his permission. Persons are not permitted to reproduce and use the MBSRQ or its items from this book. Information about obtaining the MBSRQ, its subscales, and manual for research or clinical use is available from Dr. Cash at www.body-images.com.

REFERENCES

Agras, W. S. 1995. The big picture. In *Handbook of assessment methods for eating behaviors and weight-related problems: Measures, theory, and research*, ed. D. B. Allison, 561–579. Thousand Oaks: Sage Publications.

American Psychiatric Association. 2000. *Diagnostic and statistical manual of mental disorders* (4th ed., text revision). Washington, DC: American Psychiatric Association.

Anderson, D. A., J. M. Lavender, S. M. Milnes, and A. M. Simmons. 2009. Assessment of eating disturbances in children and adolescents. In *Body image, eating disorders, and obesity in youth: Assessment, prevention, and treatment*, ed. L. Smolak and J. K. Thompson, 193–213. Washington, DC: American Psychological Association.

Avalos, L., T. L. Tylka, and N. Wood-Barcalow. 2005. The Body Appreciation Scale: Development and psychometric evaluation. *Body Image* 2: 285–297.

Basco, M. R., J. Q. Bostic, D. Davies, A. J. Rush, B. Witte, W. Hendrickse, and V. Barnett. 2000. Methods to improve diagnostic accuracy in a community mental health setting. *Am J Psychiatry* 157: 1599–1605.

Beglin, S. J. 1990. *Eating disorders in young adult women*. Unpublished doctoral dissertation. Oxford: Oxford University.

Bennett, K., and Stevens, R. 1997. The internal structure of the Eating Disorder Inventory. *Health Care Women Int* 18: 495–504.

Berrios-Hernandez, M. N., S. Rodríguez-Ruiz, M. Perez, D. H. Gleaves, M. Maysonet, and A. Cepeda-Benito. 2007. Cross-cultural assessment of eating disorders: Psychometric properties of a Spanish version of the Bulimia Test-Revised. *Eur Eat Disord Rev* 15: 418–424.

Binford, R. B., D. le Grange, and C. C. Jellar, C. C. 2005. Eating Disorders Examination versus Eating Disorders Examination-Questionnaire in adolescents with full and partial-syndrome bulimia nervosa and anorexia nervosa. *Int J Eat Disord* 37: 44–49.

Brown, T. A., T. F. Cash, and O. J. Mikulka. 1990. Attitudinal body-image assessment: Factor analysis of the Body-Self Relations Questionnaire. *J Pers Assess* 55: 135–144.

Bryant-Waugh, R., P. J. Cooper, C. L. Taylor, and B. D. Lask. 1996. The use of the Eating Disorder Examination with children: A pilot study. *Int J Eat Disord* 19: 391–397.

Callahan, S., R. Rousseau, A. Knotter, V. Bru, M. Danel, C. Cueto, M. Levasseur, F. Cuvelliez, L. Pignol, M. S. O'Halloran, and H. Chabrol, H. 2003. Les troubles alimentaires: Presentation d'un outil de diagnostic et resultats d'une etude epidemiologique chez les adolescents [Diagnosing eating disorders : Presentation of a new diagnostic test and an initial epidemiological study of eating disorders in adolescents]. *L'Encephale: Revue de psychiatrie clinique biologique et therapeutique* 29: 239–247.

Cash, T.F. 2000. Manual for the Multidimensional Body-Self Relations Questionnaire. http://www.body-images.com/ (accessed October 12, 2006).

Cash, T. F., and E. A. Deagle, E. A. 1997. The nature and extent of body-image disturbances in anorexia nervosa and bulimia nervosa: A meta-analysis. *Int J Eat Disord* 22: 107–125.

Cash, T. F., and K. Grasso. 2005. The norms and stability of new measures of the multidimensional body image construct. *Body Image* 2: 199–203.

Cash, T. F., K. Phillips, M. T. Santos, and J. I. Hrabosky. 2004. Measuring "negative body image": Validation of the Body Image Disturbance Questionnaire in a nonclinical population. *Body Image* 1: 363–372.

Cooper, Z., P. J. Cooper, and C. G. Fairburn. 1985. The specificity of the Eating Disorder Inventory. *Br J Clin Psychol* 24: 129–130.

Cooper, Z., P. J. Cooper, and C. G. Fairburn. 1989. The validity of the Eating Disorder Examination and its subscales. *Br J Psychiatry* 154: 807–812.

Cooper, Z., and C. Fairburn. 1987. The Eating Disorder Examination: A semi-structured interview for the assessment of the specific psychopathology of eating disorders. *Int J Eat Disord* 6: 1–8.

Cooper, P. J., M. J. Taylor, Z. Cooper, and C. G. Fairburn. 1987. The development and validation of the Body Shape Questionnaire. *Int J Eat Disord* 6: 485–494.

Couturier, J., J. Lock, S. Forsberg, D. Vanderheyden, and H. Y. Lee. 2007. The addition of a parent and clinical component to the Eating Disorder Examination for children and adolescents. *Int J Eat Disord* 40: 472–475.

Crowther, J. H., and N. E. Sherwood. 1997. Assessment, In *Handbook of treatment for eating disorders*, 2nd ed. D. M. Garner and P. E. Garfinkel, 34–49. New York: Guilford Press.

Cumella, E. J. 2006. Review of the Eating Disorder Inventory–3. *J Pers Assess* 87: 116–117.

Dare, C., E. Chania, I. Eisler, M. Hodes, and E. Dodge. 2000. The Eating Disorder Inventory as an instrument to explore change in adolescents in family therapy for anorexia nervosa. *Eur Eat Disord Rev* 8: 369–383.

Doll, M., G. D. C. Ball, and N. D. Willows. 2003. Rating of figures used for body image assessment varies depending on the method of figure presentation. *Int J Eat Disord* 35: 109–114.

Doninger, G., C. K. Enders, and K. F. Burnett. 2005. Validity evidence for Eating Attitudes Test scores in a sample of female college athletes. *Measurement in Physical Education and Exercise Science* 9: 35–49.

Elder, K. A., and C. M. Grilo. 2007. The Spanish language version of the Eating Disorder Examination Questionnaire: Comparison with the Spanish language version of the Eating Disorder Examination and test–retest reliability. *Behav Res Ther* 45: 1369–1377.

Espelage, D. L., S. E. Mazzeo, S. H. Aggen, A. L. Quttner, R. Sherman, and R. Thompson. 2003. Examining the construct validity of the Eating Disorder Inventory. *Psychol Assess* 15: 71–80.

Evans, C., and B. Dolan. 1993. Body shape questionnaire: Derivation of shortened "alternative forms." *Int J Eat Disord* 13: 315–321.

Fairburn, C. G., and S. J. Beglin. 1994. Assessment of eating disorders: Interview or self-report questionnaire? *Int J Eat Disord* 16: 363–370.

Fairburn, C. G., and Z. Cooper, Z. 1993. The Eating Disorder Examination (12th ed.). In *Binge eating: Nature, assessment, and treatment*, ed. C. G. Fairburn and G. T. Wilson, 317–360. New York: Guilford Press.

First, M. B., R. L. Spitzer, M. Gibbon, and J. B. W. Williams. 1994. *Structured Clinical Interview for Axis I DSM-IV Disorders Patient Edition (SCID-IL, Version 2.0)*. New York: Biometrics Research Department.

Franko, D. L., R. H. Striegel-Moore, B. A. Barton, B. C. Schumann, D. M. Garner, S. R. Daniels, B. G. Schreiber, and P. B. Crawford. 2004. Measuring eating concerns in Black and White adolescent girls. *Int J Eat Disord* 35: 179–189.

Gardner, R. M. 2003. Assessment of body image disturbance in children and adolescents. In *Body image, eating disorders, and obesity in youth: Assessment, prevention and treatment*, ed. J. K. Thompson and L. Smolak, 193–213. Washington, DC: American Psychological Association.

Garfinkel, P. E., and A. Newman. 2001. The Eating Attitudes Test: Twenty-five years later. *Eat Weight Disord* 6: 1–24.

Garner, D. M. 1991. *Eating Disorder Inventory-2 Professional Manual*. Odessa, Florida: Psychological Assessment Resources.

Garner, D. M. 2004. *The Eating Disorder Inventory-3 manual*. Odessa, FL: Psychological Assessment Resources.

Garner, D. M., and P. E. Garfinkel. 1979. The Eating Attitudes Test: An index of the symptoms of anorexia nervosa. *Psychol Med* 9: 273–279.

Garner, D. M., M. P. Olmsted, Y. Bohr, and P. E. Garfinkel. 1982. The Eating Attitudes Test: Psychometric features and clinical correlates. *Psychol Med* 12: 871–878.

Garner, D. M., M. P. Olmsted, and J. Polivy. 1983. Development and validation of a multi-dimensional Eating Disorder Inventory for anorexia nervosa and bulimia. *Int J Eat Disord* 2: 15–34.

Gross, J., J. C. Rosen, H. Leitenberg, and M. E. Willmuth, M. E. 1986. Validity of the Eating Attitudes Test and the Eating Disorders Inventory in bulimia nervosa. *J Couns Clin Psychol* 54: 875–876.

Guest, T. 2000. Using the Eating Disorder Examination in the assessment of bulimia and anorexia: Issues of reliability and validity. *Soc Work Health Care* 31: 71–83.

Hilbert, A., B. Tuschen-Caffier, A. Karwautz, H. Niederhofer, and S. Munsch. 2007. Eating Disorder Examination-Questionnaire: Psychometric properties of the German version. *Diagnotica* 53: 144–154.

House, J., I. Eisler, M. Simic, and N. Micali. 2008. Diagnosing eating disorders in adolescents: A comparison of the Eating Disorder Examination and the Development and Well-Being Assessment. *Int J Eat Disord* 41: 535–541.

Hrabosky, J. I., M. A. White, R. M. Masheb, B. S. Rothschild, C. H. Burke-Martindale, and C. M. Grilo. 2008. Psychometric evaluation of the Eating Disorder Examination-Questionnaire for bariatric surgery candidates. *Obesity* 16: 763–769.

Hurley, J. B., R. L. Palmer, and D. Stretch, D. 1990. The specificity of the Eating Disorder Inventory: A reappraisal. *Int J Eat Disord* 9: 419–424.

Kashubeck-West, S., L. B. Mintz, and K. Saunders. 2001. Assessment of eating disorders among women. *Couns Psychol* 29: 662–694.

Kashubeck-West, S., and K. Saunders. 2001. Body image. In *Eating disorders in women and children: Prevention, stress management, and treatment,* ed. J. J. Robert-McComb, 185–200. Boca Raton, FL: CRC Press.

Klemchuk, H. P., C. B. Hutchinson, and R. I. Frank, R. I. 1990. Body dissatisfaction and eating-related problems on the college campus: Usefulness of the Eating Disorder Inventory with a nonclinical population. *J Couns Psychol* 37: 297–305.

Limbert, C. 2004. The Eating Disorder Inventory: A test of the factor structure and internal consistency in a nonclinical sample. *Health Care Women Int* 25: 165–178.

Maloney, M., J. McGuire, S. Daniels, and S. Specker. 1988. Reliability testing of a children's version of the Eating Attitudes Test. *J Am Acad Child Adolesc Psychiatry* 5: 541–543.

Mintz, L. B., and S. Kashubeck-West. 2004. Trastornos de la conducta alimentaria en mujeres: Evaluación y custinones del autoinforme transcultural. *Psicología Conductural Revista Internacional de Psicología Clínica de la Salud* 12: 385–414.

Mintz, L. B., and M. S. O'Halloran. 2000. The Eating Attitudes Test: Validation with DSM-IV eating disorder criteria. *J Pers Assess* 74: 489–503.

Mintz, L. B., M. S. O'Halloran, A. M. Mulholland, and P. A. Schneider. 1997. Questionnaire for Eating Disorder Diagnoses: Reliability and validity of operationalizing DSM-IV criteria into a self-report format. *J Couns Psychol* 44: 63–79.

Mond, J. M., P. J. Hay, B. Rodgers, C. Owen, and P. J. V. Beumont. 2004a. Temporal stability of the Eating Disorder Examination Questionnaire. *Int J Eat Disord* 36: 195–203.

Mond, J. M., P. J. Hay, B. Rodgers, C. Owen, and P. J. V. Beumont. 2004b. Validity of the Eating Disorder Examination Questionnaire (EDE-Q) in screening for eating disorders in community samples. *Behav Res Ther* 42: 551–567.

Mond, J. M., T. C. Myers, R. D. Crosby, P. J. Hay, B. Rodgers, J. F. Morgan, J. H. Lacey, and J. E. Mitchell. 2008. Screening for eating disorders in primary care: EDE-Q versus SCOFF. *Behav Res Ther* 46: 612–622.

Morejón, A. J., G. Vazquez, and R. Jiménez. 2007. Psychometic characteristics of Spanish adaption of the test for bulimia (BULIT). *Actas Esp Psiquiatr* 35: 309–314.

Mulholland, A. M., and L. B. Mintz. 2001. Prevalence of eating disorders among African American women. *J Couns Psychol* 48: 111–116.

Norring, C. E. A. 1990. The Eating Disorder Inventory: Its relation to diagnostic dimensions and follow-up status. *Int J Eat Disord* 9: 685–694.

Ocker, L. B., E. T. Lam, B. E. Jensen, and J. J. Zhang. 2007. Psychometric properties of the Eating Attitudes Test. *Measurement in Physical Education and Exercise Science* 11: 25–48.

Peterson, C. B., R. D. Crosby, S. A. Wonderlich, T. Joiner, S. J. Crow, J. E. Mitchell, A. M. Bardone-Cone, M. Klein, and D. le Grange. 2007. Psychometric properties of the Eating Disorder Examination-Questionnaire: Factor structure and internal consistency. *Int J Eat Disord* 40: 386–389.

Pike, K. M., K. Loeb, and B. T. Walsh. 1995. Binge eating and purging. In *Handbook of assessment methods for eating behaviors and weight-related problems: Measures, theory, and research,* ed. D. B. Allison, 303–346. Thousand Oaks, CA: Sage Publications.

Podar, I., and J. Allik. 2009. A cross-cultural comparison of the Eating Disorder Inventory. *Int J Eat Disord* 42: 346–355.

Raciti, M. C., and J. C. Norcross. 1987. The EAT and EDI: Screening, interrelationships, and psychometrics. *Int J Eat Disord* 6: 579–586.

Reas, D. L., C. M. Grilo, and R. M. Masheb. 2005. Reliability of the Eating Disorder Examination-Questionnaire in patients with binge eating disorder. *Behav Res Ther* 44: 43–51.

Rivas, T., R. Bersabe, and S. Castro. 2001. Propiedades psicometricas del cuestionario para el diagnostico de los trastornos de la conducta alimentaria (Q-EDD) [Psychometric properties of the Questionnaire for Eating Disorder Diagnosis (Q-EDD)]. *Psicologia Conductual Revista Internacional de Psicologia Clinica de la Salud* 9: 255–266.

Rizvi, S., C. B. Peterson, S. J. Crow, and W. S. Agras. 2000. Test–retest reliability of the Eating Disorder Examination. *Int J Eat Disord* 28: 311–316.

Rusticus, S. A., and A. M. Hubley. 2006. Measurement invariance of the multidimensional body-self relations questionnaire: Can we compare across age and gender? *Sex Roles* 55: 827–842.

Schaefer, W. K., R. N. Maclennan, S. A. Yaholnitsky-Smith, and E. D. Stover, E. D. 1998. Psychometric evaluation of the eating disorder inventory (EDI) in a clinical group. *Psychol Health* 13: 873–881.

Schoemaker, C., M. Verbraak, R. Breteler, and C. van der Staak. 1997. The discriminant validity of the Eating Disorder Inventory-2. *Br J Clin Psychol* 36: 627–629.

Shedler, J., M. Mayman, and M. Manis. 1993. The illusion of mental health. *Am Psychol* 48: 1117–1131.

Stewart, T. M., H. R. Allen, H. Han, and D. A. Williamson. 2009. The development of the Body Morph Assessment version 2.0 (BMA 2.0): Tests of reliability and validity. *Body Image* 6: 67–74.

Stice, E., and E. Hoffman. 2004. Prevention of eating disorders. In *Handbook of eating disorders and obesity*, ed. J. K. Thompson, 33–57. New York: Wiley.

Sunday, S. R., K. A. Halmi, L. Werdann, and C. Levey. 1992. Comparison of body size estimation and Eating Disorder Inventory scores in anorexia and bulimia patients with obese, and restrained and unrestrained controls. *Int J Eat Disord* 11, 133–149.

Thelen, M. H., J. Farmer, S. Wonderlich, and M. A. Smith. 1991. Revision of the Bulimia Test: The BULIT-R, *Psychol Assess* 3: 119–124.

Thelen, M. H., L. B. Mintz, and J. S. Vander Wal. 1996. The Bulimia Test-Revised: Validation with DSM-IV criteria for bulimia nervosa. *Psychol Assess* 8: 219–221.

Thompson, J. K. 1995. Assessment of body image, In *Handbook of assessment methods for eating behaviors and weight-related problems: Measures, theory, and research*, ed. D. B. Allison, 119–148. Thousand Oaks: Sage Publications.

Thompson, J. K. 2004. The (mis)measurement of body image: Ten strategies to improve assessment for applied and research purposes. *Body Image* 1: 7–14.

Thompson, M. A., and J. J. Gray. 1995. Development and validation of a new body-image assessment scale. *J Pers Assess* 64: 258–269.

Thompson, K. J., M. Roehrig, G. Cafri, and L. J. Heinberg. 2005. Assessment of body image disturbance. In *Assessment of Eating Disorders*, ed. J. E Mitchell and C. B. Peterson, 175–202. New York: Gilford Press.

Wade, T. D., S. Byrne, and R. Bryant-Waugh. 2008. The Eating Disorder Examination: Norms and construct validity with young and middle adolescent girls. *Int J Eat Disord* 41: 551–558.

Warren, C. S. W., A. Cepeda-Benito, D. H. Gleaves, S. Moreno, S. Rodriguez, M. C. Fernandez, M. C. Fingeret, and C. A. Pearson. 2008. English and Spanish Versions of the Body Shape Questionnaire: Measurement equivalence across ethnicity and clinical status. *Int J Eat Disord* 41: 265–272.

Watkins, B., I. Frampton, B. Lask, and R. Bryant-Waugh. 2005. Reliability and validity of the child version of the Eating Disorder Examination: A preliminary investigation. *Int J Eat Disord* 38: 183–187.

Welch, G., A. Hall, and C. Norring. 1990. The factor structure of the Eating Disorder Inventory in a patient setting. *Int J Eat Disord* 9: 79–85.

Wertheim, E. H., S. J. Paxton, and L. Tilgner. 2004. Test–retest reliability and construct validity of Contour Drawing Rating Scale scores in a sample of early adolescent girls. *Body Image* 1: 199–205.

Williamson, D. A., D. A. Anderson, L. P. Jackman, and S. R. Jackson. 1995. Assessment of eating disordered thoughts, feelings, and behaviors. In *Handbook of assessment methods for eating behaviors and weight-related problems: Measures, theory, and research*, ed. D. B. Allison, 347–386. Thousand Oaks, CA: Sage Publications.

Williamson, D. A., B. A. Cubic, and D. H. Gleaves. 1993. Equivalence of body image disturbance in anorexia nervosa and bulimia nervosa. *J Abnorm Psychol* 102: 1–4.

Wilson, G. T., and D. Smith. 1989. Assessment of bulimia nervosa: An evaluation of the Eating Disorders Examination. *Int J Eat Disord* 8: 173–179.

Zanarini, M. C., A. E. Skodol, D. Bender, R. Dolan, C. Sanislow, E. Schaefer, L. C. Morey, C. M. Grilo, M. T. Shea, T. H. McGlashan, and J. G. Gunderson. 2000. The Collaborative Longitudinal Personality Disorders Study: Reliability of Axis I and II diagnoses. *J Pers Disord* 14: 291–299.

Part II

The Characteristics of Stress

6 The Physiology of Stress

Jacalyn J. Robert-McComb and Brett Owen Young

CONTENTS

6.1 LEARNING OBJECTIVES

After completing this chapter you should be able to

- Discuss the term "stress" as it is used in the published literature
- Describe the physiological reactions associated with the stress response, specifically the biochemical pathways most closely associated with the stress response
- Describe the physiological consequences of chronic stress
- Explain how to quantify the stress response from a physiological perspective
- Discuss the long-term physiological changes associated with effective stress management techniques
- Discuss plausible stress management techniques

6.2 BACKGROUND AND SIGNIFICANCE

If someone were to ask you to define stress, you may find it a difficult task even though you experience it on a daily basis. Your thoughts may turn to unpleasant situations, such as being berated by your boss, being stuck in traffic, or having financial difficulties. All of these certainly qualify as stressors, but why, what binds those situations together? Externally nothing, aside from all being situations we would like to avoid. Internally, however, there is an important link between them—the similar way that our body responds to each of these different situations. Within human physiology, a cascade of reactions occurs that prepares us to deal with threatening situations. What is fascinating is how general this response is. Your body responds similarly to the threat of physical harm, such as encountering an aggressive dog on the street, and to your negative thinking, whether it is realistic or not (i.e., if I mess up again I am going to be fired).

One of the first scientists to document the stress response was the endocrinologist Hans Selye (Monat and Lazarus 1991; Selye 1950b, 1974). Selye began his career studying the physiological response of rats to various physical stressors such as cold, heat, and physical injury. His discovery of a common set of responses to many and varied stressors led to his definition of stress as "the nonspecific response of the body to any demand made upon it" (Selye 1974). Further research revealed that psychological stressors also produced a similar set of reactions in the body (Selye 1950b). After those initial discoveries, both psychologists and physiologists have contributed to our understanding of the concept of stress. Richard Lazarus, a distinguished psychologist, proposed this definition of stressful situations: "any event in which environmental demands, internal demands, or both tax or exceed the adaptive resources of an individual, social system, or tissue system" (Monat and Lazarus 1991).

Regardless of the nature of the stressor (physical or psychological), certain automatic responses occur via the hypothalamus, the pituitary gland, and the adrenal gland. This pathway is referred to as the hypothalamic-pituitary-adrenal axis (HPA or HTPA axis), which is also known as the limbic-hypothalamic-pituitary-adrenal axis (LHPA axis). This set of interrelated endocrine glands initiates the signals provoking a pattern of responses that constitute to the stress response, originally called the General Adaptation Syndrome (GAS). These responses are recognized as those that allowed primitive humans (and other living organisms) to survive in hostile environments by way of accelerating the metabolic processes in the body used for either fending off or escaping from dangerous situations.

6.2.1   An Introduction to the Human Nervous System

To lay the groundwork for an understanding of the stress response, let us first briefly discuss the human nervous system with an overview that has been simplified to meet the objectives of this chapter. The basic anatomical unit of the human nervous system is the neuron. Impulses are passed within a neuron as electrical charges and are passed from neuron to neuron as chemical signals. Impulse transmission from neuron to neuron occurs via the release of a neurotransmitter substance, such as acetylcholine or norepinephrine (see Figure 6.1).

6.2.1.1   Central Nervous System

The human nervous system consists of the central nervous system (CNS) and the peripheral nervous system (PNS). The brain and the spinal cord form the CNS, and the peripheral nervous system consists of all neurons in the body exclusive of the CNS (see Figure 6.2).

6.2.1.1.1   Anatomy of the Brain

The three major parts of the brain are the cerebrum, the cerebellum, and the brainstem (see Figure 6.3). The cerebrum is responsible for thought processes including memory, interpretation of sensation, and decision making. The cerebellum is mainly involved in the control of muscular activity. The brainstem is composed of the medulla oblongata, pons, and the midbrain. The medulla oblongata is involved in the control of breathing, blood circulation, and heart rate. The pons is important in controlling several important functions, including the balance between sleep and wakefulness. The midbrain is a small region of the brainstem located between the pons and the diencephalon (hypothalamus and thalamus).

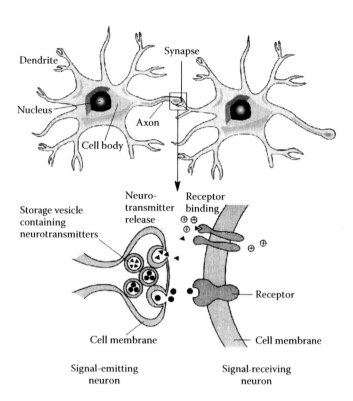

FIGURE 6.1 The neuron. (From the National Institute on Alcohol Abuse and Alcoholism http://www.niaaa.nih.gov/Resources/GraphicsGallery/Neuroscience/Pages/synapse.aspx.)

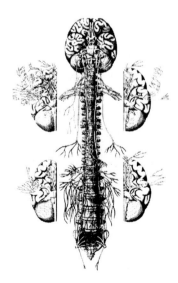

FIGURE 6.2 Central and peripheral nervous system. (From the National History of Medicine http://ihm.nlm.nih.gov/luna/servlet/detail/NLMNLM~1~1~101436592~208260:-The-brain-and-spinal-column-?qvq=q:anatomy;lc:NLMNLM~1~1&mi=17&trs=565.)

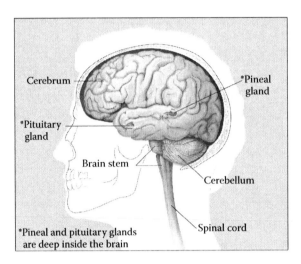

FIGURE 6.3   Anatomy of the brain. (From the National Cancer Institute http://visualsonline.cancer.gov/.)

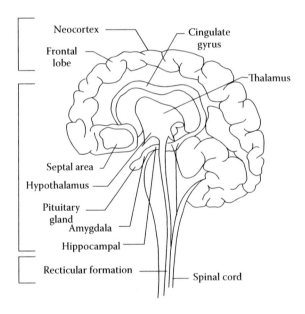

FIGURE 6.4   Hierarchical organization of the brain. (From McComb, J., et al. *Eating disorders in women and children: prevention, stress management, and treatment.* p. 124, 2000. CRC Press with permission, graphic by Robert Saar McComb.)

6.2.1.1.2   Functional Organization of the Brain

From a functional point of view, the brain can be considered to be divided into three different but interrelated levels (see Figure 6.4). There is a hierarchical organization of the brain, meaning that the functions of lower levels are influenced by the higher levels, and that higher level functions can override lower level functions.

The neocortical level (Level 1) represents the highest component of the brain. The neocortex, primarily the frontal lobe, and to a lesser degree, the temporal lobe, decodes and interprets sensory signals received from the limbic system, and processes the information and exerts control by being excitatory or inhibitory. The neocortex presides over imagination, logic, decision making, problem solving, planning, organization, and memory.

The limbic system (Level 2) represents the major component of the second level of the brain, and is the brain's emotional control center. It is composed of numerous neural structures, two of which are central to the stress response, the hypothalamus and the thalamus. The limbic system plays a significant role in the regulation of the stress response because it plays a large role in emotional regulation. The thalamus transmits information to various parts of the brain, and the hypothalamus regulates homeostatic bodily processes, such as hunger, thirst, and bodily temperature. The hypothalamus functions along with the thalamus to determine pleasure and pain and to determine a person's overall emotional state. The hypothalamus is also important in releasing neurohormones responsible for the control of endocrine functioning throughout the body. For example, the pituitary gland is controlled by hormones secreted from the hypothalamus.

The brainstem and reticular formation (Level 3) form the lowest functional level of the human brain, referred to as the vegetative level. This level is concerned with basic bodily functions, such as respiration and heart rate. The reticular formation is a diffuse network that extends from the spinal cord to the lower brain centers and is concerned with sensory and motor impulses. The reticular formation is selective, and only certain stimuli will arouse other portions of the brain through this selective pathway. Along with the spinal cord, this pathway uses neurons to send information to and from parts of the body and the brain.

6.2.1.1.3 Spinal Cord

The spinal cord is composed of tracts of nerve fibers that allow two-way conduction of nerve impulses. The sensory (afferent) fibers carry neural signals from sensory receptors, such as those located in the muscles and joints, to the upper level of the CNS. Motor (efferent) fibers from the brain and spinal cord carry neural signals down to the end organs (muscles, glands).

6.2.2 The Peripheral Nervous System

The PNS has two components—the somatic nervous system and the autonomic nervous system. The *somatic nervous system* is made up of nerves that connect to voluntary skeletal muscles and to sensory receptors. Similar to the spinal cord, it is composed of *afferent* nerves that carry information to the CNS (spinal cord) and *efferent* fibers that carry neural impulses away from the CNS.

The autonomic nervous system is further divided into two divisions: the sympathetic division and the parasympathetic division. The sympathetic and parasympathetic divisions typically function in opposition to each other in a complementary fashion in order to maintain homeostasis. Table 6.1 illustrates the opposing effects of the two branches of the autonomic nervous system.

6.2.2.1 The Sympathetic Branch of the Autonomic Nervous System

The general action of the sympathetic branch is to mobilize the body's resources under stress to induce the fight-or-flight response. The sympathetic nerves originate in the spinal cord between the thoracic and lumbar segments and innervate various organs and tissues (see Figure 6.5). The preganglion neurons (a ganglion is a group of cell bodies outside of the CNS) release the neurotransmitter, acetylcholine. The postganglion fibers of the sympathetic nervous system release norepinephrine (also known as noradrenalin) at the target organ. The end-organ response is one of excitement or activation.

6.2.2.2 The Parasympathetic Branch of the Autonomic Nervous System

The parasympathetic nervous system generally helps to conserve the body's energy. The actions of the parasympathetic nervous system can be summarized as "rest and digest." The parasympathetic nervous system is dominated by the 10th cranial nerve, known as the vagus nerve, which in turn is influenced by the brain stem. Parasympathetic nerves also originate in the sacral part of the spinal

TABLE 6.1

Opposing Yet Complementary Actions of the Autonomic Nervous System

Structure	Sympathetic Branch	Parasympathetic Branch
Adrenal medulla	Norepinephrine and epinephrine secreted	
Bladder	Wall relaxed Sphincter closed	Wall contracted Sphincter relaxed
Heart	Heart rate and force increased	Heart rate and force decreased
Iris (eye muscle)	Pupil dilation	Pupil constriction
Kidney	Decreased urine secretion	Increased urine secretion
Large Intestine	Motility reduced	Secretions and motility increased
Liver	Increased conversion of glycogen to glucose	
Lung	Bronchial muscle relaxed	Bronchial muscle contracted
Oral/Nasal Mucosa	Mucus production reduced	Mucus production increased
Salivary Glands	Saliva production reduced	Saliva production increased
Small Intestine	Motility reduced	Digestion increased
Stomach	Peristalsis reduced	Gastric juice secreted; motility increased

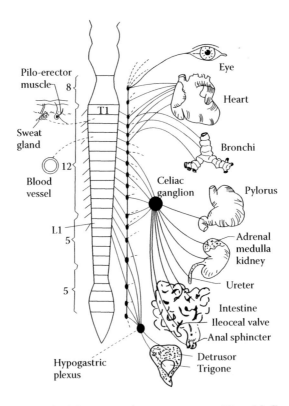

FIGURE 6.5   Sympathetic branch of the autonomic nervous system. (From McComb, J., et al. *Eating disorders in women and children: prevention, stress management, and treatment.* p. 125, 2000. CRC Press with permission, graphic by Robert Saar McComb.)

cord. Acetylcholine is the neurotransmitter that is released in both preganglion and postganglin fibers. The parasympathetic nerves generally pass uninterrupted to the organ or tissue innervated (see Figure 6.6). The end-organ response is, in general, opposite that of the sympathetic nervous system, it is one of inhibition (i.e. heart rate slows down).

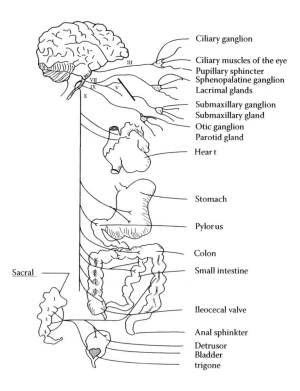

Ciliary ganglion
Ciliary muscles of the eye
Pupillary sphincter
Sphenopalatine ganglion
Lacrimal glands
Submaxillary ganglion
Submaxillary gland
Otic ganglion
Parotid gland
Heart
Stomach
Pylorus
Colon
Small intestine
Sacral
Ileocecal valve
Anal sphinkter
Detrusor
Bladder
trigone

FIGURE 6.6 Parasympathetic branch of the autonomic nervous system. (From McComb, J., et al. *Eating disorders in women and children: prevention, stress management, and treatment.* p. 126, 2000. CRC Press with permission, graphic by Robert Saar McComb.)

6.2.3 STAGES OF THE STRESS RESPONSE

In order for the stress response to be effective, it must be immediate. However, the duration of the response is short lived. If a longer response is needed, other pathways must be called into play. Table 6.2 summarizes the stages of the stress response that will be discussed in this chapter.

6.2.3.1 Immediate Stage of the Stress Response

Signals from either an internal (a cognitive state or internal physical sensation) or external (through sensory receptors of the peripheral nervous system) source are sent via sensory neural pathways toward the brain. The information is both rationally and emotionally integrated. The hypothalamus functions along with the thalamus to determine the person's emotional state and to activate autonomic nervous system activity.

If a stimulus is perceived as threatening, the stress response is elicited. During the stress response, an increased sympathetic discharge occurs. The degree of sympathetic activation depends on the perceived severity of the threat. A serious threat will result in an increased sympathetic end-organ response with a corresponding neural release of epinephrine (adrenaline) and norepinephrine. During the stress response, myocardial contractility, heart rate, and blood pressure will increase. Sympathetic stimulation causes the vasculature of the body to constrict and blood is shunted away from the periphery. In some instances, sphincter tone increases, peristaltic movement in the gastrointestinal tract is inhibited, and blood flow to the digestive organs decreases.

TABLE 6.2

Stages of the Stress Response

Stages	Pathways or Axes	Effects	Purpose
Immediate (quickest response) (2–3 s)	Autonomic Nervous System Pathway:[a] Results in the release of the neurotransmitter, norepinephrine (sympathetic) or acetylcholine (parasympathetic)	End-organ sympathetic or parasympathetic stimulation for a short duration	Overall body arousal
Intermediate (20 to 30 s)	Neuroendocrine Axis:[b] "Fight or flight"	The adrenal medulla secretes the hormones epinephrine (adrenaline) and norepinephrine (noradrenalin), prolonging the effects of sympathetic stimulation	Heightened body arousal; the effects on the physiological symptoms are more pronounced
Prolonged effects Minutes, hours, days, or weeks	Endocrine Axes Adrenal cortical axis Somatropic axis Thyroid axis General adaptation syndrome[c]	Numerous hormones are released, depending on the targeted gland.	Requires greater intensity stimulation; however, the overall metabolic effect is to mobilize energy resources in preparation for the stressful encounter

[a] See Figure 6.7.
[b] See Figure 6.9.
[c] See Figures 6.10 to 6.12.

Sympathetic activation may also dilate the bronchi and constrict blood vessels in the respiratory system, even though the effect is mild. Sympathetic activation also has an effect on the glands of the body, causing increased perspiration along with increased skin conductivity. Constriction occurs in the secretory capacity of the nasal, salivary, lacrimal, and many gastrointestinal glands. The pupil of the eye dilates during sympathetic activation, and the person exhibits increased mental alertness, muscular strength, and basal metabolic response (increased levels of glucose in blood resulting from hepatic glucose release and glycogenolysis in muscle). Conversely, activity in the ducts of the gall bladder, liver, urethra, and bladder is inhibited. All of these physiological responses are preparing the body for the increased demands that it may be called upon to meet in order to overcome the perceived threatening situation. Neural transmission during the stress response is very rapid. However, the effects do not last long because of the rapid disintegration and re-uptake of the neurotransmitters, and because the stores of the neurotransmitters can become exhausted under intense and constant stimulation.

The effects of autonomic neural activation on end organs during the stress response are immediate but not long lasting (2–3 s). In order to maintain levels of stress arousal for a longer time, the endocrine glands must be called into play. Sympathetic arousal stimulates the particular glands that are needed for the "fight-or-flight" response.

Even though there is increased sympathetic discharge during the immediate stress response, the parasympathetic nervous system also exerts an influence. Most organs of the body are innervated by both the sympathetic and parasympathetic nervous systems, and some parasympathetic end-organ stress reactions may occur. The primary role of the parasympathetic nervous system is to relax the body and return it to a restful state. Parasympathetic end-organ stress reactions include

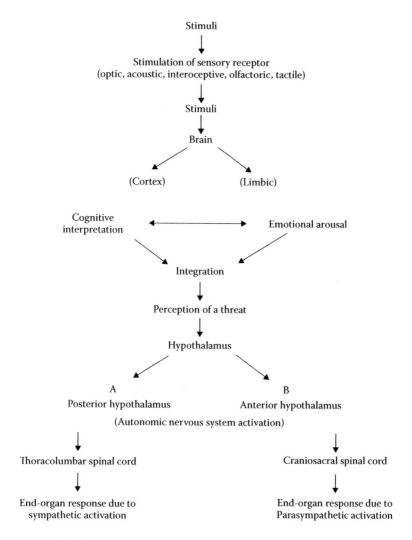

FIGURE 6.7   Initial activation of the stress response. (From McComb, J., et al. *Eating disorders in women and children: prevention, stress management, and treatment*. p. 127, 2000. CRC Press with permission.)

decreased blood pressure, heart and respiration rates, and increased vagal tone. Parasympathetic response coupled with sympathetic arousal following a stressor (i.e., shunting of blood from the periphery, a decrease in venous return) may cause a condition known as syncope or, more commonly, fainting.

6.2.3.2   Intermediate Stage of the Stress Response

Cannon was the first to describe the "fight-or-flight response" (Cannon and Paz 1911). During this response, the body is prepared for heightened muscular activity so that it may either fight or flee the perceived danger. The stress response occurs as a result of both neural and endocrine activity and is therefore neuroendocrine in nature. Figure 6.8 depicts one of the most prominent biochemical pathways during the stress response.

The flight-or-fight response has its origin in the dorsomedial–amygdalar complex. Neural impulses continue to flow through the hypothalamus, thoracic spinal cord, and eventually innervate the adrenal medulla (see Figure 6.9).

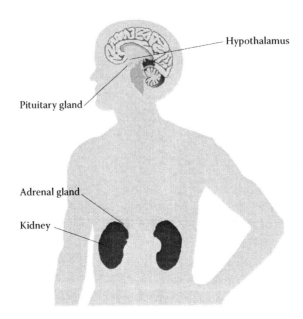

FIGURE 6.8 The hypothalamus-adrenal axis. (From the National Institute on Alcohol Abuse and Alcoholism http://www.niaaa.nih.gov/Resources/GraphicsGallery/Neuroscience/Pages/synapse.aspx with permission.)

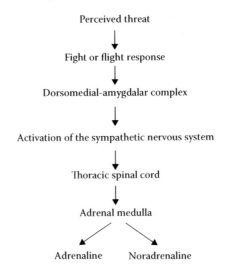

FIGURE 6.9 Intermediate activation of the stress response. (From McComb, J., et al. *Eating disorders in women and children: prevention, stress management, and treatment.* p. 129, 2000. CRC Press with permission.)

Adrenal medullary stimulation results in the release of adrenalin and noradrenalin into the bloodstream. The effects of this pathway are similar if not identical to direct sympathetic arousal. The difference between these two pathways is that adrenal medullary's measurable effects last for 20–30 s. This pathway has been termed the intermediate phase of activation in the stress response. Some of the physiological effects of adrenal medullary axis stimulation are as follows: (1) increased arterial blood pressure and cardiac output; (2) increased plasma levels of free fatty acids, triglycerides, and cholesterol; (3) increased muscular tension; and (4) decreased amount of blood flow to the kidneys and periphery of the skin. Several endocrine glands are involved in physiological response to stress.

6.2.3.3   Prolonged Stage of the Stress Response

A longer time is required both for endocrine hormonal release and for the hormones to be transported through the circulation of blood. The three main endocrine pathways that have been implicated in the stress response are termed the adrenal cortical axis, the somatotropic axis, and the thyroid axis. The most chronic and prolonged somatic response to stress is the result of these endocrine pathways.

6.2.3.2.1   The Adrenal Cortical Axis

The septal–hippocampal complex appears to be the highest point of origin for the adrenal cortical axis (see Figure 6.10). Neural impulses then descend into the median eminence of the hypothalamus. The neurosecretory cells in the median eminence of the hypothalamus release corticotropin releasing factor (CRF) into the hypothalamic hypophyseal portal system. The CRF descends into the infundibular stalk to the anterior pituitary cells. The anterior pituitary is sensitive to CRF and responds by releasing adrenocorticotropic hormone (ACTH) into the systemic circulation. ACTH then stimulates the adrenal cortex to release glucocorticoids (cortisol and corticosterone) and mineralocorticoids (aldosterone and deoxycorticosterone) into systemic circulation (Tsigos and Chrousos 1994). The physiological effects of glucocorticoids and mineralocorticoids are listed in Table 6.3.

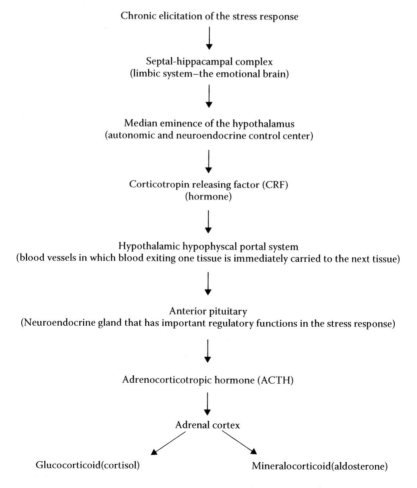

FIGURE 6.10   The adrenal cortical axis. (From McComb, J., et al. *Eating disorders in women and children: prevention, stress management, and treatment.* p. 131, 2000. CRC Press with permission.)

Table 6.3
Physiological Effects of Glucocorticoids and Mineralocorticoids

Glucocorticoids (Cortisol)	Mineralocorticoids (Aldosterone)
Increases serum glucose levels (gluconeogenesis)	Increases water retention
Increases free fatty-acid release into the systemic circulation	Promotes sodium retention
Increases ketone body production	Enhances potassium elimination
Increases arterial blood pressure	Increases blood pressure because of increased water retention
Exacerbates herpes simplex	
Suppresses the immune system	
Increases susceptibility to nonthrombotic myocardial necrosis	
Mobilizes proteins and elevates the level of amino acids in the blood, especially from muscle tissue	
Enhances amino acid transport into the liver, which contributes to gluconeogenesis	

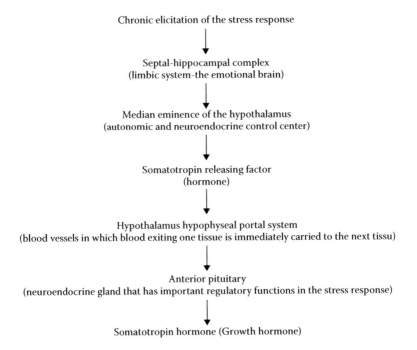

FIGURE 6.11 The somatotropic axis. (From McComb, J., et al. *Eating disorders in women and children: prevention, stress management, and treatment.* p. 133, 2000. CRC Press with permission.)

6.2.3.2.2 The Somatotropic Axis

The somatotropic axis has the same basic pathway as the adrenal cortical axis, beginning from the septal–hippocampal complex through the hypothalamic hypophyseal portal system, with the exception that the somatotropin releasing factor stimulates the pituitary to release growth hormone (somatotropin) into systemic circulation (see Figure 6.11).

Growth hormone (GH) has many metabolic effects and affects virtually every cell in the body. Secretion is influenced by the prevailing circulating levels of metabolites, such as amino acids, fatty acids, and glucose, and other hormones secreted in the stress response. The hormones secreted during the stress response have varying effects on the secretion of GH. For example, epinephrine enhances the secretion of GH, whereas high levels of circulating cortisol decrease GH secretion.

The role of GH during stress is to stimulate the uptake of amino acids by the cells and to mobilize energy resources such as fat in the body. Growth hormone enhances amino acid transfer across the cell, increasing cellular utilization of these substrates. Consequently, a reduction in cellular glucose uptake ensues, which may then result in a rise in blood sugar levels. This increase in blood sugar levels can in turn stimulate the beta cells of the pancreatic islets of Langerhans to secrete extra insulin. It has been suggested that overstimulation of GH can produce a diabetic-like insulin-resistant effect and act as a potential diabetogenic agent. Growth hormone also has an effect on many of the electrolytes in the body. GH influences the retention of sodium, potassium, phosphate, and calcium in the body. GH secretion in response to stress is not as frequent as the cortisol response. However, elevated GH levels have been found in the blood following the elicitation of the stress response in conjunction with elevated cortisol levels.

6.2.3.2.3 The Thyroid Axis

The pathway of the thyroid axis is similar to the adrenal cortical and somatotropic axes (see Figure 6.12). The difference begins at the median eminence of the hypothalamus where thyrotropin-releasing factor (TRF) is sent through the portal system to the anterior pituitary. From the anterior pituitary, thyroid-stimulating hormone or thyrotrophic hormone (TTH) is released into the systemic circulation. The target is the thyroid gland, from which thyroxine and triiodothyronine are then released.

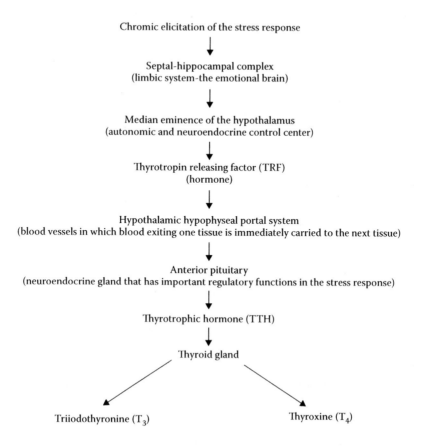

FIGURE 6.12   The thyroid axis. (From McComb, J., et al. *Eating disorders in women and children: prevention, stress management, and treatment.* p. 134, 2000. CRC Press with permission.)

Thyroid hormones have been shown to increase general metabolism, heart rate, heart contractility, peripheral vascular resistance, and the sensitivity of some tissues to catecholamines.

6.2.4 THE PHYSIOLOGICAL MEASUREMENT OF STRESS

Physiological measurement of the stress response is complex. In this section, physiological end-organ responses as well as chemical measurements will be discussed. It must be noted that because of the multifactorial nature of the stress response, several measurements are needed, psychological as well as physiological.

Physiological end-organ measurements commonly seen in the literature include heart rate, breathing rate, and blood pressure. It is important to obtain baseline measurements of these variables for each individual, since variations exist among individuals from day to day. Published norms are presented in Table 6.4. Elevation from normal in any one or any combination of these variables is an indication of sympathetic arousal and/or heightened adrenal medullary activity.

Plasma levels of catecholamines can be measured in blood samples by several techniques. Radioimmunoassay methods are frequently used. Blood levels of these hormones may vary from laboratory to laboratory and depends on test conditions, time of sampling, and the state of the individual being tested (Tietz 1976). Twenty-four hour urine samples of catecholamines are also measured in many laboratories. Typical values for total urinary catecholamines can range from 0 to 100 µg/24 sample (Asterita 1985). Under psychological stress, urine catecholamine excretions can approach 300 µg per day (Williams 1981). Table 6.5 depicts average values of the hormones epinephrine and norepinephrine in adults in normal and distressed states (Engelman and Portnoy 1970, Goodman and Gilman 1980).

Corticosteroid levels, although fairly accurately assessed, also depend on the psychological and physiological states of the individual, the test conditions, the methods used, the adequacy of the sample collection, and the means of the assay. Cortisol (adrenal cortical hormone) is secreted at an average rate of 20 mg/day (Guyton 1981). Blood concentrations of cortisol fluctuate diurnally and average 12 µg percent (Guyton 1981). A group of urinary metabolites of cortisol, the 17-hydroxycorticosteroids (17-OHCS), can be used to estimate the daily cortisol excretion rates. Table 6.5 lists 17-OHCS values observed in normal and distressed states (Tepperman 1980; Tietz 1976).

Clinical biofeedback can be used to measure the physiological response to stress. However, biofeedback is used more commonly as an educational tool to teach individuals how to listen to their bodies' physiological responses to stress and control the response through autonomic regulation. Commonly assessed variables in biofeedback include the following measurements (Fisher-Williams 1986; Miller 1989; Task Force of the European Society of Cardiology 1996):

1. Electromyographic feedback monitors electrical impulses produced by the muscles.
2. Electroencephalographic biofeedback detects and monitors brain waves.
3. Cardiovascular biofeedback, such as heart rate or heart rate variability (HRV), is often used to augment an individual's ability to control heart rate synchronously with breathing rate.

TABLE 6.4
Average Values for Heart Rate, Blood Pressure, and Respiration in Adults

Heart Rate	74 bpm (women)	72 bpm (men)
Blood Pressure	Systolic (mm Hg) <120	Diastolic (mm Hg) <80
Respiration	12 breaths per min	0.5 L per breath

Note: bpm means beats per minute.

TABLE 6.5

Catecholamine and 17-Hydroxycorticosteroid (17-OHS) Hormone Levels in Adults

Condition	Epinephrine	Norepinephrine	17-OHS
Plasma Levels (ng/mL)			
Normal	0.05	0.20	
Severe Stress	0.27	4.10	
Average 24 h			
Urinary Levels (µg)			
Normal	2 to 51	25 to 50	
Stress	>51	>51	
Plasma (µg/100 ml)			
Normal			
8:00 A.M.			5.5 to 26.3
4:00 P.M.			2.0 to 18.0
Stress			>26
Urine (µg/24-h sample)			
Normal			
8:00 A.M.			20 to 100
Stress			>100

4. Thermal biofeedback measures the flow of blood to a specific area by the heat emitted.
5. Electrodermal biofeedback measures the electrical conduction of the skin.

There has been great interest in the measurement of HRV as an indicator of stress and certain disease states. Heart rate variability is the variation in R to R intervals, in milliseconds (ms) over a period of time, usually 24 hours. An R signifies the contraction of the ventricles, you could also think of it as a heart beat. In the presence of a physiological or psychological stressor, the body will undergo a shift towards sympathetic nervous system dominance as the fight-or-flight response is activated. This shift will lead to a corresponding decrease in HRV as parasympathetic influence decreases (Carney and Freedland 2009). Therefore, clinicians can use HRV as a noninvasive way to assess a person's level of stress.

Tsuji et al. (1994) were some of the first researchers to recognize the importance of HRV as a marker of overall cardiac health, even in that absence of acute trauma (Chandola et al. 2010). They noted that HRV was lower in the vast majority of their patients following a cardiac episode, and in patients that had a significantly large low frequency component in HRV, the risk of sudden death post infarction was 5.4 times higher.

Since anorexia nervosa (AN) is often coupled with heart disease, measurement of this variable would be useful in an eating-disorder population. Depression is also common for individuals with eating disorders, and this association has clinical implications: HRV is lower in individuals with depression as opposed to nondepressed individuals (Beary and Benson 1974).

6.3 SIGNIFICANCE OF CURRENT FINDINGS

6.3.1 PHYSIOLOGICAL CONSEQUENCES OF CHRONIC STRESS

The process by which external stressors cause changes in internal bodily functions is only partially understood. However, it seems that illness occurs because of the chronic and excessive elicitation of stress hormones and the body's continual physiological attempts to overcome the perceived threat. The concept of the stress response has been around for a long time, but it was Selye (1974) who first came up with a three-component model to explain this response. His model is widely known as the

General Adaptation Syndrome (GAS). In his model, the first phase is called *alarm reaction*. The alarm reaction is characterized by the release of adrenal medullary and cortical hormones into the bloodstream. This phase parallels the fight-or-flight response proposed by Cannon in 1911 (Cannon in 1911). The second phase of GAS is termed the *stage of resistance*. Cortisol secretion is heightened and the body functions at elevated metabolic levels. The last phase is the *stage of exhaustion*. Endocrine activity is increased, and high circulatory levels of cortisol begin to produce pronounced effects on the systems of the body, such as the circulatory, digestive, immune, and other bodily systems. In this final stage of exhaustion, cardiovascular, gastrointestinal, immune, respiratory, and musculoskeletal disorders occur.

6.3.2 The Concept of Homeostasis in Health and Disease

The body is an amazingly resilient mechanism, capable of surviving in a large variety of environments, due to its ability to maintain homeostasis. However, homeostasis is only half the story because it fails to account for many processes that living organisms use for survival and propagation (McEwen and Wingfield 2009). For example, before giving birth to a calf, a cow begins to prepare physically for lactation. An example of the human body's ability to respond both to predicted demands as well as immediate concerns is that if you expected to go for a period of time without food, your last meal might exceed the volume of food that you would normally consume in order to offset future insufficiency.

For the most part, the body is fairly successful at achieving stability, even in the face of "homeostatic insult," situations in which there is some obstacle working against the body's natural, physiological balance. Suppose that a person sustains an injury, perhaps a laceration in a car accident. Without an adaptive response by the body, the continual loss of blood resulting from the injury would eventually reduce blood pressure in the body, and would then create a situation in which oxygen delivery throughout the body would drop to an unsafe level. Fortunately, as our bodies have evolved, they have developed a series of coping mechanisms needed for survival, one of which is the stress response. In the injury example, a healthy body would respond by releasing clotting factors to diminish bleeding. Meanwhile, the activation of the stress response would increase the body's immune system response, thereby decreasing the chance of foreign bacteria causing an infection. Additionally, vasoconstriction associated with the stimulation of the sympathetic nervous system would cause a decrease in the amount of blood loss. Finally, in the event of significant blood loss, the kidneys would be signaled to retain water to maintain plasma levels throughout the body.

However, it is better to prevent the damage all together instead of repairing it, and that is where the concept of *allostasis* comes into play. Allostasis refers to the ability of the body to maintain stability by making adaptive changes in response to changing circumstances and demands. If you were to encounter an aggressive dog, it would be unwise to wait until you were already under attack to start responding to the situation; by then, it might be too late. Therefore, the body predicts an expected increased demand and moves away from the homeostatic norm in order to prepare you for the future conflict. Heart rate and energy mobilization increase dramatically to prepare you in the event that you must drain your energy reserves in the escape.

The situations described above demonstrate how the allostatic response serves a valuable function in the preservation of our overall stability, even though it produces short-term departures from homeostasis. This ability is limited, as Selye (1950a) noticed in his early studies. In prolonged encounters with physiological stressors such as cold and injury, an organism may enter an exhaustion stage, where it is weaker than it was when the injury first occurred (Selye 1950a). This stage was so named due to the postulated mechanism of this stage as a depletion of the organism's "adaptation energy" reserves.

The same adaptation occurs whether we suffer psychological or physical stress. For the most part, these adaptive responses speed up the body and make the body faster and stronger to escape the threat, whether mental or physical. This altered state, while beneficial, is still by nature taxing as it requires the body to operate at above normal levels. In the short term, this allostasis is very beneficial, in that it prepares our bodies to handle upcoming physical and mental challenges. However, if the psychological stress load is too great or goes on for too long, for example, the persistent long-term stressor living in poverty and semi-starvation, the result is a situation where stress adaptations become more detrimental than beneficial. *Allostatic overload* can occur in situations in which the body produces homeostatic imbalance for a long period of time to meet challenges and demands (McEwen and Wingfield 2009). When the stressor continues for longer periods than expected, the body's physiology becomes maladaptive rather than adaptive, instead of helping the body maintain vital functioning, the changes impair healthy functioning.

Our bodies are designed to respond quickly to immediate threats, and after the threat has been removed, return to a resting state. When the stress response continues for more than just a short period of time, it hinders the healthy operation of the systems of the body. For example, in the face of a stressor, the heart begins to beat faster and arteries and arterioles constrict in order to aid in blood flow to the working muscles. These changes aid us well in a fight-or-flight situation, but when a person experiences chronic unresolved stress, blood pressure and heart rate stay elevated. This heightened state promotes the generation of atherosclerotic plaque, elevating a person's chance of having a heart attack (Tietz 1976). The cardiovascular system is thought by many investigators to be the primary target end organ for the stress response (Asterita 1985). Other cardiovascular disorders often associated with the stress response are essential hypertension, arrhythmias, migraine headaches, and Raynaud's phenomenon (vasoconstriction in the hands, fingers, feet, or toes).

Cortisol released in response to stress has different effects depending on the duration of its effects. In the short term, one of the main functions of cortisol is energy mobilization, releasing energy from its stores and getting it ready for immediate use. However, if cortisol levels remain chronically elevated, cortisol will start to modulate how fat is stored as well. Research has shown that people undergoing chronic stress tend not only to add fat mass to their bodies, but also that the fat will tend to accumulate in the abdominal region (Goodman and Gilman 1980; Williams 1981). This is a very significant finding because of the current "obesity epidemic" that the United States is experiencing. Part of the problem may be in fact that the situations that causes us stress are no longer brief and clear-cut (such as with a physical attack) but are much more prolonged and nebulous (such as chronic marital dissatisfaction). When this type of situations causes us to react hyperactively, we are more likely to experience the long-term, negative aspects of the stress response, as opposed to the short-term, beneficial adaptations.

Another potential problem with an overactivated stress response is immunosuppression, which is a decrease in the effectiveness of the immune system—the disease-fighting mechanism of the body (Engelman and Portnoy 1970). Although this may seem paradoxical given the defensive nature of the stress response, researchers have developed two plausible explanations for this phenomenon. The first explanation is that because the stress response is targeted to remediate a clear and present danger, it would be beneficial for the body to shift its resources away from long-term problems, such as disease, in order to conserve energy for meeting the current threat. The second explanation is that the body wishes to prevent autoimmune disorders. Autoimmune disorder occurs when the body's immune system becomes overactive in its response to perceived infectious threats, and actually begins attacking its own tissues. In this second way of viewing immunosuppression, the body is taking measures to prevent an overzealous response of the immune system. This decreased response occurs to make sure any local immune system activation, such as in response to mechanical injury to the body (e.g., lacerations or bone fractures), stays local to the injury. Therefore, only those areas of the body that have a heightened need for a response from the immune system will receive it.

Regardless of its potentially useful purposes, immunosuppression has obvious downfalls when it is chronic and prolonged. Several studies have reported changes in immune cells and natural killer cells important for immunity in patients with AN and BN (Vaz- Leal et al. 2010). This immunosuppression leaves individuals with eating disorders more vulnerable to illness and infections.

Every day, the body is constantly exposed to the possibility of infections from both bacteria and viruses in the environment. Our body for the most part can keep these foreign bodies from making us ill. However, we become ill if we are exposed to too many infectious agents, or if our immune system is not operating at full effectiveness. Thus, the body in a state of immunosuppression is less likely to prevent infections from gaining a foothold, making us more susceptible to everyday illnesses, such as the cold and flu.

6.3.3 Stress and Eating Disorders

Even though the relationship among stress, coping strategies, and eating disorders is not fully understood, it seems that disordered eating is often an unhealthy attempt at coping with stress (Soukup et al. 1990). Research has shown that stressful life events often precede the onset of AN and Bulimia Nervosa (BN) (Guyton 1981; Tepperman 1980).

The interpersonal stress theory states that binge eating is triggered by a stressful antecedent (Laessle et al. 1991). Support for this theory comes from observations that binge eating often occurs in frustrating and problematic situations associated with negative feelings such as anxiety (Abraham and Beumont 1982; Catteanach et al. 1988). Although individuals may use eating disorders as a method of coping, they can become caught in a negative cycle, increasingly using ineffective behaviors in attempts to cope with stress.

However, in some research studies, the eating habits of bulimic women following stressors have not been significantly different from the habits of other women. Levine and Marcus (1997) observed the eating behaviors of women with bulimic symptoms following exposure to an interpersonal stressor. They found that even though the consumption of carbohydrates increased following a stressor, the eating behaviors of these women were not significantly different from the eating behaviors of nonbulimic women. This study suggested that women with bulimic symptoms are not substantially more vulnerable to eating in response to stress than other women.

Other studies have suggested that stress is a consequence rather than a cause of eating disorders (Rosen et al. 1993). Sharpe et al. (1997) found that even though individuals with symptoms of eating disorders reported more stressful life events than individuals without those symptoms, the difference was due to the stress of disorder-specific events. Regardless of whether stress is the consequence or the cause of an eating disorder, there is an ever-increasing awareness among professionals from varied disciplines that stress, specifically chronic stress, is associated with a variety of dysfunctions, ranging from high blood pressure to immune dysfunction to eating disorders.

6.4 CONCLUDING REMARKS

Stress or more precisely, distress, is usually involved at several points in the continuum of the pathology of eating disorders. Distress may occur prior to, during, or following behaviors associated with AN, BN, or binge-eating disorder (BED). Attempts to use preventive interventions with populations at high risk for developing eating disorders should consider stress as a risk factor and incorporate stress management strategies in their interventions. Additionally, individuals who are diagnosed with eating disorders would benefit from techniques that are designed to increase parasympathetic drive and relax the body.

Herbert Benson, a researcher from Harvard Medical School, is well known for his work related to the *relaxation response*. This is a term used to describe learned techniques that are associated with parasympathetic drive or slowing down the body's metabolic processes. The regular practice of these techniques have been associated with decreased oxygen uptake, carbon dioxide production, heart rate, blood lactate, and systolic blood pressure while at rest (Benson et al. 1978). Research has also shown that the regular practice of the *relaxation response* produces a significant decrease in similar variables during submaximal exercise: oxygen uptake, rate of perceived exertion, systolic blood pressure, rate-pressure product, and frequency of breathing (Gervino and Veazey 1984; Wallace et al. 1971).

Figure 6.13 graphically displays metabolic changes related to the regular practice of meditation in which the *relaxation response* was elicited. Individuals who had been meditating anywhere from 1 month to over 9 years (20 minutes in the morning and 20 minutes in the evening) participated in data collection in which oxygen consumption was measured before, during, and after the meditation period (see Figures 6.13).

The experiments showed that during meditation, there was a marked decrease in the body's oxygen consumption (Wallace et al. 1971). This change in oxygen consumption during meditation is markedly different from the change in oxygen consumption during sleep (see Figures 6.14).

Blood lactate levels also fell rapidly during the first 10 minutes of meditation (see Figure 6.15) and remained at extremely low levels during meditation (Wallace 1970).

Illustrations of the physiological effects achieved by eliciting the *relaxation response* demonstrate how one can stimulate the parasympathetic nervous system to exert more control over the autonomic nervous system and slow down metabolic processes. A healthy body responds to the demands placed on the system yet returns to a state of rest for regeneration. A balance must be achieved between the sympathetic and parasympathetic nervous system.

Practices, such a meditation, that elicit the *relaxation response,* can also help reduce immunosuppression. As started previously, individuals with eating disorders often suffer from immunosuppression (Vaz- Leal et al. 2010). One study employing a meditative technique called mindfulness-based training examined the effectiveness of meditation on newly diagnosed breast cancer patients. This particular population experiences a very high level of chronic stress, and is therefore often included in stress intervention research. The mindfulness-based intervention not only helped to retard the immunosuppression, but also improved the participants' view of their lives, as demonstrated by the quality of life index (Witek-Janusek et al. 2008). Similar program has been developed for women with eating disorders (Proulx 2008).

While the term, meditation, is still dominant in the research literature in 2011, the term, *relaxation response,* is not widely seen in the literature. Many clinicians prefer the term *autonomic regulation* because of the skill required to achieve this response. In order to achieve the benefits

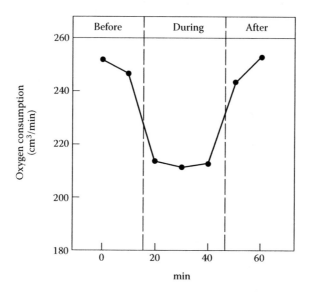

FIGURE 6.13 Changes in oxygen consumption during the practice of the relaxation response. (From McComb, J., et al. *Eating disorders in women and children: prevention, stress management, and treatment.* p. 138, 2000. CRC Press with permission.)

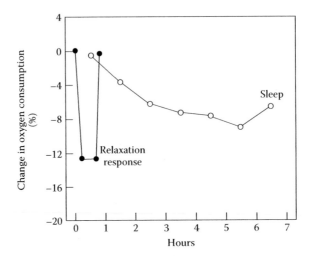

FIGURE 6.14 Comparison between the level of oxygen consumption during the practice of the relaxation response and sleep. (From McComb, J., et al. *Eating disorders in women and children: prevention, stress management, and treatment.* p. 139, 2000. CRC Press with permission.)

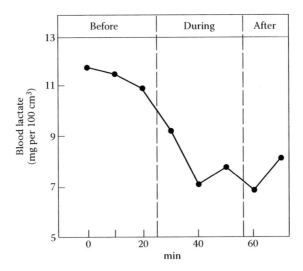

FIGURE 6.15 Changes in blood lactate during the practice of the relaxation response. (From McComb, J., et al. *Eating disorders in women and children: prevention, stress management, and treatment.* p. 140, 2000. CRC Press with permission.)

associated with the *relaxation response*, the practice must be practiced repeatedly. Improvement requires discipline. It is much different than just going to the beach to relax.

Whatever term is used, the underlying physiology for all of the practices that enable the body to slow down, get out of overdrive, and relax, are still very much needed in today's society.

6.4.1 CLOSING STATEMENT

The information in this chapter was not intended to take away any awe associated with the amazing mechanics of the human body. Indeed, only a well-designed organism would be able to preemptively respond and adapt in response to threats, and to cope later with the damage, in the manner present in human physiology. Contained within the stress response are contingencies for both the short- and long-term consequences of injury, as well as proactive measures to avoid further damage. These mechanisms are not so much flawed as they are designed for a different, earlier lifestyle. Evolution did not take into account the complex social and psychological factors that currently produce chronic stress because earlier humans did not face them.

The fact remains that in Western society, most of us will experience chronic stress. We are a future-oriented culture, and not anticipating future problems and demands is regarded as foolishness. There are some actions we can take to avoid stress, such as avoiding bad relationships and finding a job with a manageable level of demands, but it would be naïve to think that all stressful situations can be avoided. Therefore, experts in the field of stress and stress physiology are putting more emphasis on stress modulation than stress avoidance. Stress modulation is a cognitive-behavioral approach to stress management that attempts to make a person less reactive to stressing events, as opposed to attempting to avoid them all together. Two different techniques to increase parasympathetic drive can be found in Appendices 6.A and 6.B. These techniques can help readers in countering the detrimental effects of chronic stress through the practice of auto regulation and stress modulation. There are many calming techniques that if practiced regularly, can influence the autonomic nervous system and enhance the overall health of the nervous system.

APPENDIX 6.A BREATHING MEDITATION

Why Breathing Meditation?

- The techniques are easy to learn.
- Most breathing exercises can be done anywhere.
- Respiration is directly linked with the autonomic nervous system that controls (speeds up) sympathetic activation and (slows down) parasympathetic activation.

Points to Remember

- Breathing through the nose is preferred rather than breathing through the nose and mouth. The nasal passages warm and filter the air coming in.
- Breathing cycles should be natural and gentle.
- Avoid hyperventilation or artificially deep successive breathing patterns.
- Training in relaxation should never be substituted for medical treatment if needed.

Abdominal Breathing

The Practice

- Find a quiet environment.
- Lie down in a comfortable position.
- Observe the natural rhythm of your breath.
- After a couple of minutes extend your breath, making it a little longer than usual while maintaining the natural rhythm.
- Put one hand just below your rib cage on the solar plexus.
- Focus your attention on this area.
- As you breathe out, notice your hand sinking; the diaphragm is assuming its natural dome shape, pushing the air out of the lungs.
- Maintain the natural rhythm of your breathing, gently extending your breathing cycle.
- As you inhale, feel your hand rise as the diaphragm flattens out to make room for the expansion of air in your lungs.
- Let your mind follow the path of your breath.
- Be mindful of the sensations of breathing, cool air coming in, warm air going out.

- When distracting thoughts occur, acknowledge them and turn your attention back to your breathing.
- Be mindful of the slowing of your breathing pattern; in a restful state, your body does not require the oxygen content it did before you began your relaxation period.
- Continue in this deep state of relaxation just a few minutes longer.

APPENDIX 6.B   PROGRESSIVE MUSCULAR RELAXATION

Why Progressive Muscular Relaxation?

Relaxation follows tensing the muscles.
You will be asked to concentrate on the feelings that accompany the tensing and relaxing of the muscles; you may not have been aware of moments of tension in your body before.

Points to Remember

The contraction of the muscles is carried out all at once, not gradually. Tension is maintained in the muscles for 5–7 s.
Relaxation of the muscle follows contraction. The relaxation period is 30–40 s.
It is important to notice the feelings that accompany the tensing and relaxing of your muscles.
Training in relaxation should never be substituted for medical treatment if needed.

Bernstein and Borkovec's Progressive Muscular Relaxation

The Practice

Sit in a reclining chair or in a chair with a high back and arms.
There are 16 areas of concentration that will be tensed and relaxed.
The procedure is the same for each muscle group.

Procedure

Tense each area of concentration separately; however, follow this same outline.
Tense the concentrated area as tightly as possible, feel the tension, hold the tension for 5–7 s, then relax. Notice the sensations you feel in this area when you relax. Feel the relaxation flowing through the surrounding areas in your body. Compare the way this area of your body feels when it is tensed to when it is relaxed. Sequentially tense and relax the following areas of concentrations. You can alter or summarize the areas of selected concentration to fit your needs both physically (individuals with high blood pressure may need to concentrate only on the relaxation phase of the cycle) and mentally (time constraints, etc.).

Areas of Concentration

1. Make a fist with the dominant hand without involving the upper arm.
2. Using the same arm, push your elbow down on the arm of the chair.
3–4. Do the same sequence with the nondominant hand.
5. Raise your eyebrows.
6. Wrinkle your nose and squeeze your eyes shut.
7. Pull back the corners of your mouth and clench your teeth.
8. Pull the chin down and press the head against the back of the chair.
9. Bring the shoulders back.
10. Tighten the abdominal muscles.
11. Contract the thigh and hamstring muscles at the same time.

12. Point the dominant foot down.
13. Pull the dominant foot up.
14. The nondominant leg repeats the same sequence, beginning with the contraction of the thigh and hamstring.

REFERENCES

Abraham, S. F., and P. J. V. Beumont. 1982. How patients describe bulimia or binge-eating. *Psychol Med* 12: 625–635.

Asterita, M. 1985. *The physiology of stress: With special reference to the neuroendocrine system.* New York: Human Sciences Press.

Beary, J. F., and H. Benson. 1974. A simple psychophysiologic technique which elicits the hypometabolic changes of the relaxation response. *Psychol Med 36*: 115–120.

Benson, H., T. Dryer, and L. H. Hartley. 1978. Decreased VO_2 consumption during exercise with elicitation of the relaxation response. *J Human Stress* 4: 38–42.

Cannon, W. B., and D. Paz. 1911. Emotional stimulation of adrenal gland secretion. *Amer J Physiol* 28: 64–70.

Carney, R., and K. Freedland. 2009. Depression and heart rate variability in patients with coronary heart disease. *Cleve Clin J Med* 76: 13–17.

Catteanach, L., R. Malley, and J. Rodin. 1988. Psychologic and physiologic reactivity to stressors in eating disordered individuals. *Psychosom Med* 50, no. 6: 591–599.

Chandola, T., A. Haraclides, and M. Kumari. 2010. Psychophysiological biomarkers of workplace stressors. *Neurosci Biobehav Rev* 35: 51–57.

Engelman, K., and B. A. Portnoy. 1970. A sensitive double-isotope derivative assay for norepinephrine and epinephrine: Normal resting human plasma levels. *Circ Res* 26, no. 6: 53– 57.

Fisher-Williams, M. 1986. *A textbook of biological feedback.* New York: Human Sciences Press.

Gervino, E. V., and A. E. Veazey. 1984. The physiological effects of Benson's relaxation response during submaximal aerobic exercise. *J Cardiac Rehabil* 6: 10–12.

Goodman, L. S., and A. Gilman. 1980. *The pharmacological basis of therapeutics.* New York: Macmillan.

Guyton, A. C. 1981. *Textbook of medical physiology.* Philadelphia: W. B. Saunders.

Laessle, R. G., P. J. Beumont, P. Butow, W. Lennerts, M. O'Conner, K. M. Pirke, S. W. Touyz, and S. Waadt. 1991. A comparison of nutritional management with stress management in the treatment of bulimia nervosa. *Br J Psychiatry* 159: 250–61.

Levine, M. D., and M. D. Marcus. 1997. Eating behavior following stress in women with and without bulimic symptoms. *Ann Behav Med* 19: 132–138.

McEwen, B., and J. Wingfield. 2009. What is in a name? Integrating homeostasis, allostasis and stress. *Horm Behav* 57, no. 2: 105–111.

Miller, N. E. 1989. What biofeedback does (and does not) do. *Psychol Today 23*: 22–23.

Monat, S., and R. Lazarus. 1991. *Stress and coping: An anthology.* New York: Columbia Univ. Press.

Proulx, K. 2008. Experiences of women with bulimia nervosa in a mindfulness-based eating disorder treatment group. *Eat Disord* 16, no. 1: 52–72.

Rosen, J. C., B. E. Compas, and B. Tracy. 1993. The relationship among stress, psychological symptoms, and eating disorder symptoms: A prospective analysis. *Int J Eat Disord* 14: 153–162.

Selye, H. 1950a. Stress and the general adaptation syndrome. *Br Med J* 1 (no. 4667): 1384–1392.

Selye, H. 1950b. *The physiology and pathology of exposure to stress.* Montreal: Acta.

Selye, H. 1974. *Stress without distress.* Philadelphia: J. B. Lippincott.

Sharpe, T. A., E. Ryst, and H. Steiner. 1997. Reports of stress: A comparison between eating disordered and non-eating disordered adolescents. *Child Psychiatry Hum Dev* 28, no. 2: 117–132.

Soukup, V. M., M. E. Beiler, and F. Terrell. 1990. Stress, coping style, and problem-solving ability among eating-disordered inpatients. *J Clin Psychol* 46: 592 599.

Task Force of the European Society of Cardiology. 1996. Heart rate variability: Standards of measurement, physiological interpretation, and clinical use. *Circulation* 93, no. 5: 1043–1065.

Tepperman, J. 1980. *Metabolic and endocrine physiology.* Chicago: Yearbook Medical Publishers.

Tietz, N. M. 1976. *Fundamentals of clinical chemistry.* Philadelphia: W. B. Saunders.

Tsigos, C., and G. P. Chrousos. 1994. Physiology of the hypothalamic-pituitary-adrenal axis in health and dysregulation in psychiatric and autoimmune disorders. *Endocrinol Metab Clin North Am* 23: 451–466.

Tsuji, H., F. J. Venditti, E. S. Manders, J. Evans, M. Larson, L. Feldman, and D. Levy. 1994. Reduced heart rate variability and mortality risk in an elderly cohort: The Framingham Heart Study. *Circulation* 90, no. 2: 878–883.

Vaz-Leal, F. J., L. Rodriquez-Santos, J. M. Melero-Ruiz, I. M. Ramos-Fuentes, and A.M. Garcia-Herraiz. 2010. Psychopathology and lymphocyte subsets in patients with bulimia nervosa. *Nutri Neurosci* 13: 109–115.

Wallace, R. K. 1970. Physiological effects of transcendental meditation. *Science* 167: 1751–1754.

Wallace, R. K., H. Benson, and A. Wilson. 1971. A wakeful hypometabolic physiologic state. *Am J Physiol* 221, no. 3: 795–799.

Williams, R. H. 1981. *Textbook of endocrinology.* Philadelphia: W. B. Saunders.

Witek-Janusek, L., K. Albuquerque, K. R. Chroniak, C. Chroniak, R. Duzaro-Arvizu, and H. L. Mathews. 2008. Effect of mindfulness based stress reduction on immune function, quality of life and coping in women newly diagnosed with early stage breast cancer. *Brain Behav Immun* 22: 969–981.

7 The Psychology of Stress and Coping

Stephen W. Cook, Cathy L. Thompson,
and Vanessa A. Coca-Lyle

CONTENTS

7.1 LEARNING OBJECTIVES

After completing this chapter you should be able to

- Define stress and coping
- Identify the distinctions between dispositional and situational approaches to the study of coping
- Identify methods to help individuals assess their level of stress and identify various coping strategies
- Summarize the relationships among stress, coping, and psychological distress
- Describe gender differences in the experience of stress and in coping with stress
- Describe how an understanding of stress and coping can be applied to the treatment of women and children with eating disorders

7.2 BACKGROUND AND SIGNIFICANCE

Contemporary American culture has become very interested, indeed almost obsessed, with "stress" and how to "cope" with it. Self-help books, advice columns, popular magazines, and talk shows provide endless suggestions about how to assess how much stress we are currently facing, how to deal with interpersonal problems that may arise in a romantic relationship or at the workplace, and how to deal with the difficulties associated with intrapersonal problems, such as depression or anxiety. There is much we still do not know, and many people have recognized the importance of looking closely at the relationship between coping and both mental and physical health (McWilliams et al. 2003; Penley et al. 2002).

7.2.1 Stress and Coping Defined

It is important to establish a definition of the terms "stress" and "coping." Aldwin (1994) defined stress as "that quality of experience, produced through a person–environment transaction that, through overarousal or underarousal, results in psychological or physiological distress." Monat et al. (2007) described some of the complex issues when attempting to define stress, but noted that there are three general aspects of stress identified in the literature: physiological, psychological, and sociocultural. For this chapter, we will focus primarily on the psychological aspect of stress. Lazarus and Folkman (1984) defined psychological stress as "a particular relationship between the person and the environment that is appraised by the person as taxing or exceeding his or her resources and endangering his or her well-being." Put more simply, *stress* is our reaction in response to a demand. This demand or event that overwhelms us or disturbs our equilibrium is known as a *stressor*. A stressor could be physical in nature, such as a broken arm, or emotional, such as the breakup of a romantic relationship. As indicated by the previous definitions, stressors are typically considered to be aspects of the environment, but stressors could also be internal, such as the demands associated with wanting to be well-liked by others. It is important to remember that stress can be an adaptive response to stressors or demands that help us deal more effectively with problems we encounter. Just as experiencing the demands associated with lifting weights helps our muscles to become stronger, experiencing stressors in various situations can help us grow stronger psychologically (Haan 1993). Most people function best under moderate levels of stress (Yerkes and Dodson 1908). However, under conditions of persistent, high stress, people can develop a variety of damaging physical and psychological symptoms (Selye 1993).

Early research explored the relationship between stressful events and individual distress but found that stressful events accounted for only 10% of the changes in distress (Holahan et al. 1996). Obviously, there are other factors that must be considered when examining the roots of human emotional and physical distress, and some researchers have hypothesized that the coping behaviors of an individual play a central role in determining the amount of distress he or she experiences.

In their classic text on stress and coping, Lazarus and Folkman (1984) defined *coping* as "constantly changing cognitive and behavioral efforts to manage specific external and/or internal demands that are appraised as taxing or exceeding the resources of the person." Lazarus and Folkman noted that coping is limited to stressors that are consciously perceived by individuals as being especially stressful. Not everyone agrees with Lazarus and Folkman's conceptualization of coping as involving "constantly changing" behaviors, however, and there is some evidence to suggest that coping behaviors are more stable than Lazarus and Folkman theorized (Amirkhan 1994; Parkes 1994). This issue, along with the concept of appraisal, will be discussed further in this chapter. Snyder and Pulvers (2001, 4) defined coping as "thinking, feeling, or acting so as to preserve a satisfied psychological state when it is threatened." Using information from these various definitions, coping can be defined more simply as what an individual consciously does to deal with the effects of a stressor or personal problem. The coping response can include behavioral, cognitive, and affective strategies to handle a stressor (Carver and Scheier 1994).

Lazarus and Folkman's (1984) transactional model of stress and coping viewed the stressor and a person's response to that stressor as affecting each other. An individual first experiences a stressor and then must evaluate that stressor and determine its meaning for him or her. This evaluation is called *appraisal*. Appraisal is considered to be how a person cognitively evaluates the significance of a stressor and determines which coping responses could be used most effectively. Lazarus and Folkman identified three kinds of cognitive appraisal: primary, secondary, and reappraisal. Primary appraisal involves judging a situation as irrelevant, positive, or as involving harm, loss, threat, or challenge. Secondary appraisal involves a judgment about the availability and likely efficacy of coping behaviors (see Kleinke 2007, for further descriptions of primary and secondary appraisal). Reappraisal refers to "a changed appraisal based on new information from the environment ... and/or the person's own reactions" (Lazarus and Folkman 1984, 38) The appraisals of an individual change as he or she moves through a stressful situation and applies various coping strategies. Similarly, coping is seen as a process that changes over time in response to both the changing demands of the stressful situation and the individual's subjective appraisal of that situation. Other researchers have proposed similar theories of coping (Endler and Parker 1994). Common to these theories is the importance placed on both appraisals and coping strategies used by individuals as they cope with a stressor.

Several researchers (e.g., Snyder and Pulvers 2001) have emphasized the importance of considering both dispositional (i.e., personality-related) and contextual (i.e., situation-related) factors in the study of coping. Holahan et al. (1996) described dispositional variables as those having to do with a consistent, stable use of coping strategies across various situations. Contextual or situational variables were described as those concerned with how particular characteristics of a stressful event influence various coping strategies. These researchers have proposed an integrative conceptual framework, which emphasizes how both enduring personal factors as well as more changeable situational factors shape coping efforts.

Holahan et al. (1996) also distinguished between two relatively stable factors in the coping process: (1) the environmental system, which is composed of ongoing life stressors (e.g., chronic physical illness) and social coping resources (e.g., support from family members); and (2) the personal system, which includes an individual's sociodemographic characteristics and personal coping resources (e.g., self-confidence). Holahan et al. conceptualized these relatively stable variables as influencing the life crises and transitions individuals face. These events often reflect significant changes in life circumstances.

The combined influences of the environmental system, personal system, and life crises and transitions shape health and well-being both directly and indirectly through the process of cognitive appraisal and specific coping responses. For instance, if a person has relatively few ongoing life stressors, receives strong support from family members, and has a high sense of self-efficacy for dealing with personal problems, she or he will be able to more effectively cope with a life crisis (such as the death of a loved one) and will in turn exhibit relatively fewer symptoms of distress when responding to this crisis. It is important to note that the causal paths in the framework are bidirectional, indicating that reciprocal feedback can occur at each stage. For example, if someone copes effectively with a life crisis, such as the death of a loved one, this will in turn give that person a higher sense of self-efficacy for dealing with personal problems. Holahan et al. (1996, 27) pointed out that this framework "emphasizes the central mediating role of cognitive appraisal and coping responses in the stress process."

Some critics have suggested that most existing theories of coping are not fully applicable to the stressors women face and their subsequent coping strategies. Banyard and Graham-Bermann (1993) took issue with theories of coping that fail to adequately consider the unique perspective of women. They pointed out that theories portraying women as using less "healthy" coping behaviors often do not consider the ways in which a woman's social experience differs from a man's, and how a careful consideration of those differences may reveal that coping strategies previously labeled "bad" (e.g., emotion-focused coping) may be quite adaptive. The authors proposed an alternative model of coping, which acknowledges that women's experience of stress is different than men's rather than considering stress as a homogeneous concept. Additionally, this alternative model promotes an understanding "that coping occurs in a context shaped by social forces based on gender, race, class, age, and sexual orientation." The proposed theory of coping redefined the meaning of coping to include those actions "used to maximize the survival of others (such as children, family, and friends)." Descriptions of coping strategies were also revised to remove the pejorative meanings often associated with different types of coping. The implication is that a different conceptualization of coping is needed for women who are attempting to cope with an eating disorder compared to traditional conceptualizations of coping that have ignored social and cultural factors.

In addition to the consideration of gender when examining how people cope with stress, a person's religiousness or spirituality is also a useful cultural variable to consider. Folkman and Moskowitz (2004, 759) highlighted religious coping as an important new development in the study of coping with stress, noting that it is, "one of the most fertile areas for theoretical consideration and empirical research." For more than 20 years, Kenneth Pargament and his colleagues have produced a program of research that has examined the variety of ways that people incorporate religion and spirituality into their coping with stressful events (for a review, see Pargament, Ano, and Wachholtz 2005). Evidence indicates that a person's religious or spiritual orientation provides a distinctive resource for encountering, appraising, and coping with stressful events (Pargament, Magyar-Russell, and Murray-Swank 2005). Additionally, it has been argued that addressing the religious and spiritual issues of people with eating disorders is crucial for successful treatment and recovery (Richards et al. 2007). Worthington and Aten (2009) summarized Pargament's research as suggesting that people use religion and spirituality in both conservative and transformative ways to cope with stressors—attempting both to deal with stressors according to their existing religious framework, as well as modifying religious schema to most effectively cope with problems. Additionally, religious coping can be either adaptive or maladaptive (Pargament, Ano, and Wachholtz 2005). Considering religious/spiritual dimensions of coping with stress will be helpful in the assessment and treatment of women and children with eating disorders.

7.2.2 Dispositional and Situational Approaches to the Study of Coping

The dispositional approach to the study of coping assumes that individuals are predisposed to use habitual coping strategies across different types of stressful situations or at different points in time. Scientists using this approach attempt to identify basic coping styles that are relatively stable within the person. Several schools of thought provide a basis for describing person-based coping styles, including psychoanalysis with its emphasis on defense mechanisms (Kelly 1991) as well as some personality theorists who view coping styles as basic personality traits (Shevrin et al. 1996). This approach uses coping scores of the same individual aggregated over different measurement occasions, or scores collected on a single occasion to represent a stable index of the individual's coping styles, and compares that person's response with those of others. This method allows one to assess individual differences in the use of coping strategies. If one accepts the hypothesis that the basis for coping lies within the individual, it makes sense to attempt to identify and quantify individual characteristics that determine, or significantly influence, the choice and implementation of coping behaviors. However, attempts to identify person-related predictors of coping have been somewhat less than successful. Amirkhan (1994) pointed out that researchers found "only sporadic correlations between personality test scores and modes of coping," and that this has produced a "rather chaotic pattern of findings."

In a review of the research literature, Parkes (1994) stated that relatively few dimensions of personality have been found to be related to coping: locus of control, hardiness, Type A behavior, neuroticism, and dispositional optimism. Researchers subscribing to theories of coping that regard coping as a dispositional construct have attempted to relate coping to stable personality characteristics and have had moderate success. Should coping be related to stable personality characteristics, it naturally follows that individuals should be fairly consistent in the coping behaviors they use across situations. There is some evidence to suggest that this is the case, but there is also research indicating very little individual consistency in coping.

The situational approach assumes that individuals have a repertoire of coping options available to choose from depending on characteristics of the situation (e.g., the stressor's intensity, duration, and controllability) and appraisal factors. This approach is often associated with Lazarus and Folkman

(1984) who, as discussed previously, advocated a transactional view of stress and coping. A person's response to stress is seen as a continually developing process rather than a discrete behavior dependent on stable personality characteristics. According to this view, a person's response to stressful events may vary depending on situational factors and other person variables such as how the individual appraises both the stressor and his or her own coping resources. Lazarus and Folkman's contextual model relies heavily on this concept. Situational research paradigms based on this theory often study behaviors and cognitions of the same person or the same group of persons across different types of situations to determine how characteristics of those situations influence individual coping.

Appraisal is a key concept in coping theories that emphasize situational characteristics. Many environmental events have the potential to be stressful but will only become so as a function of the meaning attributed to those events by the individual (Lazarus and Folkman 1984). As stated previously, the transactional approach to coping holds that person variables, such as appraisal, can influence a person's response to stressful events. However, Cassidy and Burnside (1996) pointed out that attempts to produce a model of cognitive appraisal have met with little success. They identified several variables as contributing to psychological vulnerability including achievement motivation, attributional style, problem-solving style, emotional reactivity, hopelessness, perceived control, and perceived social support. The researchers conceptualized these variables as contributing to the ways people think about and give meaning to their experience in the process of appraisal. The researchers tested the relationship between these variables and a variety of measures of life stress, work stress, depression, anxiety, hostility, positive affect, life satisfaction, and job commitment. The data supported an explanatory role for a small set of variables associated with cognitive vulnerability and appraisal, and the researchers suggested that these variables could be used in an integrative model of cognitive appraisal of stress and could prove valuable in guiding psychotherapeutic interventions.

Transactional theorists, such as Lazarus and Folkman (1984), argued that coping behavior depends on successive processes of cognitive appraisal and reappraisal with resulting adjustments made in coping. As a stressful episode develops over time, there is a continuous interaction between appraisal, coping, and emotion, each fluctuating and evolving as the transaction unfolds. Given this constant evolution, people's coping activities may change depending on the characteristics of the situation and their appraisal of both the stressor and their own coping resources. Thus, it follows that there would be little consistency in an individual's coping behavior across situations. However, Amirkhan et al. (1995, 190) pointed out that

> it seems unlikely that people are born anew in every crisis they encounter; they must carry "person-bound" factors with them from stressor to stressor; factors that also influence the choice of a coping strategy. Whether these are personality dispositions, motivational or affective tendencies, or even accumulated coping resources, they should produce some consistency in responses across stressful situations.

The evidence regarding consistency and flexibility in coping is inconsistent, with empirical support for both dispositional and situational theories of coping.

7.2.3 Assessment of Stress and Coping

An important process in understanding stress and coping is developing effective ways to measure these concepts. The measurement of both stress and coping has been the focus of much debate (e.g., Skinner et al. 2003). In this chapter, we will focus on describing those measures of stress and coping that can best be used to assess these important dimensions in people with eating disorders. Administration and interpretation of the measures described in this section should only be done by those who have acquired relevant training in principles of psychometrics and test interpretation.

7.2.3.1 Assessment of Stress

Early attempts to measure the experience of stress for people have focused on assessing major life events, or life stressors, that people have encountered. These stimulus-oriented measures (Derogatis and Coons 1993) have been criticized for being divorced from a person's appraisal of the stressors (e.g., Lazarus 1990)—that is, while one person might appraise a particular event as threatening and stressful, another person might appraise the event as harmless and free of stress. Also, much of the recent research on measures of stress has focused on measures of stress related to trauma, particularly as related to the development or occurrence of posttraumatic stress disorder. Even though such experiences of trauma might be relevant to the assessment and treatment of eating disorders, we will limit the consideration of stress here to experiences that are more normative in nature. Therefore, measures that assess a person's subjective experience of stress will provide for more accurate assessment of stress than measures that focus solely on having respondents report the frequency of stressful life events they have experienced or report only on experiences of traumatic stress. Two such self-report measures are the Combined Hassles and Uplifts Scale and the Perceived Stress Scale.

7.2.3.1.1 Combined Hassles and Uplifts Scale

The Combined Hassles and Uplifts Scale (CHUS; DeLongis et al. 1988; Lazarus and Folkman 1989) is a 53-item measure of "the ongoing stresses and strains of daily living" (i.e., hassles; DeLongis et al. 1982, 120), as well as positive experiences in daily living (i.e., uplifts). The measure is based on the theoretical approach of Lazarus and Folkman (1984), which emphasizes the importance of appraisal when examining how people cope with stress. The CHUS is in many ways a response to the earlier efforts to measure stress by having respondents indicate how many stressful life events that have experienced (see Cooper and Dewe 2004). This scale combines the assessment of events that are considered stressful and ratings of the perceived severity of stress associated with these events, which reflect respondents' appraisals. The CHUS is a revision of earlier and longer versions of separate hassles and uplifts scales (Kanner et al. 1981). Several improvements were made in this revised version, including eliminating items that could be confounded with health outcomes.

In the instructions for the CHUS, *hassles* and *uplifts* are defined respectively as "irritants that can range from minor annoyances to fairly major pressures, problems, or difficulties," and "events that make you feel good." A time period for assessment is established (the past week or month; see Lazarus and Folkman 1989). Respondents are asked to consider how much each item served as a hassle (or uplift) during the specified time period, and then rate each item on a 4-point response scale, ranging from 0 = none or not applicable to 3 = a great deal. Two scores can be derived for hassles: frequency of occurrence (sum of the number of items with rating above 0), and severity (average of all item ratings). Previous research indicates that the hassles portion of the CHUS is an accurate measure of psychological stress (Lazarus and Folkman 1989). The manual for the measure (i.e., Lazarus and Folkman 1989) is available through mindgarden.com, and copies of the measure can be purchased through that website for $1 per administration or less, depending on how many are ordered.

7.2.3.1.2 Perceived Stress Scale

The Perceived Stress Scale (PSS) was developed by Sheldon Cohen and colleagues (Cohen et al. 1983). Cohen has produced a strong program of research focusing on how various psychological variables, including stress particularly, may influence the body's immune system. Cohen (1986) argued that the PSS provides a superior assessment of psychological stress compared to measures of hassles developed by Lazarus and colleagues, even though he also bases his assessment of stress on Lazarus's theoretical model. The PSS was originally developed as a 14-item measure to assess "the degree to which situations in one's life are appraised as stressful" (Cohen and Williamson 1988, 385). Cohen and Williamson (1988, 387) also stated that the PSS was "designed to tap the degree to which respondents found their lives unpredictable, uncontrollable, and overloading." A 10-item version of the PSS is considered preferable because of its stronger factor structure and slightly better internal consistency (Cohen and Williamson 1988). A 4-item version is available for use in telephone interviews and when administration time needs to be as brief as possible. Respondents are asked how often they have had certain feelings and thoughts during the previous month, using a 5-point response scale ranging from 0 = never to 4 = very often. Some items are reverse-scored, then all items are summed to form the scale score.

Research has provided evidence of acceptable internal consistency and strong validity of PSS scores (e.g., Cohen and Williamson 1988). The PSS was designed for use with a community adult sample and has been translated into many different languages. The scale can be used for free for research purposes. However, permission needs to be obtained if the scale is to be used for profit. Details about obtaining this permission, as well as other information about this measure (including versions in other languages) can be obtained through Sheldon Cohen's website (http://www.psy. cmu.edu/~scohen/).

7.2.3.2 Assessment of Coping

One's theoretical definition of coping influences how one identifies and measures coping behaviors. The assessment of coping has a rocky history, and a multitude of measures exist (Skinner et al. 2003). Certainly, there is much overlap between the many coping behaviors assessed by different instruments. Some researchers (Cook and Heppner 1997; Parker and Endler 1992) have provided evidence that three basic dimensions are being measured in many different coping scales: (1) problem-focused coping, which refers to strategies used to solve a problem or minimize its effects; (2) emotion-oriented coping, which refers to strategies used to manage the emotions related to the problem, including seeking social support; and (3) avoidance-oriented coping, which refers to strategies used to avoid a stressful situation. Using the combined qualitative–quantitative methodology of concept mapping, Gol and Cook (2004) identified nine clusters of coping responses organized within two dimensions: an approach–avoidance dimension and an emotional equilibrium–disequilibrium dimension. Based on an extensive analysis of many different coping measures, both empirically and rationally derived, Skinner et al. (2003) concluded that five coping categories underlie most coping measures: problem solving, support seeking, avoidance, distraction, and positive cognitive restructuring. Several other categories were considered as strong candidates (rumination, helplessness, social withdrawal, and emotional regulation) or as deserving further consideration (information seeking, negotiation, opposition). We shall describe three measures that tap into these primary dimensions of coping: the COPE Inventory, the Coping Inventory for Stressful Situations, and the Problem-Focused Styles of Coping, as well as a measure assessing religiously oriented types of coping, the RCOPE inventory.

7.2.3.2.1 COPE Inventory

The COPE Inventory (Carver et al. 1989) consists of 60 items assessing "the different ways in which people respond to stress" (p. 267). The inventory taps into a wide variety of coping strategies through 15 scales, each represented by 4 items. The COPE has been used to assess both dispositional as well as situational aspects of coping, and instructions for the measures can be changed to reflect these different orientations. Respondents report how often they use a response indicated in each item on a 4-point scale ranging from 1 = don't do this at all, to 4 = do this a lot. Item scores are summed to form scale scores. Carver et al. (1989) provided evidence supporting the validity of COPE scale scores, although it should be noted that the reliability of some of the scale scores has been less than desirable in some studies (e.g., Cronbach's alpha <.70 for several scale scores in Carver et al. 1989). A brief version of the COPE has been developed, with 14 scales consisting of only two items each (Carver 1997). Understandably, the internal consistencies of some scale scores in the brief COPE are relatively low (i.e., Cronbach's alpha coefficient below .60).

Carver et al. (1989) and others (e.g., Litman 2006) have examined how the COPE scales can be grouped into higher order factors. Findings from these studies indicate that the 15 COPE scales can be grouped generally into three or four higher order factors representing problem-focused, emotion-focused, avoidance-oriented, and social support dimensions. The COPE Turning to Religion scale often has loaded on its own distinctive factor. Carver (2007) recommended that those who want to use a higher order factor structure for the COPE should analyze their own data to determine the composition of such higher order factors. A primary advantage of the COPE is that it assesses a broad range of coping strategies when not using these higher order factors. The COPE is available for use without charge and without need for permission (see http://www.psy.miami.edu/faculty/ccarver/CCscales.html for further information on this measure).

7.2.3.2.2 Coping Inventory for Stressful Situations

The Coping Inventory for Stressful Situations (CISS; Endler and Parker 1994, 1999) consists of 48 items that assess three broad dimensions of coping: task-oriented, emotion-oriented, and avoidance-oriented. The current version of the CISS is a refinement of Endler and Parker's (1990) Multidimensional Coping Inventory. The avoidance-oriented scale can be divided into two subscales assessing distraction and social diversion. Respondents to the CISS are asked to indicate how much they engage in activities represented by the items when they "encounter a difficult, stressful, or upsetting situation" (Endler and Parker 1990, 847), using a 5-point response scale ranging from 1 = not at all, to 5 = very much. Item responses are summed to form scale scores. The original measure was designed to be a dispositional measure of coping, but a shorter, 21-item version of the CISS is available to assess coping in response to identified potentially stressful situations. Strong support exists for the psychometric properties of the CISS scale scores (see Endler and Parker 1999). The internal consistency of scores for the three primary scales is consistently high in various samples, having Cronbach's alpha coefficients greater than .80. (Cronbach's alphas for the two avoidance-oriented subscales are slightly lower but generally above .70.) Six-week test–retest correlations are statistically significant and all above .50. It is notable that the factor structure of the CISS has been empirically supported in several different studies (e.g., McWilliams et al. 2003). Evidence for the validity of scale scores is also strong, generally demonstrating expected associations with measures of psychopathology, health problems, and other measures of coping. A version of the CISS is available that is specifically designed for use with adolescents (Endler and Parker 1999).

A positive aspect of the CISS is that it assesses the three dimensions that most commonly appear in previous research on coping. Combining this conceptual strength with the existing evidence documenting the strong psychometric properties of the CISS makes it an attractive option for assessing coping. However, this measure is copyrighted and must be purchased for use. Copies of the CISS can be purchased through several internet sites, such as Multi-Health Systems, Inc. (http://www.mhs.com), where a set of 25 copies of the CISS costs $38. Also, the dispositional version of the CISS, while shorter than many available coping measures, may be longer than desired when a quick and economical assessment is desirable.

7.2.3.2.3 Problem-Focused Styles of Coping

The Problem-Focused Styles of Coping (PF-SOC; Heppner et al. 1995) is a free and relatively brief measure of coping that assesses three primary dimensions of coping. The 18-item PF-SOC was developed to assess "people's general disposition to coping with stressful events with a range of cognitive, affective, and behavioral items" (Heppner et al. 1995, 280). One specific focus during the development of this measure was to produce a measure with clearly worded items in order to decrease problems with item wording in previous coping measures. The measure was designed to provide a "broader conceptualization of problem-focused coping" (Heppner 2008, 808) and to integrate the applied problem solving and coping literatures by incorporating concepts such as adaptive coping and problem resolution (Zeidner and Saklofske 1996). Respondents are asked to indicate "how often each item describes the way you typically respond to problems," using a 5-point response scale ranging from 1 = almost never, to 5 = almost all of the time. Item responses are summed to form scale scores. The PF-SOC was originally designed to measure dispositional aspects of coping, but instructions can be modified to assess coping with specific, potentially stressful situations. Heppner et al. (1995) provided evidence for validity and reliability, including findings indicating that the PF-SOC predicted psychological distress beyond other measures of applied problem solving and coping. Instructions and a copy of the PF-SOC for use are available in an appendix at the end of this chapter. Recently, Heppner (2008) has begun work to develop valid measures of coping and applied problem solving in other cultural contexts, such as among adults in Asia (Heppner et al. 2006).

7.2.3.2.4 RCOPE

As noted earlier, as part of his research on religious and spiritual variables, Pargament has developed a comprehensive measure of religious coping, the RCOPE (Pargament et al. 2000). The 100 items from the RCOPE load onto 17 scales that assess how religiousness is involved in people's attempts to appraise, as well as cope with, stressful events. During the development of this measure, respondents were asked to identify "the most serious negative event they had experienced in the past three years" (Pargament et al. 2000, 527), and to indicate "how much or how frequently" they did what each item described on a 4-point scale ranging from 0 = not at all, to 3 = a great deal. Item responses are averaged to form scale scores.

The 17 RCOPE scales are grouped into two categories of positive and negative religious coping scales, based on previous evidence of the associations of similar scales with outcome measures. Ten scales are hypothesized to be associated with better health: religious purification/forgiveness, religious direction/conversion, religious helping, seeking support from clergy and church members, collaborative religious coping, religious focus, active religious surrender, benevolent religious reappraisal, spiritual connection, and marking religious boundaries. Seven scales are hypothesized to be associated with worse health: spiritual discontent, demonic reappraisal, passive religious deferral, interpersonal religious discontent, reappraisal of God's powers, punishing God reappraisal, and pleading for direct intercession. Pargament et al. (2000) found that the positive religious coping scales tended to be positively correlated with stress-related growth and measures of positive religious outcomes, and that the negative religious coping scales had negative correlations with measures of mental and physical health. Religious coping scales were also found to predict stress-related growth, religious outcomes, and mental and physical health variables after controlling for gender and a measure of global religiousness. Most RCOPE scale scores had good internal consistency with Cronbach's alpha coefficients greater than .80. The factor structure for the RCOPE was derived in a college student sample, but a smaller version of the RCOPE had the same factor structure confirmed in a sample of hospitalized adults.

The entire RCOPE can be overwhelming, with 100 items and 17 separate scales. However, separate scales from the RCOPE can be used by themselves or in combinations with other RCOPE scales (K. I. Pargament, personal communication). For instance, the four RCOPE scales of collaborative religious coping, active surrender, passive deferral, and pleading for direct intercession assess different religious methods to gain or relinquish control in stressful situations. These methods of religious coping are refinements of an earlier measure of religious coping, the Religious Problem Solving Scales (RPSS; Pargament et al. 1988). Pargament (2007) has noted that use of quantitatively oriented spiritual assessment, such as the RCOPE and RPSS, can provide useful information that can supplement what a therapist can learn from clients through other methods, such as interviewing or conversation.

7.3 CURRENT FINDINGS

7.3.1 STRESS, COPING, AND PSYCHOLOGICAL DISTRESS

Questions about the nature of stress and coping have relevance for the study of the development of psychopathology and the treatment of mental illness. Holahan et al. (1996) pointed out that "coping is a stabilizing factor that can help individuals maintain psychosocial adaptation during stressful periods ... " Thus, it naturally follows that under conditions of stress, when coping behaviors become inadequate, an individual may no longer be able to function adaptively. This concept is reflected repeatedly in the *Diagnostic and Statistical Manual of Mental Disorders* (Fourth Edition; Text Revision; American Psychiatric Association, 2000), which specifies that the symptoms for many disorders must "cause clinically significant distress or impairment in social, occupational, or other important areas of functioning." When adaptive functioning has been disrupted, the primary clinical goal is often re-establishing effective coping in order to reduce excessive levels of stress.

Many research studies have been conducted that examine associations between how people cope with stress and both mental and physical health outcomes. When reviewing coping research, Folkman and Moskowitz (2004, 747) noted that, "We have learned that coping is a complex, multidimensional process that is sensitive both to the environment, and its demands and resources, and to personality dispositions that influence the appraisal of stress and resources for coping." They also noted that it has been demonstrated that coping is "strongly associated with the regulation of emotion, especially distress, throughout the stress process." The only generalization these authors could make about more specific associations is that certain kinds of avoidant or escapist coping strategies have been regularly associated with psychological distress. Through a meta-analysis of several studies using an early measure of coping, Penley et al. (2002) found that several emotion-focused coping strategies had negative associations with health, a specific form of problem-focused coping (i.e., confrontive coping) had negative associations with health, and a more general form of problem-focused coping had positive associations with health. Penley et al. (2002, 591) also found that "the adaptiveness or maladaptiveness of a particular coping strategy typically depends on the type of health outcome, as well as stressor characteristics."

Kleinke (2007, 305) provided the following summary of the research on coping with stress:

- *Successful copers* respond to life challenges by taking responsibility for finding a solution to their problems. They approach problems with a sense of competence and mastery. Their goal is to assess the situation, get advice and support from others, and work out a plan that will be in their best interest. Successful copers use life challenges as an opportunity for personal growth, and they attempt to face these challenges with hope, patience, and a sense of humor.
- *Unsuccessful copers* respond to life challenges with denial and avoidance. They either withdraw from problems or react impulsively without taking the time and effort to seek the best solution. Unsuccessful copers are angry and aggressive or depressed and passive. They blame themselves or others for their problems and don't appreciate the value of approaching life challenges with a sense of hope, mastery, and personal control.

7.3.2 GENDER DIFFERENCES IN COPING

A significant area of focus in the coping research has been in the area of gender differences in coping and subsequent changes in distress. It seems particularly relevant to explore gender differences as they apply to eating disorders, since anorexia nervosa and bulimia nervosa are diagnosed more often in women than men (Fairburn et al. 2008). Therefore, it is helpful to explore how women cope with personal problems. Aldwin (1994) cited evidence indicating that gender differences in seeking social support begin to emerge between the ages of 6 and 9 years, with girls seeking more support than boys. Overall, however, some studies find that women use more emotion-focused strategies than men, yet others find that women use more problem-focused strategies (Amirkhan 1994). A few studies examining gender differences in coping are highlighted next.

McDaniel and Richards (1990) explored gender differences in how college students cope with sad mood. A small group of college students who reported experiencing depressive feelings during the last year and did not seek professional assistance to cope with those feelings were interviewed about the nature of the problem, the coping behaviors they used, and the consistency and effectiveness of coping. The results indicated that women reported sadder mood than men, both retrospectively and currently. Further, men reported using more coping techniques than women and tended to use relaxation, self-reward, and situation changes more frequently. The researchers concluded that "women profit more from more 'emotion-focused' techniques ... whereas men profit from more 'problem-focused' procedures ... "

Nolen-Hoeksema (1990) argued that one explanation for the consistent finding that approximately twice as many adult women are depressed as adult men may be found in sex differences in response to depression that stem from gender stereotypes:

> Women appear more likely to engage in ruminative responses when depressed, thereby amplifying their symptoms and extending depressive episodes. Men appear more likely to distract themselves from depressed moods, thereby dampening their symptoms ... Being active and controlling one's moods are part of the masculine stereotype; being inactive and emotional are part of the feminine stereotype. (Nolen-Hoeksema 1990, 169–171)

Ruminating can be conceptualized as an emotion-focused coping strategy. Ruminations are defined as thoughts and behaviors that focus an individual's attention inward to his or her depressed state, and the research indicates that such a response serves to exacerbate and extend a depressive episode.

Ptacek et al. (1992) explored the relationship between gender, appraisal, and coping. College undergraduates recorded daily information about the most stressful event of the day for 21 consecutive days. The researchers found evidence to support a socialization hypothesis of coping, which suggests that men and women are socialized to cope with stressful events in different ways. Sex role stereotypes and gender role expectations serve to socialize men to deal instrumentally with stress while women are socialized to express emotion, use emotion-focused coping behaviors, and seek the support of others.

Hamilton and Fagot (1988) compared college undergraduate coping strategies to test the theory that men use instrumental coping strategies more frequently than women, and that women employ more emotion-focused behaviors. With the exception of women reporting more overall stress, no gender differences emerged for frequency of stressful events or proportion of problem-solving behavior. The researchers suggested that the results of studies, which find a difference in coping behaviors between men and women (i.e., women use emotional expressiveness to a greater degree while men exhibit higher levels of active problem solving),

> may be due, in part, to differential recall of female-specific events using retrospective methods. Moreover, stressors that involve interpersonal conflict may not be addressed as effectively with instrumentality and are perhaps solved more easily by self-soothing strategies such as asking advice from friends ... the ability to use both instrumental and expressive modes of coping seems important for both men and women in daily living, and both modes are differentially applied to stressful events. (Hamilton and Fagot 1988, 822)

In sum, the researchers found no evidence to support the hypothesis that men and women differ in the actual coping behaviors they use, but they raise some interesting questions about the possibility of differential recall of stressors and the resulting effect on coping assessment.

Although many studies have produced evidence to indicate that women report more psychological distress than men (e.g., Higgins and Endler 1995), research regarding gender differences in coping remains equivocal. It has long been believed that women use emotion-focused coping to a greater extent than men, and there is some support for this belief (e.g., Ptacek et al. 1994). There is also support for the belief that men use more problem-focused coping (e.g., Ptacek et al. 1994). Other researchers have found little evidence of gender differences (e.g., Porter and Stone 1995).

7.4   APPLICATIONS

Now, we can apply what we know about stress and coping to the task of assisting someone with an eating disorder. Disordered eating can be conceptualized as a maladaptive way of coping. It follows that one way of helping someone caught in the dangerous cycle of an eating disorder is to help that individual evaluate the effectiveness of her current coping behaviors and assist the person in developing more effective coping techniques. Indeed, some psychotherapy treatment approaches to eating disorders employ specific techniques to modify coping strategies in response to high-risk situations (Fairburn et al. 2008). Following are some guidelines and suggestions based on relevant research for assisting a person exhibiting an eating disorder.

Neckowitz and Morrison (1991) investigated the coping strategies reportedly used by bulimic women when coping with a stressor involving someone known intimately and someone not known intimately. Results indicated that bulimic women differed from a comparison group in that they felt more of a sense of threat and made greater use of avoidant coping behaviors. The dilemma of using avoidance as a coping strategy is highlighted by this excerpt from Neckowitz and Morrison (1991, 1167):

> Undue reliance on escape–avoidance as a coping option can be hazardous … Over the long term, this can interfere with the processes of information seeking, anticipation, and planning that are often necessary for developing an effective response to threat or challenge. With the development of potential steps of positive action disrupted, the sense of instrumentality, interpersonal effectiveness, and agentic self-esteem would predictably be diminished, and chronic feelings of pessimism and apathy may develop … In turn, this would understandably contribute to continued reliance on avoidant coping styles rather than active responses to stressors.

It seems logical, then, that one focus of treatment of an eating disorder among women would be to assess the effectiveness of an individual's current coping behaviors and assist her in finding more adaptive coping behaviors.

In their exploration of coping behaviors in eating-disordered women, Troop et al. (1994) also found that women diagnosed with an eating disorder relied more on avoidant coping behaviors than did women in a normal comparison group. However, there was no difference between the two groups in their use of problem-focused coping strategies. There was no relationship between coping behaviors and the severity of the eating disorder; however, in women with anorexia nervosa or bulimia nervosa, avoidant coping behaviors were positively related to symptoms of depression. The researchers suggested that when treating an individual with an eating disorder, it may prove helpful to include a focus on methods to improve the efficacy of coping efforts. Perhaps, teaching women with eating disorders how to purposely avoid being avoidant could be a useful intervention. However, research in this area so far cannot produce definitive conclusions concerning whether such interventions might truly be effective.

It is important to have a good understanding of how a person copes in a variety of situations as well as how a person appraises the stressors in his or her life. An understanding of the cognitive processes involved in coping is important in planning interventions for reducing maladaptive responses to stress (Horowitz 1997). Lightsey (1996) offered several recommendations for counselors based on his review of literature concerning the psychological resources of positive thoughts, hardiness, generalized self-efficacy, and optimism. Specifically, he recommended that clinicians "help the client to develop active problem-solving skills" and "teach a variety of coping skills, because some contexts require skills other than active problem solving."

One way to explore how people cope with different problems is to ask them, very specifically, how they typically deal with common problems in a variety of domains. It should not be assumed that disordered eating is how the individual copes with *all* of the problems in her life; there is likely to be at least one stressor with which the individual deals effectively. Ask the individual how she copes with problems in her family (e.g., What do you do when your parents fight? What do you do when you fight with your brother or your sister?), at school (e.g., How do you react when you get a disappointing grade on a test or an assignment?), and with her friends (e.g., How do you cope when you have a disagreement with a friend?). It is important to thoroughly explore all areas of the individual's life, even those that do not appear to be directly related to her eating disorder, with the goal of delineating areas in which she appears to cope effectively as well as areas that appear to be plagued by problematic coping strategies.

The next step is to ask the individual how well the coping strategy she is using for any particular problem appears to be working for her. Is she accomplishing her goal? How would she like things to be different? Once she has identified areas in need of change, the task then becomes one of finding better and more effective ways of coping. One way to accomplish this is by discussing areas in which she appears to be coping well. Even effective coping with a relatively small and specific problem may be generalized to a larger, more complex problem. For example, suppose the individual states that although she makes good grades in math and actually enjoys solving complex algebra problems, she feels overwhelmed by the demands of school, a regular babysitting job, and participation in athletics. It may be possible to help her reduce her avoidant responses to these situations and draw on her more basic and logical problem-solving techniques.

However, it is important not to assume that there is one "best" style of coping. It is often tempting to consider problem-focused coping as more effective with all problems, but that is not always true. For example, it may prove more adaptive to use an avoidant or emotion-focused coping strategy when faced with a situation about which nothing can be done (e.g., a terminally ill friend), and a more problem-focused coping strategy when the problem does have a potential solution (e.g., a flat tire). More research is needed in this area to determine when certain coping strategies would be adaptive.

Once situations have been identified in which a person's coping responses do not seem adaptive and are actually increasing distress, one can work with her in generating alternative coping behaviors. Has she ever faced a similar problem in the past? How did she cope with that problem? Would those same coping behaviors work in this situation? How would she like things to be different, and how can she accomplish that objective? Educating the individual about basic problem-solving strategies (e.g., D'Zurilla and Nezu 1982) can also be helpful.

APPENDIX 7.A THE PROBLEM-FOCUSED STYLES OF COPING (PF-SOC), P. PAUL HEPPNER, STEPHEN W. COOK, DEBORAH M. WRIGHT, AND W. CALVIN JOHNSON, JR.

The Problem-Focused Styles of Coping (PF-SOC: Heppner et al. 1995) is an 18-item questionnaire that measures the degree to which adults use cognitive, behavioral, and affective strategies to resolve the variety of personal problems in their lives. The PF-SOC provides scores for the following coping styles:

Reflective Style: This is a primarily cognitive coping style that describes the tendency to plan, reflect, and examine causes when dealing with personal problems. This coping style generally conveys efforts to approach or engage in the resolution of problems.

Reactive Style: This is a coping style that includes primarily emotional and cognitive responses that deplete the individual or distort attempts to solve problems. People who score high on this factor tend to respond impulsively or be confused in response to personal problems, which tends to inhibit effective problem resolution.

Suppressive Style: This coping style describes a tendency to avoid or deny when responding to personal problems. This style portrays escapism, confusion, and a lack of persistence when coping, which inhibit successful problem resolution.

As conveyed in the definitions, the three coping scales describe both a particular style of dealing with problems and the degree to which coping responses are leading to the successful resolution of problems. The Reflective Style describes generally successful efforts to resolve problems, while the Reactive and Suppressive Styles describe generally a lack of progress toward resolving problems. Initial information about the reliability and validity of the PF-SOC can be found in Heppner et al. (1995). This questionnaire has been used primarily with college student samples. Following are the ranges of mean scores and standard deviations in three samples of women college students from two universities in the Midwest and Southwestern United States ($N = 93$ to 380; Heppner et al. 1995): *Reflective Style*: $M = 20.0$ to 22.9, $SD = 4.9$ to 5.6; *Reactive Style*: $M = 12.0$ to 14.4, $SD = 3.6$ to 4.0; and *Suppressive Style*: $M = 12.3$ to 13.1, $SD = 3.6$ to 4.2.

To score the PF-SOC, enter the responses in the corresponding blanks below and sum the responses for each scale.

Reflective: _____ + _____ + _____ + _____ + _____ + _____ + _____ = _____
             3   4   6   11   12   14   17   Total

Reactive: _____ + _____ + _____ + _____ + _____ = _____
           7   8   9   13   15   Total

Suppressive: _____ + _____ + _____ + _____ + _____ + _____ = _____
             1   2   5   10   16   18   Total

The authors would appreciate any information concerning the results you obtain using the PF-SOC. Please send such information to P. Paul Heppner, PhD, 16 Hill Hall, Department of Educational and Counseling Psychology, University of Missouri-Columbia, Columbia, MO 65211, or e-mail: HeppnerP@missouri.edu. If you would like additional information about this measure, please contact P. Paul Heppner, PhD, at the same address. Thank you.

THE PROBLEM-FOCUSED STYLES OF COPING (PF-SOC)

Directions

This inventory contains statements about how people think, feel, and behave as they attempt to resolve personal difficulties and problems in their day-to-day lives. These are personal problems that come up from time to time, such as feeling depressed, getting along with friends, choosing a career, or deciding whether to get married or divorced. In considering how you deal with such problems, think about successful and unsuccessful outcomes, and what hinders or helps you in solving these problems. Please respond to the items as honestly as possible so as to accurately portray how frequently you do what is described in each item. *Do not respond to the items as you think you should*; rather respond in a way that most accurately reflects how you actually think, feel, and behave when you solve personal problems. Some people may find that a number of these items are typical of their responses all of the time, other items are occasionally used, while others are almost never typical of their responses. For example, consider this statement: I think about past failures to help me solve my problems. If you do this often, you would indicate number 4 on the questionnaire. Please read each statement and indicate how often each item describes the way you typically respond to problems. In doing so, use the following alternatives:

1. ALMOST NEVER
2. OCCASIONALLY
3. ABOUT HALF OF THE TIME
4. OFTEN
5. ALMOST ALL OF THE TIME

Please Begin

_____ 1. I am not really sure what I think or believe about my problems.
_____ 2. I don't sustain my actions long enough to really solve my problems.

_____ 3. I think about ways that I solved similar problems in the past.

_____ 4. I identify the causes of my emotions, which helps me identify and solve my problems.

_____ 5. I feel so frustrated I just give up doing any work on my problems at all.

_____ 6. I consider the short-term and long-term consequences of each possible solution to my problems.

_____ 7. I get preoccupied thinking about my problems and overemphasize some parts of them.

_____ 8. I continue to feel uneasy about my problems, which tells me I need to do some more work.

_____ 9. My old feelings get in the way of solving current problems.

_____ 10. I spend my time doing unrelated chores and activities instead of acting on my problems.

_____ 11. I think ahead, which enables me to anticipate and prepare for problems before they arise.

_____ 12. I think my problems through in a systematic way.

_____ 13. I misread another person's motives and feelings without checking with the person to see if my conclusions are correct.

_____ 14. I get in touch with my feelings to identify and work on problems.

_____ 15. I act too quickly, which makes my problems worse.

_____ 16. I have a difficult time concentrating on my problems (i.e., my mind wanders).

_____ 17. I have alternate plans for solving my problems in case my first attempt does not work.

_____ 18. I avoid even thinking about my problems.

Source: Copyright © 1995 by the American Psychological Association. Adapted with permission. Heppner, P. P., S. W. Cook, D. M. Wright, & W. C. Johnson, Jr. 1995. Progress in resolving problems: A problem-focused style of coping. *J Couns Psychol* 42: 279–293.

REFERENCES

Aldwin, C. M. 1994. *Stress, coping, and development.* New York: The Guilford Press.

American Psychiatric Association. 2000. *Diagnostic and statistical manual of mental disorders* (4th ed.). Washington, DC: American Psychiatric Association.

Amirkhan, J. H. 1994. Seeking person-related predictors of coping: Exploratory analyses. *Eur J of Pers* 8: 13–30.

Amirkhan, J. H., R. T. Risinger, and R. J. Swickert. 1995. Extraversion: A "hidden" personality factor in coping? *J Pers* 63: 189–212.

Banyard, V. L., and S. A. Graham-Bermann. 1993. Can women cope? A gender analysis of theories of coping with stress. *Psychol Women Q* 17: 303–318.

Carver, C. S. 1997. You want to measure coping but your protocol's too long: Consider the Brief COPE. *Int J Behav Med* 4:92–100.

Carver, C. S. 2007. *COPE (complete version).* Retrieved from University of Miami website: http://www.psy.miami.edu/faculty/ccarver/sclCOPEF.html.

Carver, C. S., and M. F. Scheier. 1994. Situational coping and coping dispositions in a stressful transaction. *J Pers Soc Psychol* 66: 184–195.

Carver, C. S., M. F. Scheier, and J. K. Weintraub. 1989. Assessing coping strategies: A theoretically based approach. *J Pers Soc Psychol* 56:267–283.

Cassidy, T., and E. Burnside. 1996. Cognitive appraisal, vulnerability and coping: An integrative analysis of appraisal and coping mechanisms. *Couns Psychol Q* 9: 261–279.

Cohen, S. 1986. Contrasting the Hassles Scale and the Perceived Stress Scale: Who's really measuring appraised stress? *Am Psychol* 41:716–718.

Cohen. S., T. Kamarck, and R. Mermelstein. 1983. A global measure of perceived stress. *J Health Soc Behav* 24:385–396.

Cohen, S., and G. M. Williamson. 1988. Perceived stress in a probability sample of the United States. In *The social psychology of health: Claremont symposium on applied social psychology,* ed. S. Spacapam and S. Oskamp, 31–67. Newbury Park, CA: Sage.

Cook, S. W., and P. P. Heppner. 1997. A psychometric study of three coping measures. *Educ and Psychol Meas* 57: 906–923.

Cooper, C. L., and P. Dewe. 2004. *Stress: A brief history*. Malden, MA: Blackwell.

DeLongis, A., J. C. Coyne, G. Dakof, S. Folkman, and R. S. Lazarus. 1982. Relationship of daily hassles, uplifts, and major life events to health status. *Health Psychol* 1: 119–136.

DeLongis, A., S. Folkman, and R. S. Lazarus. 1988. The impact of daily stress on health and mood: Psychological and social resources as mediators. *J Pers Soc Psychol* 54: 486–495.

Derogatis, L. R., and H. L. Coons. 1993. Self-report measures of stress. In *Handbook of stress* (2nd ed), ed. L. Goldberger and S. Breznitz, 200–233. New York: Free Press.

D'Zurilla, T. J., and A. M. Nezu. 1982. Social problem solving in adults. In *Advances in cognitive-behavioral research and therapy*, ed. P. C. Kendall, 202–274. New York: Academic Press.

Endler, N. S., and J. D. A. Parker. 1990. Multidimensional assessment of coping: A critical evaluation. *J Pers Soc Psychol* 58: 844–854.

Endler, N. S., and J. D. A. Parker. 1994. Assessment of multidimensional coping: Task, emotion, and avoidance strategies. *Psychol Assess* 6: 50–60.

Endler, N. S., and J. D. A. Parker. 1999. *Coping Inventory for Stressful Situations (CISS)* (2nd ed). Toronto: Multi-Health Systems.

Fairburn, C. G., Z. Cooper, R. Shafran, and G. T. Wilson. 2008. Eating disorders: A transdiagnostic protocol. In *Clinical handbook of psychological disorders: A step-by-step treatment manual* (4th ed), ed. D. H. Barlow, 578–614. New York: The Guilford Press.

Folkman, S., and J. D. Moskowitz. 2004. Coping: Pitfalls and promise. *Annu Rev Psychol* 55: 745–774.

Gol, A. R., and S. W. Cook. 2004. Exploring the underlying dimensions of coping: A concept mapping approach. *J Soc Clin Psychol* 23:155–171.

Hamilton, S., and B. I. Fagot. 1988. Chronic stress and coping styles: A comparison of male and female undergraduates. *J Pers Soc Psychol* 55: 819–823.

Haan, N. 1993. The assessment of coping, defense, and stress. In *Handbook of stress: Theoretical and clinical aspects* (2nd ed), ed. L. Goldberger and S. Breznitz, 258–273. New York: The Free Press.

Heppner, P. P. 2008. Expanding the conceptualization and measurement of applied problem solving and coping: From stages to dimensions to the almost forgotten cultural context. *Am Psychol* 63: 805–816.

Heppner, P. P., S. W. Cook, D. M. Wright, and C. W. Johnson, Jr. 1995. Progress in resolving problems: A problem-focused style of coping. *J Couns Psychol* 42: 279–293.

Heppner, P. P., M. J. Heppner, D.-G. Lee, Y.-W. Wang, H.-J. Park, and L.-F. Wang. 2006. Development and validation of a collectivist coping styles inventory. *J Couns Psychol* 53: 107–125.

Higgins, J. E., and N. S. Endler. 1995. Coping, life stress, and psychological and somatic distress. *Eur J Pers* 9: 253–270.

Holahan, C. J., R. H. Moos, and J. A. Schaefer. 1996. Coping, stress resistance, and growth; Conceptualizing adaptive functioning. In *Handbook of coping: Theory, research, applications*, ed. M. Zeidner and N.S. Endler, 24–43. New York: John Wiley & Sons.

Horowitz, M. J. 1997. *Formulation as a basis for planning psychotherapy treatment*. Washington, DC: American Psychiatric Press.

Kanner, A. D., J. C. Coyne, C. Schaefer, and R. S. Lazarus. 1981. Comparison of two modes of stress measurement: Daily hassles and uplifts versus major life events. *J Behav Med* 4: 1–39.

Kelly, W. L. 1991. *Psychology of the unconscious: Mesmer, Janet, Freud, Jung, and current issues*. New York: Prometheus Books.

Kleinke, C. L. 2007. What does it mean to cope? In *Stress and coping*, ed. A. Monat, R. S. Lazarus, and G. Reevy, 289–308. Westport, CT: Praeger.

Lazarus, R. S. 1990. Theory-based stress measurement. *Psychol Inq* 1: 3–13.

Lazarus, R. S., and S. Folkman. 1984. *Stress, appraisal, and coping*. New York: Springer.

Lazarus, R. S., and S. Folkman. 1989. *Hassles and uplifts scales: Sampler set, manual, instrument, and scoring guide*. Retrieved from Mind Garden, Inc. website: www.mindgarden.com.

Lightsey, O. R. 1996. What leads to wellness? The role of psychological resources in well-being. *Couns Psychol* 24: 589–735.

Litman, J. A. 2006. The COPE inventory: Dimensionality and relationships with approach- and avoidance-motives and positive and negative traits. *Pers Individ Differences* 41: 273–284.

McDaniel, D. M., and C. S. Richards. 1990. Coping with dysphoria: Gender differences in college students. *J Clin Psychol* 46: 896–899.

McWilliams, L. A., B. J. Cox, and M. W. Enns. 2003. Use of the Coping Inventory for Stressful Situations in a clinically depressed sample: Factor structure, personality correlates, and prediction of distress. *J Clin Psychol* 59: 423–437.

Monat, A., R. Lazarus, and G. Reevy. 2007. *The Praeger handbook on stress and coping.* Westport, CT: Praeger.

Neckowitz, P., and T. L. Morrison. 1991. Interactional coping strategies of normal-weight bulimic women in intimate and nonintimate stressful situations, *Psychol Rep* 69: 1167–1175.

Nolen-Hoeksema, S. 1990. *Sex differences in depression.* Stanford, CA: Stanford Univ. Press.

Pargament, K. I. 2007. *Spiritually integrated psychotherapy: Understanding and addressing the sacred.* New York: Guilford.

Pargament, K. I., G. G. Ano, and A. B. Wachholtz. 2005. The religious dimension of coping: Advances in theory, research, and practice. In *Handbook of the psychology of religion and spirituality,* ed. R. F. Paloutzian and C. L. Park, 479–495. New York: Guilford.

Pargament, K. I., J. Kennell, W. Hathaway, N. Grevengoed, J. Newman, and W. Jones. 1988. Religion and the problem-solving process: Three styles of coping. *J Sci Study Religion* 27: 90–104.

Pargament, K. I., H. G. Koenig, and L. M. Perez. 2000. The many methods of religious coping: Development and initial validation of the RCOPE. *J Clin Psychol* 56: 519–543.

Pargament, K. I., G. M. Magyar-Russell, and N. A. Murray-Swank. 2005. The sacred and the search for significance: Religion as a unique process. *J Soc Issues* 61: 665–687.

Parker, J. D., and N. S. Endler. 1992. Coping with coping assessment: A critical review. *Eur J Pers* 6: 321–344.

Parkes, K. R. 1994. Personality and coping as moderators of work stress processes: Models, methods, and measures. *Work Stress* 8: 110–129.

Penley, J. A., J. Tomaka, and J. S. Wiebe. 2002. The association of coping to physical and psychological health outcomes: A meta-analytic review. *J Behav Med* 25: 551–603.

Porter, L. S., and A. A. Stone. 1995. Are there really gender differences in coping?: A reconsideration of previous data and results from a daily study. *J Soc Clin Psychol* 14: 184–202.

Ptacek, J. T., R. E. Smith, and K. L. Dodge. 1994. Gender differences in coping with stress: When stressor and appraisals do not differ. *Pers Soc Psychol Bull* 20: 421–430.

Ptacek, J. T., R. E. Smith, and J. Zanas. 1992. Gender, appraisal, and coping: A longitudinal analysis. *J Pers* 60: 747–770.

Richards, P. S., R. K. Hardman, and M. E. Berrett. 2007. *Spiritual approaches in the treatment of women with eating disorders.* Washington, DC: American Psychological Association.

Selye, H. 1993. History of the stress concept. In *Handbook of stress: Theoretical and clinical aspects* (2nd ed), ed. L. Goldberger and S. Breznitz, 7–17. New York: The Free Press.

Shevrin, H., J. A. Bond, L. A. W. Brakel, R. K. Hertel, and W. J. Williams. 1996. *Conscious and unconscious processes: Psychodynamic, cognitive, and neurophysiological convergences.* New York: The Guilford Press.

Skinner, E. A., K. Edge, J. Altman, and H. Sherwood. 2003. Searching for the structure of coping: A review and critique of category systems for classifying ways of coping. *Psychol Bull* 129: 216–269.

Snyder, C. R., and K. M. Pulvers. 2001. Dr. Seuss, the coping machine, and "Oh, the places you'll go." In *Coping with stress: Effective people and processes,* ed. C. R. Snyder, 3–29. Oxford: Oxford Univ. Press.

Troop, N. A., A. Holbrey, R. Trowler, and J. L. Treasure. 1994. Ways of coping in women with eating disorders. *J Nervous Ment Dis,* 182: 535–540.

Worthington, E. L., Jr., and J. D. Aten. 2009. Psychotherapy with religious and spiritual clients: An introduction. *J Clin Psychol* 65: 123–130.

Yerkes, R. M., and J. D. Dodson. 1908. The relation of strength of stimulus to rapidity of habit-formation. *J Comp Neurol Psychol* 18: 459–482.

Zeidner, M., and D. Saklofske. 1996. Adaptive and maladaptive coping. In *Handbook of coping: Theory, research, applications,* ed. M. Zeidner and N. S. Endler, 505–531. New York: Wiley.

Part III

Society and Eating Disorders

8 Family Dynamics

Annette S. Kluck, James R. Clopton, and Jan Snider Kent

CONTENTS

8.1 LEARNING OBJECTIVES

After completing this chapter, you should be able to

- Identify family characteristics thought to be of clinical significance in contributing to eating disorders
- Recognize which family variables have been empirically shown to be related to eating disorders and which have been shown to be unrelated
- Explain what is done in family therapy sessions when a girl or young woman has an eating disorder
- Discuss tools for the assessment and treatment of eating disorders from a perspective that incorporates the family

8.2   BACKGROUND AND SIGNIFICANCE

Researchers and clinicians have a long history of interest in the role that the family-of-origin plays in the development of various psychopathological conditions, including eating disorders. The interest in the potential etiological role of a young woman's family in the course of an eating disorder extends back over 200 years. In 1789, Naudeau (as cited in Minuchin et al. 1978) suggested that a patient's mother was the cause of an anorexic woman's death. Early researchers and clinicians exploring the familial determinants of eating disorders focused upon relationship-based family factors in the pathogenesis of a young woman's illness. Among the earliest well-developed etiological models grounded in family dynamics were those proposed by Salvador Minuchin (Minuchin et al. 1978) and by Hilda Bruch (1978), both of whom based their models on their clinical experiences in treating young women with anorexia. Minuchin and his colleagues (1978) identified four aspects of family relationships that seemed to differentiate the families of his anorexic patients from other families: (1) enmeshment, whereby family members have difficulty separating themselves emotionally and psychologically from one another resulting in a lack of autonomy; (2) rigidity, which is an inflexibility of family roles, restricting the ability of the family to adapt as a child develops; (3) overprotectiveness, when families are hypersensitive to potential distress and limit exposure to potential sources of distress, making it difficult for a child to develop adaptive ways of responding to stressors; and (4) lack of conflict resolution, which may involve denial of conflict or avoidance by not directly dealing with the conflict (or inclusion of the child in conflict between the parents).

Bruch's (1978) description of the families of anorexics also included enmeshment. In addition to the characteristics noted by Minuchin's group, Bruch observed that families of individuals with anorexia tended to have a strong appearance focus, to place great emphasis on achievement, and generally to avoid or to display little emotional expression. She found that the families of such individuals present themselves as being normal and happy.

Since the time that early theorists described eating disorders as a problem of the family, researchers have extended their efforts to other contextual factors outside the family (e.g., mass media) in attempts to delineate the development of eating disorders. A wide range of social factors likely contribute to the pathogenesis of these illnesses, and much of the contemporary research on sociocultural contextual risk factors for the development of disordered eating behaviors focuses on the influence of the mass media (see Chapter 9) and peers (Clemens et al. 2008; Zalta and Keel 2006). Yet, the family unit is itself a unique social context that transmits messages about how to interact in one's environment and what the ideal body type for a young woman should be.

The family can be a powerful source of influence on the development of behavior since exposure to one's family environment occurs over an extended period, and as such, affects a child during critical developmental periods. At the same time, the age of onset for the majority of individuals with eating disorders, as well as their subclinical counterparts, is before age 25 (van Hoeken et al. 2003). In other words, eating disorders are most commonly found when individuals are likely to have recent exposure to their family-of-origin, leaving a young woman open to the influence of her family in multiple domains, such as ways of relating to others, approaches to eating, and expectations about appearance. In fact, for an adolescent or young woman, it is likely that her family has had the most consistent and enduring *potential* to influence her development and psychological functioning. Thus, it is not surprising that family factors were a focus of early etiological theories and continue to receive substantial attention in research on the development, prevention, and treatment of eating disorders.

Research on the role of families in the development of eating disorders is grounded in four broad domains: (1) demographic family characteristics (genetics, social class, birth order, family structure), (2) family relationships (specifically, those between daughters and parents), (3) family behaviors associated with eating and appearance (eating patterns and problems, expectations about appearance, feedback about eating and appearance), and (4) individual problems within the family (e.g., the presence of mental or physical illness, sexual and physical assault). Given the research suggesting that the family may play a significant role in the development of eating disorders, it is not surprising that treatment of these disorders often is based on a family systems approach, particularly in the case of younger patients who still live at home (e.g., Gore et al. 2001).

8.3   CURRENT FINDINGS

8.3.1   DEMOGRAPHIC CHARACTERISTICS

8.3.1.1   Genetics, Biology, and Heritability

Eating disorders appear to congregate in families (Javaras et al. 2008; Strober et al. 2000), and many researchers and clinicians believe that biology plays a role in the development of eating disorders (Fichter and Noegel 1990; Kaye et al. 2005; Reichborn-Kjennerud et al. 2004). Although efforts to identify genetic factors have not led to an "eating disorder gene," researchers have identified some genetic markers that potentially play a role in the development of eating disorders. In particular, the search for genetic causes of eating disorders has included examination of genetic sequences associated with hormones and neurotransmitters (Eastwood et al. 2002; Gorwood et al. 2002; Urwin et al. 2002). To date, genes associated with the serotonergic system appear to have the most potential as contributors to the development of eating disorders (Klump and Gobrogge 2005). These studies, combined with brain imaging research, suggest that genetics may play a causal role in eating disorders via emotion regulation (Kaye et al. 2005). Researchers speculate that alterations in nutritional intake decrease emotional discomfort for those with eating disorders by changing the levels of serotonin, which may reduce the level of experienced anxiety (Kaye et al. 2005; Klump and Culbert 2007). As discussed later, high rates of comorbid psychopathology within families may, in part, reflect shared genetics among family members.

The research on genetics and eating disorders has yet to produce conclusive findings (Klump and Culbert 2007). However, other types of studies also support the notion that biology plays a role in the genesis of eating disorders. More broadly, twin and adopted sibling studies consistently support the notion that genetics are part of the diathesis of eating disorders (e.g., Culbert et al. 2009; Klump et al. 2009).

Attempts to delineate the effects of genetics is made difficult by the fact that genetics may influence the environmental experiences an individual selects (e.g., preferences regarding types of television shows or magazines), exposing some young women to additional eating disorder risk factors such as media that promotes dieting and thinness (Culbert et al. 2009). Moreover, the heritability of different symptoms of an eating disorder may not be uniform (e.g., Mazzeo et al. 2009), with the environmental influences, including those from the family, being more influential for some symptoms such as excessive concern about one's weight (Reichborn-Kjennerud et al. 2004). In addition, research using twin studies typically employs the assumption that the shared environment of monozygotic twins is no more alike than it is for dizygotic twins and siblings; yet, there are few studies that control for the probable increased similarity in shared environment for more closely related siblings. This potential flaw underlying most twin studies, combined with the variability in heritability of different symptoms, makes it difficult to identify the genetic factors, the environmental factors, and the genetically activated environmental factors in the etiology of eating disorders. Nevertheless, the likely, yet not fully understood, effects of genetic causes of eating disorders must be kept in mind when examining the role that the family environment plays in the development of these disorders.

8.3.1.2   Social Class

Historically, research seemed to suggest that eating disorders were more prevalent among individuals of upper socioeconomic classes. For example, one study found that in comparison to patients with general health problems, patients with anorexia nervosa were more likely to come from families with a higher socioeconomic status (Askevold 1982), and another research study found that patients with bulimia came from families with higher income levels than patients with anorexia (Herzog 1982). In addition, obesity has been linked with socioeconomic class because those individuals with fewer financial resources as children have been found to be more likely to struggle with obesity as adults (Olson et al. 2007). However, differences in socioeconomic class are not always found in research on eating disorders (Gard and Freeman 1996). In one study, dieting, but not more extreme symptoms of eating disorders, such as frequent purging or body mass index (BMI) below 17, was positively associated with socioeconomic class among adolescent girls (Rogers et al. 1997). What has yet to be determined is the manner in which correlates of socioeconomic class account for the relationship between the development of an eating disorder and greater financial resources within the family. Increased expendable income may mean that daughters have an increased opportunity for exposure to other risk factors, such as fashion magazines and dieting products. Differences in financial resources and attitudes towards treatment may also influence access to care, biasing empirical studies that rely upon clinical convenience samples (Gard and Freeman 1996).

8.3.1.3 Birth Order and Family Structure/Composition

Case studies, clinical reports, and research on birth order in the pathogenesis of eating disorders have produced inconsistent findings (Vandereycken and Van Vreckem 1992). Nearly every birth order position, including being the youngest or oldest child (Bruch 1973; Marshall and Fitch 2006), or even just being younger (e.g., Eagles et al. 2005) or older (e.g., Lacey et al. 1991) than at least one other sibling, has been speculated to place an individual at risk for developing an eating disorder. Researchers have also attempted to ascertain whether birth order can differentiate the type (anorexia vs. bulimia) or subtype (restricting vs. binge eating–purging anorexia, or purging vs. nonpurging bulimia) of eating disorder (Britto et al. 1997; Post and Crowther 1987). Much of the support for the idea that birth order plays an etiological role is based upon anecdotal reports or poorly controlled studies (see Vandereycken and Van Vreckem 1992). In fact, several studies have failed to demonstrate that birth order differentiates between presence, type, or subtype of eating disorders (Dolan et al. 1989; Gowers et al. 1985; Kent and Clopton 1992; Vandereycken and Pierloot 1983) and birth order was not shown to be related to success in treatment (Hall et al. 1984).

Research examining the potential of the presence or absence of siblings, along with their gender, has also failed to produce a definitive understanding of how family structure relates to the development of an eating disorder. Studies on the influence of sibling gender have produced mixed results. In one study, younger sisters' body image dissatisfaction and preferred level of thinness were correlated to body image dissatisfaction and preferred level of thinness in older sisters but not to other unrelated females (Tsiantas and King 2001). In another study, women with anorexia were less likely to have male siblings than other women (Eagles et al. 2005). However, several investigators have not found an effect for family size (e.g., Dolan et al. 1989) or sibling gender (Britto et al. 1997; Gowers et al. 1985; Lacey et al. 1991).

Little research has examined whether women with eating disorders are more or less likely to come from families where divorce or remarriage has occurred. Early studies seemed to suggest that the divorce rate was lower among parents of individuals with eating disorders than the general population (Bruch 1971; Halmi 1974), but in more recent studies, individuals with eating disorders did not differ from comparison groups with regard to the frequency of parental divorce (e.g., Dolan et al. 1990; Kent and Clopton 1992).

8.3.2 FAMILY RELATIONSHIPS

Family relationships among women with eating disorders have been the subject of numerous well-controlled studies. Broadly, the presence of family dysfunction appears related to the development of eating disorders and their subclinical counterparts. Among families of women with disordered eating, children and their parents tend to report more family dysfunction than do comparison families (Emanuelli et al. 2004; Humphrey 1988; McDermott et al. 2002; Pike and Rodin 1991;

Schmidt et al. 1997). The focus here will be on families of individuals with anorexia or bulimia, which will be discussed separately.

8.3.2.1 Anorexia

Much of the research on the family dynamics of individuals with anorexia builds upon the characteristics introduced by Minuchin et al. (1978) using self-report (internal perceptions) and observational studies. Early case reports described clinical observations of problematic interactions among the family members of patients with anorexia (e.g., Wold 1973). The family dynamics literature is not always consistent, and there is not one *type* of family that characterizes families of individuals with anorexia. Nevertheless, research generally supports these early case reports, and families of individuals with anorexia are marked by problems with relationships that include (1) boundary difficulties, such as enmeshment (Bailey 1991; Blitzer et al. 1961; Kog and Vandereycken 1985; Rowa et al. 2001) or detachment (Humphrey 1986a), (2) high expectations and achievement pressure for the daughter (Karwautz et al. 2001; Waller 1994), (3) problematic and mixed communication toward the daughter (Emanuelli et al. 2004; Humphrey 1989; Lattimore et al. 2000), (4) denial of conflict (Kog and Vandereycken 1985, 1989), (5) problems with structure and control (Humphrey, 1986a), and (6) overprotectiveness (Leung et al. 2000).

Although some studies have not shown expected family problems, such as conflict avoidance (Lattimore et al. 2000) or overcontrol (Attie and Brooks-Gunn 1989), among families of young women with anorexia, most studies reveal a pattern of some type of problematic family interactions. Some of the inconsistencies in family characteristics found within the literature for anorexia may reflect differences by subtype. Although research suggests that enmeshment characterizes families of individuals with anorexia (Rowa et al. 2001), studies on cohesion indicate that families differ by subtype of anorexia. In one study, individuals with the restrictive subtype of anorexia nervosa did not significantly differ from age-matched controls in their perceptions of family cohesiveness or adaptability (Vidovic et al. 2005). Families who have a daughter with this subtype have reported, often incorrectly, that little, if any, conflict among family members exists (e.g., Bruch 1971; Kog and Vandereycken 1985, 1989). Similarly, observational studies of families of individuals in treatment for anorexia suggest that such families are often conflict avoidant (Minuchin et al. 1978), and individuals with anorexia may adamantly report their families to be stable and happy. In fact, Humphrey (1988) found that families of individuals with the restrictive subtype of anorexia denied problems with nurturance and support between parents and daughters. In addition, her observations of families of individuals with the restrictive subtype revealed that parents in such families were more nurturing and comforting, but were also more neglectful and ignoring of their daughter's expression of her own feelings, than were parents of individuals without eating disorders (Humphrey 1989). As might be expected when a family denies the presence of conflict, the families of young women with restrictive anorexia have been found to have problem-solving deficits (Emanuelli et al. 2004; Humphrey et al. 1986).

Research suggests that women with the binge–purge subtype of anorexia perceived their parents as more hostile, impaired, controlling, and conflicted, as well as less cohesive, nurturing, helpful, and approachable than women who do not have eating disorders (Casper and Troiani 2001; Humphrey 1986a, 1986b, 1988; Vidovic et al. 2005). In fact, Strober (1981) found that families of girls with the binge–purge subtype of anorexia were more conflicted, less cohesive, and less organized than families of those with the restrictive subtype, and Waller (1994) found that women with anorexia who perceived their families as more cohesive engaged in episodes of binge eating less frequently. Impaired family communications has been found among families of women with the binge–purge subtype of anorexia (Emanuelli et al. 2004; Humphrey 1989; Vidovic et al. 2005). One observational study suggested that this impaired communication may more frequently include contradictory and negative messages than observed among families of women without eating disorders (Humphrey et al. 1986). Unlike women with restrictive anorexia, research on families of those with the binge–purge subtype indicates that these families may not have as great a difficulty with problem solving (Humphrey et al. 1986), but they may also be less structured than families of women without eating disorders or those of women with restrictive anorexia (Humphrey 1986a; Strober 1981).

8.3.2.2   Bulimia

As is true for anorexia, research on families of individuals with bulimia supports the notion that family relationships among individuals with bulimia are more disturbed than those of individuals without an eating disorder. Although it appears that the families of individuals with anorexia may be highly controlling, families of individuals with bulimia tend to be more openly conflicted (Bailey 1991; Casper and Troiani 2001; Kog and Vandereycken 1985). Individuals with bulimia rate their families as less cohesive, both compared to individuals with restrictive anorexia and to women without eating disorders (Vidovic et al. 2005). In contrast to the enmeshed pattern found in families of individuals with anorexia, families of women with bulimia tend to have more conflict and hostility rather than cohesion (Bailey 1991; Humphrey 1986b; Kog and Vandereycken 1985). Additionally, the families of women with bulimia tend to have poorer functioning compared to families of women with anorexia (Schmidt et al. 1997), which could be partially due to denial of conflict among families of individuals with anorexia (see Section 8.3.2.1). Moreover, families of women with bulimia may be less nurturing or caring compared to the families of women with restrictive anorexia and women who do not have eating disorders (Humphrey 1986b; Johnson and Flach 1985; Leung et al. 2000). In one study, where enmeshed family interactions were observed among women with bulimia and their parents, the enmeshed interactions were hostile in nature (Humphrey 1989). In addition, Sights and Richards (1984) found that fathers of women with bulimia differed from other fathers by being more detached from their daughters during adolescence.

Beyond relationship variables associated with caring and boundaries, research on families of individuals with bulimia suggests such families are characterized by other problematic family interactions. Vidovic and colleagues (2005) found women with bulimia rated their families as less adaptive than other women. Families of women with bulimia have also been shown to be more rejecting and emotionally disengaged than those of women without eating disorders (Humphrey 1988; Stuart et al. 1990). In fact, severity of bulimic symptomology has been associated with a lack of emotional expressiveness in the family (Bailey 1991; Crowther et al. 2002; Kent and Clopton 1992), and women with bulimia may perceive their families to be less encouraging of genuine expression of affect compared to women without eating disorders (Johnson and Flach 1985). Related to experiences of rejection, some research suggests that mothers of women with bulimia hold higher expectations for their daughters than do other mothers, and that mothers and fathers as a team may be more demanding in families of women with bulimia (Sights and Richards 1984). However, other researchers have found a link between low parental expectations and bulimic symptomology, which some have suggested may be related to perception of a lack of caring (Young et al. 2004).

Although some research suggests that a lack of organization and less structure within the family are associated with severity of bulimic behavior (Hastings and Kern 1994; Johnson and Flach 1985), a few studies have found that women with bulimia perceive both their mothers and fathers as being overly protective (Leung et al. 2000; Stuart et al. 1990). Similarly, Johnson and Flach (1985) found that women with bulimia reported lower levels of perceived parental support for the development of independence and assertiveness than did women without eating disorders, and Sights and Richards (1984) found that mothers of women with bulimia were more controlling than were mothers of women without eating disorders.

8.3.3   Family Behaviors Associated with Eating and Appearance

Although research suggests that family relationships are associated with eating disorders, problematic family relationships are not specific to eating disorders. Family dysfunction has been linked with depression (e.g., Laliberte et al. 1999; Stuart et al. 1990), anxiety (Pagani et al. 2008), and alcohol abuse (West et al. 1987). In fact, general psychiatric patients show a similar pattern in which they perceive their family relationships as low in caring (Parker 1983), more conflicted, less expressive, and less cohesive than do individuals without mental disorders (Moos and Moos 1981). It is also possible that the presence of the eating disorder, or any mental illness, changes the way family members interact. As such, research findings on family relationships and eating disorders may constitute a more common description offered by individuals with various mental disorders, and other factors may have more specific roles in the development of eating disorders.

In light of findings that problematic family relationships are not unique to eating disorders, research has suggested that behaviors among other family members that relate to appearance and weight may be more specifically related to eating disorders and dysfunctional eating (Crowther et al. 2002; Fairburn et al. 1997; Kluck 2008; Laliberte et al. 1999). In other words, it may be that within families where there are problematic dynamics, family members are more likely to display certain problematic eating behaviors and make more problematic comments (e.g., criticizing the daughter's weight or encouraging the daughter to lose weight), which are linked with problematic eating (Kluck 2008).

8.3.3.1 General Expectations Regarding Appearance

Young women and adolescent girls with disordered eating sometimes report a strong emphasis on physical appearance and attractiveness within their families (e.g., Davis et al. 2004; Laliberte et al. 1999). A family culture that emphasizes appearance may be characterized by parental admiration of thinness and encouragement to use diet and exercise as means to control one's appearance (Davis et al. 2004). The emphasis on appearance may involve a mixture of parents' concern about their own appearance and about their child's physical appearance (Striegel-Moore and Kearney-Cooke 1994). In other words, some parents seem to be more concerned about appearances in general, creating an appearance-focused environment. When daughters believe that their thinness is important to their parents, they are more likely to have dieting and weight concerns themselves (Field et al. 2001).

8.3.3.2 Family Eating Patterns and Problems

Beyond a general emphasis on appearance, specific behaviors of family members may contribute to the genesis of eating disturbances. Drawing upon behavioral theories of development, eating practices can be conceptualized as learned behaviors in which modeling helps shape the acquisition of eating behaviors. Children may adopt their attitudes toward food, weight, and shape, as well as learn eating and weight-control behaviors by watching their parents. Research suggests that problematic eating behaviors are common in the families of individuals with eating disorders and those with subclinical levels of eating pathology (Benedikt et al. 1998; Kent and Clopton 1992; Pike and Rodin 1991; Stice et al. 1999). In fact, as early as the 1960s, researchers noticed that families of individuals in treatment for eating disorders displayed problematic eating patterns (Blitzer et al. 1961).

Research on the modeling of problematic eating within families has tended to focus on the influence of mothers' eating behaviors. This research has shown that mothers' dieting and complaints or comments about their own weight and shape are associated with weight and shape concerns (Smolak et al. 1999), restrained eating (Hill et al. 1990), and use of weight management strategies in their daughters (Pike and Rodin 1991). Although there is far less research examining how fathers' eating behaviors and attitudes relate to eating disorders in offspring, some researchers have found a link between paternal modeling and eating disorders (Smolak et al. 1999). Paternal body mass has been linked with disordered eating in daughters (Stice et al. 1999). In addition, fathers' weight dissatisfaction is associated with greater weight dissatisfaction among daughters (Keel et al. 1997). However, researchers do not always find a link between paternal modeling and disordered eating behavior or other weight loss attempts in daughters (Keel et al. 1997; Moreno and Thelen 1993). As such, it appears that modeling of problematic eating from fathers may have deleterious effects, but to a lesser extent than does maternal modeling of eating and body image disturbances.

8.3.3.3 Negative Communication about Appearance

Beyond the influence that parents may exert on a young woman's eating as she observes their eating behaviors, family members may influence her eating through the comments they make. Past research suggests this is particularly true when the comments are negative or critical. Teasing from parents, particularly mothers, has often been linked with eating disturbances and body image dissatisfaction in daughters (Kluck 2008, 2010; Schwartz et al. 1999; Thompson et al. 1995). In one study, Levine and his colleagues (1994) found that parental teasing had widespread consequences. Their study suggested that parental teasing predicted disordered eating, weight-control attempts, emphasis on thinness, and body dissatisfaction in daughters. Parental criticism is another type of negative comment that is associated with eating disorders and body image dissatisfaction (e.g., Baker et al. 2000; Kluck 2010). The effect of negative comments from parents affects girls and women from middle childhood (Smolak et al. 1999; Vincent and McCabe 2000) through early adulthood (Baker et al. 2000; Crowther et al. 2002).

When parents, particularly mothers, encourage their daughters to lose weight, the daughters may be at increased risk for developing an eating disorder and body image dissatisfaction (Kluck 2010; Wertheim et al. 2002). Compared to those without eating concerns, daughters with disordered eating more frequently reported that their parents helped them diet (Moreno and Thelen 1993), and encouragement to control weight has been linked with dieting in daughters (Thelen and Cormier 1995). Although such comments might reflect genuine parental concern about a daughter's health, mothers whose daughters have an eating disorder more frequently described their daughters as less attractive (Hill and Franklin 1998). In fact, maternal encouragement to lose weight is associated with daughters' use of dieting and exercising as weight loss mechanisms regardless of body size (Benedikt et al. 1998).

8.3.4 Individual Problems within the Family

8.3.4.1 Mental and Physical Illness within the Family

Researchers have examined familial psychopathology to determine if there is a higher rate of general pathology in families of individuals with eating disorders. Affective disorders appear more prevalent in the families of individuals with eating disorders and other clinical syndromes compared to those of individuals without a mental disorder (for a review, see Kog and Vandereycken 1985). Among women with eating disorders, more severe psychopathology has been linked to the presence of alcohol problems in relatives (Redgrave et al. 2007). In some cases, higher incidences of depressive, anxiety, personality, and substance abuse disorders have been found among first-degree relatives of individuals with eating disorders than among those of normal and clinical comparison groups (Bulik 1987; Grigoroiu-Serbanescu et al. 2003; Winokur et al. 1980). Specifically, anxiety disorders were found to be more prevalent in the families of individuals with anorexia (Grigoroiu-Serbanescu et al. 2003), and alcoholism was more prevalent in family members of individuals with bulimia (Kog and Vandereycken 1985).

Despite some studies suggesting higher rates of some mental disorders in family members of individuals with eating disorders, not all studies reveal such a link. For example, some studies have found no differences between the scores for a measure of alcoholism obtained from first-degree relatives of women with eating disorders and from those of women without eating disorders (Kuntz et al. 1992), or in the presence of alcoholism in first-degree relatives across subtypes of eating disorders (Redgrave et al. 2007). The pattern of inconsistent results likely indicates that the relationship between family psychopathology and eating disorders reflects the comorbidity of other psychological disorders with eating disorders (Grigoroiu-Serbanescu et al. 2003; Redgrave et al. 2007). In other words, it may be that the higher rate of mood and alcohol disorders among family members is related to higher rates of those same disorders in individuals with eating disorders. In addition, research linking problematic family relations with a variety of psychopathologies (see Section 8.2.2) must be considered when examining the potential for psychopathology in first-degree relatives to be related to the onset or severity of eating disorders.

Research concerning the likelihood of familial physical illness in eating disorders is scant, and no clear conclusions can be made. A few studies have concluded that a higher rate of physical illness may be found in families of individuals with bulimia or the binge–purge subtype of anorexia (Herzog 1982; Strober 1981); however, when families of symptom-free individuals were used as the comparison group, there was no evidence of increased physical illness in the families of individuals with bulimia (Weiss and Ebert 1983).

8.3.4.2 Physical and Sexual Abuse/Assault

Although there is some research that suggests that a history of sexual abuse and assault, as well as physical abuse, may be more common among individuals with psychological symptoms, including those related to eating disorders (Connors and Morse 1993; Neumark-Sztainer et al. 2000; Smolak and Murnen 2002), available research typically does not involve a differentiation between abuse or assault by a family member and that experienced by a perpetrator outside the family (Smolak and Murnen 2002). The few available studies that have examined familial sexual abuse have produced mixed results, with some studies indicating that sexual abuse by a member of the family may be strongly linked with symptoms of eating disorders (Baldo et al. 1996; Waller 1992), and other studies failing to find such a link (e.g., Calam and Slade 1989). The presence of sexual abuse within the family indicates an extremely dysfunctional family environment where basic trust is not possible. In fact, women who were sexually abused by a family member have an increased risk for a range of psychological problems (Cole and Putnam 1992), and in clinical settings, the strength of the maternal bond among individuals with a history of sexual abuse by a family member predicted the degree of eating-disordered attitudes (Mallinckrodt et al. 1995). Although there may be some increased risk for the development of an eating disorder or disordered eating attitudes among individuals with a history of familial sexual abuse, the link between the abuse experience and development of an eating disorder may be quite complex and extend beyond the experiences associated with such an unstable and un-nurturing family environment (see Chapter 10 of this book).

8.3.5 SUMMARY OF RESEARCH BACKGROUND

Consistent with early clinical observations, research suggests that certain characteristics tend to distinguish families of adolescent and young adult women with eating disorders (see Table 8.1). Empirical evidence and clinical observation suggest that families of individuals with anorexia tend to be enmeshed and overly protective or controlling, whereas those of individuals with bulimia more commonly have high levels of hostility and conflict (e.g., Bailey 1991; Humphrey 1986b; Kog and Vandereycken 1985; Leung et al. 2000). In addition, a family culture that emphasizes appearance is common among individuals with eating disorders, body image dissatisfaction, and subclinical disordered eating (Benedikt et al. 1998; Kent and Clopton 1992). Both encouragement to diet and criticism or teasing about weight are associated with increased dysfunctional eating (Kluck 2010). In addition, expression of weight concern and dysfunctional eating patterns among parents are commonly found among daughters with problematic eating patterns and body image concerns (Pike and Rodin 1991; Smolak et al. 1999).

Several inconsistencies exist in the research on family factors that contribute to the development and maintenance of eating disorders. For example, not all studies find a link between parental eating patterns and eating disturbances in daughters (e.g., Thelen and Cormier 1995). In addition, there is no single pattern of family relationships among individuals with anorexia or bulimia. Rather, each family of an individual with an eating disorder has unique characteristics, including the ways in which family members relate to and support one another, which are important to understanding the eating disorder and organizing treatment (Treasure et al. 2010). Given the potential for the presence of an eating disorder among a family member to influence the way parents and other family

TABLE 8.1

Characteristics of the Families of Individuals with Eating Disorders and the Research Evidence

Confirmed Association	No Association	Inconclusive Results
Genetics	Social class	Substance abuse
Parent weight/eating problems	Birth order	Physical illness
Parental comments about weight/size	Having sisters	Sexual abuse or assault
Family conflict	Parental divorce	
Boundary concerns (e.g., enmeshment, disengagement)		
Overprotection		
Lack of mutual support		

Notes: The classification of most characteristics in this table was clear-cut. The evidence is inconclusive about the relationship between sexual abuse and eating disorders, but there are some indications that sexual abuse by a family member increases the likelihood of developing an eating disorder.

members (e.g., siblings) behave around food (e.g., resulting from the rigid eating rules of the individual with the eating disorder) and relate to the individual with the eating disorder (e.g., becoming protective of the physically frail family member), it is particularly important to consider the unique constellation of each family in working with individuals with eating disorders.

8.4   PRACTICAL APPLICATIONS

In the treatment of an individual with an eating disorder, two practical issues related to the role of the family arise: assessing the family and conducting effective treatment.

8.4.1   ASSESSMENT

Assessment of the family can aid in formulating treatment goals and identifying areas of concern. This is particularly important in the case of family therapy. Several measures are available to clinicians for assessing the way family members relate to one another. A few of the commonly used measures are described here with references to aid in accessing the measures. The Family Environment Scale– IV (Moos 2002), which contains 90 items that assess the respondent's perception of the family environment, can be completed by multiple family members, allowing the clinician to contrast parent and child perceptions of the family environment. The Parental Bonding Instrument (Parker et al. 1979) is a 25-item self-report measure for use with those under age 16. This measure assesses perceived care (including emotional expression) and overprotection from parents. The Family Adaptability and Cohesion Scales– IV (Olson et al. 2006) is a 62-item, self-report measure designed to assess family cohesion (emotional closeness within the family) and flexibility (extent to which the family structure adapts to meet new demands).

In contrast to the numerous measures available to assess the general family environment, there are few measures that assess eating-specific family experiences. The available measures have more commonly been developed for use in research. The Family Influence Scale (Young et al. 2004; See Appendix 8.A), was adapted from the Perceived Sociocultural Pressure Scale (Stice et al. 1996) and is a brief measure designed to assess the extent to which the family emphasizes thinness and appearance. The Family Experiences Related to Food Questionnaire (Kluck 2008; available from the author) measures the perceived experiences associated with negative comments about weight and size and with modeling of disordered eating from each parent. Several other general measures of behavior, such as appearance-based teasing, have been modified in research studies to focus on parents (e.g., van den Berg et al. 2002). Despite the availability of some measures for research, there is not yet sufficient documentation of the validity of these measures for use in clinical samples to warrant their use in isolation. As such, clinicians should combine the use of measures like those described above and clinical interviewing when assessing for a history of teasing and criticism about weight, as well as modeling of eating disturbances from members of the family. At the moment, none of these scales have "clinical cutoffs," so clinicians will need to rely on their own judgment about whether the client's responses indicate a particularly problematic family history of behaviors related to eating and weight. One suggestion is to consider a client's score to be problematic if it is in the top 15% (i.e., one standard deviation above the mean) of the scores in the sample used to develop that measure.

8.4.2 FAMILY THERAPIES

Historically, treatment of eating disorders focused exclusively on the individual, and in many cases the individual was treated in isolation from the family. The shift to including a family systems perspective did not occur until the 1970s, and the inclusion of the family in treatment reflected perceptions among some clinicians that the eating disorder is a response to family difficulties (e.g., Bruch 1978; Minuchin et al. 1978). Family therapy is often used in tandem with other treatments, but is sometimes used as the sole psychotherapeutic intervention. Even when a clinician does not view the family as a causal agent, work with families as part of a multimodal treatment approach is often beneficial. In addition, regardless of whether treatment involves family therapy sessions, it is important to use a family systems perspective in guiding treatment. Although inclusion of the family in treatment does not guarantee that treatment will be effective, ignoring the influence of the family is likely to reduce the effectiveness of treatment efforts, particularly when treating adolescents and young adults.

Traditional family approaches to treatment typically targeted changes in the interrelations of the family instead of directly addressing symptoms of the eating disorder (e.g., Selvini 1988). These interventions might include focusing upon improved communication, altering problematic boundaries such as the existence of inappropriate or inflexible coalitions, or strengthening the bond between parents (Selvini 1988). The eating disorder was sometimes seen as a means used by the family to maintain homeostasis and, when that view was accurate, direct attempts to reduce the eating disorder might have threatened the family's homeostasis and led to increased resistance (Selvini 1988). As such, the focus upon changing the family system was presumed to help alleviate the need for the eating disorder.

The Maudsley method is a recently developed and somewhat unique approach to family treatment of eating disorders (Dare et al. 1995). In this treatment approach, parents are encouraged to take an active role in the treatment of their child, which may include guiding what the child eats and setting limits on what the child is healthy enough to do (Lock et al. 2001). Although this approach deviates substantially from classic family systems approaches (Dare et al. 1995), research suggests that this approach is particularly effective when working with adolescents with anorexia (Lock et al. 2001), and it has been used successfully with adult patients and those with bulimia (Treasure et al. 2010).

Parents often wish they were more knowledgeable about eating disorders and want guidance in how they can help their child become well (Treasure et al. 2010). In the Maudsley approach, the parents and the child work together on a common goal of overcoming the eating disorder, allowing the parents to be active in the treatment process. The therapist, parents, siblings, and patient take the stance that the eating disorder is an illness, separate from the daughter, such that she is not blamed for her behavior. The approach also involves teaching parents basic skills such as motivational interviewing and communication. The reasoning for helping parents develop these skills is to help decrease the expressed emotion (particularly overprotectiveness and hostility) in the family since expressed emotion appears to be a maintaining factor in eating disorders as well as other forms of psychopathology (Treasure et al. 2010). In addition, raising parents' emotional intelligence allows parents to model good coping skills for their daughters.

Therapists using the Maudsley approach encourage parents to consider the seriousness of the disorder and to assume the primary responsibility for refeeding their daughter, and siblings are encouraged to support their sister as she struggles through the process of weight gain (Lock et al. 2001). The role of the therapist is to help the parents reestablish an appropriate hierarchy in the family and to support them as they take responsibility for their daughter's health. Rather than focusing upon problems within the family, weight restoration is seen as the first priority, and the therapist focuses on past parenting successes to motivate parents to assume the difficult task of their daughter's refeeding (Lock et al. 2001). Parents are incorporated as a part of the treatment team along with professionals and the patient, such that treatment views parents and family members as valuable sources of information during assessment and important resources in the treatment process (Treasure et al. 2010). Once weight stabilization has occurred, more attention is directed at processes that might maintain the eating disorder, which may involve family relationships and other developmental concerns of the adolescent.

8.5 CASE STUDY

Beverly W., an actual client whose identity has been disguised, was treated by one of the co-authors of this chapter. Beverly had the binge eating/purging type of anorexia nervosa. She was 16 years old, 5 feet, 6 inches tall, and 85 pounds. Treatment involved individual sessions and sessions with Beverly and other family members. In total, Beverly's treatment consisted of 26 sessions occurring during a 10-month period. In individual sessions, Beverly was encouraged to be less socially isolated at school, and be more direct in communicating her needs to family members.

A key strategy in family sessions was to attempt to increase closeness between Beverly and other family members. A few sessions were spent with Beverly and her three younger sisters attempting, with little success, to identify enjoyable activities they could share. Greater success was achieved in increasing the closeness between Beverly and each of her parents. Mrs. W. was overweight and found that her difficulties with weight were similar to Beverly's problems. The two of them supported and encouraged each other, and they agreed to shop for clothes together once Beverly had gained enough weight and Ms. W. had lost enough weight. The two of them enjoyed working together on weight-related issues; they achieved their goals and made the shopping trip. During a session with Mr. W. and Beverly, they mentioned a basketball game later that week between the teams of two nearby high schools—the one that Beverly attended and the one that Mr. W. had attended. Beverly usually went to the basketball games alone, but with some encouragement from the therapist, she agreed to go with her father. Attending the basketball game together was an enjoyable experience for both Beverly and her father.

At the start of treatment, Beverly was preoccupied with her weight and fearful of gaining weight. The therapist asked Beverly to put away her scales at home and to stop weighing herself. Instead, the school nurse weighed Beverly and sent weights to the therapist. Figure 8.1 shows Beverly's weight during treatment and during the 8 months after treatment ended. At the end of treatment, Beverly weighed 118 pounds and no longer had eating binges or episodes of vomiting. During the follow-up period, Beverly reached a stable weight of around 122 pounds and had no symptoms of anorexia or bulimia.

Think about the extent to which Beverly and her family exemplify characteristics of adolescents with eating disorders and their families. What were the characteristics of the W. family that are typical for families in which one member has an eating disorder? Weight and eating problems are often found in families of individuals with eating disorders, and Mrs. W. was overweight. However, few of the other characteristics listed in Table 8.1 appear to apply to the W. family. Beverly's lack of closeness to other family members suggested that she lacked support from them, but no other evidence demonstrated that mutual support among members was lacking. Conflict existed in the W. family over Beverly's binge eating, but little conflict was apparent regarding other issues.

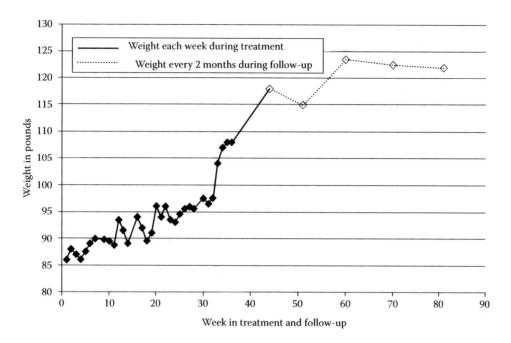

FIGURE 8.1 Beverly W.'s Weight during treatment and follow-up.

APPENDIX 8.A FAMILY INFLUENCE SCALE

Directions: In this case, the term family refers to the family that you had growing up. Please read each statement and circle the appropriate number for each item. Please answer all the questions.

    1 = Strongly Agree
    2 = Agree
    3 = Neither Agree nor Disagree
    4 = Disagree
    5 = Strongly Disagree

1. I've felt pressure from my family to lose weight.
2. I've noticed a strong message from my family to have a thin body.
3. My family members tend to make fun of people who are overweight.
4. In my family, people make favorable comments about the slender figures of other women.
5. Weight issues are frequently brought up in conversations with my family.
6. In my family, people exercise regularly as a means of weight control.
7. My family members tend to diet a lot.
8. In my family, people skip meals a lot as a means of weight control.
9. In my family, people share dieting tips with each other.
10. I feel pressured by my family to stay slim.
11. My family members often express anxiety about gaining weight.
12. My family members admire thin female models and celebrities.

Source: Adapted from Young, E. A., J. R. Clopton, and M. K. Bleckley. 2004. Perfectionism, low self-esteem, and family factors as predictors of bulimic behavior. *Eat Behav* 5: 273–283.

REFERENCES

Askevold, F. 1982. Social class and psychosomatic illness. *Psychother & Psychosom* 38: 256–259.

Attie, I., and J. Brooks-Gunn. 1989. Development of eating problems in adolescent girls: A longitudinal study. *Dev Psychol* 25: 70–79.

Bailey, C. A. 1991. Family structure and eating disorders: The family environment scale and bulimic-like symptoms. *Youth Soc* 23: 251–272.

Baker, C. W., M. A. Whisman, and K. D. Brownell. 2000. Studying intergenerational transmission of eating attitudes and behaviors: Methodological and conceptual questions. *Health Psychol* 19: 376–381.

Baldo, T. D., S. D. Wallace, and M. S. O'Halloran. 1996. Effects of intrafamilial sexual assault on eating disorders. *Psychol Rep* 79: 531–536.

Benedikt, R., E. H. Wertheim, and A. Love. 1998. Eating attitudes and weight-loss attempts in female adolescents and their mothers. *J of Youth Adolesc* 27: 43–57.

Blitzer, J. R., N. Rollins, and A. Blackwell. 1961. Children who starve themselves: Anorexia nervosa. *Psychosom Med* 23: 369–383.

Britto, D. J., D. H. Meyers, J. J. Smith, and R. L. Palmer. 1997. Anorexia nervosa and bulimia nervosa: Sibling sex ratio and birth rank—A catchment area study. *Int J Eat Behav* 21: 335–340.

Bruch, H. 1971. Family transactions in eating disorders. *Compr Psychiatry* 12: 238–248.

Bruch, H. 1973. *Eating disorders: Obesity, anorexia nervosa, and the person within*. New York: Basic Books.

Bruch, H. 1978. *The golden cage: The enigma of anorexia nervosa*. Cambridge, MA: Harvard Univ. Press.

Bulik, C. M. 1987. Drug and alcohol abuse by bulimic women and their families. *Am J Psychiatry* 144: 1604–1606.

Calam, R. M., and P. D. Slade. 1989. Sexual experience and eating problems in female undergraduates. *Int J Eat Disord* 8: 391–397.

Casper, R. C., and M. Troiani. 2001. Family functioning in anorexia nervosa differs by subtype. *Int J Eat Disord* 30: 338–342.

Clemens, H., D. Thombs, R. Scott Olds, and K. L. Gordon. 2008. Normative beliefs as risk factors for involvement in unhealthy weight control behavior. *J Am Coll Health* 56: 635–641.

Cole P. M., and F. W. Putnam. 1992. Effect of incest on self and social functioning: A developmental psychopathology perspective *J Consult Clin Psychol* 60: 174–184.

Connors, M. E., and W. Morse. 1993. Sexual abuse and eating disorders: A review. *Int J Eat Disord* 13: 1–11.

Crowther, J. H., J. C. Kichler, N. E. Sherwood, and M. E. Kuhnert. 2002. The role of familial factors in bulimia nervosa. *Eat Disord* 10: 141–151.

Culbert, K. M., S. A. Burt, M. McGue, W. G. Iacono, and K. L. Klump. 2009. Puberty and the genetic diathesis of disordered eating attitudes and behaviors. *J Abnorm Psychol* 118: 788–796.

Dare, C., I. Eisler, M. Colahan, C. Crowther, R. Senior, and E. Asen. 1995. The listening heart and the chi square: Clinical and empirical perceptions in the family therapy of anorexia nervosa. *J Family Ther* 17: 31–57.

Davis, C., B. Shuster, E. Blackmore, and J. Fox. 2004. Looking good—Family focus on appearance and the risk for eating disorders. *Int J Eat Disord* 35: 136–144.

Dolan, B. M., C. Evans, and J. H. Lacey. 1989. Family composition and social class in bulimia: A catchment area study of a clinical and a comparison group. *J Nerv Ment Dis* 177: 267–272.

Dolan, B. M., S. Lieberman, C. Evans, and J. H. Lacey. 1990. Family features associated with normal body weight bulimia. *Int J Eat Disord* 9: 639–647.

Eagles, J. M., M. I. Johnston, and H. R. Millar. 2005. A case–control study of family composition in anorexia nervosa. *Int J Eat Disord* 38: 49–54.

Eastwood, H., H. M. O. Brown, D. Markovic, and L. F. Pieri. 2002. Variation in the ESR1 and ESR2 genes and genetic susceptibility to anorexia nervosa. *Mol Psychiatry* 7: 86–89.

Emanuelli, F., R. Ostuzzi, M. Cuzzolaro, F. Baggio, B. Lask, and G. Waller. 2004. Family functioning in adolescent anorexia nervosa: A comparison of family members' perceptions. *Eat Weight Disord* 9: 1–6.

Fairburn, C. G., S. L. Welch, H. A. Doll, B. A. Davis, and M. E. O'Conner. 1997. Risk factors for bulimia nervosa: A community-based case–control study. *Arch Gen Psychiatry* 54: 509–517.

Fichter, M., and R. Noegel. 1990. Concordance for bulimia nervosa in twins. *Int J Eat Disord* 9: 255–263.

Field, A. E., C. A. Camargo, C. B. Taylor, C. S. Berkey, S. B. Roberts, and G. A. Colditz. 2001. Peer, parent and media influences on the development of weight concerns and frequent dieting among preadolescent and adolescent girls and boys. *Pediatrics* 107: 54–60.

Gard, M. C. E., and C. P. Freeman. 1996. The dismantling of a myth: A review of eating disorders and socioeconomic status. *Int J Eat Disord* 20: 1–12.

Gore, S. A., J. S. Vander Wal, and M. H. Thelen. 2001. Treatment of eating disorders in children and adolescents. In *Body image, eating disorders, and obesity in youth: Assessment, prevention, and treatment*, ed. J. K. Thompson, and L. Smolak, 293–312. Washington, D.C.: American Psychological Association.

Gorwood, P., J. Ades, L. Bellodi, E. Cellini, D. A. Collier, D. Di Belia, M. Di Bernardo, et al. 2002. The 5-HT$_{2A}$ – 1438G/A polymorphism in anorexia nervosa: A combined analysis of 316 trios from six European centres. *Mol Psychiatry* 7: 90–94.

Gowers, S., S. R. Kadambari, and A. H. Crisp. 1985. Family structure and birth order of patients with anorexia nervosa. *J Psychiatr Res* 19: 247–251.

Grigoroiu-Serbanescu, M., S. Magureanu, S. Milea, I. Dobrescu, and E. Marinescu. 2003. Modest familial aggregation of eating disorders in restrictive anorexia nervosa with adolescent onset in a Romanian sample. *Eur Child Adolesc Psychiatry* 12: 47–53.

Hall, A., E. Slim, F. Hawker, and C. Salmond. 1984. Anorexia nervosa: Long-term outcome in 50 female patients. *Br J Psychiatry* 145: 407–413.

Halmi, K. A. 1974. Anorexia nervosa: Demographic and clinical features in 94 cases. *Psychosom Med* 36: 18–26.

Hastings, T., and J. M. Kern. 1994. Relationships between bulimia, childhood sexual abuse, and family environment. *Int J Eat Disord* 15: 103–111.

Herzog, D. 1982. Bulimia: The secretive syndrome. *Psychosomatics* 23: 481–487.

Hill, A. J., and J. A. Franklin. 1998. Mothers, daughters and dieting: Investigating the transmission of weight control. *Br J Clin Psychol* 37: 3–13.

Hill, A. J., C. Weaver, and J. E. Blundell. 1990. Dieting concerns of 10-year-old girls and their mothers. *Br J Clin Psychol* 29: 346–348.

Humphrey, L. L. 1986a. Family relations in bulimic-anorexic and nondistressed families. *Int J Eat Disord* 5: 223–232.

Humphrey, L. L. 1986b. Structural analysis of parent–child relationships in eating disorders. *J Abnorm Psychol* 95: 395–402.

Humphrey, L. L. 1988. Relationships within subtypes of anorexic, bulimic, and normal families. *J Am Acad Child Adolesc Psychiatry* 27: 544–551.

Humphrey, L. L. 1989. Observed family interactions among subtypes of eating disorders using structural analysis of social behavior. *J Consult Clin Psychol* 57: 206–214.

Humphrey, L. L., R. F. Apple, and D. S. Kirschenbaum. 1986. Differentiating bulimic-anorexic from normal families using interpersonal and behavioral observation systems. *J Consult Clin Psychol* 54: 190–195.

Javaras, K. N., N. M. Laird, T. Reichborn-Kjennerud, C. M. Bulik, H. G. Pope, and J. I. Hudson. 2008. Familiality and heritability of binge eating disorder: Results of a case–control family study and twin study. *Int J Eat Disord* 41: 174–179.

Johnson, C., and A. Flach. 1985. Family characteristics of 105 patients with bulimia. *American J Psychiatry* 142: 1321–1324.

Karwautz, A., S. Rabe-Hesketh, X. Hu, J. Zhao, P. Sham, D. A. Collier, and J. L. Treasure. 2001. Individual specific risk factors for anorexia nervosa: A pilot-study using a discordant sister-pair design. *Psychol Med* 31: 317–329.

Kaye, W. H., G. K. Frank, U. F. Bailer, and S. E. Henry. 2005. Neurobiology of anorexia nervosa: Clinical implications of alterations of the function of serotonin and other neuronal systems. *Int J Eat Disord* 37: 515–519.

Keel, P. K., T. F. Heatherton, J. L. Harnden, and C. D. Hornig. 1997. Mothers, fathers, and daughters: Dieting and disordered eating. *Eat Disord* 5: 216–228.

Kent, J. S., and J. R. Clopton. 1992. Bulimic women's perceptions of their family relationships. *J Clin Psychol* 48: 281–292.

Kluck, A. S. 2008. Family factors in the development of disordered eating: Integrating dynamic and behavioral explanations. *Eat Behav* 9: 471–483.

Kluck, A. S. 2010. Family influence on disordered eating: The role of body image dissatisfaction. *Body Image* 7: 8–14.

Klump, K. L., and K. M. Culbert. 2007. Molecular genetic studies of eating disorders: Current status and future directions. *Curr Dir Psychol Sci* 16: 37–41.

Klump, K. L., and K. L. Gobrogge. 2005. A review and primer of molecular genetic studies of anorexia nervosa. *Int J Eat Disord* 37: 543–548.

Klump, K. L., J. L. Suisman, S. A. Burt, M. McGue, and W. G. Iacono. 2009. Genetic and environmental influences on disordered eating: An adoption study. *J Abnorm Psychol* 118: 797–805.

Kog, E., and W. Vandereycken. 1985. Family characteristics of anorexia nervosa and bulimia: A review of the research literature. *Clin Psychol Rev* 5: 159–180.

Kog, E., and W. Vandereycken. 1989. Family intergeneration in eating disorder patients and normal controls. *Int J Eat Disord* 8: 11–23.

Kuntz, B., V. Gorze, and W. R. Yates. 1992. Bulimia: A systemic family history perspective. *Fam Soc* 73: 604–612.

Lacey, J. H., S. G. Gowers, and A. V. Bhat. 1991. Bulimia nervosa: Family size, sibling sex and birth order: A catchment-area study. *Br J Psychiatry* 158: 491–494.

Laliberte, M., F. J. Boland, and P. Leichner. 1999. Family climates: Family factors specific to disturbed eating and bulimia nervosa. *J Clin Psychol* 55: 1021–1040.

Lattimore, P. J., H. L. Wagner, and S. Gowers. 2000. Conflict avoidance in anorexia nervosa: An observational study of mothers and daughters. *Eur Eat Disord Rev* 8: 355–368.

Levine, M. P., L. Smolak, and H. Hayden. 1994. The relation of sociocultural factors to eating attitudes and behaviors among middle school girls. *J Early Adolesc* 14: 471–490.

Leung, N., G. Thomas, and G. Waller. 2000. The relationship between parental bonding and core beliefs in anorexic and bulimic women. *Br J Clin Psychol* 39: 205–213.

Lock, J., D. Le Grange, W. S. Agras, and C. Dare. 2001. *Treatment manual for anorexia nervosa: A family-based approach.* New York: Guilford Press.

Mallinckrodt, B., B. A. McCreary, and A. K. Robertson. 1995. Co-occurrence of eating disorders and incest: The role of attachment, family environment, and social competencies. *J Couns Psychol* 42: 178–186.

Marshall, J. L., and T. J. Fitch. 2006. Adlerian perspectives on purging behavior. *J Individ Psychol* 62: 301–311

Mazzeo, S. E., K. S. Mitchell, C. M. Bulik, T. Reichborn-Kjennerud, K. S. Kendler, and M. C. Neale. 2009. Assessing the heritability of anorexia nervosa symptoms using a marginal maximal likelihood approach. *Psychol Med* 39: 463–473.

McDermott, B. M., M. Batik, L. Roberts, and P. Gibbon. 2002. Parent and child report of family functioning in a clinical child and adolescent eating disorders sample. *Aust N Z J Psychiatry* 36: 509–514.

Minuchin, S., B. L. Rosman, and L. L. Baker. 1978. *Psychosomatic families: Anorexia nervosa in context.* Cambridge: Harvard Univ. Press.

Moos, R. H. (2002) *Family Environment Scale Manual (4th ed.).* www.mindgarden.com

Moos, R. H., and B. S. Moos. 1981. *Family Environment Scale Manual* (2nd ed.). Palo Alto: Consulting Psychologists Press.

Moreno, A., and M. H. Thelen. 1993. Parental factors related to bulimia nervosa. *Addict Behav* 18: 681–689.

Neumark-Sztainer, D., M. Story, P. J. Hannan, T. Beuhring, and M. D. Resnick. 2000. Disordered eating among adolescents: Associations with sexual/physical abuse and other familial/psychosocial factors. *Int J Eat Disord* 28: 249–258.

Olson, C. M., C. F. Bove, and E. O. Miller. 2007. Growing up poor: Long-term implications for eating patterns and body weight. *Appetite* 49: 198–207.

Olson, D. H., D. M. Gorall, and J. W. Tiesel. 2006. *FACES IV package: Administration manual.* Minneapolis, MN: Live Innovations.

Pagani, L. S., C. Japel, T. Vaillancourt, S. Côté, and R. E. Tremblay. 2008. Links between life course trajectories of family dysfunction and anxiety during middle childhood. *J Abnorm Child Psychol* 36: 41–53.

Parker, G. 1983. *Parental overprotection: A risk factor for psychosocial development.* New York: Grune & Stratton.

Parker, G., H. Tupling, and L. B. Brown. 1979. A parental bonding instrument. *Br J Med Psychiatry* 52: 1–10.

Pike, K. M., and J. Rodin. 1991. Mothers, daughters, and disordered eating. *J Abnorm Psychol* 100: 198–204.

Post, G., and J. H. Crowther. 1987. Restricter–purger differences in bulimic adolescent females. *Int J Eat Disord* 6: 757–761.

Redgrave, G. W., J. W. Coughlin, L. J. Heinberg, and A. S. Guarda. 2007. First-degree relative history of alcoholism in eating disorder inpatients: Relationship to eating and substance use psychopathology. *Eat Behav* 8: 15–22.

Reichborn-Kjennerud, T., C. M. Bulik, K. S. Kendler, E. Roysamb, K. Tambs, S. Torgersen, and R. Harris. 2004. Undue influence of weight on self-evaluation: A population-based twin study of gender differences. *Int J Eat Disord* 35: 123–132.

Rogers, L., M. D. Resnick, J. E. Mitchell, and R. W. Blum. 1997. The relationship between socioeconomic status and eating-disordered behaviors in a community sample of adolescent girls. *Int J Eat Disord* 22: 15–23.

Rowa, K., P. K. Kerig, and J. Geller. 2001. The family and anorexia nervosa: Examining parent-child boundary problems. *Eur Eat Disord Rev* 9: 97–114.

Schmidt., U., H. Humfress, and J. Treasure. 1997. The role of general family environment and sexual and physical abuse in the origins of eating disorders. *Eur Eat Disord Rev* 5: 184–207.

Schwartz, D. J., V. Phares, S. Tantleff-Dunn, and J. K. Thompson. 1999. Body image, psychological functioning, and parental feedback regarding physical appearance. *Int J Eat Disord* 25: 339–343.

Selvini, M., ed. 1988. *The work of Mara Selvini Palazzoli.* Northvale: Jason Aronson Inc.

Sights, J. R., and H. C. Richards. 1984. Parents of bulimic women. *Int J Eat Disord* 3: 3–13.

Smolak, L., M. P. Levine, and F. Schermer. 1999. Parental input and weight concerns among elementary school children. *Int J Eat Disord* 28: 263–271.

Smolak, L., and S. K. Murnen. 2002. A meta-analytic examination of the relationship between child sexual abuse and eating disorders. *Int J Eat Disord* 31: 136–150.

Stice, E., W. S. Agras, and L. D. Hammer. 1999. Risk factors for the emergence of childhood eating disturbances: A five-year prospective study. *Int J Eat Disord* 25: 375–387.

Stice, E., C. Nemeroff, and H. Shaw. 1996. A test of the dual pathway model of bulimia nervosa: Evidence for restrained-eating and affect regulation mechanisms. *J Soc Clin Psychol* 15: 340–363.

Striegel-Moore, R. H., and A. Kearney-Cooke. 1994. Exploring parents' attitudes and behaviors about their children's physical appearance. *Int J Eat Disord* 15: 377–385.

Strober, M. 1981. The significance of bulimia in juvenile anorexia nervosa: An exploration of possible etiologic factors. *Int J Eat Disord* 1: 28–43.

Strober, M., R. Freeman, C. Lampert, J. Diamond, and W. Kaye. 2000. Controlled family study of anorexia nervosa and bulimia nervosa: Evidence of shared liability and transmission of partial syndromes. *Am J Psychiatry* 157: 393–401.

Stuart, G. W., M. T. Laraia, J. C. Ballenger, and R. B. Lydiard. 1990. Early family experiences of women with bulimia and depression. *Arc Psychiatr Nurs* 4: 43–52.

Thelen, M. H., and J. F. Cormier. 1995. Desire to be thinner and weight control among children and their parents. *Behav Ther* 26: 85–99.

Thompson, J. K., M. D. Coovert, K. J. Richards, S. Johnson, and J. Cattarin. 1995. Development of body image, eating disturbance, and general psychological functioning in female adolescents: Covariance structure modeling and longitudinal investigations. *Int J Eat Disord* 18: 221–236.

Treasure, J., U. Schmidt, and P. MacDonald. 2010. *The clinician's guide to collaborative caring in eating disorders: The new Maudsley Method.* New York: Routledge.

Tsiantas, G., and R. M. King. 2001. Similarities in body image in sisters: The role of sociocultural internalization and social comparison. *Eat Disord* 9: 141–158.

Urwin, R. E., B. Bennetts, B. Wilcken, B. Lampropoulos, P. Beumont, S. Clark, J. Russell, S. Tanner, and K. P. Nunn. 2002. Anorexia nervosa (restrictive subtype) is associated with a polymorphism in the novel norepinephrine transporter gene promoter polymorphic region. *Mol Psychiatry* 7: 652–657.

van den Berg, P., J. K. Thompson, K. Obremski-Brandon, and M. Coovert. 2002. The tripartite influence model of body image and eating disturbance: A covariance structure modeling investigation testing the meditational role of appearance comparison. *J Psychosom Res* 53: 1007–1020.

Vandereycken, W., and R. Pierloot. 1983. The significance of subclassification in anorexia nervosa: A comparative study of clinical features in 141 patients. *Psychol Med* 13: 543–549.

Vandereycken, W., and E. Van Vreckem. 1992. Siblings of patients with an eating disorder. *Int J Eat Disord* 12: 273–280.

van Hoeken, D., J. Seidell, and H. W. Hoek. 2003. In *Handbook of eating disorders* (2nd ed.), ed. J. Treasure, U. Schmidt, and E. Van Furth, 11–34. West Sussex, England: John Wiley & Sons.

Vidovic, V., V. Juresa, I. Begovac, M. Mahnik, and G. Tocilj. 2005. Perceived family cohesion, adaptability, and communication in eating disorders. *Eur Eat Disord Rev* 13: 19–28.

Vincent, M. A., and M. P. McCabe. 2000. Gender differences among adolescents in family, and peer influences on body dissatisfaction, weight loss, and binge eating behaviors. *J Youth Adolesc* 29: 205–221.

Waller, G. 1992. Sexual abuse and bulimic symptoms in eating disorders: Do family interactions and self-esteem explain the link? *Int J Eat Disord* 12: 235–240.

Waller, G. 1994. Bulimic women's perceptions of interaction within their families. *Psychol Rep* 74: 27–32.

Weiss, S., and M. Ebert. 1983. Psychological and behavioral characteristics of normal-weight bulimics and normal-weight controls. *Psychosom Med* 45: 293–303.

Wertheim, E. H., G. Martin, M. Prior, A. Sanson, and D. Smart. 2002. Parent influences in the transmission of eating and weight related behaviors. *Eat Disord* 10: 321–334.

West, J. D., T. W. Hosie, and J. J. Zarski. 1987. Family dynamics and substance abuse: A preliminary study. *J Couns Dev* 65: 487–490.

Winokur, A., V. March, and J. Mendels. 1980. Primary affective disorder in relatives of patients with anorexia nervosa. *Am J Psychiatry* 137: 695–698.

Wold, P. 1973. Family structure in three cases of anorexia nervosa: The role of the father. *Am J Psychiatry* 130: 1394–1397.

Young, E. A., J. R. Clopton, and M. K. Bleckley. 2004. Perfectionism, low self-esteem, and family factors as predictors of bulimic behavior. *Eat Behav* 5: 273–283.

Zalta, A. K., and P. K. Keel. 2006. Peer influence on bulimic symptoms in college students. *J Abnorm Psychol* 115: 185–189.

9 Body Image

Susan Kashubeck-West, Kendra Saunders, and Angela Coker

CONTENTS

9.1 LEARNING OBJECTIVES

After reading this chapter you should be able to

- Define body image and identify its components
- Explain the consequences of negative body image
- Understand various risk factors for body image dissatisfaction
- Describe strategies for preventing body image problems

9.2 BACKGROUND AND SIGNIFICANCE

In this chapter, body image is defined as a concept related to physical appearance, specifically, a person's size, shape, and weight. The discussion is organized as follows: (1) components of body image; (2) prevalence and consequences of body image disturbance; (3) results of research examining factors that are thought to create risk for a negative body image; and (4) information about prevention of body dissatisfaction.

9.2.1 BODY IMAGE AND ITS COMPONENTS

To put it simply, body image is a person's own evaluation of her appearance (Smolak and Thompson 2009). Most commonly, we think about body image in terms of how someone perceives her body shape and weight (Franko and Edwards George 2009). If a person perceives that her shape and weight are different than what she desires, then she is likely to experience dissatisfaction. The greater the difference between what she perceives and what she desires, the greater her dissatisfaction.

According to Thompson (1990), physical appearance-related body image is generally divided into three components: (1) a perceptual component that relates to how accurately we estimate our body size; (2) a subjective component that involves our feelings, thoughts, and attitudes toward our bodies; and (3) a behavioral component that refers to repetitive checking behavior and the tendency to avoid situations where we might feel uncomfortable about our bodies. Other researchers have defined body image in similar and different manners, and research has seldom focused on the multidimensional nature of body image described above. Rather, in trying to understand the negative body images that women often report, researchers have tended to focus on two areas: body-size distortion and body dissatisfaction (negative attitudes toward the body).

Body-size distortion occurs when a person misperceives his or her body size. Most of the focus in this field has been on overestimation of body size, and research has generally indicated that individuals who have been diagnosed with anorexia nervosa tend to overestimate their body sizes (Slade 1985; Slade and Russell 1973). Additionally, research has suggested that both individuals with bulimia nervosa and individuals without eating disorders may also overestimate their body sizes (Pasman and Thompson 1988; Thompson et al. 1986), suggesting that body-size distortion may be common for women in general. At the same time, there seems to be little relationship between body-size distortion and reports of body dissatisfaction (Thompson 1992). These findings have led some individuals to question whether the perceptual component of body image is useful (Coovert et al. 1988; Penner et al. 1991). Powell and Hendricks (1999) argued that many researchers have confused definitions of body distortion and body dissatisfaction with the assessment strategies used to measure them. They suggested that procedures for assessing body image (either distortion or dissatisfaction) be standardized. Additionally, they suggested that people be assessed with different procedures based on their gender, age, and cultural background. Furthermore, Powell and Hendricks (1999) demonstrated that many current measures of body dissatisfaction are confounded because they also contain items that assess body-size distortion. In their review of the research on body-size distortion, Powell and Hendricks (1999) reported that women tended to overestimate their body size when assessed with verbal methods (e.g., questions about whether one is underweight, normal, or overweight) but accurately estimated their body sizes when using visual methods (e.g., silhouettes). Men were accurate in their body-size estimation with either verbal or visual methods.

A significantly larger area of research involves the subjective component of body image disturbance, specifically, body image dissatisfaction, so the remainder of this chapter will focus on body image dissatisfaction. Although this component can be divided into emotional, cognitive, and behavioral factors, research has indicated that there is a great deal of overlap among these areas (Thompson et al. 1994; Williamson et al. 1995), and much of the research does not distinguish between them. Numerous studies indicate that many women report feeling dissatisfied with various body parts, their whole bodies, and their body weights (Peplau et al. 2009; Whitaker et al. 1989). Indeed, body image disturbance is so pervasive among women that it is normal, rather than unusual, for women to be unhappy with their bodies (Rodin et al. 1985). However, research indicates that women with eating disorders report much greater levels of body dissatisfaction than women without eating disorders, suggesting that they are exceptionally critical of their bodies (Cash and Deagle 1997). In addition, Cash and Deagle's (1997) summary of the research literature indicates that women with bulimia nervosa reported more body dissatisfaction than women with anorexia nervosa. Thus, severely underweight women with anorexia nervosa may experience fewer negative feelings about their bodies than women with bulimia nervosa, who tend to be of normal weight or overweight.

9.2.2 PREVALENCE AND CONSEQUENCES OF BODY IMAGE DISSATISFACTION

It is very common for women of any age to report body image disturbances, especially those related to body dissatisfaction. For example, Cash and Henry (1995) reported in a national survey that nearly half of American women had negative evaluations of their overall appearance and were preoccupied with their weights. McLaren and Kuh (2004a) found that almost 80% of middle-aged women (54-year-olds) wanted to lose weight, including more than 50% of normal-weight women. Drewnowski and Yee (1987) studied freshman college women and found that 85% of them wanted to lose weight. Alarmingly, body dissatisfaction seems to start very early in life. For example, Lowes and Tiggemann (2003) reported that 59% of girls ages 5 to 8 wanted to be thinner. DeLeel et al. (2009) reported that 35% of 9-year-old girls and 38% of 10-year-old girls wanted to be thinner than they currently were. Similarly, Thompson et al. (1997) found that 49% of fourth-grade girls indicated that an ideal figure would be thinner than their current figure. Wertheim, Paxton, and Blaney (2009) reported that more than 70% of adolescent girls want to lose weight.

One of the primary consequences of body dissatisfaction is dieting, or restricted eating based on cognitive, not physiological, control that often involves rigid dietary rules (Stice and Shaw 2002). Although maintaining a balanced diet and eating an appropriate amount of calories can be a way to lose weight, our society teaches us (inaccurately) that restrictive dieting is a good way to lose weight. Prospective evidence has linked body dissatisfaction to dieting, and a large body of data has linked dieting to eating pathology (Stice and Shaw 2002). Thus, an important consequence of body dissatisfaction is an increased risk for eating disordered behavior through dieting. A striking aspect is the age at which many girls begin to take action to lose weight. As indicated by Wertheim et al. (2009), 20% of nine-year-old girls were trying to lose weight and 35–57% of adolescent girls were using unhealthy weight loss methods such as crash dieting, vomiting, laxative use, and fasting.

A second consequence of body image dissatisfaction appears to be negative affect, such as depression and anxiety (Stice and Shaw 2002). Given that appearance, and therefore thinness, is so important for women, failure to achieve expected levels of thinness is thought to lead to negative affect. In addition, Stice and Shaw (2002) indicated that some data support the link between negative affect and eating disorder symptoms, suggesting a second pathway between body dissatisfaction and disordered eating.

9.3 CURRENT FINDINGS ON RISK FACTORS FOR BODY IMAGE DISSATISFACTION

Risk factors are characteristics of an individual or an environment that increase the likelihood of a negative or pathological outcome (Smolak 2009). To be considered causal, the risk factor has to precede in time the outcome. Additionally, it has to be shown that changing the level of the risk factor results in changes in the outcome in a predicted direction (Smolak 2009). Such data can be difficult, unethical, or impossible to collect on some variables, such as gender or race, as one cannot change levels of gender or race in participants to see if there are changes in body image. Thus, when looking at risk factors, it is important to examine whether the data on the risk factor are collected at the same time as the data on outcome (correlational), at some point in time earlier than the outcome data (prospective), and whether the data are experimental or not. If the data are prospective and experimental, then the risk factor can be considered causal (in this case, a factor that increases a person's risk for body image disturbance).

With regard to body image dissatisfaction, Smolak (2009) indicated that both correlational support and prospective support exist for the following risk factors: internalization of the thin ideal, social comparison, media influences, self-esteem, teasing from peers, peer modeling, peer conversations, body mass, and ethnicity. Correlational data support relationships between maternal comments about the daughter's body, maternal modeling, and sexual harassment with body dissatisfaction in girls. Finally, experimental data show a causal relationship between media influences and body dissatisfaction in girls. Several of these risk factors are explored in more detail in the following sections of this chapter.

9.3.1 GENDER

Many studies have investigated gender differences in body satisfaction, and the most common finding is that women report greater dissatisfaction than men (Altabe and Thompson 1993; Furnham and Greaves 1994; McCauley et al. 1988; Mintz and Betz 1986; Muth and Cash 1997; Peplau et al. 2009; Pliner et al. 1990; Rozin and Fallon 1988; Thompson 1990). For example, Muth and Cash (1997) found that, when compared to men, women had more negative evaluations of their bodies, were more concerned with their appearance, and reported negative feelings about their bodies in more situations. These gender differences also have been found in boys and girls as early as the fourth grade (Thompson et al. 1997). However, some studies indicated that men and women differ on which parts of their own bodies they regard with dissatisfaction (Gupta et al. 1993; Silberstein et al. 1988), and a few studies have found greater general body image dissatisfaction among men (Abell and Richards 1996).

To understand these conflicting findings, it is necessary to look at how studies have been conducted. For instance, many studies that investigate gender differences in total-body evaluations find that women are more dissatisfied with their bodies than men. Yet, studies that investigate attitudes toward specific body parts find that men are more dissatisfied with some parts of their bodies (e.g., often men wish to be more muscular), and women are more dissatisfied with other parts (e.g., most women wish to lose weight and have smaller body sizes) (Silberstein et al. 1988). As noted by Furnham and Greaves (1994), a discrepancy between how one perceives oneself (actual self) and how one wishes to be (ideal self) seems to be at the core of body image dissatisfaction. Studies have shown that many men (often half the sample) feel they should be more muscular and weigh more (Cash and Brown 1989; Jacobi and Cash 1994; McCauley et al. 1988; Mintz and Betz 1986; Silberstein et al. 1988). By contrast, very few women want to gain weight (Mintz and Kashubeck 1999). If studies have not taken into account the direction of men's desired weight change, it is possible that they have a pool of men, half of whom want to gain weight and half of whom want to lose weight. Average these men together, and it will seem as though this pool of men is satisfied with their current weights. Compare these men to a group of women (the vast majority of whom will wish to lose weight), and the women will show greater body dissatisfaction. Interestingly, Kashubeck-West et al. (2005) compared men and women who wanted to lose weight and found that women still showed greater dissatisfaction with their bodies. Women seem to feel more pressure from society to look a certain way than do men (Rothblum 1990), and the failure to meet these societal expectations may result in their greater body dissatisfaction.

9.3.2 RACE AND ETHNICITY

Much of the work on race and ethnicity in body dissatisfaction has focused on comparisons between African American women and white women. For example, researchers have postulated that African American women are less likely to report body dissatisfaction than white women because African American culture places less emphasis on thinness in women and has a greater range of acceptable body types (Harris 1994; Kelly et al. 2005; Nishina et al. 2006; Paxton et al. 2006). Lovejoy (2001) noted that even though African American women reported a lower incidence of anorexia nervosa than white women, they reported higher rates of overeating and obesity. Further, although it can be positive for African American women to feel good about their bodies, whatever their size, acceptance of a larger body image inadvertently may serve as a barrier to addressing life-threatening health problems, such as obesity (Lovejoy 2001).

A number of studies have found that African American girls and women are more satisfied with their bodies (Abood and Chandler 1997; Gray et al. 1987; Harris 1994; Rosen and Gross 1987; Rucker and Cash 1992; Siegel 2002; Wilfley et al. 1996) and have higher levels of self-esteem (Molloy and Herzberger 1998) than white women, despite a higher prevalence of obesity among African American women (Abood and Chandler 1997; Kuczmarski et al. 1994). However, other researchers have found comparable levels of body dissatisfaction among African American and white women (Caldwell et al. 1997; Dolan et al. 1990; Pumariega et al. 1994; Rosen et al. 1988) and have suggested that stereotypes describing women with eating disorders as white and upper class may serve to hide eating disorders in women of color (Root 1990). Lester and Petrie (1998) stated that the available data on culture and eating disorders in African American women suggest that idealization of white cultural values might increase the risk of developing an eating disorder, but that a stronger identification with African American cultural attitudes and beliefs does not seem to offer protection from eating-related problems.

Consistent with Lester and Petrie (1998), Poran (2006) found that African American women's cultural body preferences (e.g., full-figured bodies) did not serve as a protective factor against the negative consequences of media representations (both Black and mainstream media) of beauty. In Poran's (2006) study, African American women felt vulnerable to social pressures to be slim and felt misrepresented by the media, citing a plethora of African American body images (e.g., women who were thin, predominantly light skinned, had long hair, and displayed European facial features) that did not reflect the range of body types of African American women living within their communities. Thus, despite the availability of African American female images in contemporary media, many African American women did not feel empowered, but rather felt continued pressure to be thin and to conform to society's definitions of beauty.

Less work has investigated body image disturbance in women in the United States from racial and ethnic groups other than European American and African American. However, the research that has been done suggests that women from Asian American and Latina backgrounds also may be at risk for body image dissatisfaction. For example, Mintz and Kashubeck (1999) found that gender differences related to body image and disordered-eating variables in Asian American college students were similar to those seen in Caucasian college students. Phan and Tylka (2006) found that pressure to be thin was a strong predictor of body preoccupation (which was predictive of disordered eating) in Asian American women. Importantly, Yates et al. (2004) reported that women (and men) from different Asian ethnic groups had different levels of body dissatisfaction, and that combining these various ethnic groups into a single group obscured important differences between them. Similarly, George et al. (2005) found ethnic differences in ideal body image among Hispanic females and suggested that interventions need to be targeted to particular ethnic groups (e.g., Cuban, Puerto Rican) to be most effective.

The literature comparing Asian American and European American female body image is inconsistent, as some studies reported that Asian American women were more satisfied with their bodies (e.g., Akan and Grilo 1995; Franzoi and Chang 2002; Mintz and Kashubeck 1999) and other studies reported no differences in levels of body dissatisfaction (e.g., Cash et al. 2004; Story et al. 1995). Similarly, when comparing Hispanic/Latina women to European American women, many studies found no differences (e.g., Cachelin et al. 2002; McComb and Clopton 2002; Shaw et al. 2004), whereas other studies reported that Latinas had less body dissatisfaction than Anglo women (e.g., Barry and Grilo 2002; Suldo and Sandberg 2000).

Grabe and Hyde (2006) conducted a meta-analysis of the research examining body dissatisfaction and ethnicity in women. Their findings help to clarify the disparate findings in the research literature. Grabe and Hyde (2006) reported that, when comparing African American and white women, the average difference between the two groups was significant ($d = .29$). White women had higher levels of body dissatisfaction, but the size of the difference was rather small. Effect sizes were also calculated for comparisons between Asian American and white women, Hispanic and white women, African American and Hispanic women, African American and Asian women, and Asian American and Hispanic women. No differences in levels of body dissatisfaction were found when comparing Asian American and white women and when comparing Hispanic and white women. Similarly, African American and Asian American women did not differ in body dissatisfaction, and neither did Asian American and Hispanic women. African American and Hispanic women differed, in that Hispanic women reported slightly higher levels of body dissatisfaction compared to African

American women. Grabe and Hyde (2006) summarized by stating that the large differences thought to occur between white and ethnic-minority women in body dissatisfaction do not exist.

Patton (2006) emphasized the importance of understanding African American women's body image challenges within the intersections of race, gender, and class, as all three social constructs influence a woman's experience in the world. Such a perspective is important to take with regard to all women of color, and the findings outlined in this section suggest that ethnicity, not just race, is important. Further, it is important to consider the complexities of women's body concerns beyond weight, which can include other body features such as skin tone, hair texture, and facial features (e.g., Falconer and Neville 2000; Hall 1995; Patton 2006). As Grabe and Hyde (2006) noted, much more sophisticated research on body image among subgroups of women is needed. Another factor that may be important in understanding body image in racial and ethnic minority women is that of acculturation, a person's identification with one's culture of heritage and with mainstream culture (Gordon et al. 2010). Studies on the relationship of acculturation to body image have resulted in mixed findings both within and across ethnic groups and much more research in this area is needed.

9.3.3 Social Class

One confounding factor in the research examining racial and ethnic differences in body image disturbance is a failure to examine socioeconomic status (SES) or social class. Some data suggest that class differences exist in body mass, preferences for body size, and perceptions of what body sizes are attractive (Sobal and Stunkard 1989). Failure to examine class in conjunction with race and ethnicity may lead to erroneous conclusions. For example, Caldwell et al. (1997) suggested that their failure to find racial differences in body satisfaction among a sample of upper-class white women and upper-class African American women could have occurred because SES might be a more powerful factor than race in understanding body dissatisfaction. Thompson et al. (1997) reported that the effect of race was not consistent across SES levels in children's selections of ideal body size and suggested that more work be done in this area. Similarly, Snapp (2009) reported that ethnic minority girls in lower income groups had greater body satisfaction related to weight compared to ethnic minority girls in higher income groups. Thus, research is needed that focuses on the facets that comprise social class and their relation to body image and body satisfaction.

Overall, the relations between body image and social class have not been examined with the same frequency as that of eating disorders and social class. Some studies reported a relationship between higher social class and greater body dissatisfaction (e.g., Abrams and Stormer 2002; Kornblau et al. 2007; McLaren and Kuh 2004a). At the same time, other studies have found no relationship between social class and body image preferences or satisfaction (e.g., Cachelin et al. 2006; Caples 2009; DeLeel et al. 2009; Shrewsbury et al. 2009). McLaren and Kuh (2004b) examined the relations of body esteem with childhood and adult social class in a longitudinal study of middle-aged women. Their findings indicated that childhood social class and adult social class, measured as overall concepts, were not related to body esteem. However, examination of various aspects of social class, such as education level, indicated that the relationships between social class and body perceptions are complex. For example, McLaren and Kuh (2004b) found that women with higher educational levels had lower body esteem than women with lower educational levels. Given the conflation of social class with race and ethnicity, and a lack of understanding of the critical aspects of social class (such as income, education, social capital, childhood social class, and experiences of class oppression) that might be related to body image, much more work in this area is needed.

9.3.4 Sexual Orientation

The relation of sexual orientation to body image satisfaction in women has also been investigated, specifically with regard to comparisons between women who identify as heterosexual and women who identify as lesbian. However, almost nothing is known about the body image satisfaction of women who identify as bisexual. Lesbians have been thought to be more likely to reject cultural imperatives regarding female appearance, thus making them less likely to suffer from body dissatisfaction and eating disorders (Heffernan 1996). On the other hand, it has been argued that lesbians, like all other women in our culture, are exposed to the same cultural messages regarding thinness and attractiveness, and thus should show the same body dissatisfaction when they fail to meet these societal standards (Dworkin 1989).

Findings of studies comparing lesbians to heterosexual women on body image satisfaction have been quite mixed. Some studies showed that lesbians fare better than heterosexual women in terms of body satisfaction, and others showed no differences between the two groups of women. For example, Calandra (2001) reported that lesbians seemed less concerned with appearance than heterosexual women, and Share and Mintz (2002) found that lesbians indicated higher levels of body esteem concerning sexual attractiveness compared to a sample of heterosexual women. In contrast, Legenbauer et al. (2009) found no differences between heterosexual women and lesbians in weight and shape dissatisfaction. Similarly, no differences between heterosexual women and lesbians have been found for body satisfaction (Beren et al. 1996), rates of bulimia nervosa, and endorsement of social norms regarding thinness and attractiveness (Heffernan 1996).

A meta-analysis by Morrison et al. (2004) examined findings from 27 studies on body satisfaction and sexual orientation. Their results indicated no significant differences between lesbians and heterosexual women on level of body satisfaction. However, when taking into account the reported weight of participants, Morrison et al. found a significant, though small, difference, with lesbians reporting slightly greater body satisfaction. The authors indicated that the small size of the difference suggested that the norms of lesbian culture (i.e., less emphasis on weight and body shape) are not enough to counteract the large volume of messages about the importance of physical appearance that all women receive beginning in childhood. Studies show that lesbian and heterosexual women appear to be equally aware of societal standards regarding size and the importance of attractiveness, but lesbians may internalize such standards less (Bergeron and Senn 1998; Share and Mintz 2002). However, even if lesbians may internalize cultural imperatives about body shape and size less than heterosexual women, the effect of these cultural imperatives appears to be relatively similar, although not identical.

Finally, Peplau et al. (2009) used a very large sample (unlike most studies in this area) to investigate differences in body satisfaction between lesbian women and heterosexual women. Their findings indicated that lesbians and heterosexual women reported similar self-assessments of appearance and similar effects of body image on quality of life. Peplau et al. (2009) noted that all women, regardless of sexual orientation, respond to the dominant culture's powerful messages about ideal physical appearance. No information was provided regarding the racial and ethnic make-up of the participants. In sum, the results of research in this area suggest that the values of the lesbian community do not protect lesbians from body dissatisfaction, and that lesbians are not immune to the negative effects of failing to meet societal standards for thinness.

9.3.5 Developmental Factors

Several developmental factors have been identified as potential contributors to negative body images found among women. Smolak et al. (1993) noted that puberty seems to be the time when many girls develop weight concerns, body dissatisfaction, dieting habits, and eating disorders. For many adolescent girls, dieting and body dissatisfaction become commonplace (Rosen and Gross 1987). According to Smolak et al. (1993), two models have been proposed to account for the relationships among puberty, body image disturbance, and eating-disordered behavior. The first model suggests that the timing of pubertal maturation is important, in that girls who physically mature early may feel more negative about their bodies and diet more. Supporting this model is a study by Keel et al. (1997), which found that girls who achieved puberty earlier (and were heavier) were more likely to report disordered-eating attitudes and behaviors. Similarly, studies by Attie and Brooks-Gunn (1989) and by Killen and colleagues (1992, 1994) indicated that pubertal timing was associated with disordered-eating patterns.

The second model suggests that the impact of several simultaneous events, including puberty, increases the overall stress felt by adolescent girls, resulting in more eating disorder-related distress. Specifically, Levine and Smolak (1992) suggested that puberty, with its increase in fat and body size, causes girls to feel their bodies do not meet our culture's ideal of a thin and attractive body. In addition, girls may tie dating success to being thin and so choose to diet to achieve thinner and more attractive figures. If the onset of menstruation and dating occurs at the same time (within the same year), Levine and Smolak (1992) suggested that girls faced unique stresses with regard to dieting, body image, and eating-disordered attitudes. Smolak et al. (1993) investigated this theory and found that simultaneous onset of menstruation and heterosexual dating was associated with greater body dissatisfaction and stronger eating-disordered attitudes among middle-school girls. In addition, if the onset of menstruation and heterosexual dating was early, body dissatisfaction and eating-disordered attitudes were even stronger. This finding supports the second model, suggesting a synchrony in the timing of normal developmental events and the onset of eating problems. However, these results also support a hypothesis proposed by Williams and Currie (2000), who asserted that early puberty may lead adolescents to participate in activities for which they are not developmentally prepared, such as dating and sexual activity. On the other hand, platonic involvement between European American adolescent girls and boys does not appear to be related to body image satisfaction, except in less sexually mature girls, where such involvement is associated with greater body image satisfaction (Compian et al. 2004). Clearly, more research on the developmental changes associated with both puberty and dating is needed.

With regard to peer influences on body image among adolescent girls, Paxton (1996) noted that friendship environments constitute a subculture that may place more or less emphasis on thinness and weight loss behaviors. Friends talk about dieting, losing weight, disdain of fat, and similar topics that indicate the importance of being thin. Levine and colleagues (1994a, 1994b) found that how strongly friends were perceived to value dieting and how many weight loss techniques they used were related to an individual's investment in being thin and the number of weight loss strategies used. Furthermore, a study by Dohnt and Tiggemann (2006) found that perceived peer desire for thinness was a precursor to body dissatisfaction and low self-esteem among girls. In a study of peer factors and body image, Liberman et al. (2001) found that girls had a poorer body image when they were popular, teased about their bodies, encouraged to diet by peers, and when they had friends who felt negatively about their appearance. Furthermore, simple conversations with peers about appearance-related topics are associated with poor body image (Clark and Tiggemann 2006). Thus, peers appear to play a significant role in the negative body images commonly found in adolescent girls.

Family environments may also provide girls with models that emphasize thinness and encourage dieting and body dissatisfaction. For example, Levine and colleagues (1994a, 1994b) found that girls who reported peer and family investment in thinness were at higher risk for body dissatisfaction. Similarly, Vincent and McCabe (2000) found that parental remarks about their daughter's weight and encouragement to lose weight were related to dieting and a poor body image. A father's encouragement to diet has been viewed as particularly significant to a daughter's dieting and poor body image (Thelen and Cormier 1995). Rozin and Fallon (1988) reported great similarity in mothers' and daughters' levels of body dissatisfaction and dieting. Rieves and Cash (1996) found that college women's reports of maternal body images paralleled their reports of their own body images. If the mothers held negative body images, so did their daughters; positive maternal body images indicated positive body images among their daughters. Both maternal and paternal influences appear relevant to the development of a poor body image among daughters. In fact, perceived pressure to be thin from parents is believed to be one of the primary factors related to body discontent among adolescents (Ata et al. 2007; Phares et al. 2004).

Peers and family members who tease or criticize young women about their weight may also contribute to the development of negative views of their bodies. Thompson (1992) and Coovert et al. (1988) reported that teasing directly influenced body-image disturbance and overall psychological distress in adolescent females. Similarly, Thompson and colleagues (Thompson 1991; Thompson et al. 1991; Thompson and Psaltis 1988) and Cash and colleagues (Cash 1995; Rieves and Cash 1996) found that a history of teasing about appearance during adolescence was strongly related to body dissatisfaction in adults. In fact, weight teasing in adolescence was shown to influence a person's self-esteem and body dissatisfaction at a five-year follow-up (Eisenberg et al. 2006).

Recently, attention has been given to potential factors that might protect the body satisfaction of females. For example, positive family relationships, associated with spending more time together and feeling closer to one another, and parental support and acceptance can shield adolescent girls from body dissatisfaction (Barker and Galambos 2003; Boutelle et al. 2009; Byely et al. 2000; McVey et al. 2002). Healthy family relationships could protect young women from body image disturbance through support when coping with stress, and by helping them develop a healthier temperament and stable identity (Littleton and Ollendick 2003; McVey et al. 2002; Striegel-Moore and Cachelin 1999). Smolak (2009) noted that adolescent girls whose parents and friends encouraged eating healthily and exercising for fitness, not weight loss, had greater body satisfaction. Positive peer relationships could serve as a protective factor against body image disturbance by helping girls to resist societal images of beauty. Finally, research suggests that non-aesthetic and non-elite sports activities and a positive relationship with a coach also serve as protective factors against developing a negative body image (Morrison 2006; Smolak et al. 2000; Tiggemann 2001).

9.3.6 Sociocultural Factors

The most important factor thought to influence body image in women and girls is the sociocultural climate, specifically, our society's emphasis on thinness as a necessary component of beauty. Pressure to be thin comes from a number of sources, including parents, siblings, peers, mass media, and dating partners (Stice and Shaw 2002). This pressure may be communicated directly through messages that one needs to lose weight, or indirectly, such as through peers who talk about their need to diet or through the ubiquitous ads in magazines and on the internet for weight loss products. Evidence of the power of sociocultural norms comes from looking at non-Western cultures where thinness is not valued. Nassar (1988) reported that in such cultures, eating disorders are much rarer than they are in Western cultures that value thinness. Indeed, for women in Western cultures, being thin represents success, competence, sexual attractiveness, and control (Wilfley and Rodin 1995). Not surprisingly, some data suggest that in countries with increasing "westernization," there is a concomitant increase in body dissatisfaction and eating disorders (Anderson-Fye 2009). However, this data has been challenged by other findings (e.g., Abdollahi and Mann 2001), and it appears that body dissatisfaction and eating disorder risk may be associated with cultural change in more complex ways than simply westernization (Anderson-Fye 2009).

Women in our society are faced with more pressure than men to be thin and attractive (Fallon 1994). Rodin et al. (1985) discussed how the female gender-role stereotype has two central features: the pursuit of beauty and preoccupation with beauty. Thus, in order to be a real woman, a woman has to be attractive (which includes thinness) and focused on her appearance. As noted by Fallon (1990), women in many cultures across time have spent their lives attempting to modify their bodies to fit society's notions of what is attractive and acceptable. Thus, body image has a much greater role in women's self-concept than it does in men's self-concept, so that happiness and self-esteem are related to how attractive a woman feels (Wadden et al. 1991).

Objectification theory describes how (via gender role socialization) girls and women are taught that their bodies are objects to be looked at, especially with a sexual gaze (Fredrickson and Roberts 1997; Moradi et al. 2005). Girls and women internalize this gaze and engage in self-objectification, the judging and continual monitoring of their bodies to ensure that they are meeting societal standards of attractiveness (Smolak 2009). Studies have supported the existence of self-objectification and its relation to body image and eating disorders in women (e.g., Augustus-Horvath and Tylka 2009; Moradi et al. 2005; Smolak and Murnen 2008; Tylka and Hill 2004). McKinley and Hyde (1996) theorized that women who engage in self-objectification experience three components that make up what they called *objectified body consciousness*. These three components are body shame (belief that one's body does not meet cultural standards), body surveillance (experiencing one's body as an outside observer would experience it), and control beliefs (the ideas that women should be able to achieve cultural standards for beauty by controlling one's appearance, weight, and shape). Lindberg, Hyde, and McKinley (2006) posited that objectified body consciousness develops during puberty. Indeed, data from their study of 10- and 11-year-old children indicated that girls reported greater levels of body surveillance than boys.

As noted previously, the gender role socialization of females is thought to lead to their self-objectification. Experiences with family and friends, such as teasing and the modeling of dieting behavior and negative body images, are important mechanisms through which females are socialized toward self-objectification. Another critical source of gender role socialization that is thought to lead to self-objectification and body dissatisfaction is the media. Numerous studies have investigated the relationship between body dissatisfaction and exposure to media (e.g., television, movies, music videos, magazines, and the internet) depicting women who are thin and attractive. Correlational studies have established clearly that media exposure and body dissatisfaction are related (Smolak 2009), and even stronger evidence has been provided by experimental studies. These studies are based on the idea that exposure to a barrage of thin, idealized women has the effect of promoting standards for thinness that are unattainable for most women, leaving them with greater levels of body dissatisfaction (Nemeroff et al. 1994). For example, Turner et al. (1997) had undergraduate women read fashion magazines or news stories and then rate their body-image satisfaction. Women who read fashion magazines were less satisfied with their bodies, reported more frustration about their weight, were more fearful of getting fat, and were more preoccupied with wanting to be thin than women who read news magazines. Stice and Shaw (1994) asked female college students to view neutral pictures, pictures of normal-weight women, or pictures of thin women. After viewing the pictures, participants completed measures of ideal-body stereotype endorsement, body dissatisfaction, negative feelings, and bulimic symptoms. Women who saw the thin models reported more depression, guilt, shame, stress, and body dissatisfaction, and reported less self-confidence than women who saw neutral pictures or pictures of normal-weight women.

In addition to self-objectification, another important connection between media exposure and body dissatisfaction is thought to be the internalization of societal expectations about attractiveness. This internalization is often called the thin-ideal internalization (Thompson and Stice 2001). Individuals raised in our society hear and internalize messages from their families, peers, and the media that to be attractive means to be thin. Given that the level of thinness promoted by society is unattainable for most women, it is not surprising that research shows that thin-ideal internalization is a causal risk factor for body dissatisfaction (Thompson and Stice 2001). For example, perceived pressure to be thin at one point in time is associated with increases in body dissatisfaction, negative affect, dieting, and eating pathology at a later date (Stice et al. 2003). Randomized experimental data confirmed these relationships in young adult women, as exposure to media depicting the thin-ideal resulted in increases in both body dissatisfaction and negative affect (Stice et al. 2003). These findings seemed to be especially true for women who had higher initial levels of thin-ideal internalization and body dissatisfaction. Stice et al. (2003) also found that exposure to peer pressure to be thin resulted in increases in body dissatisfaction. Thus, pressure to be thin from a variety of sources is associated with increases in body dissatisfaction.

Through gender socialization (from parents, peers, and the media), girls are taught to see themselves as sexual objects and are taught that thinness is a critical part of attractiveness, and thus an important aspect of the female gender role. Self-objectification and internalization of the thin ideal lead to ongoing body surveillance, body shame, and control beliefs in women, which, in turn, are associated with disordered eating (Smolak 2009). It is clear that sociocultural forces play a large role in determining how women feel about their bodies. Unfortunately, our culture emphasizes a thin ideal that is not attainable for the vast majority of women. Consequently, the majority of women are dissatisfied with their bodies. This dissatisfaction has consequences for many women, and one of the most drastic consequences of a negative body image seems to be the development of eating disorders in some women. Research on body dissatisfaction and eating disorders has established clearly that they are linked (Cash and Deagle 1997; Nelson and Gidycz 1993; Veron-Guidry et al. 1997; Williamson et al. 1993), although not everyone with a negative body image develops an eating disorder (Smolak 2009).

9.4   SUMMARY AND CONCLUSIONS

Dissatisfaction with one's body appears to be ubiquitous for women. Factors such as age, race, ethnicity, and sexual orientation do not seem to protect women from experiencing negative body images. The relationship between social class and body image is not well understood at this point, and this area is ripe for exploration. Families and peers appear to create risk for body image disturbance through modeling, criticism, and teasing. At the same time, there is some recent research that suggests that peers and families can also protect females from experiencing dissatisfaction with their bodies. Finally, there is very strong evidence that media emphasis on thinness and attractiveness has a deleterious effect on how females think and feel about their bodies. Girls are taught at young ages that being thin and attractive is an important part of being female, and girls learn to view themselves as objects. Such self-objectification has been linked to body image disturbance and disordered eating in adolescent and adult females.

Prevention of body dissatisfaction appears to be a key way to effectively reduce or eliminate negative consequences, such as eating disorders. Levine and Smolak (2009) noted that few prevention studies meet the rigorous methodological criteria needed to demonstrate clear efficacy. Nevertheless, several meta-analyses (Fingeret et al. 2006; Stice and Shaw 2004; Stice et al. 2007) have shown that prevention efforts can be successful. Prevention programs can be divided between *targeted programs*, which focus on high-risk individuals such as those with warning signs or mild symptoms, and *universal programs*, which try to reach a wider range of people. With adolescents, targeted programs that use interactive and experiential methods are particularly effective. Teaching these adolescents about exercise, nutrition, and how to resist sociocultural pressures with regard to thinness and attractiveness has been shown to decrease thin-ideal internalization and negative body image (Stice et al. 2007). At a younger age, universal prevention programs that teach children (typically ages 4 to 7) about healthy eating, respect for differences (e.g., in size, interests, talents), and the importance of being active have been shown to be helpful (Levine and Smolak 2009). Overall, the data suggest that universal prevention programs for younger children and targeted prevention programs for high-risk individuals (especially female adolescents) are very promising avenues in the prevention of body dissatisfaction and disordered eating.

A prevention focus can be consistent with a social justice perspective on female body dissatisfaction. In recent years, there has been a steady feminist push (e.g., Russell-Mayhew 2007; Russell-Mayhew et al. 2008) urging educators, researchers, and mental health professionals to view the issue of women's body dissatisfaction and disordered eating as a social justice issue. According to Goodman et al. (2004, 798), a central principle of social justice work is "the idea that individual's struggles may be created or aggravated by oppressive systems," and that social justice workers must direct their interventions to address harmful societal values and systems that impede the full development of the human potential. Russell-Mayhew et al. (2008) asserted the importance of taking into consideration the larger sociopolitical realities women collectively face (e.g., sexism) both nationally and globally, which can translate into, for example, a social context where a women's value is measured based on her body appearance.

In using a social justice approach to address women's body image dissatisfaction, Russell-Mayhew et al. (2008) suggested the following strategies: (1) facilitating consciousness raising regarding the political, economic, and social ramifications of perpetuating an environment where women feel unhappy about their bodies, (2) encouraging youth and women to get involved and become advocates to address social issues, and (3) encouraging women to find meaning in their lives and address social justice work globally. Russell-Mayhew et al. (2008, 131) wrote:

> What if we could empower women to shift their energy and stop investing in changing their bodies through dieting, plastic surgery, and so on, AND start investing their energy into helping other mothers in the world feed their children? What if we, as a community of women with considerable social power, could mobilize others to divert attention from individual weight to global wellness?

REFERENCES

Abell, S. C., and M. H. Richards. 1996. The relationship between body shape satisfaction and self-esteem: An investigation of gender and class differences. *J Youth Adolesc* 25: 691–703.

Abood, D. A., and S. B. Chandler. 1997. Race and the role of weight, weight change, and body dissatisfaction in eating disorders. *Am J Health Behav* 21: 21–25.

Abdollahi, P., and T. Mann. 2001. Eating disorder symptoms and body image concerns in Iran: Comparisons between Iranian women in Iran and in America. *Int J Eat Disord* 30: 259–268.

Abrams, L. S., and C. C. Stormer. 2002. Sociocultural variations in the body image perception of urban adolescent females. *J Youth Adolesc* 31: 443–450.

Akan, G. E., and C. M. Grilo. 1995. Sociocultural influences on eating attitudes and behaviors, body image, and psychological functioning: A comparison of African-American, Asian American and Caucasian college women. *Int J Eat Disord* 18: 181–187.

Altabe, M., and J. K. Thompson. 1993. Body image changes during early adulthood. *Int J Eat Disord* 13: 323–328.

Anderson-Fye, E. 2009. Cross-cultural issues in body image among children and adolescents. In *Body image, eating disorders, and obesity in youth: Assessment, prevention, and treatment* (2nd ed), ed. L. E. Smolak and J. K. Thompson, 113–133. Washington, DC: American Psychological Association.

Ata, R. N., A. B. Ludden, and M. M. Lally. 2007. The effects of gender, and family, friend, and media influences on eating behaviors and body image during adolescence. *J Youth Adolesc* 36: 1024–1037.

Attie, I., and J. Brooks-Gunn. 1989. Development of eating problems in adolescent girls: A longitudinal study. *Dev Psychol* 25: 70–79.

Augustus-Horvath, C. L., and T. L. Tylka. 2009. A test and extension of objectification theory as it predicts disordered eating: Does women's age matter? *J Counsel Psychol* 56: 253–265.

Barker, E. T., and N. L. Galambos. 2003. Body dissatisfaction of adolescent girls and boys: Risk and resource factors. *J Early Adolesc* 23: 141–165.

Barry, D. T., and C. M. Grilo. 2002. Eating and body image disturbances in adolescent psychiatric inpatients: Gender and ethnicity patterns. *Int J Eat Disord* 32: 335–343.

Beren, S. E., H. A. Hayden, D. E. Wilfley, and C. M. Grilo. 1996. The influence of sexual orientation on body dissatisfaction in adult men and women. *Int J Eat Disord* 20: 135–141.

Bergeron, S. M., and C. Y. Senn. 1998. Body image and sociocultural norms: A comparison of heterosexual and lesbian women. *Psychol Women Q* 22: 385–401.

Boutelle, K., M. E. Eisenberg, M. L. Gregory, and D. Neumark-Sztainer. 2009. The reciprocal relationship between parent–child connectedness and adolescent emotional functioning over 5 years. *J Psychosom Res* 66: 309–316.

Byely, L., A. B. Archibald, J. Graber, and J. Brooks-Gunn. 2000. A prospective study of familial and social influences on girls' body image and dieting. *Int J Eat Disord* 28: 155–164.

Cachelin, F. M., T. K. Monreal, and L. C. Juarez. 2006. Body image and size perceptions of Mexican American women. *Body Image* 3: 67–75.

Cachelin, F. M., R. M. Rebeck, G. H. Chung, and E. Pelayo. 2002. Does ethnicity influence body size preference? A comparison of body image and body size. *Obes Res* 10: 158–166.

Calandra, J. M. 2001. Body image in menopausal lesbian and heterosexual women. *Dissertation Abstracts International: Section B: The Sciences and Engineering* 61: 6698.

Caldwell, M. B., K. D. Brownell, and D. E. Wilfley. 1997. Relationship of weight, body dissatisfaction, and self-esteem in African American and white female dieters. *Int J Eat Disord* 22: 127–130.

Caples, S. L. 2009. Measuring up: An examination of the impact of racial identity, schema, feminist attitudes, and socio-economic status on body image attitudes among Black women. *Diss Abstr Int: Section B: The Sciences and Engineering* 69 (9-B): 5761.

Cash, T. F. 1995. Developmental teasing about physical appearance: Retrospective descriptions and relationships with body image. *Soc Behav Pers* 23: 123–130.

Cash, T. F., and T. A. Brown. 1989. Gender and body images: Stereotypes and realities. *Sex Roles* 21: 361–373.

Cash, T. F., and E. A. Deagle III. 1997. The nature and extent of body-image disturbances in anorexia nervosa and bulimia nervosa: A meta-analysis. *Int J Eat Disord* 22: 107–125.

Cash, T. F., and P. E. Henry. 1995. Women's body images: The results of a national survey in the U.S.A. *Sex Roles* 33: 19–28.

Cash, T. F., S. E. Melnyk, and J. I. Hrabosky. 2004. The assessment of body image investment: An extensive revision of the Appearance Schemas Inventory. *Int J Eat Disord* 35: 305–316.

Clark, L. S., and M. Tiggemann. 2006. Appearance culture in 9 to 12-year-old girls: Media and peer influences on body dissatisfaction. *Soc Dev* 15: 628–643.

Compian, L., L. K. Gowen, and C. Hayward. 2004. Peripubertal girls' romantic and platonic involvement with boys: Associations with body image and depression. *Res Adolesc* 14: 23–47.

Coovert, D. L., J. K. Thompson, and B. N. Kinder. 1988. Interrelationships among multiple aspects of body image and eating disturbance. *Int J Eat Disord* 7: 495–502.

DeLeel, M. L., T. L. Hughes, J. A. Miller, A. Hipwell, and L. A. Theodore. 2009. Prevalence of eating disturbance and body image dissatisfaction in young girls: An examination of the variance across racial and socioeconomic groups. *Psychol Sch* 46: 767–775.

Dohnt, H., and M. Tiggemann. 2006. The contribution of peer and media influences to the development of body satisfaction and self-esteem in young girls: A prospective study. *Dev Psychol* 42: 929–936.

Dolan, B., J. H. Lacey, and C. Evans. 1990. Eating behaviour and attitudes to weight and shape in British women from three ethnic groups. *Br J Psychiatry* 157: 523–528.

Drewnowski, A., and D. K. Yee. 1987. Men and body-image: Are males satisfied with their body weight? *Psychosom Med* 49: 626–634.

Dworkin, S. H. 1989. Not in man's image: Lesbians and the cultural oppression of body image. *Women Ther* 8: 27–39.

Eisenburg, M. E., D. Neumark-Sztainer, J. Hanes, and M. Wall. 2006. Weight-teasing and emotional well-being in adolescents: Longitudinal finding from Project EAT. *J Adolesc Health* 38: 675–683.

Falconer, J. W., and H. A. Neville. 2000. African American college women's body image: An examination of body mass, African self-consciousness, and skin color satisfaction. *Psychol Women Q* 24: 236–243.

Fallon, A. E. 1990. Culture in the mirror: Sociocultural determinants of body image. In *Body images: Development, deviance and change*, ed. T. Cash and T. Pruzinsky, 80–109. New York: Guilford Press.

Fallon, A. E. 1994. Body image and the regulation of weight. In *Psychological perspectives on women's health*, ed. V. J. Adesso, D. M. Reddy, and R. Fleming, 127–180. Washington, DC: Taylor and Francis.

Fingeret, M. C., C. S. Warren, A. Cepeda-Benito, and D. H. Gleaves. 2006. Eating disorder prevention research: A meta-analysis. *Eat Disord: J Treat Prev* 14: 191–213.

Franko, D. L., and J. B. Edwards George. 2009. Overweight, eating behaviors, and body image in ethnically diverse youth. In *Body image, eating disorders, and obesity in youth: Assessment, prevention, and treatment* (2nd ed), ed. L.E. Smolak and J. K. Thompson, 97–112. Washington, DC: American Psychological Association.

Franzoi, S. L., and Z. Chang. 2002. The body esteem of Hmong and Caucasian young adults. *Psychol Women Q* 26: 89–91.

Fredrickson, B. L., and T. A. Roberts. 1997. Objectification theory: Toward understanding women's lived experiences and mental health risks. *Psychol Women Q* 21: 173–206.

Furnham, A., and N. Greaves. 1994. Gender and locus of control correlates of body image dissatisfaction. *Eur J Pers* 8: 183–200.

George, V. A., A. F. Erb, C. L. Harris, and K. Casazza. 2005. Psychosocial risk factors for eating disorders in Hispanic females of diverse ethnic background and non-Hispanic females. *Eat Behav* 8: 1–9.

Goodman, L. A., B. Liang, L. E. Helms, R. E. Latta, E. Sparks, and S. R. Weintraub. 2004. Training counseling psychologists as social justice agents: Feminist and multicultural principles in action. *Couns Psychol* 32: 793–837.

Gordon, K. H., Y. Castro, L. Sitnikov, and J. M. Holm-Denoma. 2010. Cultural body shape ideals and eating disorder symptoms among White, Latina, and Black college women. *Cultur Divers Ethnic Minor Psychol* 16: 135–143.

Grabe, S., and J. Hyde. 2006. Ethnicity and body dissatisfaction among women in the United States: A meta-analysis. *Psychol Bull* 132: 622–640.

Gray, J. J., K. Ford, and L. M. Kelly. 1987. The prevalence of bulimia in a black college population. *Int J Eat Disord* 6: 733–740.

Gupta, M. A., N. J. Schork, and J. S. Dhaliwal. 1993. Stature, drive for thinness and body dissatisfaction: A study of males and females from a non-clinical sample. *Can J Psychiatry* 38: 59–61.

Hall, C. C. I. 1995. Asian eyes: Body image and eating disorders of Asian and Asian American women. *Eat Disord: J Treat Prev* 3: 8–19.

Harris, S. M. 1994. Racial differences in predictors of women's body image attitudes. *Women Health* 2: 89–104.

Heffernan, K. 1996. Eating disorders and weight concern among lesbians. *Int J Eat Disord* 19: 127–138.

Jacobi, L., and T. A. Cash. 1994. In pursuit of the perfect appearance: Discrepancies among self-ideal percepts of multiple physical attributes. *J Appl Soc Psychol* 24: 379–396.

Kashubeck-West, S., L. B. Mintz, and I. Weigold. 2005. Separating the effects of gender and weight-loss desire on body satisfaction and disordered eating behavior. *Sex Roles* 53: 505–518.

Keel, P. K., J. A. Fulkerson, and G. R. Leon. 1997. Disordered eating precursors in pre- and early adolescent girls and boys. *J Youth Adolesc* 26: 203–216.

Kelly, A. M., M. Wall, M. E. Eisenberg, M. Story, and D. Neumark-Sztainer. 2005. Adolescent girls with high body satisfaction: Who are they and what can they teach us? *J Adolesc Health* 37: 391–396.

Killen, J. D., C. Hayward, I. Litt, L. D. Hammer, D. M. Wilson, B. Miner, C. B. Taylor, A. Varady, and C. Shisslak, C. 1992. Is puberty a risk factor for eating disorders? *Am J Dis Child* 146: 323–325.

Killen, J. D., C. Hayward, D. M. Wilson, C. B. Taylor, L. D. Hammer, I. Litt, B. Simmonds, and F. Haydel. 1994. Factors associated with eating disorder symptoms in a community sample of 6th and 7th grade girls. *Int J Eat Disord* 15: 357–367.

Kornblau, I. S., H. C. Pearson, and C. R. Breitkopf. 2007. Demographic, behavioral, and physical correlates of body esteem among low-income female adolescents. *J Adolesc Health* 41: 566–570.

Kuczmarski, R. J., K. M. Flegal, S. M. Campbell, and C. L. Johnson. 1994. Increasing prevalence of overweight among U.S. adults. *J Am Med Assoc* 272: 205–211.

Legenbauer, T., S. Vocks, C. Schäfer, S. Schütt-Strömel, W. Hiller, C. Wagner, C., and C. Vögele. 2009. Preference for attractiveness and thinness in a partner: Influence of internalization of the thin ideal and shape/weight dissatisfaction in heterosexual women, heterosexual men, lesbians, and gay men. *Body Image* 6: 228–234.

Lester, R., and T. A. Petrie. 1998. Physical, psychological, and societal correlates of bulimic symptomatology among African American college women. *J Couns Psychol* 45: 315–321.

Levine, M. P., and L. Smolak. 1992. Toward a developmental psychopathology of eating disorders. In *The etiology of bulimia: The individual and familial contexts*, ed. J. Crowther, S. Hobfoll, M. Stephens, and D. Tennenbaum, 59–80. Washington, DC: Hemisphere Publishers.

Levine, M. P., and L. Smolak. 2009. Recent developments and promising directions in the prevention of negative body image and disordered eating in children and adolescents. In *Body image, eating disorders, and obesity in youth: Assessment, prevention, and treatment* (2nd ed), ed. L. E. Smolak and J. K. Thompson, 215–238. Washington, DC: American Psychological Association.

Levine, M. P., L. Smolak, and H. Hayden. 1994a. The relation of sociocultural factors to eating attitudes and behavior among middle school girls. *J Early Adolesc* 14: 471–490.

Levine, M. P., L. Smolak, A. F. Moodey, M. D. Shuman, and L. D. Hessen. 1994b. Normative developmental challenges and dieting and eating disturbances in middle school girls. *Int J Eat Disord* 15: 11–20.

Liberman, M., L. Gauvin, W. M. Bukowski, and D. R. White. 2001. Interpersonal influence and disordered eating behaviors in adolescent girls: The role of peer modeling, social reinforcement, and body-related teasing. *Eat Behav* 2: 215–236.

Lindberg, S., J. S. Hyde, and N. M. McKinley. 2006. A measure of objectified body consciousness for preadolescent and adolescent youth. *Psychol Women Q* 30: 65–76.

Littleton, H. L., and T. Ollendick. 2003. Negative body image and disordered eating behavior in children and adolescents: What places youth at risk and how can these problems be prevented? *Clin Child Fam Psychol Rev* 6: 51–66.

Lovejoy, M. 2001. Disturbances in the social body: Differences in body image and eating problems among African American and white women. *Gend Soc* 15: 239–261.

Lowes, J., and M. Tiggemann. 2003. Body dissatisfaction, dieting awareness and the impact of parental influence in young children. *Br J Health Psychol* 8: 135–147.

McCauley, M. C., L. B. Mintz, and A. G. Glenn. 1988. Body image self-esteem and depression: Closing the gender gap. *Sex Roles* 18: 381–391.

McComb, J. R., and J. R. Clopton. 2002. Explanatory variance in bulimia nervosa. *Women Health* 36: 115–123.

McKinley, N. M., and J. S. Hyde. 1996. The objectified body consciousness scale: Self-objectification, body shame, and disordered eating. *Psychol Women Q* 22: 623–636.

McLaren, L., and D. Kuh. 2004a. Body dissatisfaction in midlife women. *J Women Aging* 16: 35–54.

McLaren, L., and D. Kuh. 2004b. Women's body dissatisfaction, social class, and social mobility. *Soc Sci Med* 58: 1575–1584.

McVey, G.L., D. Pepler, R. Davis, G. L. Flett, and M. Abdolell. 2002. Risk and protective factors associated with disordered eating during early adolescence. *J Early Adolesc* 22: 75–95.

Mintz, L. B. and N. E. Betz. 1986. Sex differences in the nature, realism, and correlates of body image. *Sex Roles* 15: 185–195.

Mintz, L. B., and S. Kashubeck. 1999. Body image and disordered eating in Asian and Caucasian college students: An examination of race and gender differences. *Psychol Women Q* 23: 781–796.

Molloy, B. L., and S. D. Herzberger. 1998. Body image and self-esteem: A comparison of African American and Caucasian women. *Sex Roles* 38: 631–643.

Moradi, B., D. Dirks, and A. V. Matteson. 2005. Roles of sexual objectification experiences and internalization of standards of beauty in eating disorder symptomatology: A test and extension of objectification theory. *J Couns Psychol* 52: 420–428.

Morrison, M. A., T. G. Morrison, and C. Sager. 2004. Does body satisfaction differ between gay men and lesbian women and heterosexual men and women? A meta-analytic review. *Body Image* 1: 127–138.

Morrison, C. D. 2006. The impact of sport involvement on adolescent girls' body image. *Diss Abstr Int: Section B: The Sciences and Engineering* 67: 1709.

Muth, J. L., and T. F. Cash. 1997. Body-image attitudes: What difference does gender make? *J Appl Soc Psychol* 27: 1438–1452.

Nassar, M. 1988. Culture and weight consciousness. *J Psychosom Res* 32: 573–577.

Nelson, C. L., and C. A. Gidycz. 1993. A comparison of body image perception in bulimics, restrainers, and normal women: An extension of previous findings. *Addict Behav* 18: 503–509.

Nemeroff, C. J., R. I. Stein, N. S. Diehl, and K. M. Smilack. 1994. From the Cleavers to the Clintons: Role, choices and body orientation as reflected in magazine article content. *Int J Eat Disord* 16: 167–176.

Nishina, A., N. Y. Ammon, A. D. Bellmore, and S. Graham. 2006. Body dissatisfaction and physical development among ethnic minority adolescents. *J Youth Adolesc* 35: 189–201.

Pasman, L., and J. K. Thompson. 1988. Body image and eating disturbance in obligatory runners, obligatory weightlifters, and sedentary individuals. *Int J Eat Disord* 7: 759–769.

Patton, T. O. 2006. Hey girl, am I more than my hair? African American women and their struggles with beauty, body image, and hair. *NWSA J* 18: 24–51.

Paxton, S. J. 1996. Prevention implications of peer influences on body image dissatisfaction and disturbed eating in adolescent girls. *Eat Disord: J Treat Prev* 4: 334–337.

Paxton, S. J., M.E. Eisenberg, and D. Neumark-Sztainer. 2006. Prospective predictors of body dissatisfaction in adolescent girls and boys: A five-year longitudinal study. *Dev Psychol* 42: 888–889.

Penner, L. A., J. K. Thompson, and D. L. Coovert. 1991. Size estimation among anorexics: Much ado about very little? *J Abnorm Psychol* 100: 90–93.

Peplau, L. A., D. A. Frederick, C. Yee, N. Maisel, J. Lever, and N. Ghavami. 2009. Body image satisfaction in heterosexual, gay, and lesbian adults. *Arch Sex Behav* 38: 713–725.

Phan, T., and T. L. Tylka. 2006. Exploring a model and moderators of disordered eating with Asian American college women. *J Couns Psychol* 53: 36–47.

Phares, V., A. R. Steinberg, and J. K. Thompson. 2004. Gender differences in peer and parental influences: Body image disturbance, self-worth, and psychological functioning in preadolescent children. *J Youth Adolesc* 33: 421–429.

Pliner, P., S. Chaiken, and G. L. Flett. 1990. Gender differences in concern with body weight and physical appearance over the life span. *Pers Soc Psychol Bull* 16: 263–273.

Poran, M. A. 2006. The politics of protection: Body image, social pressures, and the misrepresentation of young black women. *Sex Roles* 55: 739–755.

Powell, M. R., and B. Hendricks. 1999. Body schema, gender, and other correlates in nonclinical populations. *Genet Soc Gen Psychol Monogr* 125: 333–412.

Pumariega, A. J., C. R. Gustavson, J. C. Gustavson, P. S. Motes, and S. Ayers. 1994. Eating attitudes in African-American women: The Essence Eating Disorders Survey. *Eat Disord: J Treat Prev* 2: 5–16.

Rieves, L., and T. F. Cash. 1996. Social developmental factors and women's body-image attitudes. *J Soc Behav Pers* 11: 63–78.

Rodin, J., L.R. Silberstein, and R. H. Striegel-Moore. 1985. Women and weight: A normative discontent. In *Nebr Symp on Motivation: Psychology and Gender*, ed. T. B. Sonderegger, 267–307. Lincoln, NE: Univ of Nebr Press.

Root, M. P. 1990. Disordered eating in women of color. *Sex Roles* 22: 525–536.

Rosen, J. C., and J. Gross. 1987. Prevalence of weight reducing and weight gaining in adolescent girls and boys. *Health Psychol* 6: 131–147.

Rosen, J. C., N. T. Silberg, and J. Gross. 1988. Eating Attitudes Test and Eating Disorder Inventory: Norms for adolescent girls and boys. *J Consult Clin Psychol* 56: 305–308.

Rothblum, E. 1990. Women and weight: Fad and fiction. *J Psychol* 124: 5–24.

Rozin, P., and A. Fallon. 1988. Body image, attitudes towards weight, and misperceptions of figure preferences of the opposite sex: A comparison of men and women in two generations. *J Abnorm Psychol* 97: 342–345.

Rucker, C. E., and T. F. Cash. 1992. Body images, body-size perceptions, and eating behaviors among African American and White college women. *Int J Eat Disord* 12: 291–299.

Russell-Mayhew, S. 2007. Eating disorders and obesity as social justice issues: Implications for research and practice. *J Soc Action Couns Psychol* 1: 1–13.

Russell-Mayhew, S., M. Stewart, and S. M. MacKenzie. 2008. Eating disorders as social justice issues: Results from a focus group of content experts vigorously flapping our wings. *Can J Couns* 42: 131–146.

Share, T. L., and L. B. Mintz. 2002. Differences between lesbians and heterosexual women in disordered eating and related attitudes. *J Homosex* 42: 89–106.

Shaw, H., L. Ramirez, A. Trost, P. Randall, and E. Stice. 2004. Body image and eating disturbances across ethnic groups: More similarities than differences. *Psychol Addict Behav* 18: 12–18.

Shrewsbury, V. A., K. A. Robb, C. Power, and J. Wardle. 2009. Socioeconomic differences in weight retention, weight-related attitudes and practices in postpartum women. *Matern Child Health J* 13: 231–240.

Siegel, J. M. 2002. Body image change and adolescent depressive symptoms. *J Adolesc Res* 17: 27–41.

Silberstein, L. R., R. H. Striegel-Moore, C. Timko, and J. Rodin. 1988. Behavioral and psychological implications of body dissatisfaction: Do men and women differ? *Sex Roles* 19: 219–232.

Slade, P. D. 1985. A review of body-image studies in anorexia nervosa and bulimia nervosa. *J Psychiatr Res* 19: 255–265.

Slade, P. D., and G. G. M. Russell. 1973. Awareness of body dimensions in anorexia nervosa: Cross-sectional and longitudinal studies. *Psychol Med* 3: 188–199.

Smolak, L. 2009. Risk factors in the development of body image, eating problems, and obesity. In *Body image, eating disorders, and obesity in youth: Assessment, prevention, and treatment* (2nd ed), ed. L. E. Smolak and J. K. Thompson, 135–155. Washington, DC: American Psychological Association.

Smolak, L., M. P. Levine, and S. Gralen. 1993. The impact of puberty and dating on eating problems among middle school girls. *J Youth Adolesc* 22: 355–368.

Smolak, L., and S. K. Murnen. 2008. Drive for leanness: Assessment and relationship to gender, gender role and objectification. *Body Image* 5: 251–260.

Smolak, L., S. Murnen, and A. Ruble. 2000. Female athletes and eating problems: A meta-analytic approach. *Int J Eat Disord* 27: 371–380.

Smolak, L., and J. K. Thompson. 2009. Body image, eating disorders, and obesity in children and adolescents: Introduction to the second edition. In *Body image, eating disorders, and obesity in youth: Assessment, prevention, and treatment* (2nd ed), ed. L. E. Smolak and J. K. Thompson, 3–14. Washington, DC: American Psychological Association.

Snapp, S. 2009. Internalization of the thin ideal among low-income ethnic minority adolescent girls. *Body Image* 6: 311–314.

Sobal, J., and A. J. Stunkard. 1989. Socioeconomic status and obesity: A review of the literature. *Psychol Bull* 105: 260–275.

Stice, E., J. Maxfield, and T. Wells. 2003. Adverse effects of social pressure to be thin on young women: An experimental investigation of the effects of "fat talk." *Int J Eat Disord* 34: 108–117.

Stice, E., and H. E. Shaw. 1994. Adverse effects of the media-portrayed thin ideal on women and linkages to bulimic symptomatology. *J Soc Clin Psychol* 13: 288–308.

Stice, E., and H. E. Shaw. 2002. Role of body dissatisfaction in the onset and maintenance of eating pathology: A synthesis of research findings. *J Psychosom Res* 53: 985–993.

Stice, E., and H. Shaw. 2004. Eating disorder prevention programs: A meta-analytic review. *Psychol Bull* 130: 206–227.

Stice, E., H. Shaw, and C. N. Marti. 2007. A meta-analytic review of eating disorder prevention programs: Encouraging findings. *Annu Rev Clin Psychol* 3: 207–231.

Story, M., S. A. French, M. D. Resnick, and R. W. Blum. 1995. Ethnic/racial and socioeconomic differences in dieting behaviors and body image perceptions in adolescents. *Int J Eat Disord* 18: 173–179.

Striegel-Moore, R. H., and F. M. Cachelin. 1999. Body image concerns and disordered eating in adolescent girls: Rick and protective factors. In *Beyond appearance: A new look at adolescent girls*, ed. N. G. Johnson, M. C. Roberts, and J. Worell, 85–108. Washington, DC: American Psychological Association.

Suldo, S. M., and D. A. Sandberg, D. A. 2000. Relationship between attachment styles and eating disorder symptomatology among college women. *J College Stud Psychother* 15: 59–73.

Thelen, M. H., and J. Cormier. 1995. Desire to be thinner and weight control among children and their parents. *Behav Ther* 26: 85–99.

Thompson, J. K. 1990. *Body image disturbance: Assessment and treatment.* New York: Pergamon Press.

Thompson, J. K. 1991. Body shape preferences: Effects of instructional protocol and level of eating disturbance. *Int J Eat Disord* 10: 193–198.

Thompson, J. K. 1992. Body image: Extent of disturbance, associated features, theoretical models, assessment methodologies, intervention strategies, and a proposal for a new DSM IV diagnostic category—Body Image Disorder. In *Progress in behavior modification* (vol. 29), ed. M. Hersen, R. M. Eisler, and P. M. Miller, 3–54. New York: Sage.

Thompson, J. K., M. N. Altabe, S. Johnson, and S. Stormer. 1994. Multiple measures of body image disturbance: Are we all measuring the same construct? *Int J Eat Disord* 16: 311–315.

Thompson, J. K., N. W. Berland, P. H. Linton, and R. Weinsier. 1986. Assessment of body distortion via a self-adjusting light beam in seven eating disorder groups. *Int J Eat Disord* 7: 113–120.

Thompson, J. K., L. J. Fabian, D. O. Moulton, M. F. Dunn, and M. N. Altabe. 1991. Development and validation of the physical appearance related testing scale. *J Pers Assess* 56: 513–521.

Thompson, J. K., and K. Psaltis. 1988. Multiple aspects and correlations of body figure ratings: A replication and extension of Fallon and Rozine (1985). *Int J Eat Disord* 7: 813–818.

Thompson, J. K., and E. Stice. 2001. Thin-ideal internalization: Mounting evidence for a new risk factor for body-image disturbance and eating pathology. *Curr Dir Psychol Sci* 10: 181–183.

Thompson, S. H., S. J. Corwin, and R. G. Sargent. 1997. Ideal body size beliefs and weight concerns of fourth-grade children. *Int J Eat Disord* 21: 279–284.

Tiggemann, M. 2001. The impact of adolescent girls' life concerns and leisure activities on body dissatisfaction disordered eating, and self-esteem. *J Genet Psychol* 162: 133–142.

Turner, S. L., H. Hamilton, M. Jacobs, L. M. Angood, and D. H. Dwyer. 1997. The influence of fashion magazines on the body image satisfaction of college women: An exploratory analysis. *Adolescence* 32: 603–614.

Tylka, T. L., and M. S. Hill. 2004. Objectification theory as it relates to disordered eating among college women. *Sex Roles* 51: 719–730.

Veron-Guidry, S., D. A. Williamson, and R. G. Netemeyer. 1997. Structural modeling analysis of body dysphoria and eating disorder symptoms in preadolescent girls. *Eat Disord: J Treat Prev* 5: 15–27.

Vincent, M. A., and M. P. McCabe. 2000. Gender differences among adolescents in family and peer influences on body dissatisfaction, weight loss, and binge eating behaviors. *J Youth Adolesc* 29: 205–221.

Wadden, T. A., G. Brown, G. D. Foster, and J. R. Linowitz. 1991. Salience of weight-related worries in adolescent males and females. *Int J Eat Disord* 10: 407–414.

Wertheim, E. H., S. J. Paxton, and S. Blaney. 2009. Body image in girls. In *Body image, eating disorders, and obesity in youth: Assessment, prevention, and treatment* (2nd ed), ed. L. E. Smolak and J. K. Thompson, 47–76. Washington, DC: American Psychological Association.

Whitaker, A., M. Davies, D. Shaffer, J. Johnson, S. Abrams, T. Walsh, and K. Kalikow. 1989. The struggle to be thin: A survey of anorexic and bulimic symptoms in a non-referred adolescent population. *Psychol Med* 19: 143–163.

Wilfley, D. E., and J. Rodin. 1995. Cultural influences on eating disorders. In *Eating disorders and obesity: A comprehensive handbook*, ed. K. D. Brownell and C. G. Fairburn, 78–82. New York: Guilford Press.

Wilfley, D. E., G. B. Schreiber, K. M. Pike, R. M. Striegel-Moore, D. J. Wright, and J. Rodin. 1996. Eating disturbance and body image: A comparison of a community sample of adult black and white women. *Int J Eat Disord* 20: 377–387.

Williams, J. M., and C. Currie. 2000. Self-esteem and physical development in early adolescence: Pubertal timing and body image. *J Early Adolesc* 20: 129–149.

Williamson, D. A., S. E. Barker, L. J. Bertman, and D. H. Gleaves. 1995. Body image, body dysphoria, and dietary restraint: Factor structure in nonclinical subjects. *Behav Res Ther* 33: 85–93.

Williamson, D. A., B. A. Cubic, and D. H. Gleaves. 1993. Equivalence of body image disturbance in anorexia and bulimia nervosa. *J Abnorm Psychol* 102: 177–180.

Yates, A., J. Edman, and M. Aruguete. 2004. Ethnic differences in BMI and body/self-dissatisfaction among whites, Asian subgroups, Pacific Islanders, and African-Americans. *J Adolesc Health* 34: 300–307.

10 Sexuality and Eating Disorders

Annette S. Kluck, Sheila Garos, and Lucy Johnson

CONTENTS

10.1 LEARNING OBJECTIVES

After completing this chapter, you should be able to

- Discuss the sexual experiences that are commonly associated with eating disorders
- Recognize important variables that may influence the sexual experience of individuals with eating disorders
- Identify tools for assessing and treating eating disorders that incorporate issues pertaining to sexuality

10.2 BACKGROUND AND SIGNIFICANCE

Early conceptions of eating disorders evolved principally from the psychoanalytic perspective and asserted that eating disorders served as a means to avoid sexual intimacy and maturity (e.g., Blitzer et al. 1961; Crisp 1965). This notion continued into the early to mid-twentieth century literature, whereby eating disorders were thought of as a way for women to avoid sexual activity (e.g., Bruch 1978; Crisp 1965). Waller et al. (1940) reported that sexual urges, including masturbation, caused extreme guilt and anxiety in individuals with anorexia. Similarly, in an early case report, Janet (as cited in Russell 1997) described a young woman who, disgusted by her pubescent body, developed bulimia in an effort to maintain sexual modesty (she viewed curves as sexually provocative and sought to decrease the curvaceousness of her body). From this perspective, eating disorders allow individuals to avoid the physiological changes associated with sexual maturation and engagement in sexual relations (e.g., Bruch 1978; Crisp 1997). That is, the physiological effects of eating disorders (e.g., amenorrhea, extreme emaciation) were interpreted as a rejection of puberty itself (Bruch 1978; Crisp 1965, 1997).

Early case studies reported that some young girls believed eating and getting "fat" caused pregnancy (Blitzer et al. 1961; Rose 1943). Lorand (1943) viewed eating disorders as a fixation in Freud's oral stage of psychosexual development in which gratification occurs orally rather than genitally. It has been suggested that eating disorders act as a defense mechanism against unacceptable desires such as "penis envy," fantasies of oral impregnation, and incestuous thoughts (Lorand 1943; Rose 1943; Russell 1997; Waller et al. 1940). This link between unacceptable sexual desires and food is what Waller et al. (1940) contended causes disgust with food that is frequently observed in women with eating disorders. Thus, food refusal acts as the symbolic rejection of one's unacceptable sexual fantasies, and gorging on food is a proxy for the gratification of one's sexual fantasies.

The view that eating disorders are linked with sexual development is consistent with the tendency for eating disorders to emerge in adolescence and early adulthood (Striegel-Moore et al. 1986), the time that is associated with the development of secondary sex characteristics, such as increased breast size in women and growth of facial hair in men. In addition, adolescence and young adulthood are developmental periods that are associated with forming intimate relationships, sexual exploration, and sexual activity (Miller 2011). Not surprisingly, researchers have examined the extent to which fears of maturation, difficulties with intimacy, and problems with sexual functioning are more characteristic of individuals with eating disorders.

The notion that anorexia represents incestuous desires, impregnation fantasies, or fears of intimacy is not universal, and contemporary research has yielded more questions than answers regarding the link between sexuality and eating disorders (Coovert et al. 1989). Perhaps, most vital to understanding the eating disorder–sexuality link is research that shows that the state of starvation commonly associated with eating disorders is related to reductions in sex drive and alterations in sex hormone production (Tuiten et al. 1992, 1993; Weiner 1989). Beumont and colleagues (1981) found that 80% of their sample of women with anorexia experienced decreased libido, which the women attributed to fatigue associated with weight loss. Coovert et al. (1989) have argued that earlier observations and empirical studies of anorexic patients failed to control for the negative effects that weight can have on the timing of menarche and on sex drive. In addition, researchers have found more normal levels of sexual functioning in women with eating disorders who are in recovery (e.g. Fichter et al. 2006). Thus, differences in sexual activity among some individuals with eating disorders may be consequences of abnormal eating and abnormal weight.

Contemporary research on the role of sexuality in the development of eating disorders encompasses six broad domains: (1) maturity (timing of puberty, sex hormones and physical changes, emotional maturity), (2) patterns of sexual experience (including sexual satisfaction and achievement of sexual milestones), (3) intimacy, (4) pursuit of sexual attractiveness, (5) unwanted sexual attention, and 6) sexual orientation. However, so far, there is little research on the inclusion of sexuality in the treatment of eating disorders.

10.3 CURRENT FINDINGS

10.3.1 SEXUAL MATURITY

10.3.1.1 Timing of Puberty

As previously discussed, early psychoanalytic perspectives suggested that fears associated with physical maturation and womanhood were the causes of eating disorders. Consistent with this perspective, the onset of eating disorders often occurs during or shortly after puberty (in mid-adolescence through early adulthood), which has led many researchers to contend that adolescent sexual pressures relate to the development of these disorders (e.g., Kaltiala-Heino et al. 2001; Romeo 1984). In general, the research relating the timing of puberty to the onset of eating disorders has been inconsistent. Several studies suggest that milestones in sexual development (e.g., menarche, breast tissue development) for women diagnosed with eating disorders do not differ substantially from those experienced by women in general, and do not differ across subtypes of eating disorder (e.g., restrictive anorexia, binge–purge anorexia; e.g., Abraham et al. 1985; Pryor et al. 1996; Rothschild et al. 1991; Ruuska et al. 2003; Schmidt et al. 1995). A few studies have found some increase in body dissatisfaction and disordered eating for individuals who experienced puberty early or on time compared to individuals who experience puberty later (Keski-Rahkonen et al. 2005; McCabe and Ricciardelli 2004). However, those studies included early adolescents, such that some of the participants likely had not yet experienced puberty and its associated weight gain, both of which are risk factors for eating disorders themselves regardless of timing (Killen et al. 1992; Koff and Rierdan 1993; O'Dea and Abraham 1999). In other words, for cross-sectional studies in which women who have not yet completed puberty are compared with those who have completed puberty because they experienced it earlier, the effects of puberty itself and weight gain that accompanies puberty in women are not controlled for. Therefore, it is not possible to conclude that adolescent females who experience puberty earlier than others are at greater risk for body image dissatisfaction or eating disorders than those who have not yet experienced puberty. Despite a lack of differences in timing of pubertal development, women with eating disorders may experience puberty more negatively compared to other women (Mangweth-Matzek et al. 2007).

10.3.1.2 Sex Hormones and Physiological Changes

Although there are few differences in the timing of puberty between individuals with and without eating disorder diagnoses, ample research documents the decrease in sexual hormone levels among individuals with eating disorders and those who engage in severe dieting or other disturbed eating practices (for a review, see Goodwin 1990). Young (1991) proposed that levels of estrogen, a sexual hormone related to puberty that in high doses has been linked with decreased appetite in some women, may be a causal factor in the development of eating disorders. If so, then estrogen levels would help explain the large gender differences in prevalence rates. In addition, testosterone levels, which relate to libido, have also been found to be lower among women with anorexia than women without eating disorders (Killen et al. 1992). Young's (1991) hypothesis regarding sex hormones explains from a biological perspective rather than from a psychosexual perspective the tendency for eating disorders to emerge during adolescence and young adulthood.

Regardless of the potential for sex hormones to contribute to the development of an eating disorder, the decreased sexual interest or drive that is commonly observed with eating disorders would be expected when weight loss is sufficient to cause amenorrhea (Tuiten et al. 1992). Low body mass index has been found to predict sexual anxiety, loss of libido, and less sexual activity in relationships (Morgan et al. 1995; Pinheiro et al. 2010). Other changes in physiology that accompany starvation and subsequent weight loss include amenorrhea and de-feminizing of the female physique such that women with anorexia appear more similar to prepubescent girls with child-like body proportions (Bruch 1978; Romeo 1984). Changes in hormone levels and physical appearance make it possible, at least for a subset of women with anorexia, that the illness represents an attempt to cope with the demands associated with sexual development and attention from potential sexual partners (Tuiten et al. 1993).

10.3.1.3 Emotional Maturity

Multiple studies suggest that individuals with eating disorders are emotionally immature and develop the eating disorder as type of coping mechanism. For example, Blitzer et al. (1961) reported that all cases of eating disorders observed in his treatment group displayed regressed coping strategies. For example, some patients acted in infantile ways, such as wanting others to dress them. Lorand (1943) also described a young woman with an eating disorder as showing infantile behavior (i.e., food refusal) rather than using words to express her feelings. Later research has extended these earlier clinical reports. For example, Steiner (1990) found that adolescents with eating disorders scored higher than other adolescents on a measure of immature defense mechanisms (e.g., acting before thinking). The failure to develop emotional maturity like most adolescents may be another indication of the difficulty these patients have accepting and adapting to normal adolescent development.

10.3.2 PATTERNS OF SEXUAL EXPERIENCES

Several studies offer insight into the psychosexual experiences of women who have eating disorders. Relevant literature suggests that women with bulimia are more sexually active and experienced than women with anorexia, and women with anorexia are often characterized as more rigid and restrictive in their sexual experiences (Abraham et al. 1985; Eddy et al. 2004; Garfinkel 1981; Wiederman et al. 1996). Some research suggests that women with bulimia are more likely to have previously experienced sexual intercourse than women with anorexia, and this pattern often continues after treatment (Wiederman et al. 1996). In fact, compared to women with bulimia, women with anorexia (1) experience their first petting and coitus later in life (Schmidt et al. 1995; Wiederman et al. 1996), (2) have fewer sexual partners (Schmidt et al. 1995), (3) express more disgust toward or lack of interest in sex during and prior to the onset of their disorder (Pinheiro et al. 2010; Ruuska et al. 2003; Wiederman et al. 1996), (4) masturbate less frequently (Morgan et al. 1995; Wiederman et al. 1996), (5) have less oral sex (Beumont et al. 1981), (6) have lower sexual self-esteem (Morgan et al. 1995), and (7) date less frequently (Ruuska et al. 2003). However, differences between individuals with anorexia and bulimia are not always found for the timing of psychosexual milestones (such as the age at first coitus) and level of sexual dysfunction (e.g., Morgan et al. 1995; Rothschild et al. 1991).

Research comparing women with eating disorders to other women reveals the same general patterns. Women with anorexia were found to experience many of their psychosexual milestones (e.g., first kiss, first masturbation, first genital petting) later compared to a group of university women (Schmidt et al. 1995). In addition, compared to women in general, most women with anorexia do not report perceiving sex as enjoyable, engage in sex less frequently, and have higher rates of sexual dysfunctions (e.g., Beumont et al. 1981; Crisp et al. 1986; Schmidt et al. 1995; Tuiten et al. 1992). Research also suggests that women with anorexia lack knowledge about sex (Beumont et al. 1981). In contrast, women with bulimia were found to be similar to other women with regard to the timing of most psychosexual milestones (e.g., first date, first kiss, first coitus) and general sexual experiences (e.g., number of partners, length of longest relationship, use of sex aids; Abraham et al. 1985; Irving et al. 1990; Jagstaidt et al. 1996; Schmidt et al. 1995). However, women with bulimia or bulimic symptoms may engage in increased and more risky (i.e., unprotected) sexual activity than women who do not have eating disorders (Irving et al. 1990; Kaltiala-Heino et al. 2001; Keski-Rahkonen et al. 2005). In addition, though women with bulimia may have higher libido than other women, they do not necessarily experience sexual satisfaction with intercourse and have reported higher rates of sexual dysfunctions (Abraham et al. 1985; Garfinkel 1981; Jagstaidt et al. 1996).

Part of the reason women with eating disorders may experience more sexual dysfunctions, such as changes in sexual functioning and sex drive (Beumont et al. 1981), may relate to the physiological changes associated with eating disorders. For example, Crisp (1965) observed that for women, loss of libido was always present with amenorrhea when women with anorexia are actively restricting their caloric intake. Likewise, De Silva and Todd (1998) contended that endocrine changes associated with amenorrhea lead to reduced vaginal lubrication, making sex more painful for women with anorexia.

Despite evidence of physiological changes in women with eating disorders, these changes may not fully account for differences in sexual functioning between women with eating disorders and other women. Research suggests that women with eating disorders have more negative attitudes about sex, feel more sexual anxiety and tension, and experience their own achievement of sexual milestones more negatively than other women (Mangweth-Matzek et al. 2007; Pinheiro et al. 2010; Schmidt et al. 1995).

Except for investigations of the sexual orientation of men with eating disorders (see Section 10.3.6), research on the sexual functioning and sexual experience of men with eating disorders is lacking. The reasons for the lack of research on the sexual experiences and difficulties of men with eating disorders are not clear, but may stem from the lower prevalence rate of eating disorders among men (Buckley et al. 1991). Most available research on sexuality and eating disorders conducted with men focuses on men diagnosed with anorexia. Research suggests that men with anorexia have as much sexual anxiety as women with anorexia and, as such, may experience similar relief with the loss of libido that accompanies starvation (Fichter and Daser 1987; Herzog et al. 1984). Fichter and Daser (1987) found that only 30% of men diagnosed with anorexia had engaged in sexual intercourse with women and 15% had engaged in sexual intercourse with men, indicating that the majority of these men reported no past experience with sexual intercourse.

10.3.3 INTIMACY

The term *intimacy* is often used synonymously with sexual relationships, but intimacy also refers to emotional closeness. Research suggests that emotional intimacy is as problematic for women with eating disorders as physical intimacy (Van den Broucke et al. 1997). In a nonclinical sample of college women, those with higher levels of bulimic behavior shared information about themselves less frequently with their families and romantic partners, which may indicate some difficulty with emotional intimacy with family members and in romantic relationships (Evans and Wertheim 2002) Differences were not found in the amount of information shared with peers in this study. Women with eating disorders have also been found to be less likely to date or marry compared to women with other psychiatric diagnoses and to healthy women of similar ages (Mangweth-Matzek et al. 2007; Raboch and Faltus 1991). Furthermore, Raciti and Hendrick (1992) found that college women who endorsed more disordered eating symptoms tended to endorse possessive relationship styles and viewed relationships as "games." Additionally, women in that study who reported greater body dissatisfaction were less likely to view friendship as a part of love.

Investigations of the relationship between eating disorders and attachment also suggest problems with emotional intimacy. For example, more secure attachments, in which one is comfortable with close relationships, have been associated with lower scores on measures of disordered eating (Elgin and Pritchard 2006). Similarly, insecure attachment patterns have been linked with higher scores on measures of disordered eating in nonclinical samples (e.g., Evans and Wertheim 1998), and women with eating disorders display more problematic attachment patterns than women who do not have eating disorders (e.g., Armstrong and Roth 1989; Broberg et al. 2001). Collectively, this research suggests that intimacy may be problematic for women with eating disorders. If so, it is not surprising that women with eating disorders more often experience sexual dysfunctions (see Section 10.3.2) given the inherently "intimate" nature of sexual encounters and relations with romantic partners.

10.3.4 SEXUAL ATTRACTIVENESS STANDARDS

There is disagreement as to whether anorexia represents an attempt to avoid sexual maturity (e.g., Morgan et al. 1995). Some studies suggest that individuals with eating disorders believe being ultra thin is the standard for what is considered attractive (Silverstein and Perdue 1988; Tuiten et al. 1993). Thus, the attainment of thinness is not avoidance of sexual maturation; rather, it is an attempt to be sexually attractive to partners (Tantleff-Dunn and Thompson 1995). Tuiten et al. (1993) suggested that some women may develop disordered eating in an effort to become more sexually attractive, rather than to avoid sexual development, and that among these women, the loss of sexual desire may be an accidental by-product of extreme weight reduction. In addition, when women with bulimia are at their highest weights, they tend to avoid sexual interactions (e.g., Abraham et al. 1985; Jagstaidt et al. 1996). Keel et al.'s (2007) research lends further support to the idea that, for some women, eating less is a means to becoming more attractive. Their study found that once women became wives and mothers, their eating disorder symptoms abated. In sum, this research suggests that women may develop disordered eating in an attempt to become more appealing to the opposite sex, rather than as a means to avoid intimacy.

10.3.5 UNWANTED SEXUAL EXPERIENCES

A number of studies have examined the long-term, multifaceted consequences of childhood abuse and its association with disordered eating (e.g., Schmidt et al. 1997; Smyth et al. 2008). In addition, some research shows that men and women with a sexual assault history (e.g., rape) subsequently develop disordered eating patterns in adolescence and adulthood (e.g., Dansky et al. 1997; Laws and Golding 1996; Lock et al. 2001). However, given the complexities of the psychological effects of sexual trauma (for a review, see Cole and Putnam 1992), the increased tendency for individuals with a history of childhood sexual assault to be revictimized in adulthood (Wonderlich et al. 2001a), and methodological limitations inherent in some studies (e.g., inconsistent definitions of assault, compositions of study samples), this association may not be as simple as some research suggests (Connors and Morse 1993; Smolak and Murnen 2002). Nonetheless, most experts concede that, for some individuals, childhood sexual abuse and sexual assault later in life play a role in the development of eating disorders (Conners and Morse 1993; Smolak and Murnen 2002). However, it is likely that sexual trauma serves as a general risk factor for psychopathology, and eating disorders are only one way in which psychological problems are expressed (Connors and Morse 1993; Dansky et al. 1997).

Although a few studies have shown that rates of sexual abuse or trauma in individuals with eating disorders are similar to rates found in the general population (e.g., Finn et al. 1986), several authors suggest that eating disorders or subclinical patterns of disordered eating may develop as a means of coping for survivors of sexual trauma (e.g., Connors and Morse 1993; Wonderlich et al. 2001b). For example, women may seek to appear unappealing by gaining excessive amounts of weight in order to deter sexual attention from others (Gustafson and Sarwer 2004; Wiederman et al. 1999). Alternatively, by losing weight until they look prepubescent, women may appear less appropriate or appealing as sexual partners to a potential perpetrator (Jagstaidt et al. 1996). Tuiten et al. (1993) and Jagstaidt et al. (1996) suggested that women who experience sexual trauma might use food restriction to change their shape and "de-sexualize" their bodies as a means of neutralizing their sexuality, which they experience as having been defiled or tarnished. Research also links unwanted sexual experiences in the form of verbal comments (i.e., sexual harassment) with the development of disordered eating in women (Harned and Fitzgerald 2002). Thus, it seems that for a subgroup of women, unwanted sexual attention may be a precipitating factor in the development of disordered eating that can subsequently cause physiological changes that decrease one's sexual appeal in order to reduce unwanted sexual attention.

10.3.6 SEXUAL ORIENTATION

Adolescence is a time when young men and women begin to express romantic and sexual interests in others, whether the attraction is toward the same or opposite sex. Given that the onset of eating disorders is most common among adolescents and young adults (Striegel-Moore et al. 1986), researchers have investigated whether one's sexual orientation contributes to the etiology of eating disorders (e.g., Wichstrom 2006). Although some findings suggest that eating disorders are more common among homosexual men than heterosexual men (e.g., Feldman and Meyer 2007; Russell and Keel 2002; Wichstrom 2006), results of investigations of men do not always reveal differences in prevalence rates based on their sexual orientation (e.g., Olivardia et al. 1995). There is some evidence that a higher percentage of men than women who are receiving treatment for eating disorders identify themselves as homosexual (Herzog et al. 1984). However, Pope and colleagues (1986) found the proportion of homosexual men in treatment was similar to estimates in the general population, which can vary from 1% to 21% depending upon how investigators have defined sexual orientation (Savin-Williams 2006).

Among women, same-sex sexual experiences appear to have little bearing on the development of an eating disorder (e.g., Feldman and Meyer 2007; Jagstaidt et al. 1996). For example, a comparison of women who identify themselves as lesbian or heterosexual found that lesbian women were less likely to score above clinical cutoffs on measures of eating disorder symptoms (Siever 1996). In addition, women with eating disorders were less likely to identify themselves as homosexual or bisexual or report same-sex sexual experiences than men with eating disorders (Powers and Spratt 1994; Schneider and Agras 1987). Yet, for women, a few studies have linked bulimic eating patterns with more same-sex fantasies and a history of same-sex sexual experiences (Jagstaidt et al. 1996; Wichstrom 2006).

There is some evidence that homosexual men have higher rates of psychological problems than do their heterosexual counterparts (Cochran et al. 2003). Thus, some researchers have examined whether other psychological variables (e.g., depression) might account for the increased prevalence of disordered eating in homosexual men (e.g., Russell and Keel 2002; Wichstrom 2006). In contrast, Siever (1996) argued that it is men's tendency to value the appearance of their romantic or sexual partners more than women that accounts for both the higher prevalence rates of eating disorders in gay men and the lower rates of eating disorders in lesbian women when compared to their heterosexual counterparts. From this perspective, the association between sexuality and eating disorders is not one of avoiding sexual relations but instead is an attempt to attract sexual partners. However, little is known about the typical sexual practices and sexual development of men with eating disorders. Therefore, the findings that gay men may have higher rates of eating disturbances must be interpreted with caution. In sum, there is insufficient knowledge of how sexual orientation may relate to difficulties with eating disorders.

10.3.7 SUMMARY OF RESEARCH BACKGROUND

Research suggests that eating disorders can be associated with a range of disturbances in psychosexual development and sexual functioning for women (see Table 10.1). It is possible that these disturbances reflect hormonal changes that occur as the result of the poor nutrition that accompanies eating disorders (e.g., Tuiten et al. 1993). Though women with eating disorders generally do not differ from women without eating disorders with regard to pubertal timing, they are likely to have greater psychosexual conflict and more negative feelings about sex. Moreover, anorexia is commonly characterized by reduced sexual activity and libido. Whereas bulimia has most often

---

TABLE 10.1

Summary of Research on Sexual Experiences and Development in Women with Eating Disorders

Sexual Experiences Characteristic of	Anorexia	Bulimia
Timing of puberty	On-time	On-time
Achievement of sexual milestones	Delayed	On-time
Libido	Reduced	Potentially higher
Reduced sexual satisfaction	Yes	Sometimes
Sexual dysfunction	Yes	Yes
Reduced frequency of sexual activity	Yes	Sometimes
Increased frequency of sexual activity	No	Sometimes
Changes in sexual hormones	Yes	Under-researched
Engaged in more risky sexual activity	Under-researched	Yes

Notes: The table depicts sexual experiences of women with anorexia and bulimia compared to women without eating disorders. There is insufficient research to adequately describe the sexual experiences of men with eating disorders.

been associated with normal or higher rates of sexual activity, there is not an increase in sexual satisfaction, which is sometimes lower than found in women without eating disorders.

To understand the differences between the sexual functioning of women with eating disorders and that of normal women, researchers have examined several potential risk factors, such as difficulties with intimacy, history of sexual assault, and sexual orientation. Difficulties with emotional intimacy, pursuit of the thin cultural ideal to be more sexually appealing, and a history of sexual trauma may be part of the association between sexual functioning and eating disorders and may warrant attention when treating women with eating disorders who experience some type of sexual concern.

10.4 PRACTICAL APPLICATIONS

Despite the long history of linking sexuality to eating disorders in clinical theory, little has been written about targeting sexuality in eating disorder treatment. Research supports the inclusion of sexual concerns in treatment after the patient has achieved weight stabilization. For example, Tuiten et al. (1993) asserted that treatment for women with anorexia should initially focus on attaining a weight that is sufficient to restore hormonal levels necessary for normal sexual functioning, which often occurs subsequent to weight gain. In addition, studies suggest that individuals with eating disorders have greater difficulty with cognitive tasks, likely due to metabolic changes associated with the disorder (e.g., Laessle et al. 1990), which may impede their ability to concentrate in therapy (Zerbe 1992). Thus, most psychological aspects that warrant attention in the treatment of eating disorders, including issues pertaining to sexuality and sexual function, will need to wait to be addressed until a patient's weight and eating are sufficiently stable (and in patients who have severely restricted, wait until sufficient weight gain has occurred) to maximize cognitive function and subsequently enable engagement in treatment (De Silva and Todd 1998). Sexual dysfunction is a negative predictor of long-term treatment outcomes for eating disorders (Fichter et al. 2006). Thus, it is important to address issues pertaining to sexuality and sexual function once weight gain or weight stabilization has occurred. Moreover, given the psychological factors associated with sexual function, it is important to remember that weight restoration and weight stabilization are often not sufficient to restore sexual functioning (De Silva and Todd 1998; Morgan et al. 1995).

To adequately address sexual concerns in the treatment of eating disorders, the therapist will need to explore sexual concerns and sexual development during the initial sessions of therapy. For some individuals with eating disorders, sex is considered a taboo topic, and shyness or shame about one's sexual "self" will prevent a patient from broaching the subject (Zerbe 1992). In other cases, fears about sexuality or difficulties with intimacy may be precipitating factors in the development of the eating disorder (Guile et al. 1978). Although the questions that are necessary to obtain a thorough sexual history are explicit and may provoke anxiety in the clinician and patient, the clinician will need to broach the subject and explain the importance of obtaining an accurate sexual history, which may give patients a "license" to talk about subjects they would otherwise be reluctant to discuss. When possible, the clinician should involve the patient's spouse or partner in the evaluation and treatment of the patient, including his or her concerns pertaining to sex and intimacy (Van den Broucke et al. 1997).

When initially exploring the sexual history and concerns of a patient, the therapist may wish to use a structured interview on sexual functioning such as the *Derogatis Interview for Sexual Functioning* (DIFS; Derogatis 1997), which can be used with both men and women. The clinical interview should include information about the patient's sexual fantasies and dreams, attitudes and values related to sex and sexuality, and developmental information (e.g., timing of menses). When exploring sexual concerns for patients with eating disorders, the clinician should also explore the early recognition of changes in one's physical appearance, recollections of emotional reactions to physiological signs of maturity, and changes in appearance of sexual characteristics through the course of the eating disorder. In addition, clinicians should inquire about (1) the course, duration and nature of any sexual difficulties (including pain during sex), (2) patterns of sexual initiation and foreplay, (3) types of sexual acts the patients engages in, (4) age of first sexual experience, (5) how sexual knowledge was acquired, and (6) the use of any prescription, recreational, or illicit drugs that may affect sexual function. Two measures are available for clinicians who wish to use standardized measures of sexual functioning to understand whether the patient's sexual functioning represents a clinical concern: the *Profile of Female Sexual Function* (Derogatis et al. 2004, Sarti et al. 2004), a measure developed to assess level of sexual desire in women, and the *Female Sexual Distress Scale* (Derogatis et al. 2002), a measure designed to assess subjective distress regarding sexual concerns for women. The therapist will also want to ask the patient about her (or his) past and current romantic relationships along with the effect of the patient's illness on these relationships (Van den Broucke et al. 1997).

In addition, the clinicians should collaborate with the patients' medical providers (i.e., gynecologist or urologist) to rule out medically based etiologies (e.g., physical abnormalities, illnesses, medications) underlying any sexual concerns. When treatment of sexual disorders extends beyond one's competency, a referral to a sex therapist is needed.

Given that many eating disorder patients have a history of sexual trauma (see Section 10.3.5), exploration of the patient's history should include questions concerning unwanted sexual experiences and adult–child sexual contact. When present, a history of sexual abuse or other sexual trauma should be considered a comorbid concern with specific interventions to address those concerns. Clinicians should keep in mind that a history of sexual assault may make discussion of sexual development and current sexual concerns more difficult until the patient is sufficiently able to manage anxiety about the past abuse (Zerbe 1992).

Morgan et al. (1995) recommended that clinicians be prepared to help patients address sexual and relationship concerns and suggested that clinicians use behavior modification techniques commonly employed in sex therapy. Such techniques include directed masturbation, cognitive-behavioral interventions, and sensate focus. With directed masturbation, women who have never experienced orgasm are given explicit instructions on how to stimulate themselves (Heiman 2000; McMullen and Rosen 1979). Cognitive-behavioral interventions used to effectively treat sexual dysfunctions include psychoeducation, cognitive restructuring of maladaptive thoughts, and anxiety-reduction techniques (e.g., systematic desensitization; Brotto et al. 2008). Sensate focus, which involves a series of structured touching exercises that progress to genital touching and intercourse at the patient's pace, is designed to help improve communication, pleasure, and intimacy between sexual partners (DeVillers and Turgeon 2005; Masters and Johnson 1970) and has been recommended for use with eating disorder patients (De Silva and Todd 1998; Simpson and Ramberg 1991). In cases in which the onset of an eating disorder appeared to be related to severe guilt about one's past sexual activity, desensitization to touch, comfort with one's genitals, and autoerotic stimulation can be incorporated as part of treatment (e.g., Guile et al. 1978; Simpson and Ramberg 1991).

At present, information on sex therapy specifically for individuals with eating disorders is sparse. In the few available published articles, a variety of approaches including individual, group, and couple's work are discussed. For example, Van Vreckem and Vandereycken (1994) used a group setting that included a significant psychoeducational component for women with eating disorders in an inpatient treatment facility. Several aspects of their approach are noteworthy. First, groups were divided based upon the degree of past sexual experience. Second, when issues of sexual trauma were revealed, those issues were explored further in other group and individual sessions. Third, the sexual component included exercises that focused upon accepting one's body shape, and the focus on sexuality was connected with other treatment goals (e.g., acceptance of one's physical appearance). Fourth, groups were patient directed (e.g., patients decided what types of topics they wished to discuss). Finally, the sex education groups were part of a larger treatment protocol, which signified the importance of addressing such issues without ignoring other important aspects of treatment. De Silva and Todd (1998) suggested clinicians use the same types of cognitive interventions commonly used in the treatment of eating disorders (e.g., challenging negative thoughts) to address problematic cognitions about sex and sexuality with patients. De Silva and Todd (1998) also suggested that clinicians provide ample opportunities for self-exploration before partners are included in treatment.

10.5   CASE STUDY

Ms. X was a patient whose identity has been disguised. She was treated in an outpatient clinic, using a cognitive-behavioral approach, by one of this chapter's co-authors. Ms. X was a 34-year-old, Caucasian, heterosexual woman. She was 5' 3" tall and had a reported weight of less than 85 pounds. She was previously diagnosed with anorexia nervosa, binge eating/purging type. Ms. X struggled with an eating disorder for about 15 years and was hospitalized repeatedly during this time. Throughout the course of her illness, Ms. X did not date or engage in sexual activity, and she rarely interacted with men. Due to her low weight, she was amenorrheic. Ms. X wore oversized clothing and dressed in conservative attire because she was concerned about her physical appearance. Her physique lacked any visible signs of secondary sex characteristics, such as breast development or fat tissue associated with rounded or "womanly" hips. Ms. X had not experienced coitus prior to the onset of her illness but had started menstruation before she had lost weight. At the age of 34, Ms. X lived alone, but she maintained semiregular contact with her family via email messages, phone conversations, and visits for special events. She described herself as being somewhat socially isolated, stating that most of her social support came from treatment professionals and other patients with eating disorders.

Ms. X saw a female, psychodynamically oriented therapist every week for two years. Treatment focused principally on Ms X's interpersonal difficulties, which her therapist believed were due largely to Ms. X's history of sexual trauma by a male relative — a relative who provided financial support for her treatment, but whom she rarely saw because he lived several states away. Though the focus of therapy was on resolving issues related to the abuse, the therapist insisted that Ms. X maintain a weight of at least 85 pounds to remain a patient. Despite substantial gains in treatment with the therapist (e.g., setting boundaries with the relative who had sexually assaulted her as a child, maintaining a job, engaging in occasional social activities), Ms. X continued to struggle to maintain her goal weight of 85 pounds.

In addition to the her individual therapy, Ms. X participated in an open, outpatient, process group for women with eating disorders under the guidance of two therapists (one being the co-author who treated her). Multiple times during the course of treatment with her primary therapist, Ms. X sought additional treatment from another therapist (one of the chapter co-authors) for help with weight maintenance. Individual therapy with the second therapist (the co-author) involved a brief (less than 5 months) cognitive-behavioral approach to weight management. In addition to working on comfort with calorie-dense foods, resisting urges to purge after eating, and consuming sufficient calories, the therapy included challenging the patient's belief that she would not recover, providing her with other skills to manage stressful situations (e.g., relaxation techniques), and helping her fully process her feelings. Upon gaining an increased sense of control over her eating and maintaining a weight of 86 lbs. for several weeks, Ms. X terminated treatment with the co-author and continued treatment with her primary therapist to further address other therapeutic issues, such as a desire for a romantic relationship.

In considering this case, Ms. X had several characteristics that are common in individuals who develop an eating disorder shortly after puberty. In fact, Ms. X's experiences with sexual development were typical for someone whose difficulties with anorexia began during adolescence (see Table 10.1). Specifically, amenorrhea, social isolation, lack of a romantic relationship, and lack of sexual interactions are common among women who develop anorexia prior to marriage. In addition, she was sexually assaulted by a relative during childhood. Ms. X incurred significant medical expenses to cover the costs of her illness, and she had received financial assistance from the perpetrator of her sexual abuse though she very rarely saw him. Given these factors, exploration of her early sexual experiences, evaluation of her fears of intimacy in both friendships and romantic relationships, and the establishment of boundaries were necessary aims of treatment. However, Ms. X required additional help of another type to deal directly with her eating disorder, as her difficulties in maintaining a weight of 85 pounds often resulted in repeated hospitalizations and lapses in therapy.

This case illustrates that targeting immediate psychological concerns of a patient may be necessary but not sufficient to ensure stabilization of weight or healthier eating behavior. Likewise, targeting weight restoration and modification of eating behaviors is necessary but is not sufficient to ensure treatment success. Thus, the most effective treatments are those that target both the psychosexual and psychological factors that underlie the development and maintenance of disordered eating behavior as well as the thoughts, feelings, and behaviors that are typical in eating disorder patients (Bruch 1978). Ms. X's therapies addressed underlying issues, such as her difficulties expressing emotions, her lack of boundaries, her struggles with sex and intimacy, and her difficulties more closely tied to her eating behaviors, including her anxiety concerning food, lack of effective stress reduction skills, and need for weight stabilization and subsequent weight gain.

REFERENCES

Abraham, S. F., N. Bendit, C. Mason, H. Mitchell, N. O'Connor, J. Ward, S. Young, and D. Llewellyn-Jones. 1985. The psychosexual histories of young women with bulimia. *Aust N Z J Psychiatry* 19: 72–76.

Armstrong, J. G., and D. M. Roth. 1989. Attachment and separation difficulties in eating disorders: A preliminary investigation. *Int J Eat Disord* 8: 141–155.

Beumont, P. J. V., S. F. Abraham, and K. G. Simson. 1981. The psychosexual histories of adolescent girls and young women with anorexia nervosa. *Psychol Med* 11: 131–140.

Blitzer, J. R., N. Rollins, and A. Blackwell. (1961). Children who starve themselves: Anorexia nervosa. *Psychosom Med* 23: 369–383.

Broberg, A. G., I. Hjalmers, and L. Nevonen. 2001. Eating disorders, attachment and interpersonal difficulties: A comparison between 18024 year old patients and controls. *Eur Eat Disord Rev* 9: 381–396.

Brotto, L. A., R. Basson, and M. Luria. 2008. A mindfulness-based group psychoeducational intervention targeting sexual arousal disorder in women. *J Sex Med* 5: 1646–1659.

Bruch, H. 1978. *The golden cage: The enigma of anorexia nervosa.* Cambridge, MA: Harvard University Press.

Buckley, P., A. Freyne, and N. Walsh. 1991. Anorexia nervosa in males. *Irish J Psychol Med* 8: 15–18.

Cochran, S. D., J. G. Sullivan, and V. M. Mays. 2003. Prevalence of mental disorders, psychological distress, and mental health services use among lesbian, gay, and bisexual adults in the United States. *J Consult Clin Psychol* 71: 53–61.

Cole, P. M., and F. W. Putnam. 1992. Effect of incest on self and social functioning: A developmental psychopathology perspective. *J Consult Clin Psychol* 60: 174–184.

Connors, M. E., and W. Morse. 1993. Sexual abuse and eating disorders: A review. *Int J Eat Disord,* 13: 1–11.

Coovert, D. L., B. N. Kinder, and J. K. Thompson. 1989. The psychosexual aspects of anorexia nervosa and bulimia nervosa: A review of the literature. *Clin Psychol Rev* 9: 169–180.

Crisp, A. H. 1965. Clinical and therapeutic aspects of anorexia nervosa—A study of 30 cases. *J Psychosom Res* 9: 67–78.

Crisp, A. H. 1997. Anorexia nervosa as flight from growth: Assessment and treatment based on the model. In *Handbook of treatment for eating disorders* (2nd ed.), eds. David. M. Garner and Paul. E. Garfinkel, 248–277. New York: Guilford.

Crisp, A. H., T. Burns, and A. V. Bhat. 1986. Primary anorexia nervosa in male and female: A comparison of clinical features and prognosis. *Brit J Med Psychol* 59: 123–132.

Dansky, B. S., T. D. Brewerton, D. G. Kilpatrick, and P. M. O'Neil. 1997. The national women's study: Relationship of victimization and posttraumatic stress disorder to bulimia nervosa. *Int J Eat Disord* 21: 213–228.

Derogatis, L. R. 1997. The Derogatis Interview for Sexual Functioning (DISF/DISF-SR): An introductory report. *J Sex Marit Ther* 23: 291–304.

Derogatis, L. R., R. Rosen, S. Leiblum, A. Burnett, and J. Heiman. 2002. The Female Sexual Distress Scale (FSDS): Initial validation of a standardized scale for assessment of sexually related personal distress in women. *J Sex Marit Ther* 28: 317–330.

Derogatis, L., J. Rust, S. Golombok, C. Bouchard, L. Nachtigall, C. Rodenberg, J. Kuznicki, and C. A. McHorney. 2004. Validation of the Profile of Female Sexual Function (PFSF) in surgically and naturally menopausal women. *J Sex Marit Ther* 30: 25–36.

De Silva, P., and G. Todd. 1998. Sexual dysfunction in women with anorexia nervosa: Nature and treatment. *Sex Marital Ther* 13: 21–36.

De Villers, L., and H. Turgeon. 2005. The uses and benefits of "sensate focus" therapy. *Contemp Sex* 39: i–vii.

Eddy, K. T., C. M. Novotny, and D. Westen. 2004. Sexuality, personality, and eating disorders. *Eat Disord* 12: 191–208.

Elgin, J., and M. Pritchard. 2006. Adult attachment and disordered eating in undergraduate men and women. *J College Stud Psychother* 21: 25–40.

Evans, L., and E. H. Wertheim. 1998. Intimacy patterns and relationship satisfaction of women with eating problems and mediating effects of depression, trait anxiety and social anxiety. *J Psychosom Res* 44: 355–365.

Evans, L., and E. H. Wertheim. 2002. An examination of willingness to self-disclose in women with bulimic symptoms considering the context of disclosure and negative affect levels. *Int J Eat Disord* 31: 344–348.

Feldman, M. B., and I. H. Meyer. 2007. Eating disorders in diverse lesbian, gay, and bisexual populations. *Int J Eat Disord* 40: 218–226.

Fichter, M. M., and C. Daser. 1987. Symptomatology, psychosexual development and gender identity in 42 anorexic males. *Psychol Med* 17: 409–418.

Fichter, M. M., N. Quadflieg, and S. Hedlund. 2006. Twelve-year course and outcome predictors of anorexia nervosa. *Int J Eat Disord* 39: 87–100.

Finn, S. E., M. Hartman, G. R. Leon, and L. Lawson. 1986. Eating disorders and sexual abuse: Lack of confirmation for a clinical hypothesis. *Int J Eat Disord* 5: 1051–1060.

Garfinkel, P. E. 1981. Some recent observations on the pathogenesis of anorexia nervosa. *Can J Psychiatry* 26: 218–223.

Goodwin, G. M. 1990. Neuroendocrine function and the biology of eating disorders. *Hum Psychopharmacol* 5: 249–253.

Guile, L., M. Horne, and R. Dunston. 1978. Anorexia nervosa, sexual behavior modification as an adjunct to an integrated treatment programme. *Aust N Z J Psychiatry* 12: 165–167.

Gustafson, T. B., and D. B. Sarwer. 2004. Childhood sexual abuse and obesity. *Obes Rev* 5: 129–135.

Harned, M. S., and L. F. Fitzgerald. 2002. Understanding a link between sexual harassment and eating disorder symptoms: A mediational analysis. *J Consult Clin Psychol* 70: 1170–1181.

Heiman, J. R. 2000. Orgasmic disorders in women. In Sandra R. Leiblum, and Raymond C. Rosen Eds.), *Principles and Practice of Sex Therapy* (3rd ed; pp. 118–153). New York: Guilford.

Herzog, D. B., D. K. Norman, C. Gordon, and M. Pepose. 1984. Sexual conflict and eating disorders in 27 males. *Am J Psychiatry* 141: 989–990.

Irving, L. M., K. McCluskey-Fawcett, and D. Thissen. 1990. Sexual attitudes and behavior of bulimic women: A preliminary investigation. *J Youth Adolesc* 19: 395–411.

Jagstaidt, V., A. Golay, and W. Pasin. 1996. Sexuality and bulimia. *New Trends Exp Clin Psychiatry* 12: 9–15.

Kaltiala-Heino, R., M. Rimpela, A. Rissanen, and P. Rantanen. 2001. Early puberty and early sexual activity are associated with bulimic-type eating pathology in middle adolescence. *J Adolesc Health* 28: 346–352.

Keel, P. K., M. G. Baxter, T. F. Heatherton, and T. E. Joiner, Jr. 2007. A 20-year longitudinal study of body weight, dieting, and eating disorder symptoms. *J Abnorm Psychol* 116: 422–432.

Keski-Rahkonen, A., C. M. Bulik, B. M. Neale, R. J. Rose, A. Rissanen, and J. Kaprio. 2005. Body dissatisfaction and drive for thinness in young adult twins. *Int J Eat Disord* 37: 188–199.

Killen, J. D., C. Hayward, I. Litt, L. D. Hammer, D. M. Wilson, B. Miner, C. B. Taylor, A. Varady, and C. Shisslak. 1992. Is puberty a risk factor for eating disorders. *Arch Pediatr Adolesc Med* 146: 323–325.

Koff, E., and J. Rierdan. 1993. Advanced pubertal development and eating disturbance in early adolescent girls. *J Adolesc Health* 14: 433–439.

Laessle, R. G., S. Bossert, G. Hank, K. Hahlweg, and K. M. Pirke. 1990. Cognitive performance in patients with bulimia nervosa: Relationship to intermittent starvation. *Biol Psychiatry* 27, 549–551.

Laws, A., and J. M. Golding. 1996. Sexual assault history and eating disorder symptoms among white, Hispanic, & African American women and men. *Am J Public Health* 86: 579–582.

Lock, J., B. Reisel, and H. Steiner. 2001. Associated health risks of adolescents with disordered eating: How different are they from their peers? Results from a high school survey. *Child Psychiatry Hum Dev* 31: 249–265.

Lorand, S. 1943. Anorexia nervosa: Report of a case. *Psychosom Med* 5: 282–292.

Mangweth-Matzek, B., C. I. Rupp, A. Hausmann, G. Kemmler, and W. Biebl. 2007. Menarche, puberty, and first sexual activities in eating disordered patients as compared with a psychiatric and nonpsychiatric control group. *Int J Eat Disord* 40: 705–710.

Masters, W. H., and V. E. Johnson. 1970. *Human sexual inadequacy.* Boston: Little Brown and Company.

McCabe, M. P., and L. A. Ricciardelli. 2004. A longitudinal study of pubertal timing and extreme body change behaviors among adolescent boys and girls. *Adolesc* 39: 145–166.

McMullen, S., and R. C. Rosen. 1979. Self-administered masturbation training in the treatment of primary orgasmic dysfunction. *J Consult Clin Psychol* 47: 912–918.

Miller, P. H. 2011. *Theories of developmental psychology* (5th ed.). New York: Worth Publishers.

Morgan, C. D., M. W. Wiederman, and T. L. Pryor. 1995. Sexual functioning and attitudes of eating-disordered women: A follow-up study. *J Sex Marit Ther* 21: 67–77.

O'Dea, J. A., and S. Abraham. 1999. Onset of disordered eating attitudes and behaviors in early adolescence: Interplay of pubertal status, gender, weight, and age. *Adolesc* 34: 671–679.

Olivardia, R., H. G. Pope, B. Mangweth, and J. I. Hudson. 1995. Eating disorders in college men. *Am J Psychiatry* 152: 1279–1285.

Pinheiro, A. P., T. J. Raney, L. M. Thornton, M. M. Fichter, W. H. Berrettini, D. Goldman, K. A. Halmi et al. 2010. Sexual functioning in women with eating disorders. *Int J Eat Disord* 43: 123–129.

Pope, H. C., J. A. Hudson, and J. M. Jonas. 1986. Bulimia in men: A series of fifteen cases. *J Nerv Ment Dis* 174: 117–119.

Powers, P. S., and E. G. Spratt. 1994. Males and females with eating disorders. *Eat Disord* 2: 197–214.

Pryor, T., M. W. Wiederman, and B. McGilley. 1996. Clinical correlates of anorexia nervosa subtypes. *Int J Eat Disord* 19: 371–379.

Raboch, J., and F. Faltus. 1991. Sexuality of women with anorexia nervosa. *Acta Psychiatr Scand* 84: 9–11.

Raciti, M., and S. S. Hendrick. 1992. Relationships between eating disorder characteristics and love and sex attitudes. *Sex Roles* 27: 553–564.

Romeo, F. F. 1984. Adolescence, sexual conflict, and anorexia nervosa. *Adolesc* 19: 551–555.

Rose, J. A. 1943. Eating inhibitions in children in relation to anorexia nervosa. *Psychosom Med* 5: 117–124.

Rothschild, B. S., P. J. Fagan, C. Woodall, and A. E. Anderson. 1991. Sexual functioning of female eating-disordered patients. *Int J Eat Disord* 10: 389–394.

Russell, C. J., and P. K. Keel. 2002. Homosexuality as a specific risk factor for eating disorders in men. *Int J Eat Disord* 31: 300–306.

Russell, G. F. M. 1997. The history of bulimia nervosa. In *Handbook of treatment for eating disorders* (2nd ed.), eds. David. M. Garner and Paul. E. Garfinkel, 11–24. New York: Guilford.

Ruuska, J., R. Kaltiala-Heino, A. Koivisto, and P. Rantanen. 2003. Puberty, sexual development and eating disorders in adolescent outpatients. *Eur Child Adolesc Psychiatry* 12: 214–220.

Sarti, C. D., J. Kuznicki, C. Rodenberg, L. Derogatis, C. A. McHorney, J. Rust, S. Golombok et al. 2004. Profile of Female Sexual Dysfunction: A patient-based, international, psychometric instrument for the assessment of hypoactive desire in oophorectomized women. *Menopause* 11: 474–483.

Savin-Williams, R. C. 2006. Who's gay? Does it matter? *Curr Dir Psychol Sci* 15: 40–44.

Schmidt, U., K. Evans, J. Tiller, and J. Treasure. 1995. Puberty, sexual milestones and abuse: How are they related in eating disorder patients? *Psychological Med* 25: 413–417.

Schmidt, U., H. Humfress, and J. Treasure. 1997. The role of general family environment and sexual and physical abuse in the origins of eating disorders. *Eur Eat Disord Rev* 5: 184–207.

Schneider, J. A., and W. S. Agras. 1987. Bulimia in males: A matched comparison with females. *Int J Eat Disord* 6: 235–242.

Siever, M. D. 1996. The perils of sexual objectification: Sexual orientation, gender, and socioculturally acquired vulnerability to body dissatisfaction and eating disorders. In *Gay and lesbian mental health: A sourcebook for practitioners*, ed. C. J. Alexander, 223–247. Binghampton: The Hawood Press.

Silverstein, B., and L. Perdue. 1988. The relationship between role concerns, preferences for slimness, and symptoms of eating problems among college women. *Sex Roles* 18: 101–106.

Simpson, W. S., and J. A. Ramberg. 1991. Sexual dysfunction in married female patients with anorexia and bulimia nervosa. *J Sex Marit Ther* 18:44–54.

Smolak, L., and S. K. Murnen. 2002. A meta-analytic examination of the relationship between child sexual abuse and eating disorders. *Int J Eat Disord* 31: 136–150.

Smyth, J. M., K. E. Heron, S. Wonderlich, R. D. Crosby, and K. M. Thompson. 2008. The influence of reported trauma and adverse events on eating disturbance in young adults. *Int J Eat Disord* 41: 195–202.

Steiner, H. 1990. Defense styles in eating disorders. *Int J Eat Disord* 9: 141–151.

Striegel-Moore, R. H., L. R. Silberstein, and J. Rodin. 1986. Toward an understanding of risk factors for bulimia. *Am Psychol* 41: 246–263.

Tantleff-Dun, S., and J. K. Thompson. 1995. Romantic partners and body image disturbance: Further evidence for the role of perceived-actual disparities. *Sex Roles* 33: 589–605.

Tuiten, A., G. Panhuysen, W. Everaerd, E. Laan, H. Koppeschaar, E. Te Velde, and M. Smeets. 1992. Anorexia nervosa and sexuality. *Neuro Endocrinol Lett* 14: 259.

Tuiten, A., G. Panhuysen, W. Everaerd, H. Koppeschaar, P. Krabbe, and P. Zelissen. 1993. The paradoxical nature of sexuality in anorexia nervosa. *J Sex Marital Ther* 19: 259–273.

Van den Broucke, S., W. Vandereycken, and J. Norre. 1997. *Eating disorders and marital Marital relationships*. New York: Routledge.

Van Vreckem, E., and W. Vandereycken. 1994. A sexual education programme for women with eating disorders (new updated edition). In *Why women? Gender issues and eating disorders*, ed. B. Dolan and I. Gitzinger, 110–116. Atlantic Highlands, NJ: Athlone Press.

Waller, J. V., M. R. Kaufman, and F. Deutsch. 1940. Anorexia nervosa: A psychosomatic entity. *Psychosom Med* 11: 3–16.

Weiner, H. 1989. Psychoendocrinology of anorexia nervosa. *Psychiatr Clin North Am* 12: 187–206.

Wichstrom, L. 2006. Sexual orientation as a risk factor for bulimic symptoms. *Int J Eat Disord* 39: 448–453.

Wiederman, M. W., T. Pryor, and C. D. Morgan. 1996. The sexual experience of women diagnosed with anorexia nervosa or bulimia nervosa. *Int J Eat Disord* 19: 109–118.

Wiederman, M. W., R. A. Sansone, and L. A. Sansone. 1999. Obesity among sexually abused women: An adaptive function for some? *Women Health* 29: 89–100.

Wonderlich, S. A., R. D. Crosby, J. E. Mitchell, K. M. Thompson, J. Redlin, G. Demuth, J. Smyth, and B. Haseltine. 2001a. Eating disturbance and sexual trauma in childhood and adulthood. *Int J Eat Disord* 30: 401–412.

Wonderlich, S. A., R. D. Crosby, J. E. Mitchell, K. M. Thompson, J. Redlin, G. Demuth, and J. Smyth. 2001b. Pathways mediating sexual abuse and eating disturbance in children. *Int J Eat Disord* 29: 270–279.

Young, J. K. 1991. Estrogen and the etiology of anorexia nervosa. *Neurosci Biobehav Rev* 15: 327–331.

Zerbe, K. J. 1992. Why eating-disordered patients resist sex therapy: A response to Simpson and Ramberg. *J Sex Marital Ther* 18: 55–64.

Part IV

Prevention of Eating Disorders

11 Factors Associated with Eating Disorders in Children

John L. Rohwer

CONTENTS

11.1 LEARNING OBJECTIVES

After reading this chapter you should be able to

- Recognize eating disorders as a significant problem among children and youth, especially girls and young women
- Comprehend the complex relationship between the onset of eating disorders and the transition from childhood to adolescence
- Identify the risks that lead to increased vulnerability to eating disorders

11.2 BACKGROUND AND SIGNIFICANCE

Eating disorders and unhealthy eating practices among children and youth are of serious public health concern due to their adverse effects on psychosocial (Johnson, Cohen, Kasen et al. 2002; McKnight Investigators 2003; Strauss et al. 1984) and physical health (Fagot-Campagna et al. 2000,

Herzog et al. 1992; McKnight Investigators, 2003; Zipfel et al. 2000). A common explanation for the development of eating disorders is society's preoccupation with thinness, and this certainly plays a part. However, most clinicians believe that there are many other contributing factors, including psychological, social, family, spiritual, and at times biological.

Risk factors are also referred to as potential "causes" of an eating disorder. Eating disorders can occur across all ages and socioeconomic groups; however, there are certain groups, such as young teenage girls, who demonstrate a higher incidence of eating disorders. Below is a list of potential risk factors for the development of an eating disorder, which are standard across all age groups and genders. Individuals who display a number of these risk factors are considered to be at a higher risk of developing an eating disorder.

11.2.1 DIETING AND EATING DISORDERS

A high number of children and youth report dieting for weight loss. In population-based surveys with youth, dieting is often assessed using a single item (e.g., how often have you been on a diet to lose weight), which may or may not provide a brief definition of dieting (e.g., by diet, we mean change the way you eat to lose weight; Haines et al. 2006; Neumark-Sztainer et al. 2002).

While eating disorders affect a smaller percentage of children and youth (1–3%) (Agras 2001; American Psychiatric Association [*DSM-IV*] 2004), the Youth Risk Behavioral Surveillance System (YRBSS) found that less than 11% of high school girls and 7% of high school boys in the United States reported taking diet pills, powders, or liquids to lose weight (Grunbaum et al. 2004). Eight percent of girls and close to 4% of boys reported vomiting or taking laxatives in the past month (Grunbaum et al. 2004). According to the same report, almost 60% of female and 29% of male school-aged students were trying to lose weight. Prevalence estimates for dieting among children aged 6–11 range from 20% to 56% for girls and from 31% to 39% for boys (Schreiber et al. 1996).

Research suggests that dieting behavior may be causally linked to eating disorders (Field et al. 2003). A number of studies involving clinical samples have found that the majority of individuals with eating disorders report that they started to diet before they initiated their disordered eating behaviors (Bulik et al. 1997; McKnight Investigators, 2003). Further evidence of the association is provided by prospective studies within community samples of adolescents. Among adolescents, self-reported dieting has been shown to predict increased risk of disordered eating behavior (Agras 1998; Field et al. 1999; Killen et al. 1996; Stice, 2001) and subthreshold eating disorders (Leon et al. 1999; Patton et al. 1990; Santonastaso et al. 1999). These suggest that self-reported dieting among adolescents may lead to more severe eating disorders.

11.2.2 MEDIA AND EATING DISORDERS

Media use and the internalization of the messages promoted by the media have been explored as possible risk factors for eating disorders (Gordon 1988). Due to the ever-present nature of media in our culture and its relentless promotion of the thin beauty ideal, media has long been identified as a potential risk factor for eating disorders (Garner and Garfinkel 1980; Gordon 1988; Haines et al. 2006; McKnight Investigators 2003). A key tenet of sociocultural theories of eating disorders is that society through avenues including mass media pressures individuals to conform to the cultural ideal for size and shape (Heinberg 1996; McKnight Investigators 2003). This cultural ideal has changed throughout history, becoming increasingly thin for females (Wiseman et al. 1992) and increasingly lean and muscular for males (Leit et al. 2001). Theoretically, media's pressure to conform to the ideal promotes internalization of this ideal (Stice 1994; Thompson et al. 1999). Internalization, in turn, leads to body dissatisfaction because the cultural ideal is unattainable for most people (Thompson et al. 1999). Body dissatisfaction then leads to disordered eating and negative affect, which may lead to an increased risk for eating disorders (Stice 1994).

Several cross-sectional surveys have found a positive association between media use and body dissatisfaction and disordered eating behavior among both children and adolescents (Harrison 2000a, 2000b; Levine et al. 1994; Utter et al. 2003). Evidence from a recent prospective study providing further support for this association (Vaughan and Fouts 2003) found that decreases in magazine reading over 16 months were associated with decreases in eating disorder symptoms among a sample of adolescent girls. Findings from prospective research provide evidence for the hypothesized association between thin-ideal internalization and eating disorder symptoms. Thin-ideal internalization has been shown to predict body dissatisfaction (Stice 2001) and disordered eating behaviors (Field et al. 1999; Stice and Agras 1998). In one study, researchers (Field et al. 1999) found that girls who reported at baseline trying to look like females in the media were almost two times more likely to report purging behavior 1 year later than those that did not report trying to look like figures in the media, after adjustment for age and BMI.

11.2.3 BODY DISSATISFACTION AND EATING DISORDERS

Body dissatisfaction is common among children and adolescents. Approximately 50% of girls and 30% of boys report that they are dissatisfied with their bodies (Keel et al. 1997; Neumark-Sztainer, Story et al. 2002; Ricciardelli and McCabe 2001). Body-image dissatisfaction may have relevance for the development of eating disorders (Stice 2002). Research findings suggest that body dissatisfaction leads to an increased risk of eating disorders in three ways. The first suggests that body dissatisfaction leads to elevated attempts to reach the thin ideal using dieting behaviors, which in turn increases the risk for eating disorders (Field et al. 1999; Patton et al. 1990). The second hypothesized means is that body dissatisfaction contributes to negative affect (anxiety or depression), which, in turn, is thought to increase the risk of binge eating and the use of radical compensatory behaviors, such as purging behavior (Stice 2001). Third, body dissatisfaction may directly promote the development of eating disorders (Davison and Birch 2004; Dohnt and Tiggemann 2006). The following quote on this issue may be heard from time to time:

> "My whole childhood I heard, 'You'll never make anything of yourself if you grow up fat.' So I was always dieting to look good for others."

There is substantial support for the role of body dissatisfaction in the development of dieting behaviors. Cross-sectional studies have shown that children and adolescents with higher levels of body dissatisfaction also engage more frequently in dieting behaviors (Hill and Bhatti 1995; Hill et al. 1994; Thelen et al. 1992). Prospective studies involving adolescent girls have found that elevated body dissatisfaction at baseline were significantly associated with dieting behaviors at follow-up 8 months later (Wertheim et al. 2001), 9 months later (Stice et al. 1998) and 20 months later (Stice 2001). There is also evidence from prospective studies that body dissatisfaction predicts negative affect (Cole et al. 1998; Stice and Bearman 2001; Stice et al. 2000, Stice and Bearman 2001). Numerous prospective studies have found body dissatisfaction to predict bulimic behaviors (Field et al. 1999; Killen et al. 1994; Stice and Agras 1998) and eating pathology (Leon et al. 1999; Wertheim et al. 2001). A more recent longitudinal study (Neumark-Sztainer et al. 2006) found that lower levels of body satisfaction are associated with more health-compromising behaviors, such as unhealthy weight control behaviors and binge eating, and fewer health-promoting behaviors, such as physical activity. The same study indicated the importance of body satisfaction for the overall well-being of children and youth. Body satisfaction was predictive of health-related behaviors even after a 5-year period. The researchers also suggest the importance of avoiding messages or interventions that may, inadvertently, lead to lower levels of body satisfaction in teens.

11.2.4 Weight-Related Teasing and Eating Disorders

Weight-related teasing is prevalent among children and adolescents with overweight youth reporting higher levels of weight-related teasing compared with their average weight peers (Haines et al. 2006; Hayden-Wade et al. 2002; Janssen et al. 2004; Neumark-Sztainer et al. 2002; Stormer and Thompson 1996). The following expressions are typical for body dissatisfaction:

> "I was very overweight and I got teased. I was so lonely and always felt left out. No one wanted to be my friend. I decided early on that I'd better not stay fat."

> "My family made fun of fat people. All of us did. It was like a sport for us. Now I'm ashamed of how we acted. But it did not drive home to us kids that being large was not something good to be, not something to be proud of."

Weight-related teasing has been shown to be associated with both binge eating and other disordered eating behaviors (e.g. purging, restricting), suggesting that it may have a potential relevance for the development of eating disorders. Among adult populations, studies have examined the relation of retrospective reports of teasing and use of disordered eating behaviors and found that women who were teased about their appearance as children demonstrate higher levels of restrictive eating patterns than women who did not report being teased (Myers and Rosen 1999; Stormer and Thompson 1996).

Among children and adolescents, cross-sectional research has shown that being teased about weight is associated with higher levels of disordered eating behaviors (Fabian and Thompson 1989; Keery et al. 2005; Levine et al. 1994; Neumark-Sztainer et al. 2002). Fewer prospective studies have examined the effects of teasing on the development of disordered eating behaviors. Cattarin and Thompson (1994) followed a sample of adolescent girls for 3 years and found that teasing was directly associated with the level of appearance dissatisfaction, which in turn predicted use of restrictive and bulimic behaviors. Wertheim and others (2001) found that weight-related teasing predicted subsequent levels of bulimic behaviors among adolescent girls. Conversely, Field and colleagues (2003) found that weight-related teasing was not related to subsequent purging behaviors, after accounting for other relevant factors.

Gardner and others (2000) followed a sample of children aged 6–14 for 3 years, and observed that teasing predicted higher eating disorder scores among males but not females. Similar gender differences were seen in longitudinal analyses of a large sample of adolescents (Eisenberg et al. 2006; Haines et al. 2006). It is possible that because females receive more messages about achieving the "thin ideal" from a larger range of sources than their male counterparts, weight teasing does not independently explain as much of the variance in these behaviors in females as it does in males.

Taken together, the cross-sectional and prospective research on the impact of teasing on dieting and disordered eating behaviors suggests that being teased about weight may function directly or indirectly through body/appearance dissatisfaction to influence the use of dieting and disordered eating behaviors. As discussed previously, dieting and use of unhealthy weight control behaviors may increase the risk for developing an eating disorder (Field et al. 1999; McKnight Investigators 2003; Neumark-Sztainer, Story et al. 2002).

11.2.5 Ethnicity and Eating Disorders

Most studies of individuals with eating disorders have been conducted using Caucasian middle-class females. Studies are now reporting, however, that minority populations, including Hispanics and African Americans, are significantly affected. There is some indication that African-American girls and young women may be at particular risk for eating disorders because of poor body images caused by cultural attitudes that denigrate the physical characteristics of minorities.

Members of certain ethnic groups such as Asians, Native Americans, and African Americans appear less likely to have eating disorders than other ethnic groups. The finding that a factor reflecting high weight/shape and other concerns and issues (including dieting) predicts onset of eating disorders is consistent across longitudinal studies in less diverse populations (Killen et al. 1994, 1996). Smolak and Striegel-Moore (2001) argue, however, that where there is inconsistency in the research findings, that ethnicity is actually a summary variable capturing diverse experiences and elements such as immigration status, gender roles, discrimination, socioeconomic disparities, and acculturation. For example, Hispanic girls in some parts of the United States are more likely to identify themselves as being Latin Americans while those in another part of the country may be identified as Latinos. In addition, studies routinely find African American girls to be more satisfied with their bodies and to show fewer eating problems and disorders than white or Hispanic girls (Striegel-Moore et al. 2000). African Americans have lower rates of anorexia than do white populations, but there may be less of a difference in the disorders involving binge eating (Smolak and Striegel-Moore 2001; Striegel-Moore et al. 2000).

11.3 CURRENT FINDINGS

It is possible to develop an eating disorder with or without the risk factors listed below. However, the more risk factors one has, the greater the likelihood of developing an eating disorder. What factors may make individuals vulnerable, then, to eating disorders?

Risk factors can be defined as circumstances or predispositions that result in increased levels of vulnerability to harmful health behaviors (Kraemer et al. 1997). While eating disorders have been considered purely social or psychological (as evidenced above), they are now viewed as more complex, resulting from the interaction of biological, psychological, and social factors. In fact, it appears that risk factors leading to the onset of eating disorders cross social, environmental, biological, and psychological lines. While a number of empirical studies have attempted to isolate various risk factors associated with eating disorders, this section describes each category detailing how current scientific research supports how intricate and varied they really are.

11.3.1 PHYSIOLOGICAL/BIOLOGICAL FACTORS

Research provides strong evidence for an inherited predisposition (tendency) toward developing an eating disorder. In other words, eating disorders are often biologically inherited and tend to run in families.

11.3.1.1 Genetic Factors

Research in this area has been initiated in part by the observation that anorexia can run in families, and that bulimia repeatedly occurs in families where members suffer from depression or alcoholism. Many questions about the relationship between genetics and eating disorders remain to be answered and deserve additional study.

Studies examining shared genetic and environmental influences in the development of an eating disorder, have suggested that genetic factors play the larger role in the etiology of the disorder (Klump et al. 2001; Wade, Bulik et al. 2000). Individuals who have a mother or a sister with anorexia nervosa are approximately 12 times more likely to develop anorexia and four times more likely to develop bulimia than other individuals without a family history of these disorders. Studies of twins have shown a higher rate of eating disorders when they are identical (compared to fraternal twins or other siblings). Samples of DNA, the substance inside cells that carries genetic information, from pairs of siblings with eating disorders are now being analyzed to determine if they share genetic characteristics that are different from pairs of siblings without these disorders (Bulik 2005).

11.3.1.2 Neurobiological Factors

Research has also focused on abnormalities in the structure or activity of the hypothalamus, a brain structure responsible for regulating eating behaviors (Carlson 2007; Kaye, Frank et al. 2005). Studies suggest that the hypothalamus of bulimics may not trigger a normal satiation (feeling full or finished) response (Long 2009; Kalat 2006). So, even after a meal, these individuals do not feel full. Several research studies suggest that different neurotransmitters are involved in eating disorders (Long 2009; Uher and Treasure 2005). The neurotransmitter serotonin affects bingeing behavior in bulimics. These individuals often crave (and gorge) on foods rich in carbohydrates. The body converts sugars from carbohydrates into tryptophan. Tryptophan is then used to create serotonin, which is partially responsible for the regulation of appetite, creating a sense of satiation, and regulating emotions and judgment. Thus, the bingeing behavior of bulimics may also be a response to low serotonin levels in the brain (Yager and Anderson 2005). While bulimics may have low levels of serotonin, other studies indicate that anorexics have high levels of neurotransmitters in some areas of the brain (Yager and Anderson 2005). The exact relationship between serotonin and anorexia has yet to be clarified, however.

Numerous other hormones in the brain have also been linked to eating disorders (Södersten et al. 2006). Stress triggers the production and release of a hormone called cortisol; chronically elevated cortisol levels have been observed in patients with both anorexia and bulimia. Cortisol also inhibits the release of a powerful appetite stimulant. This process may serve as a link between stressful conditions and the later development of eating disorders (Kalat 2006; Södersten et al. 2006).

Leptin is another hormone produced by the body's adipose tissue. This hormone travels to the brain, where it tells the body how much energy is available. This information plays a part in the regulation of reproduction, appetite, metabolism, and bone formation. If individuals with eating disorders lose extreme amounts of body fat, leptin levels drop (Kalat 2006; Södersten et al. 2006).

New research suggests that women who develop anorexia nervosa may have altered levels of dopamine in their brains. Improper levels of dopamine may explain why anorexics feel intensely driven to lose weight yet feel little pleasure in shedding pounds (Kalat 2006; Södersten et al. 2006).

One of the difficulties in deciphering a biological component in eating disorders is determining whether an imbalance in neurotransmitters precipitates the development of the illness or whether the imbalance occurs as a result of the disorder. This depends on the individual and is best discussed with a medical professional. There is evidence, however, that both personality characteristics (such as anxiety and perfectionism) and disturbances to the serotonin system are still apparent after patients have recovered from anorexia (Kaye et al. 2005), suggesting that these disturbances are likely to be causal risk factors.

11.3.2 SOCIOCULTURAL/ENVIRONMENTAL FACTORS

11.3.2.1 Media Influences

Eating disorders tend to be more common in industrialized countries; however, this is changing as less developed parts of the world have access to new technology and become Westernized. Sociocultural studies have highlighted the role of cultural factors, such as the promotion of thinness as the ideal female form in Western industrialized nations, particularly through the media. Western culture is blamed for being obsessed with the human body and a lean and lithe appearance. Beauty is sold as the key to happiness and the ultimate goal. Such images of beauty are delivered in a daily barrage in numerous women's magazines, on television, film, and other forms of mass media. A classic study by Garner and Garfinkel (1980) demonstrated that those in professions where there is a particular social pressure to be thin (such as models and dancers) were much more likely to develop an eating disorder during the course of their career, and further research (Toro et al. 2006) has suggested that those with anorexia have much higher contact with cultural sources that promote weight loss.

Although anorexia nervosa is usually associated with Western cultures, exposure to Western media is thought to have led to an increase in cases in non-Western countries. However, it is notable that other cultures may not display the same "fat phobia" worries about becoming fat as those with the condition in the West, and instead may present low appetite with the other common features (Simpson 2002). However powerful these influences may be, sociocultural factors should not be considered to be the only cause of eating disorders, but one ingredient in a complicated formula.

11.3.3 PSYCHOLOGICAL FACTORS

11.3.3.1 Personality Traits

There has been a significant amount of study on psychological factors that suggest how biases in thinking and perception help maintain or contribute to the risk of developing an eating disorder. Anorexic eating behavior, for example, is thought to originate from feelings of fatness and unattractiveness (Rosen et al. 1995) and is maintained by various cognitive biases that alter how the affected individual evaluates and thinks about their body, food, and eating.

One of the most well-known findings is that people with an eating disorder tend to overestimate the size of fatness of their own bodies. Research in this area (Skrzypek et al. 2001) suggests that this is not a perceptual problem, but one of how the perceptual information is evaluated by the affected person. More recent research (Jansen et al. 2006), however, suggests people with an eating disorder may lack a type of overconfidence bias in which the majority of people feel themselves more attractive than others would rate them. In contrast, people with an eating disorder seem to more accurately judge their own attractiveness compared to unaffected people, meaning that they potentially lack this self-esteem boosting bias.

People with eating disorders tend to share similar personality and behavioral traits, including low self-esteem, dependency, and problems with self-direction. Specific psychiatric personality disorders may put people at higher risk for eating disorders (Johnson, Cohen, Kotler et al. 2002; Wonderlich et al. 2005). These might include:

1. Avoidant personalities characterized by being perfectionistic, emotionally and sexually inhibited, being perceived as always being good rather than being rebellious, and being terrified of ridicule, criticism, or humiliation.
2. Obsessive-compulsive personality defines certain character traits, such as being morally rigid or preoccupied with rules and order.
3. Narcissistic personality is exemplified with one having a need for admiration, hypersensitive to criticism, and an inability to empathize with others.

As one examines the personality characteristics of individuals prone to developing eating disorders, the following quotes are commonplace:

"I care too much about what everyone thinks about me, I want to make everyone happy all of the time. I don't care how that makes me feel."

"People always say how compulsive I am. How driven I am all the time. But, I can't sit still. I have to be moving and doing things all the time."

"I've always been fear-based. I'm afraid of everything. Especially change. Even good kinds of changes terrify me. I hate being so insecure."

11.3.3.2 Family Influences

Significant attention has been paid to the family dynamics of people with eating disorders. In discussing the issue, it is important to remember the integral relationship between psychological and familial factors. The individual is part of the family system and develops within it. Thus, individual and family psychology has been implicated, and theories of causation tend to be related to this interaction. Nevertheless, some studies have produced the following observations and theories regarding family influence (Davison and Birch 2001; Meyer and Russell 1998; Park et al. 2004; Sharpe et al. 1998; Taylor et al. 1998; Troisi et al. 2005):

Insecure Infancy. Some experts theorize that parents who fail to provide a safe and secure foundation in infancy may foster eating disorders. In such cases, children experience so-called insecure attachments. They are more likely to have greater weight concerns and lower self-esteem than are those with secure attachments.

Parental Behaviors. Poor parenting by both mothers and fathers has been implicated in eating disorders. One study found that 40% of 9- and 10-year-old girls are trying to lose weight generally with the urging of their mothers. Some studies have found that mothers of anorexics tend to be overinvolved in their child's life, while mothers of people with bulimia are critical and detached. Overly critical fathers, brothers, or both may play a factor in the development of anorexia in both girls and boys.

Family History of Addictions or Emotional Disorders. Studies report that people with either anorexia or bulimia are more likely to have parents with alcoholism or substance abuse than are those in the general population. Parents of people with bulimia appear to be more likely to have psychiatric disorders than parents of patients with anorexia.

History of Abuse. Women with eating disorders, particularly bulimia, appear to have a higher incidence of sexual abuse. Studies have reported sexual abuse rates as high as 35% in women with bulimia.

Family History of Obesity. People with bulimia are more likely than others to have an obese parent or to have been overweight themselves during childhood.

Here are several reflections from young women on the influence of family members' attitudes and beliefs regarding weight:

"My family doesn't know what to do with feelings. We just pretend they don't exist. I don't know what to do with them either, so I throw them up."

"In my family you always had to act pretty. You could never be mad or loud. You could never make noise. I learned to not show what I was really feeling. Sometimes, I'm still not even sure what I'm feeling."

"My father was really volatile. He could get really mad and yell. I hated it. I felt so unsafe and out of control. I hate that I could have feelings in me that might be scary and out of control."

Although there has been quite a lot of research into psychological factors, there are relatively few hypotheses that attempt to explain the condition as a whole.

In conclusion, it is important to consider all factors in the etiology of eating disorders. It has roots in the biological, psychological, and sociocultural. All these complex factors interact and are interrelated. One must consider individual differences in assessing an individual with a possible eating disorder.

11.4 CASE STUDIES

Read the following case scenario and then identify those behaviors/risk factors that are specific to that eating disorder.

Jennifer appears, from the outside, to be an average female teenager; she stands 5 ft, 4 in tall and weighs 115 pounds. Up until recently, however, she had weighed 155 pounds. Overweight since childhood, she was frequently taunted and ostracized by her peers and has few friends. About 6 months ago, Jennifer joined *Weight Watchers* and lost 45 pounds. She really stuck with it initially and felt good about her success; so good, in fact, that she stopped attending the meetings and felt she could now regulate her eating on her own. It did not take long for the weight to creep back on—one pound here, two pounds there. Jennifer was becoming quite discouraged until she found a way to eat all the food she wanted while maintaining her trim figure. One day, like every other, Jennifer returned home quickly from school because she knew the house would be empty; she had been planning this all day! Once inside, she headed straight for the kitchen where she consumed one quart of cookies and cream ice cream, two bags of chocolate chip cookies, four chocolate bars, a bag of potato chips, and a quart bottle of cola. Finished with her "snack" she removed herself from the table and went to the bathroom to vomit. She felt calm, cleansed, and relieved. She now had control of herself. Half an hour later, she was back in the kitchen eating again. This time she snacked on cold leftover spaghetti, a quart of milk, two peanut butter and jelly sandwiches, and a box of crackers. Uncomfortably full (again) and disgusted with herself, she returned to the bathroom for a second purging. The only thing that stood in the way of a third binge–purge episode was the return of her mother from work. Jennifer would often perform this sequence of overeating and then making herself vomit ten to 12 times per day. Sometimes, this would result in headaches and sore throat, but she just could not make herself stop; after vomiting, she felt like a new person.

Next, read the following case scenario and then identify the behaviors/risk factors associated with this eating disorder.

Marie is 5 feet, 5 inches tall and somewhat thin for her height. If she could lose just ten pounds more, she would no longer feel fat. The first thing she does every morning is run over to her full-length mirror and lift up her nightgown to see if her stomach is flatter than it was before she went to bed; it usually is, but not enough to satisfy her. Marie cannot comprehend why she is continually bloated. Just to be sure she has lost at least a little weight, she moves quickly from the full-length mirror to the bathroom scale. She weighs in at 99; immediately, she jumps off the scale, lets it return to "0," and steps back on, hoping the first reading was an error. It is not. She thinks it over in her mind: "I didn't even eat that much yesterday. At this rate, I'll never lose those ten pounds!" She plans her day very carefully from what she will eat to how and when she will exercise and what she will cook for the other family members for dinner; she loves to cook extravagant meals for other people. While Marie is eating her breakfast of one glass of water and one hard-boiled egg, she reads a new cookbook her mother has just purchased. She delights in reading the section of desserts and other baked goods and selects a new recipe for tonight's meal. With breakfast completed, it is time for a good, long run of about six miles. With the run behind her and the hour hand on the clock approaching noon, Marie insists to herself that she is not hungry. To take her mind off her hunger pains, she volunteers to do the dusting, vacuuming, and laundry for her mother. About 2:00 p.m., she grabs an apple on the way out the door to her aerobics class where she exercises vigorously for at least an hour and then lifts weights. At home, she prepares dinner and serves it. While everyone else is eating, Marie makes excuses for not having to eat what is on her plat: "I'm not really hungry since I ate a late lunch"; "I'll go out to the kitchen and start the coffee"; "I didn't think it would taste like this"; "I had so much on my plate to start … "

11.5   SUMMARY AND CONCLUSIONS

The cause of an eating disorder is quite a bit more complicated than, say, that of a bacterial infection, which can be directly traced to the presence of a particular organism. With an eating disorder, though, several factors are usually involved, and no two cases are exactly alike. Sometimes, it is more useful to think in terms of risk factors that might predispose someone to the development of an illness. One person can have every possible risk factor for an eating disorder and remain perfectly healthy. Someone else may have only one, but because of the particular circumstances of events that make up his/her life and how it affects him/her, he/she may go on to develop a full-blown eating disorder.

Risk factors leading to eating disorders appear to cross biological, social, and psychological lines, and they are extremely intricate, varied and complex. Table 11.1 summarizes the risk factors discussed in this chapter; however, the identification of risk factors in eating disorders does not necessarily provide a clear sense of what particular strategies are needed to reduce the risks. The determination of those factors that can be most effectively targeted for prevention, however, offers a key challenge that still needs to be answered.

TABLE 11.1
Risk Factors Associated with Eating Disorders

Category	Trait
Biological/physiological	• Genetic predisposition
	• Runs in families
	• Biochemical changes
	• Imbalance of certain chemicals
Sociocultural	• Value placed on thinness
	• Emphasis on "perfect body"
	• Valuing outward appearance
	• Media portrayal of men's and women's shapes
	• Pressure to achieve or succeed
	• Professions with an emphasis on body shape and size
Psychological	• Low self-esteem
	• Feelings of inadequacy
	• Incidence of depression and anxiety
	• Fear of responsibility
	• Difficulty in expressing emotions and feelings
	• Ineffective coping strategies
	• Perfectionism
	• Fear or avoidance of conflict
	• Competitiveness
	• Impulsive or obsessive behaviors
	• Need to please others
	• Concerned about the opinions of others
	• Prone to extremes
	• Poor communication between family members
	• Fear of avoidance of conflict

11.6 GLOSSARY OF TERMS

Risk factor—a characteristic, experience or event that, if present, is associated with an increase in the probability (risk) of a particular outcome over the base rate of that outcome in the general population.

Sociocultural risk factors—influences due to the prevailing societal conditions and norms, especially with respect to accepted beliefs, attitudes, and practices, but also including economic and cultural conditions.

Psychological risk factors—cognitive, emotional, and behavioral characteristics of individual people (i.e., knowledge, beliefs, attitudes, concepts, values, skills, experiences, habits, and feelings).

REFERENCES

Agras, W. S. 2001. The consequences and costs of the eating disorders. *Psychiatr Clin N Am* 24: 371–379.

American Psychiatric Association. 2004. *Diagnostic and Statistical Manual of Mental Disorders: DSM-IV-TR*. Washington, DC: American Psychiatric Association.

Bulik, C. M. 2005. Exploring the gene-environment nexus in eating disorders. *J Psychiatry Neurosci* 30: 335–339.

Bulik, C. M., P. F. Sullivan, F. A. Carter, and P. R. Joyce. 1997. Initial manifestations of disordered eating behavior: Dieting versus binging. *Int J Eat Disord* 22: 195–201.

Carlson, N. 2007. *Physiology of behavior.* Boston, MA: Pearson.

Cattarin, J., and J. Thompson. 1994. A three-year longitudinal study of body image, eating disturbance, and general psychological functioning in adolescent females. *Eat Disord* 2: 114–125.

Cole, D. A., J. M. Martin, L. G. Peeke, A. D. Seroczński, and K. Hoffman. 1998. Are cognitive errors of underestimation predictive or reflective of depressive symptoms in children: A longitudinal study. *J Abnorm Psychol* 107: 481–496.

Davison, K. K., and Birch, L. L. 2004. Predictors of fat stereotypes among 9-year-old girls and their parents. *Obes Res* 12: 86–94.

Davison, K. K., and Birch, L. L. 2001. Weight status, parent reaction, and self-concept in five-year-old girls. *Pediatrics* 107: 46–53.

Dohnt, H., and Tiggemann, M. 2006. The contribution of peer and media influences to the development of body dissatisfaction and self-esteem in young girls: A prospective study. *Dev Psychol* 42: 929–936.

Eisenberg, M. E., D. Neumark-Sztainer, J. Haines, and M. Wall. 2006. Weight-teasing and emotional well-being in adolescents: Longitudinal findings from Project EAT. *J Adolesc Health* 38: 675–683.

Fabian, L. J., and J. K. Thompson. 1989. Body image and eating disturbance in young females. *Int J Eat Disord* 8: 63–74.

Fagot-Campagna, A., D. J. Pettitt, M. M. Engelgau, N. R. Burrows, L. S. Geiss, R. Valdez, G. L. Beckles, J. Saaddine, E. W. Gregg, D. F. Williamson, and K. M. Narayan. 2000. Type 2 diabetes among North American children and adolescents: An epidemiologic review and a public health perspective. *J Pediatr* 135: 664–672.

Field, A. E., S. B. Austin, C. B. Taylor, S. Malspeis, B. Rosner, H. R. Rockett, M. W. Gillman, and G. A. Colditz. 2003. Relation between dieting and weight change among preadolescents and adolescents. *Pediatrics* 112: 900–906.

Field, A. E., C. A. Camargo, Jr., C. B. Taylor, C. S. Berkey, and G. A. Colditz. 1999. Relation of peer and media influences to the development of purging behaviors among preadolescent and adolescent girls. *Arch Pediatr Adolesc Med* 153: 1184–1189.

Gardner, R. M., K. Stark, B. N. Friedman, and N. A. Jackson. 2000. Predictors of eating disorder scores in children ages 6–14: A longitudinal study. *J Psychosom Res* 49: 199–205.

Garner, D. M., and P. E. Garfinkel. 1980. Socio-cultural factors in the development of anorexia nervosa. *Psychol Med* 10: 647–656.

Gordon, R. A. 1988. A socio-cultural interpretation of the current epidemic of eating disorders. In *The Eating Disorders*, ed. B. J. Blinder, B. F. Chaiting, and R. Goldstein, 151–163. Great Neck, NY: PMA.

Grunbaum, J., A., L. Kann, S. Kinchen, J. Ross, J. Hawkins, R. Lowry, W. A. Harris, T. McManus, D. Chyen, and J. Collins. 2004. Youth Risk Behavior Surveillance-United States, 2003. *MMWR Surveillance Summary* 53: 1–96.

Haines, J., D. Neumark-Sztainer, M. E. Eisenberg, and P. J. Hannan. 2006. Weight-teasing and disordered eating behaviors in adolescents: Longitudinal findings from Project EAT (Eating among Teens). *Pediatrics* 117: 209–215.

Harrison, K. 2000a. Television viewing, fat stereotying, body shape standards, and eating disorder symptomatology in grade school children. *Communic Res* 27: 617–640.

Harrison, K. 2000b. The body electric: Thin-ideal media and eating disorders in adolescents. *J Commun* 50: 119–143.

Hayden-Wade, H. A., R. I. Stein, A. Ghaderi, B. E. Saelens, M. F. Zabinski, and D. E. Wilfley. 2002. Prevalence, characteristics, and correlates of teasing experiences among overweight children vs. non-overweight peers. *Obes Res* 13: 1381–1392.

Heinberg, L. J. 1996. Theories of body image disturbance: Perceptual, developmental, and socio-cultural models. In *Body Image, Eating Disorders, and Obesity*, ed. J. K. Thompson, 27–47. Washington, DC: American Psychological Association.

Herzog, D. B., M. B. Keller, N. R. Sacks, C. J. Yeh, and P. W. Lavori. 1992. Psychiatric co-morbidity in treatment-seeking anorexics and bulimics. *J Amer Acad Child Adolesc Psychiatry* 31: 810–818.

Hill, A. J., and R. Bhatti. 1995. Body shape perception and dieting in preadolescent British Asian girls: links with eating disorders. *Int J Eat Disord* 17: 175–183.

Hill, A. J., E. Draper, and J. Stack. 1994. A weight on children's minds: Body shape dissatisfactions at 9-years old. *Int J Obes Relat Metab Disord* 18: 383–389.

Jansen, A., T. Smeets, C. Martijn, and C. Nederkoorn. 2006. I see what you see: The lack of a self-serving body-image bias in eating disorders. *Br J Clin Psychol* 45: 123–135.

Janssen, I., W. M. Craig, W. F. Boyce, W. Pickett. 2004. Associations between overweight and obesity with bullying behaviors in school-aged children. *Pediatrics* 113: 1187–1894.

Johnson, J. G., P. Cohen, S. Kasen, and J. S. Brook. 2002. Childhood adversities associated with risk for eating disorders or weight problems during adolescence or early adulthood. *Am J Psychiatry* 159: 394–400.

Johnson, J. G., P. Cohen, L. Kotler, S. Kasen, and J. S. Brook. 2002. Psychiatric disorders associated with risk for the development of eating disorders during adolescence and early adulthood. *J Consult Clin Psychol* 70: 1119–1128.

Kalat, J. W. 2006. *Biological psychology* (8th ed.). Houston, TX: Wadsworth.

Kaye, W. H., U. F. Bailer, G. K. Frank, A. Wagner, and S. E. Henry. 2005. Brain imaging of serotonin after recovery from anorexia and bulimia nervosa. *Physiol Behav* 86: 15–17.

Kaye, W. H., G. K. Frank, U. F. Bailer, S. E. Henry, C. C. Meltzer, J. C. Price, C. A. Mathis, and A. Wagner. 2005. Serotonin alterations in anorexia and bulimia nervosa: New insights from imaging studies. *Physiol Behav* 85: 73–81.

Keel, P. K., J. A. Fulkerson, and G. R. Leon. 1997. Disordered eating precursors in pre- and early adolescent girls and boys. *J Youth Adolesc* 26: 203–206.

Keery, J., K. Boutelle, P. van den Berg, and J. K. Thompson. 2005. The impact of appearance-related teasing by family members. *J Adolesc Health* 37: 120–127.

Killen, J. D., C. B. Taylor, C. Hayward, D. M. Wilson, K. F. Haydel, L. D. Hammer, B. Simmonds, T. N. Robinson, I. Litt, A. Varady, and H. Kraemer. 1994. Pursuit of thinness and onset of eating disorder symptoms in a community sample of adolescent girls: A three-year prospective analysis. *Int J Eat Disord* 16: 227–238.

Killen, J. D., C. B. Taylor, C. Hayward, K. F. Haydel, D. M. Wilson, L. Hammer, H. Kraemer, A. Blair-Greiner, and D. Strachowski. 1996. Weight concerns influence the development of eating disorders: A 4-year prospective study. *J Consult Clin Psychol* 64: 936–940.

Klump, K. L., W. H. Kaye, and M. Strober. 2001. The evolving genetic foundation of eating disorders. *Psychiatr Clin N Am* 24: 215–225.

Kraemer, H. C., A. E. Kazdin, D. R. Offord, R. C. Kessler, P. S. Jensen, and D. J. Kupfer. 1997. Coming to terms with the terms of risk. *Arch Gen Psychiatry* 54: 337–343.

Leit, R. A., H. G. Pope, Jr., and J. J. Gray. 2001. Cultural expectations of muscularity in men: The evolution of playgirl centerfolds. *Int J Eat Disord* 29: 90–93.

Leon, G. R., J. A. Fulkerson, C. L. Perry, P. K. Keel, and K. L. Klump. 1999. Three to four year prospective evaluation of personality and behavior risk factors for later disordered eating in adolescent girls and boys. *J Youth Adolesc* 28: 181–196.

Levine, M. P., L. Smolak, and H. Hayden. 1994. The relation of socio-cultural factors to eating attitudes and behaviors among middle-school girls. *J Early Adolesc* 14: 471–490.

Long, P. W. 2009. Eating disorders. Retrieved from the National Institute of Mental Health website: http:www. mental health.com/book/p45-eat1.html (accessed November 5, 2009).

McKnight Investigators. 2003. Risk factors for the onset of eating disorders in adolescent girls: Results of the McKnight longitudinal risk factor study. *Am J Psychiatry* 160: 248–254.

Meyer, D. F., and R. K. Russell. 1998. Caretaking, separation from parents and the development of eating disorders. *J Couns Dev* 76: 166–173.

Myers, A., and J. Rosen. 1999. Obesity stigmatization and coping: Relation to mental health symptoms, body image, and self-esteem. *Int J Obes Relat Metab Disord* 23: 221–230.

Neumark-Sztainer, D., N. Falkner, M. Story, C. Perry, P. J. Hannan, and S. Mulert. 2002. Weight-teasing among adolescents: Correlations with weight status and disordered eating behaviors. *Int J Obes Relat Metab Disord* 26: 123–131.

Neumark-Sztainer, D., S. J. Paxton, P. J. Hannan, J. Haines, and M. Story. 2006. Does body satisfaction matter? Five-year longitudinal associations between body satisfaction and health behaviors in adolescent females and males. *J Adolesc Health* 39: 244–251.

Neumark-Sztainer, D., M. Story, P. J. Hannan, C. L. Perry, and L. M. Irving. 2002. Weight-related concerns and behaviors among overweight and non-overweight adolescents: Implications for preventing weight-related disorders. *Arch Pediatr Adolesc Med* 156: 171–178.

Park, L. E., J. Crocker, and K. D. Mickelson. 2004. Attachment styles and contingencies of self-worth. *Pers Soc Psychol Bull* 30: 1243–1254.

Patton, G. C., E. Johnson-Sabine, K. Wood, A. H. Mann, and A. Wakeling. 1990. Abnormal eating attitudes in London school-girls—a prospective epidemiological study: Outcome at twelve month follow-up. *Psychol Med* 20: 383–394.

Ricciardelli, L. A., and M. P. McCabe. 2001. Dietary restraint and negative affect as mediators of body dissatisfaction and bulimic behavior in adolescent girls and boys. *Int J Behav Consult Ther* 39: 1317–1328.

Rosen, J. C., J. Reiter, and P. Orosan. 1995. Assessment of body image in eating disorders with the Body Dysmorphic Disorder Examination. *Behav Res Ther* 33: 77–84.

Santonastaso, P., S. Friederici, and A. Favaro. 1999. Full and partial syndromes in eating disorders: A 1-year prospective study of risk factors among female students. *Psychopathology* 32: 50–56.

Schreiber, B., M. Robins, R. Striegel-Moore, E. Obarzanek, J. A. Morrison, and D. J. Wright. 1996. Weight modification efforts reported by black and white preadolescent girls: National Heart, Lung, and Blood Institute Growth and Health Study. *Pediatrics* 98: 63–70.

Sharpe, T. M., J. D. Killen, S. W. Bryson, C. M. Shisslack, L. S. Estes, N. Gray, M. Crago, and C. B. Taylor. 1998. Attachment style and weight concerns in preadolescent and adolescent girls. *Int J Eat Disord* 23: 39–44.

Simpson, K. J. 2002. Anorexia nervosa and culture. *J Psychiatr Ment Health Nurs* 9: 65–71.

Skrzypek, S., P. M. Wehmeier, and H. Remschmidt. 2001. Body image assessment using body size estimation in recent studies on anorexia nervosa. *J Am Acad Child Adolesc Psychiatry* 10: 215–221.

Smolak, L. and R. H. Striegel-Moore. 2001. Challenging the myth of the golden girls: Ethnicity and eating disorders. In *Eating Disorders: Innovative Directions in Research and Practice*, ed. R. H. Striegel-Moore and L. Smolak, 67–98. Washington, DC: American Psychological Association.

Södersten, P., C. Bergh, and M. Zandian. 2006. Understanding eating disorders. *Horm Behav* 50: 572–578.

Stice, E. 1994. Review of the evidence for a socio-cultural model of bulimia nervosa and an exploration of the mechanisms of action. *Clin Psychol Rev* 14: 633–661.

Stice, E. 2001. A prospective test of the dual-pathway model of bulimic pathology: Mediating effects of dieting and negative affect. *J Abnorm Psychol* 110: 124–135.

Stice, E. 2002. Risk and maintenance factors for eating pathology: A meta-analytic review. *Psychol Bull* 128: 825–848.

Stice, E., and W. S. Agras. 1998. Predicting onset and cessation of bulimic behaviors during adolescence: A longitudinal grouping analysis. *Behav Ther* 29: 257–276.

Stice, E. and S. K. Bearman. 2001. Body-image and eating disturbances prospectively predict increases in depressive symptoms in adolescent girls: A growth curve analysis. *Dev Psychol* 37: 597–607.

Stice, E., C. Hayward, R. P. Cameron, J. D. Killen, and C. B. Taylor. 2000. Body-image and eating disturbances predict onset of depression among female adolescents: A longitudinal study. *J Abnorm Psychol* 109: 438–444.

Stice, E., L. Mazotti, M. Krebs, and S. Martin. 1998. Predictors of adolescent dieting behaviors: A longitudinal study. *Psychol Addict Behav* 12: 195–205.

Stormer, S., and J. Thompson. 1996. Explanations of body image disturbance: A test of maturational status, negative verbal commentary, social comparison, and socio-cultural hypotheses. *Int J Eat Disord* 19: 193–202.

Strauss, C. C., K. Smith, C. Frame, and R. Forehand. 1984. Personal and interpersonal characteristics associated with childhood obesity. *J Pediatr Psychol* 10: 337–347.

Striegel-Moore, R., D. Wilfley, K. Pike, F. Dohm, and C. Fairburn. 2000. Recurrent binge eating in black American women. *Arch Fam Med* 9: 83–87.

Taylor, C. B., T. Sharpe, C. Shisslak, S. Bryson, L. S. Estes, N. Gray, K. M. McKnight, M. Crago, H. C. Kraemer, and J. D. Killen. 1998. Factors associated with weight concerns in adolescent girls. *Int J Eat Disord* 24: 31–42.

Thelen, M. H., A. L. Powell, C. Lawrence, and M. E. Kuhnert. 1992. Eating and body image concerns among children. *J Clin Child Adolesc Psychol* 21: 41–46.

Thompson, J. K., L. J. Heinberg, M. Altabe, and S. Tanleff-Dunn. 1999. *Exacting beauty: Theory, assessment, and treatment of body image disturbance.* Washington, DC: American Psychological Association.

Toro, J., M. Salamero, and E. Marinez. 2006. Assessment of socio-cultural influences on the aesthetic body shape model in anorexia nervosa. *J Psychiatr Ment Health Nurs* 89: 146–151.

Troisi, A., P. Massaroni, and M. Cuzzolaro. 2005. Early separation anxiety and adult attachment style in women with eating disorders. *Br J Clin Psychol* 44: 89–97.

Uher, R., and J. Treasure. 2005. Grain lesions and eating disorders. *J Neurol Neurosurg Psychiatry* 76: 852–857.

Utter, J., D. Neumark-Sztainer, M. Wall, and M. Story. 2003. Reading magazine articles about dieting and associated weight control behaviors among adolescents. *J Adolesc Health* 32: 78–82.

Vaughan, K. K., and G. T. Fouts. 2003. Changes in television and magazine exposure and eating disorder symptomatology. *Sex Roles* 49: 313–320.

Wade, T. D., C. M. Bulik, M. Neale, and K. S. Kendler. 2000. Anorexia nervosa and major depression: Shared genetic and environmental risk factors. *Am J Psychiatry* 157: 469–471.

Ward, A., R. Ramsay, S. Turnbull, M. Benedettini, and J. Treasure. 2000. Attachment patterns in eating disorders: Past in the present. *Int J Eat Disord* 28: 370–376.

Wertheim, E., J. Koerner, and S. Paxton. 2001. Longitudinal predictors of restrictive eating and bulimic tendencies in three different age groups of adolescent girls. *J Youth Adolesc* 30: 69–81.

Wiseman, C. V., J. J. Gray, J. E. Mosimann, and A. H. Ahrens. 1992. Cultural expectations of thinness in women: An update. *Int J Eat Disord* 11: 85–89.

Wonderlich, S. A., L. R. Lilenfeld, L. P. Riso, S. Engel, and J. E. Mitchell. 2005. Personality and anorexia nervosa. *Int J Eat Disord* 37: 68–71.

Yager, J., and A. E. Anderson. 2005. Anorexia nervosa. *N Engl J Med* 353: 1481–1488.

Zipfel, S., B. Lowe, D. L. Reas, H. Deter, and W. Herzog. 2000. Long-term prognosis in anorexia nervosa: Lessons from a 21-year follow-up study. *Lancet* 355: 721–722.

12 Educational Programs Aimed at Primary Prevention

John L. Rohwer

CONTENTS

12.1 LEARNING OBJECTIVES

After completing this chapter you should be able to

- Identify the various dimensions of prevention and determine when they are most appropriately applied in program development
- Recognize how the comprehensive prevention model can be incorporated into an eating disorder prevention program
- Understand the various components for an effective primary prevention education program model

12.2 BACKGROUND AND SIGNIFICANCE

Eating disorder prevention is a topic that has received little attention in the literature. This is ironic because many researchers and health care workers suggest eating disorders are more difficult to treat the more deeply rooted anorexic or bulimic behaviors become in an individual's lifestyle. Furthermore, most would agree that helping individuals avoid being affected by the factors perpetuating eating disorders is a crucial factor in preventing eating problems from occurring in the first place.

12.2.1 LEVELS OF PREVENTION

"Prevention" is a term that can refer to either the elimination of factors causing eating disorders, called primary prevention, or the early detection and treatment of eating problems, known as secondary prevention. Primary prevention refers to programs or efforts that are designed to prevent the occurrence of eating disorders before they begin (Cook-Cotton and Scime 2006). Its objective is to help individuals avoid problems before signs or symptoms occur. Primary prevention is intended to help promote healthy development.

The goal of primary prevention is to reduce the incidence of anorexia nervosa and bulimia nervosa. Finding effective ways of approaching primary prevention is a problem since the causes of eating disorders are not fully understood. However, it is possible to minimize common social, familial, and individual factors, which are generally recognized as leading to eating disorders. This implies eliminating or reducing the sociocultural factors (such as the stigma attached to being overweight or misconceptions about weight reduction) that increase the risk of eating disorders. It also involves changing the behaviors that influence body image, self-esteem, eating habits, and coping skills. Therefore, one of the reasons for designing elementary school primary prevention programs is the relatively low prevalence of serious eating problems in that environment, and hence the opportunity to prevent their onset, or at the very least decrease their rate and severity.

A number of strategies can be developed to minimize the impact of social pressures, especially pressures to be thin. For example, children can be taught not to be preoccupied with their weight. This means learning to accept a broad range of body sizes, including their own. It also means placing less emphasis on appearance and more on personality and individuality. Schools provide an ideal location for prevention programs at this level. Teachers and school counselors should become educated about the causes of eating disorders, especially those who are in contact with high-risk groups. Teachers should also educate students about accepting a wide range of weights and the dangers of dieting. These themes can easily be incorporated into health, science, or physical education classes. Health professionals, parents, peers, and siblings can all contribute by not focusing on body size, appearance or weight loss, as well as by refusing to endorse dieting or the pursuit of thinness as healthy.

As far as primary prevention efforts in minimizing family factors go, it is important for parents to guard against transmitting harmful attitudes to their children. Parents should make sure that lines of communication are open among family members. Parents should also educate themselves about eating disorders so that they become aware of changing attitudes around food and weight and can recognize symptoms. Parents, too, are in a good position to help by learning how to accept their children and teaching them to respect and like themselves. Finally, family members should be encouraged to examine their own attitudes around food, weight, and shape since parental attitudes do become the attitudes of their children.

Individual factors, like low self-esteem and perfectionism, often develop as a result of both family interactive patterns and larger cultural values. Teachers can contribute by educating students about self-esteem and adaptive ways of relating with others. Teachers can initiate discussions focusing on ways of achieving a sense of self-worth and role-play exercises to develop assertiveness skills. Teachers identifying low self-esteem or family problems should recommend counseling. Both health professional and teachers can assist by encouraging those with low self-esteem or other individual issues to seek counseling.

Secondary prevention (sometimes called "targeted prevention") refers to programs or efforts that are designed to identify and correct eating disorder attitudes and behaviors in the very early stages, before a full clinical disorder is manifested (Cook-Cotton and Scime 2006). The earlier an eating disorder is discovered and addressed, the better the chance of recovery. Secondary prevention focuses on reducing the duration of an eating disorder through early diagnosis and effective treatment. The objective is to facilitate identification and correction of a disorder in its early stages when it is less likely to be a lifestyle and associated with other significant problems, such as depression. For this reason, early detection and intervention are important aspects of secondary prevention. Secondary prevention involves knowing the (1) warning signs, (2) effective ways to reach out to people in distress, and (3) sources of treatment.

It is difficult to implement strategies for early detection because individuals with eating problems often attempt to conceal their behavior. An advantage of secondary prevention is that limited time and resources may be directed towards those at greatest risk for eating disorders. Parents, peers, and siblings are all in a good position to detect changing attitudes around food, weight, and shape. However, the nature of their relationship with the individual at risk or frequency of contact may prevent them from perceiving a problem until it has developed into a "full-blown" eating disorder. Parents, peers, and siblings should know the warning signs and high-risk groups and know how to approach the individual and where to get help. Often, teachers are in an excellent position to detect developing eating problems. Not only do teachers spend a lot of time with children and youth, they have a more objective picture of student behavior and attitude changes.

Tertiary prevention directs efforts at the stage when a disorder has become established or an unwanted behavior has become fixed. These prevention efforts are directed at reducing the consequences in case a disorder or negative behavior cannot be completely controlled. The appropriate levels of prevention with regard to eating disorder are diagrammed in Table 12.1.

12.2.2 Research on Primary Prevention for Eating Disorders

Given the incidence of eating disorders, their serious physical and psychological consequences, and the difficulties and high costs of treatment, it is not surprising that primary and secondary prevention programs for eating disorders are receiving attention in the scientific literature (Pearson et al. 2002). Yet, prevention in this field continues to be controversial. Although some authors consider it to be an essential part of health promotion policy (Huon 1996), others have warned that our

TABLE 12.1
Three Levels of Prevention

Levels	Distinctions	Examples
Primary—attempts to forestall the onset of unwanted behavior	Precedes the earliest signs of a disease or disorder and involves efforts directed at a time before the unwanted behavior occurs.	Educational efforts encourage students to understand the determinants of body size and weight; develop healthy, balanced eating and activity patterns as well as social and cultural resiliency skills.
Secondary—attempts to reduce the extent of the unwanted behavior	Identifies disorder at its earliest stage and when the unwanted behavior manifests itself or is believed to be a threat.	The early identification via the DSM-IV diagnostic criteria; accurate referral; emphasis on social alternatives.
Tertiary—attempts to prevent relapse following recovery in a treatment program	Maintains appropriate treatment through its full course to complete rehabilitation. Efforts are directed at reducing the consequences of the disorder or behavior.	Full scale treatment of severe eating disorders, including psychotherapy; hospitalization; re-education on body image; dieting and exercise.

knowledge of etiology is inadequate, and that, in some cases, prevention is potentially dangerous (Carter 1997; Mann et al. 1997). Such discrepant views are not surprising, given that published accounts have yielded inconsistent findings (Pratt and Woolfenden 2002; Stice and Shaw 2004). Being able to demonstrate the effectiveness of cost-effective preventive interventions is, however, an important research objective.

The question that requires answering is: "Are eating disorder prevention programs effective?" The clinical questions that assist in answering this basic question are the following:

(a) Does presenting educational material on eating disorders produce iatrogenic (harmful because of the intervention) effects on eating attitudes and behaviors?

(b) Are eating disorder prevention programs effective in promoting healthy eating attitudes and behaviors?

(c) Do eating disorder prevention programs have a long-term, sustainable, and positive impact on the mental and physical health of children and youth?

(d) Do eating disorder prevention programs promote psychological factors that protect children and youth from developing eating disorders?

Research conducted by Langmesser and Verscheure (2009) recently looked at 46 studies focusing on reducing the risk of eating disorders. All of the studies had to meet certain qualifying features including a nonclinical sample and a comparison group. The researchers categorized each study on certain features: population targeted, length of intervention and follow-up, and intervention strategies. Population targets included those with no risk factors associated with eating disorders, at-risk population, and a symptomatic group. The intervention strategies looked at the amount of information related to eating disorders included in the prevention program. In addition, the authors categorized the intervention strategies as being (1) purely educational, (2) enhanced educational with elements of cognitive-behavioral therapy, or (3) purely interactive cognitive-behavioral therapy with no educational component. All eating disorder prevention programs produced the largest positive change in participant knowledge without regard to the targeted population. The biggest gains in knowledge occurred right after completion of the prevention program. During follow-up, the gains in knowledge decreased but still remained higher than knowledge before the program. General eating abnormalities, such as dieting and thin-ideal internalization, showed small positive changes. Even though the changes were relatively small at posttest for all the outcomes, they seemed to last, because the follow-up studies showed results very similar to those obtained at posttest. Body dissatisfaction was the most frequently measured outcome but had the smallest change. No differences were noted between educational and enhanced educational interventions concerning dieting behaviors, thin-ideal internalizations, or body dissatisfaction. From these studies, the authors determined that while no firm conclusions can be made about the effect of prevention programs for eating disorders, no harmful effects occurred as a result of including educational information about eating disorders in an eating disorder prevention program. One thing that was learned is that longer-term effects of the intervention approaches will need to be monitored across development to demonstrate a decline in the incidence of eating disorders and associated risk factors.

12.3 CURRENT FINDINGS

Traditional primary prevention programs may be most effective in the lower elementary years before the crystallization of the preoccupation with body shape and weight within the construct of self (Piran 2001). For many years, prevention efforts have been aimed at later middle school and high school students because it was believed that eating-disordered behaviors and beliefs were rare among prepubertal children (Thelen et al.1992). While evidence of dieting, body dissatisfaction, and fear of fat is present among elementary school children (ages 6–11), data suggest that these attitudes and behaviors are not as interconnected or ingrained as they are in adolescence (Smolak and Levine 1994). However, research reveals that eating-disordered behaviors and risk factors associated with their development may emerge as early as fourth grade (Thelen et al. 1992). If indeed, these attitudes and behaviors are not yet fully developed in elementary school children, then it is possible that early intervention may prevent the onset of eating disorders. The focus in such intervention might, for example, place an emphasis on developing a positive body image, as well as identifying the dangers of caloric-restrictive dieting.

Regarding older students, there is an increasing likelihood of internalization of the thin ideal, dieting, and experimentation with eating-disordered behaviors. Accordingly, the notion of a pure primary prevention program is not realistic. It may be effective to combine primary and secondary prevention efforts (Piran 2001). To illustrate, a yoga and wellness group run as part of the school's wellness program is open to all interested students (primary prevention). However, teachers, staff, and parents are also encouraged to refer students with whom they are concerned (secondary prevention). Health and physical education curriculums might include: self-care (e.g., yoga/relaxation), life skills (e.g., assertiveness, problem-solving and decision-making skills), and community-based skills (e.g., media literacy and how to locate healthy resources).

Traditionally, eating disorder prevention programs have relied on didactic presentation of factual information targeting risk factors and defining eating disorders, showing little effect (Littleton and Ollendick 2003; Stice et al. 2007). Over the years, positive innovations have included educational sessions that offer information on healthy bodies, eating, and exercise (Baranowski and Hetherington 2001). Despite content changes, meta-analyses have demonstrated that it is extremely difficult to demonstrate effects in knowledge, attitude, and behavior utilizing universal, psychoeducational methods for prevention of eating disorders, especially in children and younger adolescents (Fingeret et al. 2006; Stice et al. 2007).

The current trend in newer curricular models is an interactive, experiential approach (Dalle Grave et al. 2001; Stice et al. 2007). Preliminary results are promising, demonstrating an increase in knowledge, as well as some decreases in dysfunctional eating attitudes and behaviors (Dalle Grave et al. 2001; Stewart et al. 2001; Stice et al. 2007; Varnado-Sullivan et al. 2001). Programs employing a constructivist approach (i.e., student-centered, problem/project-based learning) demonstrate impressive and lasting results (Piran 2001). Further, several researchers suggest adopting a positive psychology framework as a replacement for the traditional approach of solely targeting risk factors (Seligman and Csikszentmihalyi 2000; Steck et al. 2004). Although the findings of O'Dea and Abraham (2000) and Phelps and others (1999) are promising, subsequent efforts to replicate and expand these findings have been less successful (McVey and Davis 2002; Wade et al. 2003). Recently there has been very compelling evidence supporting the use of dissonance techniques to prevent the internalization of the thin ideal (Stice et al. 2007). Findings also reveal a greater emphasis on enacting change in the social environment (Littleton and Ollendick 2003) and Piran's (2001) work supports this contention. Logistical recommendations for improving the impact of prevention efforts include utilizing experts to implement programs and increasing the length of time groups spend together (Littleton and Ollendick 2003).

Recent meta-analyses by Fingeret (2006) and Stice and others (2007; Stice and Shaw 2004) provide further support for a distinct combination of components. In Stice and Shaw (2004), examination of effect sizes for the various programs revealed that larger effects were found for interactive programs with no psychoeducational content that were directed at high-risk participants, lasted for multiple sessions, and were carried out with solely females.

Collectively, research trends suggest seven core components have been found to show the most promise in terms of primary prevention groups targeting eating disorders (Scime and Cook-Cottone 2008):

(a) An interactive format
(b) The use of constructivism
(c) A positive psychology framework

(d) Dissonance-induction content (e.g., an emphasis on enacting media or social change and/ or helping other avoid thin-ideal internalization)
(e) Experts as facilitators
(f) Multiple session interventions
(g) All female participants

Unfortunately, to date, there are no known programs that have combined all of these components.

12.3.1 PROGRAM CONTENT

Specific topics suggested for primary prevention education for eating disorders include information about (Austin et al. 2005; Neumark-Sztainer 2005) the following:

(a) Normal physiological, social, and psychological changes during puberty, the increased deposition of fat tissue, and the diversity among individuals
(b) Nutrition, meal skipping and other eating habits, and the connection between food and emotions
(c) Physical activity, its importance, and appropriate levels
(d) Weight control, including an understanding of the physiological and psychological effects of food restriction and chronic dieting, discouragement of drastic weight-loss techniques, an understanding of the facts and myths of dietary fads, realistic and safe methods of weight control, and realistic goals for weight change and maintenance
(e) Body image, including discussions of the role of the media in suggesting slimness as the answer to social concerns and of student images of the ideal body, and an offer to help in determining one's appropriate body weight
(f) Women-related issues, including the role of women in society, media portrayal of women, and the balance between femininity and competence/autonomy
(g) Self-esteem and personal identity
(h) Activities focused on skills for coping with stress and with social pressures (i.e. being assertive)
(i) Anorexia and bulimia nervosa in a manner that discourages their glamorization

12.3.2 LEARNING STRATEGIES

For the most effective learning to take place, program implementers should seek student-centered strategies that provide for group involvement, and use more than one strategy or activity for each major concept to address the full variety of student abilities and aptitudes. The objective should be to select those strategies that are most appropriate and effective with the target audience, based on student learning styles (i.e. auditory, kinesthetic, or visual).

Learning strategies include the following, which have been incorporated into many of the current eating disorder prevention curricula:

(a) Conflict resolution skill training, which can help ease the tensions children experience during the transition to adolescence
(b) Peer group involvement, especially the use of older peer facilitators who can correct unrealistic attitudes and misperceptions regarding weight and appearance
(c) Group exercises utilizing role-playing techniques to learn to cope with teasing
(d) Assertiveness training, which can teach coping skills, as well as how to deal with increased peer pressures to diet
(e) Problem-solving and time-management skills, which can help children and youth to set realistic goals balancing achievement and relaxation

The goal, therefore, of prevention intervention should be to help each child or youth develop a strong, positive sense of self-worth, self-respect, and integrity regarding body image. The strategies should be used to assist youngsters in recognizing the importance of eating for health and satisfaction of hunger, not to manipulate weight. Children and youth should learn that choices can be made about which, when, and how food will be eaten, and about a sedentary versus active lifestyle. Children and youth should also learn how healthy bodies progress through puberty. They should learn critical thinking skills, how to resist messages contradicting realistic body diversity, and how to select positive role models.

12.3.3 School-Based Primary Prevention Programs

According to the National Eating Disorder Information Centre (NEDIC; McVey and Davis 2002), a recent trend in the primary prevention of disordered eating and eating disorders involves adopting health promotion programs designed to promote overall wellness, and alter some of the predisposing risk factors (e.g., low self-esteem) related to disordered eating. This approach contrasts the traditional health education approach of teaching traits, behaviors, and dangers associated with eating disorders. The Centre suggests that school-based education programs change their focus from highlighting negative, problem-based issues (e.g., glamorization of eating disorders, suggestive information about weight control techniques, negative language around food messages). Rather, their focus should turn to helping young people enjoy healthy, active lifestyles without developing a fear of food, and to build self-esteem as well as become media literate. It is the opinion that using the self-esteem approach, for example, can have a positive effect on other health-related outcomes (e.g., depression, anxiety, sexual risk taking, substance abuse, and obesity).

Schools are an important arena for health promotion and prevention efforts. Best practices principles recommend that comprehensive health education programs match the developmental level of students. Ideally, health promotion programs in the area of eating disorders would be introduced with students as early as grade four and continue throughout high school (e.g., booster sessions incorporating the prevention material into the school curriculum across various topics). In addition, peer support groups would be offered to students approaching the high-risk period of early adolescence (grades 5–7) to help combat weight and shape teasing and pressure from peers to diet.

Although many recommendations have been made with regard to the implementation of school-based programs, and although various primary prevention eating disorder programs have been integrated into school curricula, published results and evaluations of their effects have been scant. As stated earlier, Scime and Cook-Cottone (2008) remarked that there are no known programs to date that have combined all seven components of effective primary prevention. The following, however, are a list of the most promising primary prevention school-based programs based on best practice principles.

12.3.3.1 Teaching Kids to Eat and Love Their Bodies Too!

"Healthy Body Image: Teaching Kids to Eat and Love Their Bodies Too!" (HBI), a 10-lesson curriculum for grades four through six, includes age-appropriate activities, cross-curricular program based on widely recognized prevention principles. The HBI curriculum is based on the Model for Healthy Body Image (Kater 2005). This curriculum assists teachers in empowering students to form a foundation for acceptance of their bodies, based on recognition of what they can and cannot control with regard to body size and shape. Through stories and activities, students are prepared and empowered to resist unhealthy and unrealistic cultural pressures regarding body image, and are inspired to develop a practical understanding of healthy eating. Four of the ten lessons emphasize the biology of what cannot be controlled regarding body size, shape, and hunger. Four additional lessons emphasize factors influencing weight and body image that offer choices; eating well to satisfy hunger, energy, and nutritional needs, limiting sedentary activities, embracing a balanced sense of identity (vs. placing undue focus on any single aspect, such as appearance), and choosing realistic role models. Two lessons are sociocultural in nature.

Evaluation results demonstrated knowledge about the biology of body size and shape, and the counterproductive nature of dieting, improved dramatically for students receiving the HBI lessons. Boys and girls also demonstrated a significant increase in the ability to think critically about media messages regarding appearance. Outcomes for boys also reflected a significant decrease in prejudicial attitudes about body size, and improved choices regarding eating and physical activity. All scores for girls in the test group reflected a trend in the desired direction regarding self-image, body size prejudices, and lifestyle behaviors endorsed. Body image did not change significantly during the intervention for either boys or girls, but this result would not be expected because dissatisfaction was not a great concern initially. This result is consistent with the thesis that primary prevention programs like HBI should be implemented before problems like body dissatisfaction develop, and that the goal is to maintain health (Rohwer et al. 2002).

12.3.3.2 Girls' Group

"Girls' Group" is an eating disorder prevention program built on the most recent findings in school-based eating disorder prevention, while simultaneously incorporating innovative practices that have demonstrated preliminary efficacy (Scime et al. 2006). Specifically, the "Girls' Group" utilizes an interactive format, a positive psychology orientation (including yoga as a guided-practice body component), facilitators with expertise in eating disorders and wellness, and a multisession format implemented with all female fifth graders. The last several sessions of the group lessons are allocated to the completion of an entirely student-centered project designed to promote feelings of empowerment to affect media and social change and a counterthin ideal cognitive stance (Pratt and Woolfenden 2002). Specifically, following the earlier group activities and content including activities on assertiveness, self-care, nutrition, gender roles, and the exploration of media image and media literacy, the girls are asked to create their own magazine that is healthy and will help girls learn from what they have learned.

Research findings indicated that the "Girls' Group" was efficacious in reducing body dissatisfaction, the most robust risk factor associated with eating disorders. In fact, while body dissatisfaction significantly decreased over time for the participants, it slightly increased for the control group. Participants in the experimental group also reported significantly decreased tendencies to think about and engage in uncontrollable eating whereas these tendencies remained constant for the comparison group. Social self-concept also increased significantly more for participants in the "Girls' Group" compared with those in the comparison group. Increased social self-esteem may protect against various weight-related pressures and potentially subsequent eating-disordered behaviors (Strong and Huon 1998). It is also important to note that there were also several factors that were not significantly impacted by the "Girls' Group." For example, drive for thinness and current methods and future intentions related to eating-disordered behavior were not impacted.

Both "Teaching Kids to Eat and Love their Bodies" and the "Girls' Group" curricula have similar significant limitations, namely (1) Sample sizes were relatively small and participants were not randomly assigned to condition; (2) The lack of follow-up study eliminates making conclusions about the maintenance of gains or the long-term impact of the intervention; and (3) The ability to generalize findings is questionable.

12.3.3.3 Eating Smart/Eating for Me

"Eating Smart/Eating for Me" is a 10-lesson primary prevention school-based curriculum for fourth and fifth graders. The lessons, aimed at reducing the influence of risk factors and introducing the impact of protective factors, addresses the following concepts: (1) healthy eating without counting calories or fat; (2) exercising for fun, fitness, and friendship; (3) reduction of ignorance and prejudice toward body fat and fat people; (4) greater acceptance of natural diversity in weight and shape;

(5) development of a positive body image; (6) the dangers of calorie-restricted dieting; and (7) a critical evaluation of media messages pertaining to body image and nutrition.

The research results indicated that 2 years after the initial intervention, students were not only more knowledgeable, but had higher body self-esteem and used fewer unhealthy weight management techniques than students in a control group (Smolak and Levine 2001). Since the point of primary prevention is not to reverse unhealthy behaviors and attitudes but to create a foundation that will stop them from occurring in the first place, these are hopeful results. Interventions introduced at the upper elementary level promoting increased knowledge, critical thinking skills, and realistic attitudes may counteract unhealthy pressures about appearance, weight, and eating during the vulnerable middle school years.

12.3.3.4 Giving Our Girls Inspiration and Resources for Lasting Self-esteem

"GO GIRLS" is a high school prevention program and curriculum created by the National Eating Disorders Association (National Eating Disorder Association 1999). The program provides young women with the tools, confidence, and self-esteem they need to impact one of the major influences in their lives, the media, on one of the most pressing teen health issues, body image! Through facilitated discussions, students in the program explore their own body image issues, general principles about eating disorders and prevention, and the connection between media and body image. "GO GIRLS" teams take an in-depth look at how advertisements are developed, and, in the process, gain an ability to analyze their underlying messages. Team members learn how to construct effective letters and presentations to voice their support or concern to advertisers who either responsibly or irresponsibly impact youth body image. By becoming "critical viewers" of the media and by discovering effective means of self-expression, "GO GIRLS" participants are better able to develop and maintain healthy self-esteem and body image.

12.3.3.5 Growing Together: Watch Me Grow

"Growing Together" is a curriculum kit that addresses and promotes healthy eating and body images in elementary grade level children. The curriculum consists of a video, a video guidebook, and a four-lesson curriculum on healthy eating. The curriculum features a 50-page teacher workbook, complete with ready-to-use lesson plans, examples, and student handouts. "Growing Together" is about healthy eating and not about a particular weight or body shape. The goal is to prevent and counteract nutritional, emotional, and physical issues that cause disordered eating and eating disorders (Film Media Group 2003).

12.3.3.6 Full of Ourselves

"Full of Ourselves" a health and wellness education program created by Catherine Steiner-Adair addresses critical issues of body preoccupation and reducing risks for disordered eating in girls ages 8–13. Emphasizing girls' personal power and overall mental and physical well being, each unit ends with a "Call to Action" to help girls make positive action at school, home, and in their community. Evaluated with more than 800 girls, this primary prevention curriculum demonstrates positive and sustained changes in girls' body image, body satisfaction, and body esteem (Steiner et al. 2006).

12.3.3.7 Positive Body Image

"Positive Body Image: Healthy Bodies" is a curriculum for grades 1–6 covering the topics on healthy eating, physical activity, self-esteem, body image, and body shapes. Using age-appropriate language and concepts, the lessons promote realistic body image and prevent eating disorders through interactive engaging lessons. The curriculum includes a lesson book, teacher background information with video, posters illustrating lesson topics, and parent newsletters. The kits are designed to help children and youth feel better about their bodies. Developed and piloted, the curriculum illustrates the benefits of integrating health, education, research, and prevention. Each level addresses body image in its broadest sense by focusing on behaviors and attitudes that support wellness (Russell-Mayhew 2005).

12.3.3.8 Girls on the Run International

The "Girls on the Run" program is a 12-week (two 1-h sessions per week) experiential learning program for 8–12-year-old girls that combines running with curriculum-based activities that encourage emotional, social, mental, and physical health in addition to character development. The mission of the program is to educate and prepare girls for a lifetime of self-respect and healthy living. The objectives of the curriculum include increasing self-esteem, body image, and healthy eating attitudes. The program is implemented by a trained "Girls on the Run" educator.

Program evaluation employed a cross-sectional pretest/posttest design to examine the effectiveness of the 12-week program. Questionnaires were administered before the first program session and again at the end of the last session. Measures were obtained relative to self-esteem, body size satisfaction, and general eating attitudes and behaviors. Findings of the evaluation indicated that over the 12-week study, period significant changes in all three of the noted areas occurred. Researchers concluded that programs that positively impact self-esteem in young females do improve self-concept, body image, and also prevent eating disorders (*Girls on the Run International* 2007).

12.4 SUMMARY AND CONCLUSIONS

Both program evaluation research and the prevalence of dieting and body dissatisfaction in children and youth emphasize the need for additional primary prevention programs. As can be seen from the chapter research studies, most of the programs show mixed results. From a clinical perspective, the development and refinement of prevention programs are complicated by a lack of knowledge about risk factors associated with eating disorders and considering the potential to cause harm. From a research perspective, longer-term effects of any intervention approaches will need to be monitored across development in order to demonstrate a decline in the incidence of eating disorders and associated risk factors. It should also be remembered that even the best prevention efforts will fail unless adults are simultaneously educated, impassioned, and empowered to join students in resisting and challenging a cultural environment that creates body image problems, unhealthy weight concerns, and eating disorders.

12.5 CASE STUDY

Megan is working with a group of young girls between the ages of 9 and 11 at her local middle school. She has designed a unit to improve general levels of health, particularly related to nutrition and eating disorders. As she begins her introductory lesson on the benefits of good food, proper exercise, and weight management, she notices some whispering and laughter occurring among the group members. Megan stops the lesson to inquire as to the students' reactions. To Megan's dismay, a number of them comment on how often they have dieted in the last 3 months and expressed their desire to look like the models they see on MTV and in the teen magazines. Besides, they say, in their opinion, there is nothing harmful in dieting. The students argue that their parents do nothing to discourage them from dieting and other students in the school make comments to them about their weight. In addition, some of the girls in the group have formed a support group to encourage each other to continue a regimen of dieting and exercising. After several minutes of discussion, what becomes clear to Megan is that many of the young girls in the class have a distorted sense of thinness. Instead of continuing on with the planned unit, she decides to rethink her original unit of instruction and make some modifications in the program instruction.

12.5.1 Your Response

What approach should Megan take in redesigning an intervention program that not only includes factual information related to nutrition, eating disorders, and exercise, but also includes strategies to address the students' unrealistic attitudes and misperceptions regarding weight and appearance?

12.5.2   APPROPRIATE RESPONSE (THERE MAY BE MORE THAN ONE CORRECT ANSWER)

Based on the information provided in this chapter, Megan might find the following suggestions helpful:

(a) Acceptance of diverse body shapes. This requires discussion of the causes of body size and shape and of prejudice against heavy people. It should also include, especially among older elementary school-aged children, information concerning pubertal changes.

(b) Understanding that body shape is not infinitely mutable.

(c) Understanding proper nutrition, including the importance of dietary fat and of a minimum caloric intake.

(d) Discussion of the negative effects of dieting, as well as the lack of long-term positive effects.

(e) Consideration of the positive effects of moderate exercise and the negative effects of excessive or compensatory exercise.

(f) Development of strategies to resist teasing, pressure to diet, propaganda about the importance of slenderness.

In essence, Megan's intervention program should model those same prevention framework principles recognized by experts in the field; namely (1) providing accurate information regarding normal weight gain during prepubertal development; (2) teaching about genetic diversity of body shapes and the limits of "weight management," (3) emphasizing the predictable, counterproductive efforts of dieting while providing incentives for healthy eating and activity habits, (4) encouraging students to develop interests and competencies not based on appearance, and (5) teaching skills for resisting unhealthy cultural pressures regarding weight and dieting. As with any primary prevention program that challenges cultural factors, an initial inoculation is not sufficient to sustain resiliency. Subsequently, teachers in the upper grade levels may wish to follow up on Megan's educational wellness program by providing occasional 'booster' lessons. Megan may also consider talking with her local school health education director as to the possibility of implementing a prevention program in the junior and senior high levels using any of a number of age-appropriate research-based best practices curricula.

12.6   GLOSSARY OF TERMS

Prevention—a process of creating conditions and/or developing personal attributes and skills to promote the wellness of individuals, families, and communities.

Primary Prevention—a process aimed at reducing the incidence of a disorder through the reduction or elimination of those risk factors that cause or contribute to its occurrence before symptoms are evident.

Secondary Prevention—action that is taken to enable early detection of a health problem and to stop or modify the severity or extent of illness and disease.

Tertiary Prevention—action aimed at reducing the impairment that may result from an established disorder.

REFERENCES

Austin, S. B., A. E. Field, J. Wiecha, K. E. Peterson, and S. L. Gortmaker. 2005. The impact of a school-based prevention trial on disordered weight control behaviors in early adolescent girls. *Arch Pediatr Adolesc Med* 159: 225–230.

Baranowski, M. J., and M. M. Hetherington. 2001. Testing the efficacy of an eating disorder prevention program. *Int J Eat Disord* 29: 119–124.

Carter, J. C., A. Stewart, N. V. J. Dunn, and C. G. Fairburn. 1997. Primary prevention of eating disorders: Might it do more harm than good? *Int J Eat Disord* 22: 167–172.

Cook-Cottone, C. P., and M. Scime. 2006. The prevention and treatment of eating disorders: An overview for school psychologists. *The Communiqué* 34: 38–40.

Dalle Grave, R., L. de Luca, and G. Campello. 2001. Middle school primary prevention program for eating disorders: A controlled study with a twelve-month follow-up. *Eat Disord* 9: 327–337.

Film Media Group. 2003. *Growing Together: Watch Me Grow.*

Fingeret, M. C., C. S. Warren, A. Cepeda-Benito, and D. H. Gleaves. 2006. Eating disorder prevention research: A meta-analysis. *Eat Disord* 14: 191–213.

Girls on the Run International (GOTR). 2007. Charlotte, NC: GOTR International. www.girlsontherun.org (accessed October 21, 2009).

Huon, G. G. 1996. Health promotion and the prevention of dieting-induced disorders. *Eat Disord* 4: 27–32.

Kater, K. 2005. *Teaching kids to eat, and love their bodies too!* (2nd ed.). Seattle, WA: National Eating Disorders Association (NEDA).

Langmesser, L., and S. Verscheure. 2009. Are eating disorder prevention programs effective? *J Athl Train* 44: 304–305.

Littleton, H. L., and T. Ollendick. 2003. Negative body image and disordered eating behavior in children and adolescents: What places youth at risk and how can these problems be prevented? *Clin Child Fam Psychol Rev* 6: 51–66.

Mann, T., S. Nolen-Hoeksema, K. Huang, D. Burgard, A. Wright, and K. Hanson. 1997. Are two interventions worse than none: Joint primary and secondary prevention of eating disorders in college females. *Health Psychol* 16: 215–125.

McVey, G. What we have learned about primary prevention of food and weight preoccupation. *National Eating Disorder Information Centre* M5G 2C4 www.nedic.ca.

McVey, G. L., and R. Davis. 2002. A program to promote positive body image: A one-year follow-up evaluation. The *J Early Adolesc* 22: 96–108.

National Eating Disorder Association (NEDA). 1999. *Giving our girls inspiration and resources for long-lasting self-esteem.* Seattle, WA: NEDA.

Neumark-Sztainer, D. 2005. Can we simultaneously work toward the prevention of obesity and eating disorders in children and adolescents? *Int J Eat Disord* 38: 220–227.

O'Dea, J., and S. Abraham. 2000. Improving the body image, eating attitudes, and behaviors of young male and female adolescents: A new educational approach that focuses on self-esteem. *Int J Eat Disord* 28: 43–57.

Pearson, J., D. Goldklang, and R. H. Striegel-Moore. 2002. Prevention of eating disorders: Challenges and opportunities. *Int J Eat Disord* 31: 233–239.

Phelps, L., M. Dempsey, J. Sapia, and L. Nelson. 1999. The efficacy of a school-based eating disorder prevention program: Building physical self-esteem and competencies. In *Preventing eating disorders: A handbook of interventions and special challenges*, ed. N. Piran, M. P. Levine, and C. Steiner-Adair, 163–174. New York: Taylor & Francis.

Piran, N. 2001. The body logic program: Discussions and reflections. *Cogn Behav Pract* 8: 259–264.

Pratt, B. M., and S. R. Woolfenden. 2002. Interventions for preventing eating disorders in children and adolescents. *Cochrane Database Syst Rev* http://onlinelibrary.wiley.com/o/cochrane/clsysrev/articles/CD002891/frame.html (accessed December 8, 2010).

Rohwer, J., K. Kater, and K. Londre. 2002. Evaluation of an upper elementary school program to prevent body image, eating and weight concerns. *J School Health* 72: 199–204.

Russell-Mayhew, S. 2005. *Body image works.* Carlsbad, CA: Gürze Books.

Seligman, M.E.P., and M. Csikszentmihalyi. 2000. Positive psychology: An introduction. *Am J Psychol* 55: 5–14.

Scime, M., and C. Cook-Cottone. 2008. Primary prevention of eating disorders: A constructivist integration of mind and body strategies. *Int J Eat Disord* 41:134–142.

Scime, M., C. Cook-Cottone, L. Kane, and T. Watson. 2006. Group prevention of eating disorders with fifth-grade females: Impact on body dissatisfaction, drive for thinness, and media influence. *Eat Disord* 14: 143–55.

Smolak, L., and M. Levine, M. 1994. Toward an empirical basis for primary prevention of eating problems with elementary school children. *Eat Disord* 2: 293–307.

Smolak, L., and M. P. Levine. 2001. A two-year follow-up of a primary prevention program for negative body image and unhealthy weight regulation. *Eat Disord* 20: 75–90.

Steck, E. L., L. M. Abrams, and L. Phelps. 2004. Positive psychology in the prevention of eating disorders. *Psychol Sch* 41: 111–117.

Steiner-Adair, C., and L. Sjostrom, L. 2006. *Full of ourselves: A wellness program to advance girl power, health, and leadership.* New York, NY: Teachers College Press.

Stewart, D. A., J. C. Carter, J. Drinkwater, J. Hainsworth, and C. G. Fairburn. 2001. Modification of eating attitudes and behavior in adolescent girls: A controlled study. *Int J Eat Disord* 29: 107–118.

Stice, E., and H. Shaw. 2004. Eating disorder prevention programs: A meta-analytic review. *Psychol Bull* 130: 206–227.

Stice, E., H. Shaw, and C. N. Marti. 2007. A meta-analytic review of eating disorder prevention programs: Encouraging findings. *Annu Rev Clin Psychol* 3: 233–257.

Strong, K.G., and G. F. Huon. 1998. An evaluation of a structural model for studies of the initiation of dieting among adolescent girls. *J Psychosom Res* 44: 315–326.

Thelen, M. H., A. L. Powell, C. Lawrence, and M. E. Kulnert. 1992. Eating and body image concerns among children. *J Clin Child Psychol* 21: 41–46.

Varnado-Sullivan, P. J., N. Zucker, D. A. Williamson, D. Reas, J. Thaw, and S. B. Netemeyer. 2001. Development and implementation of the body logic program for adolescents: A two-stage prevention program for eating disorders. *Cogn Behav Pract* 8: 248–259.

Wade, T. D., S. Davidson, and J. A. O'Dea. 2003. A preliminary controlled evaluation of a school-based media literacy program and self-esteem program for reducing eating disorder risk factors. *Int J Eat Disord* 33: 371–383.

13 An Ecological Approach to the Prevention of Eating Disorders in Children and Adolescents

Marilyn Massey-Stokes, Barbara A. Barton,
Mandy Golman, and Deidre J. Holland

CONTENTS

13.1 LEARNING OBJECTIVES

After completing this chapter, the reader will be able to

- Examine the importance of primary prevention in the consideration of eating disorders
- Discuss important considerations for primary prevention programs targeting children and adolescents

- Explain how the ecological approach can be used in eating disorder prevention targeting children and adolescents
- Analyze how media literacy can be used to promote healthy body image among youth
- Examine the role of cultural competence in eating disorder prevention among youth
- Describe primary prevention interventions that can be implemented with children and adolescents in school and community settings
- Analyze how an integrated approach can effectively address both eating disorder prevention and obesity prevention among youth

13.2 BACKGROUND AND SIGNIFICANCE

13.2.1 PRIMARY PREVENTION

Prevention of eating disorders can occur on three different levels: primary, secondary, and tertiary. The goal of primary prevention is to prevent an eating disorder from occurring, which can be accomplished by reducing risk factors and increasing protective factors (Levine and Maine 2005; Piran 2005). Secondary prevention efforts focus on the early detection of precursors and implementation of interventions to prevent full-blown clinical eating disorders (Levine and Maine 2005; Piran 2005). Tertiary prevention includes the proper identification of and treatment for those who already have developed an eating disorder (Piran 2005; Piran et al. 1999). Historically, primary prevention programs have been educational, relaying information about eating disorders, including symptoms and warning signs of these disorders (Scime et al. 2006). However, simply disseminating information may not be enough to prevent the development of eating disorders. Levine and Maine (2005) suggested moving beyond educating individuals about warning signs and symptoms of eating disorders and incorporating multiple primary prevention components, such as learning activities to promote self-esteem, positive body image, and media awareness and advocacy. Furthermore, newer prevention programs have been specifically designed to be interactive and student-centered to help foster self-esteem and self-efficacy (Kater et al. 2000, 2002; McVey et al. 2003, 2004; O'Dea 2005; O'Dea and Abraham 2000), both of which may be protective against eating disorders (O'Dea 2005; Shisslak and Crago 2001; Wiser and Telch 1999).

13.2.1.1 Universal versus Targeted Programs

Neumark-Sztainer, Levine et al. (2006) also discussed moving towards *universal* prevention programs that are aimed at all youth, not just those who have been identified as particularly at risk for body image and eating difficulties. These universal programs can foster protective factors, including self-esteem, self-efficacy, media literacy, social-emotional learning, stress management, creative problem solving, and overall resilience. They can also prevent risk factors, such as body dissatisfaction, dieting, and unhealthy weight-control practices (Kater et al. 2002; Massey-Stokes 2008; McVey et al. 2004; Neumark-Sztainer, Levine et al. 2006; O'Dea 2007). A distinct advantage of a universal approach is that children and adolescents do not feel "singled out" and are not teased or bullied for a particular problem, including body dissatisfaction or disordered eating (Holt and Ricciardelli 2008; McVey et al. 2004). Furthermore, the promotion of life skills, youth development, and overall resilience also can help prevent other health-risk behaviors among youth, such as violence, early sexual activity, and the use of tobacco, alcohol, and other drugs (Catalano et al. 2002; Kahn et al. 2010; McVey et al. 2004; Resnick et al. 1997).

Parallel to universal prevention programs are "covert prevention programs" (Stice and Ragan 2002). Through meta-analysis, Stice and Shaw (2004) found that 10 out of 15 prevention programs that produced significant effects for disordered eating were described as "body acceptance interventions" as opposed to eating disorder prevention programs. According to Stice and Shaw (2004, 222), "individuals may be less defensive about their body image and eating disturbances and thus more willing to entertain alternative perspectives when they are not aware that they are in an intervention focusing on these outcomes."

On the other hand, there are also those who believe that targeted prevention programs—those programs designed for children and adolescents who are identified as at risk for body image and eating concerns—may be more effective than universal programs (Holt and Ricciardelli 2008). Proponents for targeted programs have argued that young people who are at risk are generally more distressed and therefore more motivated to engage in behavioral change. Plus, targeted programs are generally smaller and easier to fund, simpler to implement, and require fewer resources (Stice and Ragan 2002). Nonetheless, research has shown that targeted programs aimed at recruiting high-risk participants through eating disorder screening were ineffective (Varnado-Sullivan et al. 2001).

13.2.1.2 Age of Participants

Age is an important factor when planning eating disorder primary prevention programs. Results of a meta-analysis supported the implementation of prevention programs targeting adolescents over the age of 15, suggesting that older youth are at higher risk for eating disorders; thus, they may be more cognitively mature and more motivated to participate in an intervention than younger girls (Stice and Shaw 2004). However, body dissatisfaction, drive for thinness, and other weight concerns have been exhibited in younger children; plus, unhealthy body image attitudes and eating behaviors are difficult to reverse once they are ingrained. Therefore, numerous researchers have argued the importance of beginning prevention efforts earlier, such as during the later elementary school years (Agras et al. 2007; Dohnt and Tiggemann 2005; Gehrman et al. 2006; Ghaderi et al. 2005; Kater et al. 2000, 2002; Levine and Smolak 2001; McCabe, Ricciardelli, and Salmon 2006; Neumark-Sztainer et al. 2000; Paxton 1993; Scime et al. 2006; Smolak et al. 1998). Then, too, Dohnt and Tiggemann (2008) suggested starting prevention programs as early as the age of school entry, citing that girls as young as 6 years of age have indicated that they desire to be thinner (Dohnt and Tiggemann 2005). According to Dohnt and Tiggemann (2008), starting prevention at the age of school entry makes sense because this is around the age that weight-related attitudes and beliefs are less established, and unhealthy weight-control behaviors have not yet been developed. Similarly, Shunk and Birch (2004, 7) argued that childhood obesity prevention programs should begin during the preschool years because "girls' weight status at age 5 [appears to be] a risk factor for the emergence of dietary restraint, disinhibited overeating, weight concern, and body dissatisfaction during middle childhood." Regardless of the exact age that prevention programs target, it is extremely important that these programs address the relevant skills and challenges for each stage of development (Compas 1993; Holt and Ricciardelli 2008; Society for Adolescent Medicine 2003).

13.2.1.3 Program Characteristics

In addition to questions about whom to target with these prevention programs, there also are questions regarding characteristics of prevention programs that would be most effective. For example, multiple-session health promotion programs employing diverse strategies are widely considered more effective than single-dose approaches (McKenzie et al. 2009; Stice and Shaw 2004). Although it may be useful to design relatively brief intervention programs (e.g., three to four sessions) because they are more easily implemented, less expensive, and more logistically attractive to both adolescents and school administrators (Stice and Shaw 2004), other interventions with 10 or more sessions have been successfully implemented as well (e.g., Kater et al. 2000, 2002). Furthermore, program delivery (e.g., interactive format vs. didactic format) may be more important than program content in producing more positive attitudinal and behavioral outcomes (Piran 2004, as cited in Piran 2005; Holt and Ricciardelli 2008; Stice and Shaw 2004). More specifically, the most promising outcomes have occurred through interventions aimed at changing unhealthy attitudes (e.g., body thin-ideal internalization and body dissatisfaction) and promoting healthy weight-management practices (Stice and Shaw 2004).

13.2.1.4 Program Evaluation

Clearly defined program goals and objectives are prerequisites for meaningful primary prevention program evaluations (Levine and Smolak 2001; McKenzie et al. 2009). Although process, impact, and outcome evaluations are all critical to the overall evaluation process, program evaluation remains a major challenge for primary prevention efforts. One hindrance is that the full impact of primary prevention often does not emerge until several years later, and many primary prevention programs do not match well within experimental evaluation frameworks (Kelly et al. 2005). Then, too, several prevention programs have demonstrated positive results in the short term (e.g., increases in knowledge), but results were not maintained or were difficult to measure in follow-up evaluations (Levine and Smolak 2001; O'Dea 2005; Stice and Shaw 2004). Additionally, although changes in knowledge are important, these changes do not necessarily lead to sustainable attitudinal and behavioral changes. Therefore, evaluations that include follow-up measurements that occur months or even years after the initial intervention are useful in determining whether program effects have been sustained over time. For example, Stice and Shaw (2004, 224) reported that the effects of certain eating disorder prevention programs "persisted as long as 2 years and were superior to minimal-intervention control conditions." Likewise, others have asserted that quality prevention studies should include long-term follow-up of at least one year, and preferably longer (Piran 2005; World Health Organization [WHO] 2000). Also, Stice and Shaw (2004, 223) found that many prevention studies did not assess eating pathology, which "is troublesome because the defining feature of a successful eating disorder prevention program is that it reduces current or future eating disorder symptoms or syndromes—otherwise it should not logically be considered an eating disorder prevention program." Therefore, to obtain more significant program outcomes, program evaluations must assess both risk factors and protective factors with validated outcome measures, both in the short term and the long term (Stice and Shaw 2004).

13.2.1.5 Primary Prevention Studies

In the past, some eating disorder prevention programs resulted in nonsignificant or even negative findings. For example, some of these programs actually caused harm in girls who were at risk for developing eating disorders because these types of programs served as instruction on how to have an eating disorder rather than preventing the development of one (Killen et al. 1993). On the other hand, more current studies have reported that children appeared to experience no adverse effects from participating in prevention programs addressing issues related to eating disorder prevention (Gehrman et al. 2006; Kater et al. 2000, 2002; McVey et al. 2003, 2004 Neumark-Sztainer et al. 2000; O'Dea and Abraham 2002). More specifically, research with children has revealed some promising results. According to Piran (2005), a majority of the reviewed studies in children aged 9–14 showed changes in children's knowledge, particularly their knowledge about nutrition, exercise, and the natural and expected body weight and shape changes that accompany puberty. Also, in a controlled study with a large sample of boys and girls between the ages of 9 and 13, Kater et al. (2002, 203) found that students in the intervention groups gained knowledge about the "biology of body size and shape, and the counterproductive nature of dieting." They also increased their ability to think critically about media messages concerning physical appearance. Additionally, Holt and Ricciardelli (2008) reported that the elementary school prevention programs in their review were effective in improving children's knowledge, but showed little evidence for promoting self-esteem and no evidence for decreasing body image concerns or dieting and eating problems. However, there were limitations to these studies that should be considered. For example, 8 out of the 13 studies only conducted a post-test evaluation, and four of the other studies may not have included follow-up assessments that were long enough to reveal possible prevention effects (Holt and Ricciardelli 2008).

In summary, health promotion professionals must carefully plan and implement eating disorder prevention programs (Killen et al. 1993; Levine and Smolak 2001; Paxton 1993) so that the benefits outweigh any risks and harm is minimized (Daníelsdóttir et al. 2010; O'Dea 2007; Society for Nutrition Education 2003). While additional research and improvements still need to be pursued, body dissatisfaction and eating disorder prevention programs have made significant improvements over the past decade (Neumark-Sztainer, Levine et al. 2006). Addressing the concerns and building upon these improvements will result in the continued advancement of primary prevention in the study of body image and eating disorders. In addition, an ecological perspective calls for prevention research to include more studies regarding the efficacy of multilevel interventions that target individual and broader, systemic changes along with longer term follow-up (Piran 2005).

13.2.2 The Ecological Framework

13.2.2.1 Overview of the Ecological Model

The ecological framework for health behavior, modification, promotion, and prevention encompasses comprehensive and multidimensional approaches to health issues. The ecological model places emphasis on systematically assessing and targeting behavioral factors that influence health at multiple levels (Sallis et al. 2008; U.S. Department of Health and Human Services [USDHHS] 2005a). The core principles of the ecological approach to health behavior changes recommend behavior-specific, interactive strategies and multilevel interventions (Sallis et al. 2008). The ecological perspective is vital for considering various facets that both influence body image and prevent eating disorders in girls (Evans et al. 2008; Kater et al. 2000; Neumark-Sztainer 2007; Smith et al. 2004). The ecological model underscores the interconnectedness of individual and environmental factors that affect health because it signifies a "reciprocal causation" between individual behavior and the social environment (USDHHS 2005a). This perspective emphasizes the interactive roles of individuals, groups, organizations, policies, and the environment within the larger context of community prevention strategies (Stokol 1996). Moreover, a primary assumption of ecological models is that it generally requires "the combination of *both* individual-level and environmental/policy-level interactions to achieve substantial changes in health behaviors" (Sallis et al. 2008, 467).

Within the ecological model, the five levels of influence (Battle and Brownell 1996; Sallis et al. 2008; Stokol 1996; USDHHS 2005a; WHO 2000) include the following:

1. Intrapersonal/individual factors—Individual characteristics influencing behavior (e.g., knowledge, beliefs, attitudes, personal traits)
2. Interpersonal factors—Relationships with primary social groups that provide social identity (e.g., family, friends, peers, neighbors, coworkers)
3. Organizational/institutional factors—Attributes, regulations, and policies/procedures supporting or hindering behavior change (e.g., coordinated school health programs)
4. Community factors—Social environments and informal or formal networks that provide social identities and resources (e.g., faith communities, schools, worksites)
5. Public policy factors—Local, state, and federal policies, procedures, and laws that protect the health of communities or support healthy behaviors (e.g., media regulations)

13.2.2.2 Application of the Ecological Model

Application of the ecological model has also developed through research and practice regarding behavior modification because of the comprehensive, interactive, and systematic approach to primary prevention. In the last few decades, prevention strategies and research have focused on promoting healthy body image and preventing eating disorders in children and adolescents using the ecological framework (Cook-Cottone 2006; Elder et al. 2007; Evans et al. 2008; Haines and Neumark-Sztainer 2006; Keca and Cook-Cottone 2005; Levine and Smolak 2001; Loth et al. 2009; McVey et al. 2003, 2004; Neumark-Sztainer 2007; O'Dea and Abraham; 2002; O'Dea and Maloney 2000; Smith et al. 2004). This perspective has been successfully applied in other child and adolescent prevention programs as well, such as those targeting dietary behaviors, physical activity, cardiovascular health promotion, alcohol and other drug use, youth violence, and youth diversion (Booth et al. 2001; Elder et al. 2007; Fraser 1996; Kubic et al. 2003; Perry et al. 1997, 2002).

Within the ecological framework, prevention programs should be tailored for adolescents because the model does not place emphasis on specific, individual factors; however, it encompasses various domains that affect adolescent behavior (Banister and Begoray 2004; Elder et al. 2007; Haines and Neumark-Sztainer 2006; Kater et al. 2000; Smith et al. 2004; Stock et al. 2007). For instance, environmental and social factors play an integral role in shaping adolescent behavior. Therefore, it is important to implement multiple prevention strategies to target these influences (Booth et al. 2001; Haines and Neumark-Sztainer 2006; O'Dea 2005; Neumark-Sztainer 2007).

Then, too, incorporating other theories and models of health behavior within the ecological framework can provide methods to address specific behaviors as well as environmental factors. For example, Social Cognitive Theory (Bandura 1986) posits that a person's behavior "is the product of the dynamic interplay of personal, behavioral, and environmental influences" (McAlister et al. 2008, 170). Therefore, it can serve as a helpful theory to guide program development that accounts for varying backgrounds and influences, including various interpersonal interactions and numerous media influences (Banister and Begoray 2004; Booth et al. 2001; Dohnt and Tiggemann 2008; USDHHS 2005b). Because coordinated efforts facilitate change at all levels, integration of prevention efforts at multiple levels significantly increases the capacity to develop and apply prevention programs that work effectively (Haines and Neumark-Sztainer 2006; Piran 2005; Shunk and Birch 2004).

Body dissatisfaction, dieting, unhealthy weight-control practices, and eating disorders in children and adolescents present public health concerns that need to be addressed with an ecological approach. The premise of the ecological model provides a foundation to implement strategies to target the diverse factors that affect body image and eating disorders at each level of influence. As depicted in Figure 13.1, some examples of the factors within each level include the following:

1. *Individual Factors*—self-esteem and self-acceptance, self-efficacy, body image and body satisfaction, eating attitudes and behaviors, physical activity, and weight-control behaviors (Dohnt and Tiggemann 2008; Elder et al. 2007; Feinberg-Walker et al. 2009; Golman 2009; Haines and Neumark-Sztainer 2006; Kater 2005; McVey et al. 2003, 2004; O'Dea 2005; Shunk and Birch 2004).

2. *Interpersonal Factors*—relationships with family members; eating patterns within the family system; the influence of friends and adult role models; social support from family and peers; and weight-related comments, teasing, and bullying (Eisenberg and Neumark-Sztainer 2010; Evans et al. 2008; Hayden-Wade et al. 2005; Loth et al. 2009; McVey et al. 2003; Neumark-Sztainer 2007; Neumark-Sztainer et al. 2007; Shomaker and Furman 2009; Shunk and Birch 2004; Steese et al. 2006; Wertheim et al. 1997).

3. *Organizational/Institutional Factors*—health promoting schools (WHO 2000), such as those providing coordinated school health programs with interrelated components, including health education, physical education, health services, mental health and social services, nutrition services, healthy and safe environment, family and community involvement, and staff wellness (Centers for Disease Control and Prevention [CDC] 2010; Elder et al. 2007; Evans et al. 2008; Keca and Cook-Cottone 2005; Massey-Stokes 2008; Neumark-Sztainer 2007; O'Dea 2005; O'Dea and Maloney 2000; Skemp-Arlt 2006).

4. *Community Factors*—media messages, cultural norms for body shape and size, community prevention programs, health services, relationships between school and community, and accessibility of safe and affordable recreation facilities (ADA 2002; Elder et al. 2007; Evans et al. 2008; Keca and Cook-Cottone 2005; Neumark-Sztainer 2009).

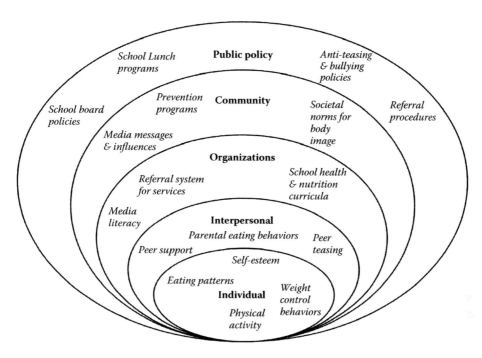

FIGURE 13.1   The ecological model: Application for the prevention of eating disorders in children & adole cents. (Adapted from Booth et al. 2001; Elder et al. 2007; Evans et al. 2008; Neumark-Sztainer 2005, 2007.)

5. *Public Policy Factors*—state and federal statutes for nutrition and health; state mandates for curricula; referral procedures for health and social services; federal and international policies guiding standard definitions of eating disorders and accepted standards of care, media regulations; and coordinated school health program policies, including no-tolerance teasing and bullying policies and policies for school food services (Battle and Brownell 1996; CDC 2010b; Evans et al. 2008; O'Dea 2005; Haines and Neumark-Sztainer 2006; Klump et al. 2009; Neumark-Sztainer 2007).

13.3   CURRENT FINDINGS

13.3.1   Media Literacy

13.3.1.1   Media Influences on Body Image and Eating Problems

No girl is immune from experiencing the widespread societal endorsement of the thin ideal through media, which has assumed a ubiquitous role in homes across America. According to a Kaiser Family Foundation Study, young people consume media approximately 7½ hours per day, seven days a week. Furthermore, because they often use more than one medium at a time, youth cram a total of 10 hours and 45 minutes of media into their daily usage, resulting in "an increase of almost 2¼ hours of media exposure per day over the past five years" (Rideout et al. 2010, 2).

Mass media has been shown to have a pervasive influence on both preadolescent and adolescent girls and their body satisfaction (Dohnt and Tiggemann 2005; McCabe, Ricciardelli, and Ridge 2006; USDHHS 2005b). Dohnt and Tiggemann (2005) reported that girls as young as 5 years old were already being influenced by peers and the media. Additionally, numerous interviews with adolescent girls have exemplified the media's influence on their body dissatisfaction, such as the pressure to be thin from magazines and the fashion industry (Tiggemann et al. 2000; Wertheim et al. 1997). In a study examining mass media exposure and weight concerns among adolescent girls, 69% reported that magazine pictures influenced their idea of the perfect body shape; and 47% reported wanting to lose weight because of magazine pictures showing the perfect body (Field et al. 1999). Another study of high-school-aged girls revealed that the girls were influenced by the media's promotion of the thin ideal. However, these media influences were mediated by the strong influence of family and friends. For example, many girls reported that they dieted in response to teasing, friends' dieting behaviors, the desire to "fit in," and both positive and negative family influences (Wertheim et al. 1997). Therefore, it appears that awareness and internalization of the sociocultural thin ideal may lead to disordered eating, especially when girls receive negative comments from parents and peers (Cordero and Israel 2009; Rodgers et al. 2009).

The types of television programs that adolescent girls watch also influence their body satisfaction. Watching movies, soap operas, and music videos where women are portrayed in stereotypical roles (i.e., thin, beautiful, and scantily dressed) has been correlated with increased body dissatisfaction among adolescent girls (Tiggemann and Pickering 1996). More specifically, Tiggemann (2005) found that adolescents who watched television programs such as soap operas have higher rates of negative body image and disordered eating. Additionally, adolescent girls, especially those who are overweight, feel "particularly bad about not conforming to the ideal" that is continually portrayed in the media (McCabe, Ricciardelli, and Ridge 2006, 416). Moreover, increased media exposure to ultra-thin ideals increases the risk of developing an eating disorder among adolescent girls who already buy into the thin ideal as the socially defined and desired norm (Stice, Spangler, and Agras 2001).

Media influence on body image and eating behaviors has become a global health issue, as it extends beyond the United States and affects developed countries as well as developing countries (Klump et al. 2009; Levin Institute 2009; Shuriquie 1999; WHO 2003). For example, in Fiji, where eating disorders used to be extremely scarce, a study of adolescent girls showed that eating disturbances and weight concerns dramatically increased after prolonged television exposure (Becker et al. 2002). In addition, body image disturbances and eating disorders have increased among Asian and Arab teens, indicating that the influence of Western media and the thin ideal is making a global impact (Levin Institute 2009; Shuriquie 1999).

Internet websites that encourage youth to practice disordered eating warrant attention as well. Websites that support disordered eating often promote eating disorders as lifestyles rather than serious illnesses, and these websites reinforce people who are engaging in disordered eating behaviors or are vulnerable to developing disordered eating. These websites often include photo galleries of emaciated girls and women; tips on how to starve, purge, and hide an eating disorder; lists of "safe foods" that do not contain many calories; and blogs, forums, and chat rooms that promote favorable views of disordered eating and unhealthy weight-control methods (Giles 2006; Society for Adolescent Medicine 2003; Wilson et al. 2006). Unfortunately, these websites appear to function like a type of social network by providing participants with a sense of community and belonging (Giles 2006). Because these sites can strongly influence vulnerable young girls and have the potential to cause serious harm, increased awareness among parents, teachers, health care providers, and other caring adults who work with youth is needed.

13.3.1.2 Media Literacy for Promoting Healthy Body Image

The Center for Media Literacy (2007b, p. 1) has defined *media literacy* as "a framework to access, analyze, evaluate and create messages in a variety of forms—from print to video to the Internet." Media literacy has been increasingly recognized as an integral educational component for addressing a wide range of health issues facing youth, including violence, drug use, sexuality, and eating disorders (Center for Media Literacy 2007a; Kaiser Family Foundation 2003). Given the pervasive influence of media on our culture and the ubiquitous sociocultural messages promoting the thin ideal, media literacy is an essential tool for helping girls develop the knowledge and skills to think critically, analyze media messages, and challenge messages that promote unhealthy and unrealistic body weight and shape (Kater et al. 2000, 2002; O'Dea 2007; O'Dea and Abraham 2002; USDHHS 2005b). Such media literacy program components have been effective in decreasing the internalization of the thin ideal, as well as improving knowledge, attitudes, and self-efficacy regarding healthy lifestyle behaviors related to eating disorder prevention (Kater et al. 2000, 2002; McVey et al. 2003; Neumark-Sztainer et al. 2000; O'Dea and Abraham 2002; Scime et al. 2006; Wade et al. 2003; Wilksch et al. 2006). According to O'Dea (2005, 22), it is unclear exactly how media literacy skills help to improve body image. For instance, critical thinking that is required for media literacy may help improve body image via a cognitive route perhaps "by helping young people reject social norms for the thin ideal." Or, perhaps media literacy serves as a springboard for increased self-acceptance and self-esteem by "encouraging young people to accept themselves and reject cultural stereotypes."

Tiggemann (2005, 376) asserted that media literacy programs should move beyond teaching youth about "image distortion techniques" to a more sophisticated approach that examines underlying messages. For example, "adolescents need to be able to recognize and think critically about the pervasive but more complex and subtle messages that link appearance and body type with success and happiness" that are commonly communicated to the teen market. Additionally, in keeping with the ecological perspective, media literacy programs are most effective when the school environment is supportive in rejecting the thin ideal and fostering self-acceptance (O'Dea 2007).

13.3.2 Cultural Competence in Eating Disorder Prevention

Cultural competence has been defined as "the ability of an individual to understand and respect values, attitudes, beliefs, and mores that differ across cultures, and to consider and respond appropriately to these differences in planning, implementing, and evaluating health education and promotion programs and interventions" (2000 Joint Committee on Health Education and Promotion Terminology 2002, 5). Cultural competence is a key factor in effectively addressing eating and weight-related concerns within minority populations, yet very few eating disorder prevention programs have addressed the issues of minorities and eating disorders.

13.3.2.1 Eating Disorders among Different Ethnic Groups

Although eating disorders historically have been considered to affect largely an upper-middle-class Caucasian population, eating disorders cross all cultural and ethnic boundaries (O'Dea 2007). For example, Hispanic/Latina girls are at increased risk for engaging in several health-risk behaviors, including disordered eating (Zurn 2006). In their study of ninth grade girls, Croll et al. (2002) reported that Hispanic/Latina girls and American Indian girls had a high level of disordered eating behaviors, such as fasting, bingeing and purging, and laxative abuse. Negative body image also has been associated with higher levels of substance abuse, especially among Mexican American teens (Nieri et al. 2005). Additionally, Kelly et al. (2005) reported that Asian, Hispanic/Latina, and American Indian girls experienced as much—if not more—body dissatisfaction than Caucasian girls. Another study found the association between overweight and body dissatisfaction was highest among Asian children (Duncan et al. 2006).

In addition, studies have shown that Caucasian girls continually report higher body dissatisfaction rates when compared to African American girls (Franko and Striegel-Moore 2002; Nishina et al. 2006; Siegel et al. 1999). Caucasian girls also report a thinner body size ideal and are more likely to report themselves "overweight" and "trying to lose weight" than African American girls, even though African American girls are often larger (Franko and Striegel-Moore 2002). Neumark-Sztainer et al. (2002) also found that African American girls were less likely to internalize the thin ideal and reported fewer weight-related concerns than girls from Caucasian, Hispanic/Latina, Asian, or American Indian backgrounds. However, Gentles and Harrison (2006) discussed the importance of not discounting African American girls' drive for thinness and body dissatisfaction. Using a sample of African American adolescent girls, they found that the girls still had negative body image based on peer influence and perception. The smaller girls believed that their friends thought they should be larger, and the larger girls believed that their friends thought they should be smaller (Gentles and Harrison 2006).

13.3.2.2 Culture and Prevention

Because sociocultural factors play a key role in the development of body image and eating disorders, it is important to study how these factors may differ across different ethnic and cultural groups. These differences can be studied *between* as well as *within* groups to provide a better knowledge base for developing more culturally relevant prevention programs that reflect unique cultural factors (Franko and George 2008; Smolak 2004). Prevention efforts must identify and accurately reflect the central role of popular culture and traditional values across diverse ethnic and socioeconomic populations to be effective (Black and Young-Hyman 2007; Neumark-Sztainer et al. 2002).

13.3.3 PRIMARY PREVENTION INTERVENTIONS

Culturally relevant primary prevention strategies that are directed at enhancing body image and preventing eating disorders and other weight-related concerns can occur through a variety of channels, including public or private schools, health care settings, nonprofit organizations, and faith-based settings. Therefore, school and community educators, health care providers, and leaders of faith communities play a major role in the prevention process by working closely with children, adolescents, and their families.

13.3.3.1 School-based Prevention

Although health promotion programs that are aimed at promoting healthy body image and preventing eating disorders can occur in a variety of settings, schools can be particularly effective intervention sites (McKenzie et al. 2009; O'Dea 2005; O'Dea and Maloney 2000; Stice and Shaw 2004; WHO 2000). Health promoting schools foster collaboration among schools, families, and entire communities to positively influence both health and learning (WHO 2000). This comprehensive approach facilitates the "implementation of policies, procedure, activities, and structures required to promote a healthy body image and healthy eating behaviors in children, teachers, parents, and community members" (O'Dea and Maloney 2000, 20). Those who are responsible for implementing school-based prevention programs should be stakeholders in the process, such as school personnel (e.g., administrators, teachers, nurses, counselors/psychologists, social workers, food service workers, and other staff), students, families, and the larger community (Massey-Stokes 2008). Moreover, school-based prevention programs "can serve as catalysts for broader societal changes" (Skemp-Arlt 2006, 49).

13.3.3.1.1 Selected School-Based Primary Prevention Programs

In a scholarly review of 21 school-based body image and eating disorder prevention programs, O'Dea (2005) found that the most effective programs were student-centered and interactive, incorporated parent involvement, fostered self-esteem, and provided education in media literacy. For a more thorough overview of those programs along with ecological considerations that involve school environment, curriculum, and policy, see O'Dea (2005). For the purposes of this chapter, three selected examples of school-based prevention programs are briefly discussed next.

Shapesville (Mills and Osborn 2003) is a developmentally appropriate children's picture book that promotes positive body image and also includes information about healthy eating, physical activity, sense of uniqueness, unrealistic media messages, and the hurtfulness of weight-related teasing. Results from an evaluation study showed that *Shapesville* was effective in producing short-term improvements in young girls' body image (Dohnt and Tiggemann 2008, 232). In addition, young girls experienced improvements in "media internalisation, and knowledge of their own special talents and healthy eating, [which] remained significantly greater at follow-up than prior to reading *Shapesville*." However, the girls' appearance satisfaction and awareness of weight stereotyping were not maintained at follow-up. Nevertheless, *Shapesville* can serve as a viable curriculum tool to help prevent the early development of body image difficulties and eating disturbances (Dohnt and Tiggemann 2008).

Healthy Body Image: Teaching Kids to Eat and Love Their Bodies Too! (HBI; Kater 2005) is a curriculum for grades 4–6 that includes 10 age-appropriate and interactive lessons about normal development, body acceptance, media literacy, healthy eating, and being physically active (see Appendix 13.B). The HBI curriculum is based on the Model for Healthy Body Image (Kater 1998, see Appendix 13.C) and is now in its second edition. The underlying prevention concepts of the curriculum are taught experientially (e.g., through games, hands-on activities, stories, and discussions) and reflect "an approach not found in traditional health and nutrition curriculum" (Kater et al. 2002, 201). When compared to a control group, students who experienced the HBI curriculum showed positive, short-term improvements in self-image; increased knowledge about the biology of size, shape, and dieting; awareness of body-size prejudice; increased media literacy; and awareness of healthy eating and physical activity behaviors. It is recommended that future studies use more ethnically diverse samples and incorporate follow-up surveys to determine long-term changes (Kater et al. 2002).

Everybody's Different (O'Dea 2007) is another student-centered, interactive program designed to promote positive self-esteem and body image in relation to health, puberty, nutrition, and obesity prevention. The activities that comprise this program are adaptable and can be used with a wide range of age groups, spanning from elementary school children to undergraduate students in the college or university setting (O'Dea 2007). According to O'Dea (2007, 57), "the self-esteem approach is a relevant and appropriate approach to take in both the prevention of body image and eating problems and the prevention of child obesity, because the two issues are inextricably entwined." In the original research study using a large sample of male and female adolescents between the ages of 11 and 14, results showed that *Everybody's Different* significantly improved the body image of participants compared to those in the control group (O'Dea and Abraham 2002). Adolescent girls and those at high risk for eating problems particularly showed improvements in "Body Dissatisfaction, Drive for Thinness, physical appearance ratings, reduced dieting and less unhealthy weight loss after the intervention" (O'Dea 2007, 58). Furthermore, many of the positive changes were still significant at the 12-month follow-up (O'Dea 2007).

13.3.3.1.2 Peer Support Groups

Another primary prevention component that can be used in school or community settings is the use of peer support groups (McVey et al. 2003; Piran 1998, 1999, 2001; Steese et al. 2006). These support groups center around empowering relationships that help girls counter peer pressure to diet and creatively solve problems, such as how to deal with media pressure to attain the thin ideal. Use of peer support groups has been found to decrease dieting behaviors and enhance body image and self-efficacy (McVey et al. 2003; Steese et al. 2006). Furthermore, peer support groups can empower girls to take leadership and advocacy roles in creating positive health communication messages and lobbying for changes to the environment to decrease disordered eating (McVey et al. 2003; Piran 2001; Scime et al. 2006).

13.3.3.1.3 Peer-Led Health Education

Likewise, peer-led educational sessions have been suggested as useful primary prevention program components (Paxton 1993; Stock et al. 2007). For example, older students were paired with younger students in an innovative program called *Healthy Buddies*, which was designed for students in grades K–7. The pilot study revealed that peer-led teaching can be effective for increasing health knowledge, attitudes, and behaviors in both older and younger children (Stock et al. 2007), which adds to the evidence that peer-led health education may be more effective than teacher-led interventions (Story et al. 2002).

13.3.3.1.3.1 Girls in Motion® Girls in Motion® (GIM 2010) is a program that incorporates a primary prevention program in which college-aged females mentor preadolescent girls between the ages of 9 and 11 (GIM 2010; Golman 2009). The goals of GIM focus on promoting positive body image and self-esteem, preventing obesity and eating disorders, and training young adult women to serve as positive role models and mentors for younger girls (GIM 2010). The GIM program is flexible and can function as an 8-week curriculum or a summer camp. It also can be implemented within nonprofit organizations and after-school programs to maximize resources and community involvement (Golman 2009). In an evaluation study of the GIM program, Golman (2009) found a significant decrease in drive for thinness and body dissatisfaction among the participants. In addition, African American girls had more significant reductions in their drive for thinness (from pre- to posttest) compared to Caucasian and Hispanic/Latina girls. Also, girls who were in fourth grade had significant reductions in their body dissatisfaction (from pre- to posttest) compared to fifth-grade girls. Appendices 13.D and 13.E are the GIM 2010 Day 4 Curriculum and the Worsheet 4 Magazine Cover Design.

13.3.3.2 Community-Based Prevention

13.3.3.2.1 Health Care Settings

Health care providers, including dieticians, play an important role in the prevention of weight-related problems, such as obesity, disordered eating, and eating disorders. These providers are in a unique position to educate children, adolescents, parents, and entire communities in a variety of settings. These interactions with children, adolescents, parents, and community members must occur in a safe and supportive environment in order to facilitate open communication. For example, a clinic visit provides an excellent opportunity to screen children and adolescents for disordered eating attitudes and behaviors, as well as discuss body image and weight concerns (Hautala et al. 2008; Rome et al. 2003). Furthermore, health care providers are in "the unique position to detect subtle clues to an eating disorder early on in its course," which can contribute to greater treatment outcomes (Rome et al. 2003, 100).

Some health care providers may be uncomfortable discussing body image and weight-related problems with children and adolescents because of concern that such conversations could spark sensitivity and possibly even deter youth from returning to the clinic for further care. However, given the health risks associated with obesity and eating disorders, particularly during the formative preteen and teen years, such conversations are imperative. The overarching message of all interactions should focus on promoting self-acceptance along with healthy eating and physical activity behaviors that can be sustained over time to promote overall wellness, as opposed to focusing on body weight and shape. It is very important to help youth understand that dieting and unhealthy weight-control behaviors increase the risk for weight gain and eating disorders (Neumark-Sztainer, Wall et al. 2006), both of which are harmful to one's health. It also is important for health care providers to ask youth about their friends' eating and dieting practices to better understand the "peer culture" and help adolescents effectively deal with peer behaviors such as dieting and unhealthy weight control (Eisenberg and Neumark-Sztainer 2010).

13.3.3.2.1.1 Recommendations for Health Care Providers Neumark-Sztainer (2009) described key recommendations for health care providers regarding the prevention of eating disorders and obesity. These recommendations are based upon the results of *Project EAT* and other research studies (Neumark-Sztainer et al. 2004; Neumark-Sztainer, Wall et al. 2006). Although they are research-based, these recommendations are not intended to represent a complete and comprehensive list, but rather should be used as a general framework for approaching prevention.

1. *Encourage positive eating behaviors and regular physical activity that can be maintained over time.* Health care providers should discuss healthy nutrition and physical activity with all of their patients, not just those who are underweight or overweight (Sokol et al. 2005). Also, it is important to encourage parents to consistently model healthy eating and physical activity behaviors to their children (Loth et al. 2009). Inform parents and adolescents that, over time, dieting often results in weight gain instead of weight loss because dieting rarely leads to sustained behavior change. Dieting adolescents are particularly at risk for weight gain as their eating behaviors swing between food deprivation and binge eating (Neumark-Sztainer, Wall et al. 2006; Haines et al. 2007).

2. *Promote a positive body image.* Body dissatisfaction has been identified as a major risk factor for eating disorders (Jacobi et al. 2004). Therefore, it is strongly recommended to avoid using body dissatisfaction as the motivator for weight loss. Instead, facilitate the development of a positive body image through the use of positive self-talk and teaching adolescents to value and care for their bodies through healthy eating and physical activity.

3. *Eat together as a family and make mealtime fun.* The results of *Project EAT* indicated that more frequent family meals and greater enjoyment at mealtime were associated with lower risks of extreme weight-control behaviors, especially in adolescent girls (Neumark-Sztainer et al. 2004; Loth et al. 2009). Overall, parental support (e.g., love, acceptance, encouragement, and quality time) appears to be protective against eating disorders (Loth et al. 2009).

4. *Instruct parents to minimize discussions about weight and instead talk about healthy eating and physical activity.* Potentially damaging discussions about weight include parents commenting about their own weight, encouraging adolescents to lose weight, talking about other people's weight, and teasing. Research findings suggest that talking about weight at home is associated with increased risk of eating disorders and of being overweight during adolescence (Agras et al. 2007; Haines et al. 2007; Loth et al. 2009; Rodgers et al. 2009). Although both maternal and paternal influences on girls' body weight and shape have been deemed significant, the father's influence may become more critical as girls mature (Agras et al. 2007).

5. *Health care providers should assume that overweight children and adolescents have experienced mistreatment and/or stigmatization related to being overweight, and discuss this with them and their parents.* Project EAT and other research studies have repeatedly demonstrated associations between weight teasing by family and peers and the resulting negative effects on overall health and well-being of youth (Hayden-Wade et al. 2005; Neumark-Sztainer et al. 2007). Children and adolescents must be educated that they do not deserve to be ridiculed or mistreated because of their weight, and health care providers are often in a unique position to talk about these issues.

In addition to one-on-one patient–provider interactions, health care providers can also play an important role in health communication and health education to broader groups. For example, dieticians and other health care providers can deliver positive media messages about healthy eating and body image, as well as plan and implement school- and community-based programs targeting healthy body image and eating disorder prevention (Neumark-Sztainer et al. 2000). Health care providers can also work to increase health literacy among young people and their families regarding issues linked with body image and eating disorders. In addition, providers can serve as critical linkage agents for young people and their families to access necessary health-related resources within the community, including those providing screening and treatment services for eating disorders.

13.3.3.2.1.2 Diabetes and Eating Disorders   Another challenge facing health care providers is that girls with type 1 diabetes are almost twice as likely to develop eating disorders when compared to girls without diabetes (ADA 2002; Jones et al. 2000). Prevalence rates of comorbid type 1 diabetes and clinical eating disorders have been estimated to range from 3.8% to 16% (Affenito et al. 1997 and Pollock et al. 1995, as cited in Howe et al. 2008). Furthermore, comorbid type 1 diabetes and anorexia nervosa is a deadly combination, with mortality at much higher rates than in either condition alone (Nielsen et al. 2002). The most common factors associated with eating disorders in girls with type 1 diabetes include body dissatisfaction, binge eating, dieting, and insulin manipulation to control weight (ADA 2002). Because significant weight gain can occur with insulin treatment, some teens with diabetes skip or manipulate insulin doses to purge calories and lose weight (Howe et al. 2008), a condition known as diabulima (Juvenile Diabetes Research Foundation International [JDRF] 2007). It is estimated that 10%–20% of mid-adolescent girls and 30%–40% of older adolescent girls and young adult women with diabetes skip or alter insulin doses to manage their weight (ADA 2002).

All health care providers should be aware of warning signs of eating disorders in their young female diabetes patients, including: extremely high hemoglobin A1C test results (indicating poor blood sugar management); recurring, severely low blood sugar; unexplained, fluctuating blood sugar levels; anxiety about or avoidance of weighing; frequent requests to switch meal-planning strategies; and excessive exercise (ADA 2002). Other risk factors include changes in eating habits (i.e., eating more, but still experiencing weight loss), unexplained weight loss, low energy levels, and frequent urination (JDRF 2007).

Screening and prevention programs for this high-risk group should begin in the preteen years (Colton et al. 2004) and include parents (Howe et al. 2008). Prevention programs should incorporate education about the importance of healthy, balanced nutrition and insulin use (JDRF 2007), as well as information about the risks involved with unhealthy weight-management behaviors (Howe et al. 2008). Additionally, Coordinated School Health personnel (e.g., school health educators, school nurses, and school psychologists/counselors) play important roles in the prevention and recognition of diabulimia (Hasken et al. 2010). More research is needed to assess whether brief interview methods or more formal screening tools are more effective in determining which children and adolescents with type 1 diabetes are at risk for body dissatisfaction and unhealthy weight-control practices. The benefits of prevention and early treatment programs for this group need to be evaluated as well (Howe et al. 2008).

13.3.3.2.2 Nonprofit Organizations

Nonprofit organizations that engage children, adolescents, and parents provide an important setting for community-based primary prevention of eating disorders and obesity. These organizations have considerable capacity to influence behavior through activities and programming that are not subjected to the pressures of competition and grading that are often found in the school setting (Elder et al. 2007). Nonprofit organizations can also provide children and adolescents with healthy messages about body image and weight that challenge societal norms that glamorize thinness, particularly in girls. This type of programming can involve members of the community serving as role models to promote positive body image and self-esteem, improved nutrition, and healthy physical activity. These positive role models may include educators, coaches, older students, athletes, business professionals, and health professionals. Selected nonprofit prevention programs are described next.

13.3.3.2.2.2 Prevention Programs for Girl Scouts The Girl Scouts of the United States of America (GSUSA) is another nonprofit organization that has incorporated primary prevention initiatives into the activities of the organization. The GSUSA has formally recognized that a strong community social environment, in combination with individual-level behavior change, is needed to address children's overall health and wellness (Schoenberg et al. 2004). As a result, this organization has implemented a variety of programs designed to encourage healthy eating, physical activity, body satisfaction, and self-efficacy among prepubescent and adolescent girls (Schoenberg et al. 2004).

Research supports the feasibility of implementing eating disorder and obesity prevention programs within nonprofit organizations, such as the GSUSA. In a group-randomized controlled trial, the effectiveness of the Scouting Nutrition and Activity Program (SNAP) was evaluated among Girl Scouts in fourth and fifth grades (Rosenkranz et al. 2010). SNAP was created to promote the adoption of healthy troop meeting environments and increase obesity prevention behaviors at home. The results showed that girls exposed to SNAP were more physically active and had greater opportunities for healthy eating during troop meetings compared to girls in the control group troops. Also, troop leaders demonstrated a high level of fidelity in the implementation of the SNAP curriculum and supporting policies, indicating that wide-scale implementation of this health promotion program was feasible. However, no measurable effect was observed in obesity prevention behaviors at home among the girls and parents, indicating that additional work is needed to understand how to transfer health promotion from troop meetings to the home environment (Rosenkranz et al. 2010).

In an earlier study, Girl Scout troops were involved in the evaluation of a community-based program entitled *Free to Be Me*, which was uniquely designed to prevent disordered eating by addressing media literacy, body image attitudes, and dieting behaviors among Girls Scout members (Neumark-Sztainer et al. 2000). The results demonstrated the feasibility of using the GSUSA framework for the delivery of primary prevention programming aimed at enhancing protective factors and preventing risk factors for disordered eating. In addition, a significant positive effect was reported on media-related and weight-related attitudes and behaviors among girls, their parents, and troop leaders. Not all positive effects were sustained, however, which supports the need for longer, more intensive community interventions in this area (Neumark-Sztainer et al. 2000). While clearly additional research is needed, all of these studies provide evidence of the significant role that community-based nonprofit organizations can play in the primary prevention of eating disorders and obesity.

13.3.3.2.3 Faith-Based Prevention

During the past two decades, churches and other faith-based organizations have been recognized as important avenues for health promotion programming (Campbell et al. 2007). For example, prevention programming incorporated into African American churches has demonstrated promise in reducing cardiovascular risk factors, including obesity, among African American adults who tend to be at high risk for these diseases (Campbell et al. 2007; DeHaven et al. 2004). Many churches view promoting the health and well-being of the congregation as an essential part of the church's mission and service, and therefore have hired parish nurses to support and lead these health promotion efforts. While the potential for churches to impact the health of their congregations is apparent, they have largely not been used to address the primary prevention of eating disorders in children and adolescents. This represents a missed opportunity for primary prevention in this area and is also a noticeable gap in the prevention literature regarding eating disorders.

13.3.4 An Integrated Approach for Eating Disorder and Obesity Prevention

In order to address the increasing prevalence and harmful effects of eating disorders and obesity among children and adolescents, researchers in both fields of eating disorder and obesity prevention have argued the importance of adopting an integrated prevention approach to address these issues (Haines and Neumark-Sztainer 2006; Neumark-Sztainer 2005, 2007; Neumark-Sztainer, Wall et al. 2006; O'Dea 2007; Shaw et al. 2007; Stock et al. 2007). There are clear reasons why an integrated prevention approach makes sense. For example, eating disorders and obesity share some common risk factors, such as internalization of the thin ideal, body dissatisfaction, disordered eating, dieting, unhealthy weight-control behaviors, and weight-related teasing (Haines and Neumark-Sztainer 2006; O'Dea 2007; Shaw et al. 2007). In addition, there is evidence that eating disorders and obesity can co-occur in the same individuals (e.g., bulimia nervosa and obesity; Haines and Neumark-Sztainer 2006; Neumark-Sztainer 2005, 2007; Neumark-Sztainer, Wall et al. 2006; O'Dea 2007; Shaw et al. 2007; Stock et al. 2007). Over time, one problem may intertwine with another problem, and minor problems might lead to more serious problems (e.g., dieting and unhealthy weight-control behaviors may serve as precursors to obesity and eating disorders; Neumark-Sztainer 2005, 2007; Neumark-Sztainer, Wall et al. 2006). There also are some practical reasons for using an integrated prevention approach, such as efficient use of resources by addressing two issues within a single program and decreasing the probability of inadvertently causing an eating disorder while trying to prevent obesity (Haines and Neumark-Sztainer 2006; Neumark-Sztainer 2005, 2007; O'Dea 2007). As such, it is important to address both eating disorders and obesity along a continuum of disordered eating.

An integrated approach targeting eating disorder and obesity prevention focuses on healthy behaviors and critical life skills that can benefit *all* youth, not just those struggling with weight-related concerns. These programs can occur in a wide variety of settings, such as schools, community-based after-school programs, summer camps, community youth organizations, places of worship, and health care clinics. In these programs, health promotion professionals can promote healthy knowledge, attitudes, and behaviors in areas like self-esteem, body image, media literacy, balanced nutrition and physical activity, and stress management and coping. Examples of integrated prevention programs that incorporate lessons addressing some combination of two or more of these critical topics include *Everybody's Different* (O'Dea 2007), *Free to Be Me* (Neumark-Sztainer et al. 2000), *Girls in Motion*® (Golman 2009), *Healthy Body Image* (Kater 2005), *Healthy Buddies* (Stock et al. 2007), and *Shapesville* (Mills and Osborn 2003), all of which are addressed elsewhere in this chapter.

To increase the effectiveness of prevention programs, it is imperative to enlist supportive persons who have the potential to influence youth. First, it is essential to involve the family in prevention efforts as they "play a key role in the development of their children's eating behaviors, physical activity patterns, and attitudes toward their own bodies and those of others" (Neumark-Sztainer 2007, 13). Furthermore, the ecological perspective can be employed in terms of developing physical and social environments that are conducive to promoting healthy eating and physical activity, as well as fostering acceptance of diverse body shapes and sizes. Additionally, important policies to prevent eating disorders and obesity can be implemented within schools, communities, and the media (Neumark-Sztainer 2009; O'Dea 2005; Shaw et al. 2007).

13.4 SUMMARY AND CONCLUSIONS

Negative body image and eating disorders are serious health issues that exert a heavy blow to individuals, families, and the broader society. Therefore, culturally relevant primary prevention programs that target children and adolescents must become a public health priority. Although interventions aimed at youth can produce positive outcomes in knowledge, body esteem, self-acceptance, and eating behaviors, it is largely unknown whether these effects can be sustained in the long term. Positive long-term effects of prevention programs will likely require booster sessions with children and adolescents, behavioral change among adults and peers of influence, and fundamental changes in contextual factors that impact young people's lives (Levine and Smolak 2001). As Kater et al. (2002, 204) aptly observed, " … even the best of prevention efforts will fail unless adults are simultaneously educated, impassioned, and empowered to join students in resisting and challenging a cultural environment that creates body image problems, unhealthy weight concerns, and disordered eating."

As such, the ecological framework can be effective for planning and implementing eating disorder prevention programs because the model accounts for multiple influences on behavior. For example, prevention efforts have proven successful when environmental and policy reinforcements are in place that provide support for and promote opportunities for behavior modification (Booth et al. 2001; Cook-Cottone 2006; Elder et al. 2007; Evans et al. 2008; Haines and Neumark-Sztainer 2006; Keca and Cook-Cottone 2005; Loth et al. 2009; Neumark-Sztainer 2007; O'Dea 2005; Smith et al. 2004). Children and adolescents are our most valuable natural resource (WHO 2003). Therefore, it is imperative that individuals, families, schools, communities, and society as a whole proactively work in tandem to enhance child and adolescent health and prevent body image and eating disturbances.

APPENDIX 13.A

Lesson 9

Media Awareness

Facilitator's Note

Middle school students can be quite vulnerable to the influences of peers and the media, making them susceptible to over-focusing on their outside appearance. For this reason, we have opted to include a second lesson on the topic of "Fairly Comparing," with this one dedicated to media influences regarding our appearance, our bodies, and ourselves in general.

In this lesson we want to increase students' awareness of how magazines, movies, and TV shows can give messages that often are not in our best interest. Learning how to examine advertisements for their subtle and direct messages, and how to read and view media with a critical eye, will help students reflect, evaluate, and make healthy choices for themselves.

We want students to understand that advertising permeates almost all media sources and that it is in the economic interest of advertisers to create insecurity and a sense of inadequacy, thereby generating a perceived need for the product they wish to sell. When any of us falls prey to the direct or subtle messages suggesting that we "should" look certain ways in order to be acceptable to our peers, our self-esteem becomes at risk, self-doubt increases, and we lose confidence in ourselves. It is important for young people to understand that in the interest of boosting sales, advertisers purposefully increase viewers' dissatisfaction with themselves. They falsely promise that we will feel better if we purchase their product—be it shampoo, jeans, perfume, cigarettes, or diet foods.

We believe that it is also essential for students to begin to consider the cultural messages about gender that are conveyed by the media. For example, attention to the models' body position gives information about character traits such as powerful, dominant, passive, vulnerable, submissive, or subservient. There is a growing trend amongst advertisers to sexualize young girls, both in the design of clothing and the words used for slogans on clothes. For additional interpretations of these messages and multimedia presentations for use with students, we suggest viewing the following sites.

JeanKilbourne.com

campaignforrealbeauty.com

youtube.com

video.google.com

loveyourbody.nowfoundation.org/presentations/ SexStereotypesBeauty/flash.html

achancetoheal.org

As students go through magazines, they are likely to see messages about diets and losing weight. Research shows that the majority of people who diet gain their weight back within two years and that dieting is the number one predecessor to developing an eating disorder. The diet industry spends billions of dollars trying to convince children and adults to diet despite overwhelming evidence that they don't work. Kathy Kater, in her book *Real Kids Come in All Sizes,* offers an excellent child-oriented explanation of why diets don't work (New York: Broadway Books, 2004, Chapter 6, pages 137–151).

What Is Media Literacy?

By Sherri Hope Culver, Director of the Media Education Lab at Temple University, and Advisory Board Member, A Chance to Heal Foundation

Media Literacy is the act of asking questions about the media we are exposed to and consume. It is most often defined as a series of competencies, including the ability to *access, analyze, evaluate,* and *communicate* information in a variety of forms. Media Literacy isn't about TV bashing or demanding that you tune out or turn off your source of media. It's about developing the skills of critical inquiry needed in a world loaded with media messages.

Key Questions of Media Literacy

- Who is the author and what is the purpose of the message?
- What techniques are used to attract your attention?
- What lifestyles, values, and points of view are represented?
- How might people interpret the message differently?
- What is omitted from the message?

Resources

National Association for Media Literacy Education: amlainfo.org/

Media Education Lab—Temple University: mediaeducationlab.com/

My Pop Studio: mypopstudio.com/

Company Logo Quiz: money.aol.com/special/company-logos-brand-awareness

Retail Alphabet Game: www.joeykatzen.com/alpha/

Kids Corner (See Sherri's Podcasts—suitable for young children): www.kidscorner.
   org/html/audio.php

Center on Media and Child Health: www.cmch.tv/

National Institute on Media and the Family: www.mediafamily.org/

Fat Talk Video: http://www.youtube.com/watch?v=RKPaxD61lwo (This is the most
stable link at time of publication.)

Helping Women Achieve Healthy Mind, Body and Spirit: www.bodyimageprogram.org/

Troubleshooting

In the activity for this lesson, we provide enough magazines for students to look at in small groups of three or four. An alternative would be for the group leader to go through magazines and select images to illustrate main points for discussion. (These could be cut out and glued to construction paper.) If you have an excitable group, you may wish to try this alternative, as students can get immersed in the magazines, which can diminish the purpose of the lesson.

These magazines can be stimulating for students and they can easily get off topic. We recommend setting up a clear structure for this lesson: It is important to lay the groundwork for each lesson. Be sure each group has a list of questions to answer and set clear time limits. Although we include typical teen magazines for this activity, we *choose these magazines carefully and screen for appropriateness of content for students at this age* (i.e., we do not purchase *Teen Cosmo, Jane,* or *Sports Illustrated* swimsuit issue). We suggest looking for teen sport magazines and health magazines as well. Some may find it useful to share specific adult–oriented magazine ads to illustrate particular images, such as ultra-muscular male models and ultra-thin female models.

It is important to help students consider how easily "Photo-shopping" (using Photoshop or other image-adjusting software) allows an image to be manipulated or changed, creating a finished image that is not real. Dove.com has an excellent video that shows the process of making up a model whose image eventually appears on a billboard.

In the recommended Warm Up for this lesson, we introduce some simple yoga poses. Students will need space to stand, sit, and lie on the floor for some of the poses. You may want to provide mats for this activity.

Sources

Lesson 9 Vocabulary: Adapted from Gary VandenBos, ed., *APA Dictionary of Psychology* (Washington, DC: APA, 2007).

A Chance to Heal ACTH newsletter article from Sheri Hope Culver (Spring, 2008)

Lesson 9: Media Awareness

Goals

Students will:

- recognize messages presented by the media (including the advertising and fashion industries) that generate feelings of insecurity and increase self-criticism

- become more aware that advertisers are concerned with making money, not the well-being of others

- consider how to make healthy choices in the face of these influences

Objectives

Students will be able to:

- identify messages that can be generated by media images

- identify qualities that the media presents as attractive

- identify the "should" messages that might be taken from the media's use of images and language

- identify cultural stereotypes about gender

Materials and Preparation

Prepare:

Arrange for space and mats to teach yoga, if possible; if not available, students may use the floor.

Use these Internet sites to directly show the videos that are recommended for activities in this lesson. If you will not have access to the Internet, you may want to download the videos and save them on a DVD that can be used on a DVD player.

www.campaignforrealbeauty.com click on features, then click on videos

www.youtube.com type in Dove Evolution or Dove Onslaught

video.google.com type in Dove Evolution or Dove Onslaught

We recommend that you download the video "Onslaught" to show how children are bombarded with images from the media and "Evolution" to show how the media manipulates our perception of beauty.

> http://www.BodyImageProgram.org Reflections Program website "Stopping Fat Talk"

Materials Needed:

- teen fashion, teen sport, and/or teen health magazines; catalogs from popular stores for teens, also L.L. Bean, Wal-Mart, Sears—enough to allow students to look at magazines in small groups

Copy one for each student:

- **Lesson 9 Vocabulary**
- **Media Awareness: Media Friends and Media Foes**

Review:

- **Lesson 9 Vocabulary** terms and definitions

Warm Up

10 minutes

We recommend Simple Yoga Stretches as a Warm Up for this lesson.

See Warm-Up Activities section for complete directions.

Brief Presentation

10 minutes

Say to students:

> Today we are going to explore how the media influences us to compare ourselves unfairly by using standards that are extreme and unattainable by the majority of people. In the interest of boosting sales, advertisers purposefully try to make us feel dissatisfied and unacceptable. They falsely promise that we will feel better if we purchase their product—be it shampoo, jeans, shoes or foods. The media also conveys messages about gender via body positions that suggest character traits such as powerful, vulnerable, or courageous, to name a few.

Today we are going to become media literate and learn how to ask questions that help us evaluate and analyze the messages we are being given. Let's start by looking at a video created by the Dove company.

www.campaignforrealbeauty.com/

www.youtube.com (type in Dove Evolution or Dove Onslaught)

video.google.com (type in Dove Evolution or Dove Onslaught)

View the video.

Say to students:

- What did you see?

- What is surprising to you?

When we look at a person in a magazine, television or billboard advertisement, we generally don't stop to think about how long it took for the person to get made up and we don't consider that the computer manipulated her or his features. It is important to think about the purpose of messages and the techniques used to attract our attention.

We've talked about our negative self-talk, and how we can at times slip into "feeding our monster." One of the ways many of us feel unhappy with ourselves is when we criticize ourselves for how we look. Research tells us that:

- Advertising in teen magazines and on television typically glamorizes skinny models who do not resemble the average real woman.

- The average person in the United States sees approximately three thousand ads in magazines, on billboards, and on television every day.

- Media directed at teenage girls emphasizes the ideal of thinness as a standard for beauty and increasingly emphasizes a standard of extreme fitness for males.

- Stop and think about the fact that the average height and weight for an adult female model is 5'10" and 110 lbs, while the height and weight for the average woman is 5'4" and 145 lbs. Most fashion models are thinner than 98 percent of American women. If girls and women think that they should be able to look like a model, they could risk their emotional and physical health.

- The diet industry spends billions of dollars trying to convince children and adults to diet despite overwhelming evidence that diets don't work—that in fact the majority of people who diet to lose weight (rather than change their behaviors and learn to have a balance approach to eating) gain their weight back within a few years.

Activity

5 minutes

Inoculation Exercise

Say to students:

Before we take a look at these magazines and catalog ads, let's think a minute about times when we feel happy and like being who we are (being ourselves). Please write a few examples of these times.

Pause to let students write.

Then say:

We encourage you to remember these pleasant and meaningful times at any point when you might start to feel critical of yourself.

Ask students:

- Do you think it's possible to believe that you are okay as you are—that you don't need or want to change your looks, your body, or any other aspect of yourself—no improvements necessary?

- When does it make sense to try to improve ourselves? *(striving to improve our long shot in basketball or to play a piece of music without error or to speak up more directly when you are upset with someone)*

- When does the message make us feel that, in order to be acceptable, attractive, or "ok," we need to change something about who we are? How might this impact our sense of confidence?

Activity

20 minutes

Media Friends and Media Foes

Allow about ten minutes to search magazines and ten minutes to discuss students' findings. You may prefer to do this activity in small groupings of students or as a class, exploring the questions together. Alternatively, you might want to use pictures you have found in magazines, mount them on construction paper, and pass them out to small groups of two to four students, who will critique them.

If this program is being adapted for a mixed gender group, consider first asking the group to identify messages that might be more oriented toward targeting girls and then ask them to identify messages that might be oriented toward targeting boys. This can be followed up with asking "how are the media foes for girls and boys different? How are they similar" (encourage them to be specific). Do the differences have to do with appearance, weight, or fitness? Are there some messages that would "feed the monster" regardless of one's gender? Be sure to help students to recognize that boys also experience social pressures and "should" messages about being masculine and attractive.

Say to students:

> Most media sources depend on advertising dollars to pay their bills and stay in business. It is important to understand how to decode the messages we receive from advertisements because many of the messages used in ads are intentionally designed to make us feel bad about ourselves. Advertisers have discovered that they sell more products if they get us to feel that we aren't good enough and that we could feel better about ourselves if we spend our money to buy their products.

> In a moment we are going to look at magazine ads in order to see which messages are "media friends" and which ones are "media foes." We could think about media foes as those messages that are likely to feed our monsters.

> Use the student handout (or take a piece of paper) and write down the magazine and page number, and the ideas that come to mind for the questions to follow (if there are enough magazines, you might allow students to tear out the advertisements and separate them in to stacks for the two categories—"media friends" and "media foes").

> • Pay close attention and ask yourself: what message might they be suggesting?

- Notice if there are any differences in the messages being sent to girls and boys about how they "should" and "shouldn't" be?

- Note whether you think that the message or the images used have anything to do with the product that is being sold.

- Ask yourself if you agree with the message, for example, will having peppermint breath ensure that we are popular with the opposite sex?

- Notice the words used in the ad and (think about how they make you feel).

Additional Activity if Time Permits

10 minutes

Don't Let Friend's Fat-Talk

Stopping Fat Talk

Note to facilitator: The video Stopping Fat Talk, created by Dr. Carol Becker in conjunction with Tri Delta National Sorority, is an excellent tool for helping students understand the damaging impact of the "thin ideal." Examples of fat talk include: "I'm so fat," "I need to lose weight," "I don't look so fat," "Do I look fat in this?" "She's too fat to be wearing that," and "You look great, have you lost weight?" Fat talk statements might seem positive but they undermine self-esteem by reinforcing the drive to be "thin" and "perfect."

When using this exercise you might add to the video by brainstorming with the group about those words that are commonly used to make fun of others. Some words to include in this discussion are: stupid, ugly, dumb, giant, shrimp, etc. Ask students if they think that there are different ways that girls and boys are put down or made to feel bad about themselves.

Materials Needed:

Review the powerful video

https://secure.pursuantgroup.net/pursuant4/deltadeltadelta/fall08/dddselect/flashstory.asp developed by Dr. Carolyn Becker, an associate professor of psychology at Trinity University, in conjunction with Tri Delta National Sorority.

Activity

10 minutes

Say to Students:

> We have been discussing the impact that the media has on the words we use to describe ourselves and others. Let's look at a video that was designed to get us to think about the impact of our language when it comes to calling ourselves fat.

Following the video, ask students to respond to the following questions:

- What did you notice in this video?
- Why do you think that the creators of the video chose to only use words?
- What do you think about their message that: "Friends Don't Let Friends Fat Talk?"
- What kinds of things can we do to resist saying "fat talk?"

Tell students about Fat Talk Free Week, a national, 5-day public awareness effort initiated by Reflections, a body image education and eating disorders prevention program, developed by a college professor, Carol Becker, PhD, in conjunction with the Tri Delta National Sorority. Consider having students organize a fat talk free event at your school. For more information on ideas for activities go to http://www.BodyImageProgram.org.

Wrap Up

5 minutes

Say to students:

> We have discovered that the advertising industry has its own agenda, and this agenda, which is to make as much money as it can, may or may not be in our best interest. Despite thinking that we are not influenced by the media, all of us (including parents and teachers) are. According to media expert Jean Kilbourne, we are exposed to three thousand ads on an average day (television, magazines, Internet, billboards, etc.). That's a lot of ads.
>
> Often, the messages that advertisers send our way strengthen misconceptions and irrational beliefs.

These irrational beliefs include:

- Everybody should like us and that we would be liked more if we dress a certain way or have the "right" product.

- If we don't have/do these things, we will be unhappy, unattractive, and without friends.

- We have to be good at everything in order to be accepted.

- We have to look just right at all times. You can never relax and just be yourself.

- There's only one right way to look and act in order to appear attractive.

Ask students if they have anything to add to this list.

Then ask students:

- What ways do you think advertisers say we need to be or should be?

- Why don't they show us more realistic images?

- Why don't they show different kinds of body shapes and sizes ("body diversity")?

Say to students:

If we believe these irrational messages, we will feed our monster and feel bad about ourselves. Advertisers of certain products will be glad, because we will keep spending money in a never-ending quest to feel and look better.

Thoughts/Self-Discoveries for the Week

2 minutes

Say to students:

Be on the lookout this week for examples of helpful media friends and unhelpful media foes. Bring some examples to class next week. You may discover that some advertisers are beginning to use more realistic images (e. g., Dove Campaign for Real Beauty) while others are not.

Lesson 9 Vocabulary

Body Image: The mental picture you form of how you look and how you imagine others perceive your body and appearance.

Body Image Ideals: Your personal standards of the best appearance for various body features; idealized features as opposed to actual features or appearance.

Body Esteem: The degree of positiveness with which you regard and accept the parts of your body and your physical appearance in general.

Body Ideal: The body type considered most attractive or most appropriate to one's age and sex by a particular individual, culture, or generation.

Media Friends and Media Foes

Directions: Look at magazine advertisements. Select an ad and answer the following question to determine if the ad is a "media friend" or a "media foe." Write down the Magazine Name and Page Number for each ad you select.

Magazine Name _____ Page _____

- Is this ad a "media friend" or "media foe?"

  _____

- What message might this ad suggest?

  _____

  _____

- Do you notice any difference in the messages being sent to girls and boys about how they "should" and "shouldn't" be?

  _____

  _____

- Do you think that the message or the images used have anything to do with the product that is being sold?

  _____

  _____

- Do you agree with the message, for example, will having peppermint breath ensure that we are popular with the opposite sex?

  _____

  _____

- Notice the words that are used and think about the words that the ad gets you to think.

  _____

  _____

APPENDIX 13.B   HEALTHY BODY IMAGE TABLE OF CONTENTS

APPENDIX 13.C   HEALTHY BODY IMAGE MODEL

UNIT INTRODUCTION: The way we look will change as we grow up.

LESSON 6: Hardly anyone looks as perfect as the models in advertisements. I will be careful not to compare myself or others to them.

LESSON 1: People become unhappy trying to control something that is not in their power to control. As for looks, it's best to make the most of who we were born to be.

LESSON 7: Weight-loss diets are not a good idea. We can hold back hunger for a while but will eat more to make up for it later.

LESSON 2: The way we look is only one part of us. We need to pay attention to *all* of who we are.

LESSON 8: Satisfy hunger completely with enough wholesome food at regular meals and snacks.

LESSON 3: There are many different normal ways for looks to change in puberty. Sooner or later, most girls and boys will gain weight and fill out.

LESSON 9: It's important not to sit too much in our free time. Being active is one of the best things we can do for our health and self-confidence.

LESSON 4: Most of the way we look is determined before we are even born: taller, shorter, fatter, thin– all are normal, all built in!

LESSON 10: Choose role models you admire for things deep inside and who make you feel good about who you are.

LESSON 5: Each person's body works to grow and maintain a weight that is natural for him or her.

ALL LESSONS: Support each other in having a healthy body image, in eating well, and in being active.

APPENDIX 13.D   GIRLS IN MOTION DAY 4 CURRICULUM

MEDIA MESSAGES & POPULAR BODY IMAGE

Objectives:

Students will ..
- Begin to analyze and evaluate media messages
- Discuss media messages and the influence of the media on behaviors and values
- Acknowledge their own power in accepting or rejecting media messages

Supplies:

1) Worksheet 3: Media Messages Discussion Questions
2) Worksheet 4: Modern Images of Beauty/Magazine cover
3) Teen magazines
4) Pencils
5) Water bottles

Outline:

1. `Warm-up Game
2. Stretching
3. We will walk/run for 30 minutes today with 5 minutes walking–5 minutes running inter-vals. Make sure that the girls that are choosing to run are pacing themselves in a comfort-able jog so they can continue for 5 minutes. Mentors should follow up discussion from last week. In addition, begin discussion about advertisements, media images and popular culture. Discuss some of the points in "Tips to becoming a Critical Viewer of the Media," such as touch-ups, etc. When finished with the walk/run come back and sit down and men-tor will assist student in looking at magazines and filling out "Worksheet 3—Discussion Questions and Worksheet 4—Modern Images of Beauty
4. Wrap-up

WORKSHEET 3—MEDIA MESSAGES

Discussion Questions:

1. How do you think the average person feels after looking through this magazine?

2. What message do these ads send (other than "buy my product")?

3. Does this magazine celebrate/honor the differences in people? How or how not?

4. Think of a person you admire. Below, list the characteristics about this person that makes him/her a "beautiful person."

5. List your best characteristics.

6. How do you think the average person feels after looking through this magazine?

7. What message do these ads send (other than "buy my product")?

8. Does this magazine celebrate/honor the differences in people? How or how not?

9. Think of a person you admire. Below, list the characteristics about this person that makes him/her a "beautiful person."

10. List your best characteristics.

Source: From Girls in Motion Day 4 Curriculum worksheets provided by
© Copyright Girls in Motion, Inc. 2006. With permission.

WORKSHEET 4   MODERN IMAGE OF BEAUTY—MAGAZINE COVER

OK, on the next page, please design a magazine cover you would like to see targeting girls your age. Draw a picture and then add the side advertisements or articles included in the magazine.

Source: From Girls in Motion Day 4 Curriculum worksheets provided by
© Copyright Girls in Motion, Inc. 2006. With permission.

APPENDIX 13.E   WORKSHEET 4 MAGAZINE COVER DESIGN

July 2010
Volume 1 Issue 1

Girls in Motion

#1
Best Seller!

REFERENCES

Agras, W. S., S. Bryson, L. D. Hammer, and H. C. Kraemer. 2007. Childhood risk factors for thin body preoccupation and social pressure to be thin. *J Am Acad Child Adolesc Psychiatry* 46: 171–178.

American Diabetes Association. 2002. Diabetes and eating disorders. *Diabetes Spectr* 15: 106.

American Psychiatric Association. 2000. *Diagnostic and statistical manual of mental disorder—Fourth Edition
Text Revision (DSM-IV-TR)*. Washington, DC: Author.

Bandura, A. 1986. *Social foundations of thought and actionm*. Englewood Cliffs, NJ: Prentice all.

Banister, E., and D. L. Begoray. 2004. Beyond talking groups: Strategies for improving adolescent health education. *Health Care Women Int* 25: 481–488.

Battle, E. K., and K. D. Brownell. 1996. Confronting a rising tide of eating disorders and obesity: Treatment vs.
prevention and policy. *Addictive Behav* 21: 755–765.

Becker, A. E., R. A. Burwell, S. E. Gilman, D. B. Herzog, and P. Hamburg. 2002. Eating behaviours and attitudes following prolonged exposure to television among ethnic Fijian adolescent girls. *Br J Psychiatry* 180: 509–514.

Black, M. M., and D. Young-Hyman. 2007. Introduction to the special issue: Pediatric overweight. *J Pediatr
Psychol* 32: 1–5.

Booth, S. L., J. F. Sallis, C. Ritenbaugh, J. O. Hill, L. L. Birch, L. D. Frank, K. Glanz et al. 2001. Environmental
and societal factors affect food choice and physical activity: Rationale, influences, and leverage points.
Nutr Rev 59: S21–S36.

Campbell, M. K., M. A. Hudson, K. Resnicow, N. Blakeney, A. Paxton, and M. Baskin. 2007. Church-based
health promotion interventions: Evidence and lessons learned. *Annu Rev Public Health* 28: 213–234.

Catalano, R. F., M. L. Berglund, J. A. M. Ryan, H. S. Lonczak, and J. D. Hawkins. 2002. Positive youth development in the United States: Research findings on evaluations of positive youth development programs.
ANNALS Amer Acad Pol Soc Sci 591: 98–124.

Center for Media Literacy. 2007a. Health/prevention. http://www.medialit.org/focus/prev_home.html (accessed
May 28, 2010).

Center for Media Literacy. 2007b. Media literacy: A definition … and more. http://www.medialit.org/reading_
room/rr2def.php (accessed June 17, 2010).

Centers for Disease Control and Prevention. 2010. Healthy youth! Coordinated school health program. http://
www.cdc.gov/HealthyYouth/CSHP/ (accessed December, 8, 2010).

Colton, P., M. Olmsted, D. Daneman, A. Rydall, and G. Rodin. 2004. Disturbed eating behavior and eating
disorders in preteen and early teenage girls with type 1 diabetes: A case-controlled study. *Diabetes Care*
27: 1654–1659.

Compas, B. E. 1993. Promoting positive mental health during adolescence. In *Promoting the health of adolescents*, ed. S. G. Millstein, A. C. Petersen, and E. O. Nightingale, 159–179. New York: Oxford.

Cook-Cottone, C. 2006. The attuned representation model for the primary prevention of eating disorders: An
overview for school psychologists. *Psychol Sch* 43: 223–230.

Cordero, E. D., and T. Israel. 2009. Parents as protective factors in eating problems of college women. *Eat
Disord* 17: 146–161.

Croll J., D. Neumark-Sztainer, M. Story, and M. Ireland. 2002. Prevalence and risk and protective factors
related to disordered eating behaviors among adolescents: Relationship to gender and ethnicity. *J Adolesc
Health* 2: 166–75.

Daníelsdóttir, S., D. Burgard, and W. Oliver-Pyatt. 2010. AED guidelines for childhood obesity prevention
programs. American Academy of Eating Disorders. http://www.aedweb.org/Content/NavigationMenu/
ResourcesFor/ResourcesforthePress/Guidelines.htm (accessed June 14, 2010).

DeHaven, M. J., I. B. Hunter, L. Wilder, J. W. Walton, and J. Berry. 2004. Health programs in faith-based organizations: Are they effective? *Am J Public Health* 94: 1030–1036.

Dohnt, H. K., and M. Tiggemann. 2005. Body image concerns in young girls: The role of peer and media prior
to adolescence. *J Youth Adolesc* 35: 135–145.

Dohnt, H. K., and M. Tiggemann. 2008. Promoting positive body image in young girls: An evaluation of
"Shapesville." *Eur Eat Disord Rev* 16: 222–233.

Duncan, M. J., Y. Al-Nakeeb, A. M. Nevill, and M. V. Jones. 2006. Body dissatisfaction, body fat and physical
activity in British children. *Int J Pediatr Obes* 1: 89–95.

Eisenberg, M. E., and D. Neumark-Sztainer. 2010. Friends' dieting and disordered eating behaviors among
adolescents: Five years later: Findings from Project EAT. *J Adolesc Health* 47: 67–73.

Elder, J. P., L. Lytle, J. F. Sallis, D. R. Young, A. Steckler, D. Simons-Morton, E. Stone, J. B. et al. 2007. A
description of the socio-ecological framework used in the trial of activity for adolescent girls (TAAG).
Health Educ Res 22: 155–165.

Ethnic/racial differences in weight-related concerns and behaviors among adolescent girls and boys: Findings from project EAT. *J Psychosom Res* 53: 963–974.

Evans, R. E., J. Roy, B. F. Geiger, K. A. Werner, and D. Burnett. 2008. Ecological strategies to promote healthy body image among children. *J Sch Health* 78: 359–367.

Feinberg-Walker, H., S. Barrett, and J. Shure. 2009. *Inside/outside self-discovery for teens: Strategies to promote resilience, relationships, and positive body image*. Santa Cruz, CA: ToucanEd.

Field, A. E., L. Cheung, A. M. Wolf, D. B. Herzog, S. L. Gortmaker, and G. A. Colditz. 1999. Exposure to the mass media and weight concerns among girls. *Pediatr* 103: E36.

Franko, D. L., and J. B. E. George. 2008. A pilot intervention to reduce eating disorder risk in Latina women. *Eur Eat Disord Rev* 16: 436–441.

Franko, D. L., and R. H. Striegel-Moore. 2002. The role of body dissatisfaction as a risk factor for depression: Are the differences black and white? *J Psychosom Res* 53: 975–983.

Fraser. M. W. 1996. Aggressive behavior in childhood and early adolescence: An ecological developmental perspective on youth violence. *Soc Work* 41: 347–361.

Gehrman, C. A., M. F. Hovell, J. F. Sallis, and K. Keating. 2006. The effects of a physical activity and nutrition intervention on body dissatisfaction, drive for thinness, and weight concerns in pre-adolescents. *Body Image* 3: 345–351.

Gentles, K. A., and K. Harrison. 2006. Television and perceived peer expectations of body size among African American adolescent girls. *Howard J Communications* 17: 39–55.

Ghaderi, A., M. Martensson, and H. Schwan. 2005. "Everybody's different": A primary prevention program among fifth grade school children. *Eat Disord* 13: 245–259.

Giles, D. 2006. Constructing identities in cyberspace: The case of eating disorders. *Br J Soc Psychol* 45: 463–477.

Girls in Motion. 2010. *About the program*. http://www.girlsinmotion.org/7.html (accessed July 5, 2010).

Golman, M. 2009. A study to evaluate the effectiveness of the Girls in Motion program in improving body satisfaction in preadolescent girls. PhD diss., Texas Woman's Univ.

Haines, J., and D. Neumark-Sztainer. 2006. Prevention of obesity and eating disorders: A consideration of shared risk factors. *Health Educ Res* 21: 770–782.

Haines, J., D. Neumark-Sztainer, M. Wall, and M. Story. 2007. Personal, behavioral, and environmental risk and protective factors for adolescent overweight. *Obes* 15: 2748–2760.

Hasken, J., L. Kresl, T. Nydegger, and M. Temme. 2010. Diabulimia and the role of school health personnel. *J Sch Health* 80: 465–469.

Hautala, L. A., J. Junnila, H. Helenius, A-M Väänänen, P-R Liuksila, H. Räihä, M. Välimäki, and S. Saarijärvi. 2008. Towards understanding gender differences in disordered eating among adolescents. *J Clin Nurs* 17: 1803–1813.

Hayden-Wade, H. A., R. I. Stein, A. Ghaderi, B. E. Saeleens, M. F. Zabinski, and D. E. Wilfley. 2005. Prevalence, characteristics, and correlates of teasing experiences among overweight children vs. non-overweight peers. *Obes Res* 13: 1381–1392.

Holt, K. E., and L. A. Ricciardelli. 2008. Weight concerns among elementary school children: A review of prevention programs. *Body Image* 5: 233–243.

Howe, C. J., A. J. Jawad, S. D. Kelly, and T. H. Lipman. 2008. Weight-related concerns and behaviors in children and adolescents with type 1 diabetes. *J Am Psychiatr Nurses Assoc* 13: 376–385.

Jacobi, C., C. Hayward, M. Zwaan, H. C. Kraemer, and W. S. Agras. (2004). Coming to terms with risk factors for eating disorders: Application of risk terminology and suggestions for a genera taxonomy. *Psychol Bull* 130: 19–65.

2000 Joint Committee on Health Education and Promotion Terminology. 2002. Report of the 2000 Joint Committee on health education and promotion terminology. *J Sch Health* 72: 3–7.

Jones, J. M., M. L. Lawson, D. Daneman, M. P. Olmsted, and G. Rodin. 2000. Eating disorders in adolescent females with and without type 1 diabetes: Cross sectional study. *Br Med J* 32: 1563–1566.

Juvenile Diabetes Research Foundation International. 2007. "*Diabulimia.*" http://www.jdrf.org/index.cfm?fuseaction=home.viewPage&page_id=FDF69313-1279-CFD5-A79B429F10056B6F (accessed July 5, 2010).

Kahn, A., J. Max, and P. Paluzzi. 2010. Engaging youth on their turf: Creative approaches to connecting youth through community. Healthy Teen Network. http://healthyteennetwork.org/vertical/Sites/%7BB4D0CC76-CF78-4784-BA7C-5D0436F6040C%7D/uploads/%7B3EE4600A-02E4-47B5-AC27-0A1B2CB543D3%7D.PDF (accessed June 21, 2010).

Kaiser Family Foundation. 2003. Key facts — media literacy. http://www.kff.org/entmedia/upload/Key-Facts-Media-Literacy.pdf (accessed May 28, 2010).

Kater, K. 1998. *Healthy body image: Teaching kids to eat and love their bodies too!* Seattle WA: Eating Disorders Awareness and Prevention, Inc.

Kater, K. 2005. *Healthy body image: Teaching kids to eat and love their bodies too!* (2nd ed.). Seattle, WA: National Eating Disorders Association.

Kater, K. J., J. Rohwer, and M. P. Levine. 2000. An elementary school project for developing healthy body image and reducing risk factors for unhealthy and disordered eating. *Eat Disord* 8: 3–16.

Kater, K., J. Rohwer, and K. Londre. 2002. Evaluation of an upper elementary school program to prevent body image, eating and weight concerns. *J Sch Health* 72: 199–205.

Keca, J., and C. Cook-Cottone. 2005. Middle-school and high-school programs help beat eating disorders. *Educ Dig* 71: 33–39.

Kelly, A. M., M. Wall, M. E. Eisenberg, M. Story, and D. Neumark-Sztainer. 2005. Adolescent girls with high body satisfaction: Who are they and what can they teach us? *J Adolesc Health* 37: 391–396.

Killen, J. D., C. B. Taylor, L. D. Hammer, I. Litt, D. M. Wilson, T. Rich, and C. Hayward. 1993. An attempt to modify unhealthful eating attitudes and weight regulation practices of young adolescent girls. *Int J Eat Disord* 13: 369–384.

Klump, K. L., C. M. Bulik, W. H. Kaye, J. Treasure, and E. Tyson. 2009. Academy for Eating Disorders position paper: Eating disorders are serious mental illnesses. *Int J Eat Dis* 42: 97–103.

Kubic, M. Y., L. A. Lytle, P. J. Hannan, C. L. Perry, and M. Story. 2003. The association of the school food environment with dietary behaviors of young adolescents. *Am J Public Health* 93: 1168–1173.

Levin Institute, State University of New York. 2009. Globalization and eating disorders. http://www.globalization101. org/news1/eating_disorders (accessed June 13, 2010).

Levine, M., and M. Maine. 2005. Eating disorders can be prevented. http://www.nationaleatingdisorders.org/nedaDir/files/documents/handouts/EDsPrev.pdf (accessed November 22, 2010).

Levine, M. P. and L. Smolak. 2001. Primary prevention of body image disturbances and disordered eating in childhood and early adolescence. In *Body image, eating disorders, and obesity in youth*, eds. J. K. Thompson and L. Smolak, 237–260. Washington, DC: American Psychological Association.

Loth, K. A., D. Neumark-Sztainer, and J. K. Croll. 2009. Informing family approaches to eating disorder prevention: Perspectives of those who have been there. *Int J Eat Disord* 42: 146–152.

Massey-Stokes, M. 2008. Body image and eating disturbances in children and adolescents. In *The active female*, ed. J. J. Robert-McComb, R. Norma, and M. Zumwalt, 57–79. Totowa, NJ: Humana Press.

McAlister, A. L., C. L. Perry, and G. S. Parcel. 2008. How individuals, environments, and health behaviors interact: Social cognitive theory. In *Health behavior and health education: Theory, research, and practice* (4th ed.), ed. K. Glanz, B. K. Rimer, and K. Viswanath, 169–188. San Francisco, CA: Jossey-Bass.

McCabe, M. P., L. A. Ricciardelli, and D. Ridge. 2006. "Who thinks I need a perfect body?" Perceptions and internal dialogue among adolescents and their bodies. *Sex Roles* 55: 409–419.

McCabe, M. P., L. A. Ricciardelli, and J. Salmon. 2006. Evaluation of a prevention program to address body focus and negative affect among children. *J Health Psychol* 11: 589–598.

McKenzie, J. F., B. L. Neiger, and R. Thackeray. 2009. *Planning, implementing, and evaluating health promotion programs: A primer* (5th ed.). San Francisco, CA: Benjamin Cummings (Pearson).

McVey G. L., R. Davis, S. Tweed, and F. Shaw. 2004. Evaluation of a school-based program designed to improve body image satisfaction, global self-esteem, and eating attitudes and behaviours: A replication study. *Int J Eat Disord* 36: 1–11.

McVey, G. L., M. Lieberman, N. Voorberg, D. Wardrope, and E. Blackmore. 2003. School-based peer support groups: A new approach to the prevention of disordered eating. *Eat Disord* 11: 169–185.

Mills, A., and B. Osborn. 2003. *Shapesville*. Carlsbad, CA: Gürze Books.

Neumark-Sztainer, D. 2005. Can we simultaneously work toward the prevention of obesity and eating disorders in children and adolescents? *Int J Eat Disord* 38: 220–227.

Neumark-Sztainer, D. 2007. Addressing the spectrum of adolescent weight-related problems: Engaging parents and communities. *Prev Res* 14: 11–14.

Neumark-Sztainer, D. 2009. Preventing obesity and eating disorders in adolescents: What can health care providers do? *J Adolesc Health* 44: 206–213.

Neumark-Sztainer, D., J. Croll, M. Story, P. J. Hannan, S. A. French, and C. Perry. 2002.

Neumark-Sztainer, D., M. P. Levine, S. J. Paxton, L. Smolak, N. Piran, and E. H. Wertheim. 2006. Prevention of body dissatisfaction and disordered eating: What next? *Eat Disord* 14: 265–285.

Neumark-Sztainer, D., M. Wall, J. Guo, M. Story, J. Haines, and M. Eisenberg. 2006. Obesity, disordered eating, and eating disorders in a longitudinal study of adolescents: How do dieters fare five years later? *J Am Diet Assoc* 106: 559–568.

Neumark-Sztainer, D., M. Wall, J. Haines, M. Story, N. E. Sherwood, and P. A. van den Berg. 2007. Shared risk and protective factors for overweight and disordered eating in adolescents. *Am J Prev Med* 33: 359–369.

Neumark-Sztainer, D., M. Wall, M. Story, and J. A. Fulkerson. 2004. Are family meal patterns associated with disordered eating behaviors among adolescents? *J Adolesc Health* 35: 350–359.

Neumark-Sztainer, D., N. E. Sherwood, T. Coller, and P. J. Hannan. 2000. Primary prevention of disordered eating among preadolescent girls: Feasibility and short-term effect of a community-based intervention. *J Am Diet Assoc* 100: 1466–1473.

Nielsen, S., C. Emborg, and A. G. Molbak. 2002. Mortality in concurrent type 1 diabetes and anorexia nervosa. *Diabetes Care* 15: 309–312.

Nieri, T., S. Kulin, V. M. Keith, and D. Hurdle. 2005. Body image, acculturation, and substance abuse among boys and girls in the Southwest. *Am J Drug Alcohol Abuse* 31: 617–639.

Nishina, A., N. Y. Ammon, A. D. Bellmore, and S. Graham. 2006. Body dissatisfaction and physical development among ethnic minority adolescents. *J Youth Adolesc* 35: 179–191.

O'Dea, J. A. 2005. School-based health education strategies for the improvement of body image and prevention of eating problems: An overview of safe and successful interventions. *Health Educ* 105: 11–33.

O'Dea, J. 2007. *Everybody's different: A positive approach to teaching about health, puberty, body image, nutrition, self-esteem and obesity prevention.* Camberwell, Victoria, Australia: ACER Press.

O'Dea, J., and S. Abraham. 2002. Improving the body image, eating attitudes and behaviours of young male and female adolescents: A new approach that focuses on self-esteem. *Int J Eat Disord* 28: 43–57.

O'Dea, J., and D. Maloney. 2000. Preventing eating and body image problems in children and adolescents using the health promoting schools framework. *J Sch Health* 70: 18–21.

Paxton, S. J. 1993. A prevention program for disturbed eating and body dissatisfaction in adolescent girls: A 1-year follow-up. *Health Educ Res* 8: 43–51.

Perry, C. L., D. E. Sellers, C. Johnson, S. Pedersen, K. J. Bachman, G. S. Parcel, E. J. Stone, R. V. Luepker, M. Wu, P. R. Nader, and K. Cook. 1997. The Child and Adolescent Trial for Cardiovascular Health (CATCH): Intervention, implementation, and feasibility for elementary schools in the United States. *Health Ed Behav* 24: 716–735.

Piran, N. 1998. A participatory approach to the prevention of eating disorders in a school. In *The prevention of eating disorders*, ed. W. Vandereycken and G. Noordenbos, 166–179. New York: New York Univ. Press.

Piran, N. 1999. Eating disorders: A trial of prevention in a high risk school setting. *J Prim Prev* 20: 75–90.

Piran N. 2001. Re-inhabiting the body from the inside out: Girls transform their school environment. In *From subjects to subjectivities: A handbook of interpretative and participatory methods*, ed. D. L. Tolman and M. Brydon-Miller, 218–238. New York: New York Univ. Press.

Piran, N. 2005. Prevention of eating disorders: A review of outcome evaluation research. *Isr J Psychiatry Relat Sci* 42: 172–177.

Piran, N., M. P. Levine, and C. Steiner-Adair. 1999. *Preventing eating disorders: A handbook of interventions and special challenges.* Philadelphia, PA: Brunner/Mazel.

Resnick M. D., P. S. Bearman, R. W. Blum, K. E. Bauman, K. M. Harris, J. Jones, J. A. Tabor, et al. 1997. Protecting adolescents from harm: Findings from the National Longitudinal Study on Adolescent Health. *JAMA* 278: 823–832.

Rideout, V. J., U. G. Foehr, and D. F. Roberts. 2010. *Generation M²: Media in the lives of 8- to 18-year-olds.* Menlo Park, CA: The Henry J. Kaiser Family Foundation. http://www.kff.org/entmedia/upload/8010.pdf (accessed June 11, 2010).

Rodgers, R. F., S. J. Paxton, and H. Chabrol. 2009. Effects of parental comments on body dissatisfaction and eating disturbance in young adults: A sociocultural model. *Body Image* 6: 171–177.

Rome, E. S., S. Ammerman, S. Rosen, R. J. Keller, J. Lock, K. A. Mammel, J. O'Toole, et al. 2003. Children and adolescents with eating disorders: The state of the art. *Pediatr* 111: 98–108.

Rosenkranz, R. R., T. K. Behrens, and D. A. Dzewaltowski. 2010. A group-randomized controlled trial for health promotion in Girl Scouts: Healthier troops in a SNAP (Scouting Nutrition & Activity Program). *BMC Public Health* 10: 1–13.

Sallis, J. F., N. Owen, and E. B. Fisher. 2008. Ecological models of health behavior. In *Health education and health behavior: Theory, research, and practice* (4th ed.), ed. K. Glanz, B. K. Rimer, and K. Viswanath, 465–485. San Francisco: Jossey-Bass.

Schoenberg, J., K. Salmond, and P. Fleshman. 2004. Weighing in: Helping girls be healthy today, health tomorrow. Retrieved from the Girl Scout Research Institute at http://www.girlscouts.org/research/publications/reviews/weighing_in.asp (accessed December 5, 2010).

Scime, M., C. Cook-Cottone, L. Kane, and T. Watson. 2006. Group prevention of eating disorders with fifth-grade females: Impact on body dissatisfaction, drive for thinness, and media influence. *Eat Disord* 14: 143–155.

Shaw, H., J. Ng, and E. Stice. 2007. Integrating eating disorder and obesity prevention programs for adolescents. *Prev Res* 14: 18–20

Shisslak, C. M., and M. Crago. 2001. Risk and protective factors in the development of eating disorders. In *Body image, eating disorders, and obesity in youth*, ed. J. K. Thompson and L. Smolak, 103–125. Washington, DC: American Psychological Association.

Shomaker, L. B., and W. Furman. 2009. Interpersonal influences on late adolescent girls' and boys' disordered eating. *Eat Behav* 10: 97–106.

Shunk, J. A., and L. L. Birch. 2004. Girls at risk for overweight at age 5 are at risk for dietary restraint, disinhibited overeating, weight concerns, and greater weight gain from 5 to 9 years. *J Am Diet Assoc* 104: 1120–1126.

Shuriquie, N. 1999. Eating disorders: A transcultural perspective. *East Mediterr Health J* 5: 354–360.

Siegel, J. M., A. K. Yancey, C. S. Aneshensel, and R. Schuler. 1999. Body image, perceived pubertal timing, and adolescent mental health. *J Adolesc Health* 25: 155–165.

Skemp-Arlt, K. M. 2006. Body image dissatisfaction and eating disturbances among children and adolescents: Prevalence, risk factors, and prevention strategies. *J Phys Educ Rec Dance* 77: 45–51.

Smith, E. P., A. M. Wolf, D. M. Cantillon, O. Thomas, and W. S. Davidson. 2004. The adolescent diversion project: 25 years of research on an ecological model of intervention. *J Prev Interv Community* 27: 29–47.

Smolak, L. 2004. Body image in children and adolescents: Where do we go from here? *Body Image* 1: 15–28.

Smolak, L., M. P. Levine, and F. Schermer. 1998. A controlled evaluation of an elementary school primary prevention program for eating problems. *J Psychosom Res* 44: 339–353.

Society for Adolescent Medicine. 2003. Eating disorders in adolescents: Position paper of the Society for Adolescent Medicine. *J Adolesc Health* 33: 496–503.

Society for Nutrition Education. 2003. Guidelines for childhood obesity prevention programs: Promoting healthy weight in children. *J Nutr Educ Behav* 35: 1–4.

Sokol, M. S., T. K. Jackson, C. T. Selser, H. A. Nice, N. D. Christiansen, and A. K. Carroll. 2005. Review of clinical research in child and adolescent eating disorders. *Prim Psychiatry* 12: 52–58.

Steese, S., M. Dollette, W. Phillips, E. Hossfeld, G. Matthews, and G. Taormina. 2006. Understanding Girls' Circle as an intervention on perceived social support, body image, self-efficacy, locus of control, and self-esteem. *Adolesc* 41: 55–74.

Stice, E., K. Presnell, and S. K. Bearman. 2001. Relation of early menarche to depression, eating disorders, substance abuse, and comorbid psychopathology among adolescent girls. *Dev Psychol* 37: 608–619.

Stice, E., and J. Ragan. 2002. A preliminary controlled evaluation of an eating disturbance psychoeducational intervention for college students. *Int J Eat Disord* 31: 159–171.

Stice, E., and H. Shaw. 2004. Eating disorder prevention programs: A meta-analytic review. *Psychol Bull* 130: 206–227.

Stice, E., D. Spangler, and W. S. Agras. 2001. Exposure to media-portrayed thin-ideal images adversely affects vulnerable girls: A longitudinal experiment. *J Soc Clin Psychol* 20: 270–288.

Stock, S., C. Miranda, S. Evans, S. Plessis, J. Ridley, S. Yeh, and J. Chaoine. 2007. Healthy buddies: A novel, peer-led health promotion program for the prevention of obesity and eating disorders in children in elementary school. *Pediatr* 120: e1059–e1068.

Stokol, D. 1996. Translating social ecological theory into guidelines for community health promotion. *Am J Health Promot* 10: 282–298.

Story, M., L. A. Lytle, A. S. Birnbaum, and C. L. Perry. 2002. Peer-led, school-based nutrition education for young adolescents: Feasibility and process evaluation of the TEENS study. *J Sch Health* 72: 121–127.

Tiggemann, M. 2005. Television and adolescent body image: The role of program content and viewing motivation. *J Soc Clin Psychol* 24: 361–381.

Tiggemann, M., M. Gardiner, and A. Slater. 2000. "I would rather be size 10 than have straight A's": A focus group study of adolescent girls' wish to be thinner. *J Adolesc* 23: 645–659.

Tiggemann, M., and A. S. Pickering. 1996. Role of television in adolescent women's body dissatisfaction and drive for thinness. *Int J Eat Disord* 20: 199–203.

U.S. Census Bureau. (2002). *Voting and registration in the election.*

U.S. Department of Health and Human Services, National Cancer Institute. 2005a. *Theory at a glance: A guide for health promotion practice* (2nd ed.). NIH Pub. No. 05-3896. Washington DC: U.S. Government Printing Office.

U.S. Department of Health and Human Services, Office on Women's Health. 2005b. *BodyWise handbook.* http://www.athealth.com/consumer/disorders/bodyimage.html (accessed November 21, 2010).

Varnado-Sullivan, P. J., N. Zucker, D. A. Williamson, D. Reas, J. Thaw, and S. B. Netemeyer. 2001. Development and implementation of the Body Logic Program for adolescents: A two-stage prevention program for eating disorders. *Cogn Behav Pract* 8: 248–259.

Wade, T. D., S. Davidson, and J. A. O'Dea. 2003. A controlled evaluation of a school-based media literacy program and self-esteem program for reducing eating disorder risk factors: A preliminary investigation. *Int J Eat Disord* 33: 371–383.

Wertheim E. H., S. J. Paxton, H. K. Schutz, and S. L. Muir. 1997. Why do adolescent girls watch their weight? An interview study examining sociocultural pressures to be thin. *J Psychosom Res* 42: 345–355.

Wilksch, S. M., M. Tiggemann, and T. D. Wade. 2006. Impact of interactive school-based media literacy lessons for reducing internalization of media ideals in young adolescent girls and boys. *Int J Eat Disord* 39: 385–393.

Wilson, J. L., R. Peebles, K. K. Hardy, and I. F. Litt. 2006. Surfing for thinness: A pilot study of pro-eating disorder web site usage in adolescents with eating disorders. *Pediatr* 188: e1635–e1643.

Wiser, S., and C. F. Telch. 1999. Dialectical behavior therapy for binge-eating disorder. *J Clin Psychol* 55: 755–768.

World Health Organization. 2003. Caring for children and adolescents with mental disorders: Setting WHO directions, http://www.who.int/mental_health/media/en/785.pdf (accessed November 22, 2010).

World Health Organization. 2000. Local action: Creating health promoting schools. http://www.who.int/school_youth_health/media/en/88.pdf (accessed June 27, 2010).

Zurn, L. 2006. *The Women's Sports Foundation Report: The status of health and physical activity of girls in Texas.* East Meadow, NY: Women's Sports Foundation.

Part V

Developing Healthy Attitudes
and Behaviors to Manage
Stress and Eating Disorders

14 Behavior Modification

Anna M. Tacón

CONTENTS

14.1 LEARNING OBJECTIVES

After reading this chapter you should be able to

- Understand what behavior and behavior modification are
- Comprehend the research bases of behavior modification
- Be able to apply basic principles used in behavior modification
- Understand basic procedures used in modifying behavior

14.2 BACKGROUND AND SIGNIFICANCE

Behavior is the most basic component of any process of change, and the transition to healthy behaviors best occurs in increments as a gradual process of achieving short-term goals within an overarching, long-term goal. In this way, modification of the behavior will be reinforced, incorporated into one's behavioral repertoire, and successfully maintained. Positive reinforcement at each point in the process can provide motivation to achieve the next short-term goal. Thus, the acquisition of a series of small units of behavior can form new and healthier patterns of eating behaviors.

14.2.1 Behavior Modification

Behavior modification, with its historical roots grounded in the behaviorist tradition, is an important option for treating various eating disorders. The perspective that behaviors form the malleable or modifiable building blocks with which to effect positive change in the individual—behavior modification—is an approach in psychology that focuses on altering maladaptive behaviors rather than focusing on internal characteristics, such as attitudes, values, and other personality characteristics. Thus, in the context of eating disorders, the behaviorist tradition would focus on a client's external actions rather than focusing on his or her internal processes. When dealing with individuals diagnosed with eating disorders, behavior modification emphasizes changing the eating behaviors—not altering unrealistic body-size expectations or dealing with the construct of appetite. Overt behavior is considered to play a major role in clinical dysfunction, but the etiology of such behavior is not central to treatment. The behaviorist approach emphasizing the primacy of behavior in developing adaptive strategies for daily functioning was derived from experimental research with laboratory animals (Kazdin 1989; Skinner 1938). Additionally, behavior modification strategies include attention to specific environmental contingencies that elicit the maladaptive behavior or alter the frequency of the specific behavior. For example, being in public places tends to decrease the frequency of binge eating episodes in a client.

14.2.2 Behavior Modification: Distinctions and Features

Human behavior, as it is conceptualized in behavior modification, has several important properties. First, behaviors are overt, meaning that they can be observed and defined as actions and can therefore be objectively described by others. Third, the interaction between behavior and environment must be determined. For example, which environments and environmental cues or triggers are present that maintain the maladaptive behaviors (Skinner 1966). Essentially, the behaviorist approach is about what people overtly do and say, rather than about invisible individual characteristics or personality traits and flaws. An advantage of taking the behaviorist approach in treating eating disorders is its simplicity and directness. The overt components of dysfunctional eating are identified for modification because they are the maladaptive behaviors that are essential to the diagnostic presentation of eating disorders.

There are several other central features of behavior modification (Miltenberger 1997). The first basic characteristic of any behavior modification regimen is the focus on behavior and associated behavioral principles derived from many years of research in applied behavior analysis. The scientific study of behavior is called the experimental analysis of behavior or behavior analysis (Skinner 1938), and the scientific study of human behavior frequently is referred to as applied behavior analysis (Baer et al. 1968). The behavior to be modified is known as the *target behavior*, which can be further identified as either a behavioral excess or deficit. Behavioral *excess* is an undesirable target behavior that one seeks to decrease in frequency, duration, or intensity. Binge eating and purging would be examples of behavioral excess. A behavioral *deficit* is a desirable target behavior that one seeks to increase in frequency, duration, or intensity. Retaining a meal after eating would be an example of a behavioral deficit.

Another important feature of behavior modification is the emphasis on current environmental factors that are functionally related to the target behavior. Any goal of behavior modification must identify and modify the reciprocal influences between the immediate environment and the behavior. Therefore, environmental factors that contribute to the individual's eating disorder symptoms, such as restrictive eating, binge eating, or purging, must be identified. For example, a common environmental factor related to these symptoms could be exposure to photographs of very thin models in magazines that the adolescent frequently purchases. Once the environmental contingencies related to the maladaptive behavior are identified, a plan to modify that relationship can be designed and implemented so that desired change can occur. In the last example, part of the treatment plan would be to restrict the client's access to certain magazines in her immediate environment. This could be achieved by removing transportation or financial resources to purchase such magazines, and also by removing similar image sources of very thin models from the home.

Another basic aspect of behavior modification is specificity. *Specificity* in behavior modification involves a precise description of the behavior to be changed and the procedure or technique to be implemented to insure that the desired changes occur. The effectiveness of a modification program is assessed by measuring behavior before and after intervention to determine the behavior change resulting from a given modification technique. Once the procedure is operationally defined and training of a behavior modification strategy has been conducted, the treatment frequently is implemented by someone in the client's life, such as a parent or spouse, rather than being implemented solely by a professional (Kazdin 1994).

14.2.3 OPERANT CONDITIONING: BASIC PRINCIPLES AND PROCEDURES

In his laboratory experiments with animals, Skinner (1938, 1966, 1969, 1974) concluded that many behaviors are emitted and influenced primarily by their consequences, and he explored the effect of various consequences that influenced behavior. Such behaviors he termed "operants" to specify that operants were behaviors that operated on the environment to produce certain outcomes. Operant conditioning, also known as instrumental conditioning, refers to the Skinnerian principle that such behaviors are considered instrumental in determining consequences or outcomes. Thus, operants are regarded as being controlled, motivated, or influenced by consequences that are contingent on such operant behaviors.

Basic principles to be discussed in this chapter are positive and negative reinforcements, extinction, punishment, and stimulus control. Basic procedures in behavior modification include shaping and chaining, prompting and fading, contingency contracts, self-management, alternate response training, and systematic desensitization.

14.2.4 REINFORCEMENT

Reinforcement is a major concept in operant conditioning. Essentially, reinforcement refers to an increase in the frequency or likelihood of a behavior when that behavior is immediately followed by a specific consequence. The consequence that is contingent upon a given behavior strengthens the probability that the behavior will occur again, and the consequence that increases the frequency of an operant behavior is known as a reinforcer (Skinner 1969). For example, after purging, the individual feels less full. Every time the individual purges, she feels less full, and feeling less full is reinforcing.

Another example of reinforcement is the constant negative attention the person with anorexia receives when she does not eat during mealtime. Even though the parent might reprimand the adolescent in an effort to get the adolescent to eat, such reprimanding actually may increase the adolescent's dysfunctional eating behavior. Therefore, a reinforcer is not an inherently "good" or "bad" event; it is simply an environmental event that increases the likelihood that a specific behavioral response will occur with greater frequency.

Positive reinforcement occurs when a behavior is followed by the addition of a desired stimulus or event immediately after the response. Such stimuli are commonly known as rewards; however, the defining feature of a reinforcer is its ability to increase the frequency of a behavior, hence not all reinforcers are rewards. An example of a positive reinforcer for a child or an adolescent with an eating disorder might be taking the person to the movies after he or she eats a balanced meal.

Negative reinforcement refers to an increase in the frequency of a response by removing or avoiding an aversive stimulus immediately after the behavior. This escape or avoidance of an aversive stimulus strengthens the behavior. In escape behavior, the aversive stimulus or event is already present. In avoidant behavior, the person avoids the aversive stimulus before its occurrence, often because of a signal or warning cue prior to the aversive event. For example, criticism or reprimand-ing by the adolescent's parents could serve as a negative reinforcer for an adolescent to begin eating appropriately at meal times.

Reinforcement effectiveness is influenced by the schedule of reinforcement used, that is, by the timing and frequency with which the reinforcer is administered. The schedule of reinforcement specifies whether a reinforcer will be given every time the desired response is exhibited (*continuous reinforcement*) or only after a specific interval or after a specific number of desired responses occurs (*intermittent reinforcement*) (Skinner 1969). For example, at the beginning of a behavior modifica-tion program, the individual might be praised every time a meal is eaten. Once eating regularly is accomplished, praise continues but is not given every time.

14.2.5 EXTINCTION

Extinction is a principle of behavior modification that suggests that the absence of reinforcement will gradually reduce the frequency of a behavior, which may result in complete cessation of the behavior. Thus, if a behavior no longer produces the reinforcing consequences, the behavior will stop. Numerous studies have demonstrated the effectiveness of extinction for decreasing problem behaviors (Kazdin 1994; Lerman and Iwata 1995; Mazaleski and Iwata 1993; Rincover 1978). For an adolescent girl with bulimia, for example, the behaviors to be extinguished are binge eating and purging. Groups of adolescent girls might reinforce her purging behavior by praising her for having the courage to vomit, and such praise from her peers maintains her purging behavior. This rein-forcement for the maladaptive eating behavior thus needs to be removed from the adolescent girl's environment. In this specific example, a behavior modification plan could include educating the girl's peers so that they do not continue to reinforce her purging behavior by praising her. If edu-cating her peers fails to eliminate the reinforcement, then the person with bulimia may need to be discouraged or restricted from associating with the peers who are reinforcing her purging behavior. Incorporating either of these strategies into the behavior modification plan should help reduce the purging behavior since she is no longer being reinforced for vomiting.

A behavior modification procedure that combines reinforcement and extinction is *differential reinforcement*. Specifically, this procedure is intended to increase the frequency of a desired behav-ior via reinforcement while also decreasing the frequency of an undesired behavior that may inter-fere with the desired behavior via extinction. Several behavior modification studies have supported the use of differential reinforcement for various behaviors (Reed 1989; Sulzer-Azaroff 1988). For a person who severely restricts her food intake, for example, the behavior modification plan should include positive reinforcement when she eats a balanced meal and the elimination of praise when she loses weight or skips meals.

14.2.6 PUNISHMENT

Most proponents of behavior modification typically avoid the use of punishment because there are a wide range of positive reinforcers available and because there are undesirable associations connected with the use of punishment (Kazdin 1989). In behavior modification, the application of *punishment* refers to a process in which the consequence of a behavior results in the decreased performance of the specific behavior in the future. Thus, punishment is similar to reinforcement because it is contingent on the consequences of a behavior but is different because, unlike reinforce-ment, the consequences decrease the likelihood of the behavior occurring in the future.

Just as the distinction between positive and negative reinforcement deals with either the presenta-tion or the removal of a consequent stimulus, positive and negative punishments also have similar distinctions. *Positive punishment* refers to the presentation of a stimulus that the individual consid-ers aversive or unpleasant following the occurrence of the specified behavior in order to decrease the probability of that behavior in the future. After an episode of purging, for example, parents might use positive punishment by criticizing that behavior or by adding extra chores, duties, or assignments to their child's list of responsibilities for a week. *Negative punishment*, on the other hand, is the removal of something that is considered a positive reinforcer following a behavior. Again, the intended result is to decrease the likelihood of that behavior occurring in the future. For example, parents might withdraw the privilege of going to the mall with her friends when their daughter restricts her diet or refuses to eat.

14.2.7 STIMULUS CONTROL: DISCRIMINATION AND GENERALIZATION

A behavior is under *stimulus control* when the probability of its occurrence increases in the presence of a specific stimulus. This increase often occurs because reinforcement is administered only when that specific stimulus is present. This principle specifies that responses will vary depending upon the presence of different stimuli. When an individual responds one way in the presence of one stimulus and another way in the presence of a different stimulus, that individual has made a *discrimination* (Kazdin 1989). An antecedent stimulus that is present when a behavior is reinforced is termed a discriminative stimulus, and when a behavior is differentially controlled by such antecedent stimuli, the behavior is said to be under stimulus control. *Generalization,* on the other hand, takes place when a behavior occurs in the presence of stimuli that are similar to the discriminative stimulus.

Principles of stimulus control are important for behavior modification because the goal is to change target behaviors by altering the existing relationship among (1) the conditions prior to the behavior (antecedent context), (2) the target behavior, and (3) the consequences of the behavior. In a behavior modification plan for an adolescent with anorexia, for example, eating can be deliberately reinforced when she sits down to eat at her parents' dining room table. Whenever she enters her parents' dining room, she expects to be rewarded and therefore is more likely to eat her meal. Later on, when she is invited by her friend's parents to eat at their dining room table, she might generalize her behavior and thus eat her meal.

14.2.8 SHAPING AND CHAINING

Frequently, the development of a new behavior cannot be achieved by reinforcement of current responses because the desired behavior may be so complex that the elements making up that behavior do not currently exist in the individual's repertoire. To establish a new, complex behavioral response, shaping is used. *Shaping* is a procedure where successive approximations of a target behavior are reinforced. Therefore, the final goal behavior is achieved by reinforcing the small steps toward the final, desired response rather than by waiting to reinforce the final response itself (Kazdin 1989). Shaping has been applied in medical settings (O'Neill and Gardner 1983) and has been used in studies to modify maladaptive behavior (Howie and Woods 1982; Jackson and Wallace 1974). For example, eating a full meal will be a difficult task at the beginning of treatment for an adolescent with anorexia nervosa. Instead of waiting to reinforce the adolescent until she eats a full meal, her eating behavior may be shaped. That is, initially, the eating of any amount of food could be reinforced. Gradually, reinforcement is given only when she eats more and more, and eventually she will be able to eat a full meal.

Most behaviors are made up of a sequence of several responses, and a complex behavior consisting of many component behaviors occurring in a certain sequence is called a behavioral chain (Miltenberger 1997). *Chaining* procedures teach an individual to incorporate a sequence of behaviors into her behavioral repertoire of responses. An example of chaining for an adolescent girl with anorexia would be (1) sitting at the table, (2) placing a napkin on her lap, (3) holding utensils, (4) bringing food to mouth, (5) chewing the food, (6) swallowing the food, and (7) repeating the last three behaviors until an adequate amount of food has been eaten. At first, reinforcement would be given when each step in the chain is completed. Gradually, reinforcement would follow only after the all of the units in the chain of behavior are completed and the adolescent has completed her meal.

Another strategy to assist in teaching behavioral chains is known as written task analysis. This objective, documented format helps to guide the sequence of component behaviors in a desired behavioral chain. The analysis clearly lists every instruction or component in the chain in the proper sequence, and a detailed list of instructions helps the individual to perform the task correctly (Miltenberger 1997). Both shaping and chaining demonstrate the significance of identifying and reinforcing small steps or components in behavior modification programs. Achievement of small or short-term goals can be critically important to the achievement of long-term goals.

14.2.9 PROMPTING AND FADING

Prompting is a behavior modification method that is used to develop appropriate stimulus control for a specific behavior. Prompts or cues are used during discrimination training so that the individual will produce the desired behavior in the presence of the discriminative stimulus. Essentially, *prompting* refers to stimuli that help initiate a response, such as instruction, reminders, or guidance during a behavioral action or when modeling a behavior (Kazdin 1989). When a prompt results in the desired response, the behavior can then be reinforced. As behavioral training progresses and the need for prompting decreases, *fading* (i.e., the gradual removal of the prompt) occurs. Fading is a way to transfer stimulus control from the facilitating prompts to the discriminative stimulus and the reinforcers (Miltenberger 1997).

A behavior modification program for a person with anorexia nervosa, for example, could include reinforcing her whenever she eats at her parent's dining room table. While eating in this setting, she might be given a prompt such as a comment like, "This is a new recipe, so I'm interested in what you think of it" or "I hope you like the asparagus." Every time she eats in the dining room after being prompted, she is reinforced. Later, she can go to a restaurant and be prompted to eat. Eventually, when prompting is no longer needed, fading is initiated.

14.2.10 CONTINGENCY CONTRACTS

Contingencies of reinforcement are often designed in the form of *contingency contracts,* which are behavioral contracts between individuals who design behavior modification plans (i.e., the professional) and the individual whose target behavior is the goal for change (i.e., the client). The procedure of behavioral contracting precisely specifies the consequences for certain behaviors. That is, contracts specify the reinforcers that are available and that are contingent on certain behaviors (Kazdin 1989; Skinner 1969). Contracts have been used in studies for a variety of target behaviors, including weight loss and weight maintenance in adults and academic performance in children, adolescents, and college students (Jeffery and Bjornson-Benson 1984; Kelly and Stokes 1984; Kramer et al. 1986; Miller and Kelly 1994).

Contingency contracts have five basic components (Miltenberger 1997). First, the target behaviors are clearly defined in objective, operational terms. Target behaviors can include desirable behaviors to be increased, undesirable behaviors to be decreased, or both. Next, specific statements about when a target behavior is to be performed are included so that a timeframe for the contracted contingencies can be determined. Third, the target behaviors must be observable so that they can be measured objectively. Fourth, the contract specifies the reinforcement for the target behavior as well as sanctions or punishment for failure to meet the agreed upon terms. Last, the contract clearly identifies the roles of all persons involved, including the person who will be responsible for implementing the contingencies based on the behaviors, such as a parent. One of the greatest advantages of such contracts is the participation of several people, most importantly, the individual with the targeted behaviors. Taking an active role in negotiation and creation of the contract, rather than having a behavior modification program imposed without any input from her, may lead to an enhanced sense of control in the individual.

14.2.11   SELF-MANAGEMENT

Self-management occurs when an individual engages in a behavior at one point to increase the likelihood of the occurrence of another behavior—the target behavior—at a later point in time (Watson and Tharp 1993; Yates 1986). Self-management strategies include a variety of controlling behaviors to increase the future occurrence of a controlled behavior (target behavior). Examples of self-management strategies include appropriate goal setting, self-monitoring, self-reinforcement, self-punishment, positive self-talk, self-instruction, arranging social support, and developing a behavioral contract (Kazdin 1989; Miltenberger 1997). Of these, appropriate goal setting and self-monitoring are perhaps the most crucial techniques. Self-management strategies enhance self-control, as people exert more effective control of their behavior in their everyday lives. These strategies advance the person to the ultimate goal of behavior modification, which is training individuals to control their behaviors and to achieve their self-selected goals (Kazdin 1989).

The most self-defeating goal is one that is unrealistic, inappropriate, or unachievable, for such goals lead to inevitable failure. *Appropriate goal setting*, therefore, identifies a desirable and achievable target behavior. The goal should be written down, the target behavior should be precisely described, and a reasonable timeframe for achieving the goal should be established. Intermediate or short-term goals are to be identified and specified within the global goal setting. These intermediate goals build upon a baseline level of behavior and indicate progress toward the final goal (Miltenberger 1997).

Goal setting is best implemented in conjunction with self-monitoring techniques because monitoring behavior provides a record of effectiveness to use in evaluating progress toward the goal. *Self-monitoring* consists of systematic observation of one's own behavior. Since many behaviors are automatic, they usually go unrecognized. Self-monitoring devices, such as daily log sheets for recording behaviors, can increase awareness of the behavior. Variations of self-monitoring used in conjunction with behavioral recording may also provide motivation and reinforcement. Although self-monitoring strategies alone do not alter behavior directly, such techniques often initiate other behaviors that do alter behavior, such as self-reinforcement or self-punishment.

14.2.12   ALTERNATE RESPONSE TRAINING

A form of self-control or self-management is that of *interference*, specifically, replacing an undesired behavior with another, more appropriate behavior. In order to give up an undesired response, the individual may need an alternative to the undesired response. For example, instead of binge eating when anxious, a young woman could replace binge eating with an anxiety-reduction strategy, such as deep breathing, progressive muscle relaxation, meditation, exercise, or thinking positive thoughts. Forms of relaxation have been widely used as an alternative to maladaptive behavior because relaxation is incompatible with anxiety—one cannot be anxious or stressed and also be relaxed (Kazdin 1989). Whatever alternate behavior is chosen, the behavior needs to be an acceptable option for the individual and effective in interfering with or replacing the undesired behavior.

14.2.13   SYSTEMATIC DESENSITIZATION

Systematic desensitization is one of the most effective and widely employed procedures in behavioral approaches to treatment. The basic assumption is that anxiety is a learned or conditioned response that can be inhibited by a response that is incompatible with anxiety. *Systematic desensitization* involves repeated pairing of the anxiety-producing stimuli with relaxation until the connection between those stimuli and the anxious response is eliminated (Wolpe 1990).

Systematic desensitization involves three basic steps: relaxation training, development of an anxiety hierarchy, and desensitization "proper" (Morris 1986). The client is taught to relax and is encouraged to practice this skill daily outside of sessions. Following this phase, the client and therapist work together to create an anxiety hierarchy, which involves increments of stimuli that produce anxiety or fear in the client. For example, an adolescent may be fearful about eating a normal meal. The anxiety hierarchy for this adolescent might have this target behavior, described in detail, at the top of the anxiety hierarchy. At the bottom of the hierarchy might be taking a sip of water. In between these two hierarchy points, there would be gradual increments of eating increased amounts of food.

Once the first two steps are completed, each stimulus in the hierarchy is paired with relaxation. Specifically, in a relaxed state, the client is asked to visualize the least arousing stimuli in the hierarchy. After this stimulus can be visualized without anxiety, the client proceeds up the anxiety hierarchy to levels that are associated with greater anxiety. Every time the client reports experiencing anxiety, the visualization of that stimulus is halted and relaxation is induced. Once a relaxed state is achieved, movement up the anxiety hierarchy continues and relaxation is induced as needed. Thus, the original association of each stimulus and anxiety is eventually replaced with a new connection between that stimulus and relaxation. For example, as the client proceeds up the hierarchy visualizing different stimuli, she starts becoming anxious and physiologically aroused from the image. At that moment, the client shifts her focus back to a stimulus that no longer produces significant anxiety and concentrates remaining relaxed while visualizing that stimulus. When her anxiety dissipates, she resumes her attempt to visualize more challenging items on the anxiety hierarchy while remaining relaxed.

14.3 CURRENT FINDINGS

14.3.1 Reinforcement

Reinforcement continues to be an essential element in behavior modification as evidenced by research investigating the roles of negative and positive reinforcements in disordered eating. Several studies have indicated that client expectations of negative consequences from eating play an important role in the development of eating disorders (Epstein, Leddy et al. 2007; Nassar et al. 2009). Recent research on eating disorders also highlights the powerful role of positive consequences. For example, one study investigated eating expectancies, emotion dysregulation, and symptoms of bulimia nervosa in undergraduate women (Hayaki 2009). The results suggested that individuals who are especially susceptible to disordered eating are those who expect that eating will provide emotional relief.

Research also has documented the positively reinforcing value of food itself as being an influential factor in caloric intake or increased food consumption. According to Epstein, Leddy, et al. (2007), the reinforcing value of food is evidenced by a method of food regulation, specifically the amount of work one is willing to do to gain access to food. The reinforcing value of a certain food is exhibited when applying progressive ratio schedules of reinforcement. For example, the specific schedule of reinforcement increases after each designated episode of food reinforcement occurs. For example, at the beginning of behavior modification, the number of times that the desired behavior needs to be performed in order to obtain the reinforcer may be five times. Then, proceeding with a progressive ratio schedule of reinforcement, the number of times that the desired behavior needs to be performed for reinforcement to occur might be increased to ten times, and later to twenty times, etc. An example of this procedure is an adolescent with binge eating disorder who likes pizza and is working on specified goals to earn a slice of pizza (reinforcer). The amount of work this adolescent is required to do to earn the same amount of pizza can be steadily increased.

Several reinforcement strategies have been developed to target pediatric obesity. Specifically, a research study using a family-based behavioral treatment investigated the effects of reinforcement and stimulus control on reducing sedentary behavior in a sample of obese children (mean age, 9 years; Epstein et al. 2000). The goals of the treatment were to reduce sedentary behaviors, encourage physical activity, and decrease food intake. Specifically, physical activity was substituted for the sedentary behaviors, and consequently, the behavioral changes resulted in weight loss. Consistent with earlier studies, these behavioral strategies produced significant effects leading to the conclusion that stimulus control and reinforcement are behavioral options for decreasing sedentary behavior in obese children (Epstein et al. 1995, 2002; Epstein and Saelens 2000; Lambiase 2009).

Another example from Epstein, Beecher et al. (2007) involved the use of interactive game programs. Specifically, they evaluated the reinforcing value and activity levels of interactive dance and bicycle race games in overweight and nonoverweight children between the ages of 8 and 12. A behavioral choice paradigm was used to assess the reinforcing value of the games by providing children the opportunity to respond on progressive ratio schedules of reinforcement for options of playing either the video dance or bicycle game using a handheld video game controller or one of three options: dancing or bicycling alone, dancing or bicycling while watching a video, or playing the interactive dance or bicycle game. Data showed that the interactive dance game was more reinforcing than dancing alone or dancing while watching the video but no differences were found across bicycling conditions. Additionally, healthy weight youth were more active when given the opportunity to play the interactive dance game than overweight children. These findings suggest that children may be motivated to be physically active when given the option of playing an interactive activity game, such as a dance game.

14.3.2 Binge Eating and Obesity

The complexity of disordered eating behaviors also has been investigated within the context of behavioral modification. Investigations and interventions have produced a debate regarding the relationship between binge eating and obesity, since binge eating and obesity are frequently comorbid behaviors. These debates have also raised concern and produced disagreements about appropriate weight loss treatments for obese, binge eating individuals (Bulik et al. 2002; Manson et al. 2002; Munsch and Beglinger 2005; Pi-Sunyer 2003; Rapps et al. 2009; Rieger et al. 2005; Yanovski 2002).

A growing body of literature indicates that binge eating is associated with eating distress, body image distress, and other psychopathology (Telch and Stice 1998; Wilfley et al. 2000). However, increasing evidence shows that binge eating is not a barrier to behavioral treatment for weight loss among obese clients (Raymond et al. 2002). For example, a recent study by Delinsky and colleagues (2006) involving obese individuals with BED, found that binge eating did not interfere with weight loss for these participants who were enrolled in a self-help, behavior modification program. Binge eating is frequent among obese populations because 23% to 46% of obese patients who are seeking weight loss treatments also have BED (Delinsky et al. 2006).

The purpose of the Delinsky et al. (2006) study was to assess the influence of binge eating behavior on weight loss, but not to eliminate any psychopathology associated with binge eating disorder. The entire sample consisted of participants with varying degrees of binge eating behavior, and a significant subsample (17%) had objective bulimic episodes averaging twice a week— the frequency criterion for binge eating disorder. Participants who reported at least eight objective bulimic episodes in the past month on the Eating Disorder Examination or Eating Disorder Examination Questionnaire (see Chapter 5) were classified as binge eaters, and participants with fewer than eight objective bulimic episodes in the past month were categorized as non-binge eaters. When binge eating participants were compared with non-binge eating participants, those who reported eight or more objective bulimic episodes during the past month reported greater concerns about eating and weight, body shape, and also were more depressed. These findings are consistent with growing data that binge eating is associated with more eating and body image-related distress and psychopathology (Delinsky et al. 2006). Even though objective bulimic episodes were documented for 41% of the sample, the point is that weight loss still occurred despite the binge eating episodes. Specifically, the mean weight loss after 12 months for those who completed the program was 28.2 kg or 18.8% of original weight, and 10.3 kg or 10.5% of original weight for the entire sample. Thus, initial data indicate that binge eating is not an automatic deterrent to weight loss in behavioral modification programs. Even if obese clients are able to lose weight in behavioral modification programs, it might still be necessary to address the binge eating and the psychological problems that contribute to binge eating. Losing weight by itself is unlikely to reduce or eliminate the binge eating.

14.3.3 TECHNOLOGY IN BEHAVIORAL MODIFICATION PROGRAMS

In an effort to reduce the time-consuming nature of behavior modification programs and to expand intervention options, new technologies in the treatment of eating disorders have been explored (Myers et al. 2004). For example, some of these investigations have included computerized internet treatment programs (Harvey-Berino et al. 2002; Tate et al. 2001), telecommunications (Harvey-Berino 1998), virtual environments (Ferrer-Garcia et al. 2009), or completely computerized treatment trials (Wylie-Rosett et al. 2001). One advantage of using advanced technology is that it allows a large population to be monitored over a period of time at relatively low cost. One such program is known as E[S]SPRIT.

E[S]SPRIT is a computer-based program for preventing or intervening early in the development of eating disorders among college students. E[S]SPRIT was implemented at Heidelberg University in 2007 and is still being evaluated (Bauer et al. 2009). Monitoring is used to track information related to participants' eating behavior throughout their participation. For example, participants receive email reminders to fill out a short questionnaire that includes questions about dieting, nutrition, body dissatisfaction, concern with weight and shape, and disordered eating behaviors, such as binge eating and compensatory behaviors. Chat technology can also be used to interact with students individually or as a group. This approach shows promise in identifying students who have the potential for developing an eating disorder and in helping them avoid future trouble.

Another innovative application of technology involves the traditional components of journaling and self-monitoring to modify eating behaviors. Dietary self-monitoring has been referred to as the "cornerstone" of all behavioral weight-control interventions (Foreyt and Goodrick 1993). Yon and colleagues (2007) investigated the efficacy of personal digital assistants (PDAs) and traditional paper diary and journal entries in weight loss programs by comparing findings from their study using PDAs with a previous study's use of the traditional paper method. No significant differences were found in either weight loss or dietary self-monitoring. Specifically, weight loss in both the traditional group and the PDA group was correlated with the amount of self-monitoring. The researchers concluded that PDAs were comparable to traditional diaries for self-monitoring purposes in a weight loss program, and therefore can be used without compromising the effectiveness of a traditional weight loss program.

In Japan, a randomized clinical trial investigated the effectiveness of a new, 1-month, behavioral weight-control program that used computer-tailored individual advice for behavior modification and participants' treatment needs (Adachi et al. 2007). At the beginning, participants provided personalized information for three to five behaviors that were targeted for modification. This information was then loaded into a computer system, and personalized advice was presented to each participant. Consistent with previous findings (Adachi and Yamatsu 2004), significant weight loss was found, which suggested that computer-tailored personal advice programs may be a useful mechanism for future behavioral weight-control programs.

14.4 SUMMARY AND CONCLUSION

Behavior modification is an important therapy option in the treatment of eating disorders, as shown by recent research in this area. The use of novel modification strategies in weight loss programs for overweight children, including reducing sedentary behaviors and increasing activity with interactive game choices, are important contributions given the growing epidemic of pediatric obesity. In addition, the field of behavior modification remains contemporary by incorporating technology into behavioral intervention programs. For example, research showing the use of PDA devices to be equivalent to traditional diaries, as well as comprehensive online intervention programs such as E[S]SPRIT, are advances that may increase the ease of self-monitoring and can provide effective and low-cost interventions to large numbers of people.

REFERENCES

Adachi, Y., C. Sato, K. Yamatsu, S. Ito, K. Adachi, and T. Yamagami. 2007. A randomized control trial on the long-term effects of a one month behavioral weight control program assisted by computer tailored advice. *Behav Res Th* 45: 459–470.

Adachi Y., and K. Yamatsu. 2004. The structured computer tailored behavior change program for obesity. *J Japan Soc Study Obes* 10: 31–36

Baer, D., M. Wolf, and T. Risley. 1968. Some current dimensions of applied behavior analysis. *J Appl Behav Anal* 1: 91.

Bauer, S., M. Moessner, and M. Wolf. 2009. ES[S]PRIT—an Internet-based program for the prevention and early intervention of eating disorders in college students. *Brit J Guid & Couns* 37: 327–336.

Bulik, C., P. Sullivan, and K. Kendler. 2002. Medical and psychiatric morbidity in obese women with and without binge eating. *Int J Eat Disord* 32: 72–78.

Delinsky, S., J. Latner, and T. Wilson. 2006. Binge eating and weight loss in a self-help behavior modification program. *Obesity* 14: 1244–1249.

Epstein, L., Beecher, M., Graf, J., and Roemich, J. 2007. Choice of interactive dance and bicycle games in overweight and nonoverweight youth. *Ann Behav Med* 33: 124–131.

Epstein, L., R. Paluch, A. Consalvi, K. Riordan, and T. Scholl. 2002. Effects of manipulating sedentary behaviour on physical activity and food intake. *J Ped* 140: 334–339.

Epstein, L., Paluch, R., Gordy, C., and Dorn, J. 2000. Decreasing sedentary behaviors in treating paediatric obesity. *Arch Ped Adol Med* 154: 220–226

Epstein, L., J. Leddy, and J. Temple. 2007. Food reinforcement and eating: A multilevel analysis. *Ann Behav Med* 33: 124–131.

Epstein, L., A. Valoski, and L. Vara. 1995. Effects of decreasing sedentary behavior and increasing activity on weight change in obese children. *Health Psychol* 14:*Health Psychol,14,*109–115.

Epstein, L., and B. Saelens. 2000. Behavioral economics of obesity: Food intake and energy expenditure. In *Reframing health behavior change with behavioral economics*, ed. W. K. Bickel and R. E. Vunchinich, 293–311. Mahwah, NJ: Erlbaum.

Ferrer-Garcia, M., J. Gutierrex-Maldonado, A. Caqueo-Urízar, and E. Moreno. 2009. The validity of virtual environments for eliciting emotional responses in patients with eating disorders and in controls. *Behav Modif* 33: 830–854.

Foreyt, J., and G. Goodrick. 1993. Evidence of success of behavior modification in weight loss and control. *Ann Intern Med* 119: 698–701.

Harvey-Berino, J. 1998. Changing health behavior via telecommunications technology: Using interactive television to treat obesity. *Behav Ther* 29(3): 505–519.

Harvey-Berino, J., S. Pintauro, and P. Buzzell. 2002. Does using the internet facilitate the maintenance of weight loss. *Int J Obes* 26: 1254–1260.

Hayaki, J. 2009. Negative reinforcement eating expectancies, emotion dysregulation, and symptoms of bulimia nervosa. *Int J Eat Disord* 42: 552–6.

Howie, P., and C. Woods. 1982. Token reinforcement during the instatement and shaping of fluency in the treatment of stuttering. *J Appl Behav Anal* 15: 55.

Jackson, D.A., and R. F. Wallace. 1974. The modification and generalization of voice loudness in a fifteen-year-old retarded girl. *J Appl Behav Anal* 7(3): 461–471.

Jeffery, R., and W. Bjornson-Benson. 1984. The effectiveness of monetary contracts with two repayment schedules on weight reduction in men and women from self-referred and population samples. *Behav Ther* 15: 273.

Kazdin, A. 1989. *Behavior modification in applied settings* (4th ed.). Pacific Grove, CA: Brooks-Cole.

Kazdin, A. 1994. *Behavior modification in applied settings* (5th ed.). Pacific Grove, CA: Brooks-Cole.

Kelly, M.L., and T.F. Stokes 1984. Student–teacher contracting with goal setting for maintenance. *Behav Modif* 8(2): 223–224.

Kramer, F., R. Jeffery, M. Snell, and J. Forster. 1986. Maintenance of successful weight loss over one year: Effects of contracts for weight maintenance or participation in skills training. *Behav Ther* 17: 295.

Lambiase, M. 2009. Treating pediatric overweight through reductions in sedentary behavior: A review of the literature. *J Pediatr Health Care* 23: 29–36.

Lerman, D., and B. Iwata. 1995. Prevalence of extinction burst and its attenuation during treatment. *J Appl Behav Anal* 28: 93.

Manson, J., P. Skerrett, and W. Willett. 2002. Epidemiology of health risks associated with obesity. In *Eating disorders and obesity: A comprehensive handbook*, ed. C. Fairburn and K. Browenell, 127–143. New York: The Guilford Press.

Mazaleski, J., and B. Iwata. 1993. Analysis of the reinforcement and extinction components in contingencies with self-injury. *J Appl Behav Anal* 26: 143.

Miller, D., and M. Kelly. 1994. The use of goal setting and contingency contracting for improving children's homework. *J Appl Behav Anal* 27: 73.

Miltenberger, R. 1997. *Behavior modification*. Pacific Grove, CA: Brooks-Cole.

Morris, R. 1986. Fear reduction methods. In *Helping people change: A textbook of methods*, ed. F. Kanfer and A. Goldstein, 231–256. New York: Pergamon Press.

Munsch S., and C. Beglinger. 2005. *Obesity and binge eating disorder*. Basel, Switzerland: S. Karger.

Myers, T., L. Swan-Kremeier, and S. Wonderlich. 2004. The use of alternative delivery systems and new technologies in the treatment of patients with eating disorders. *Int J Eat Disord* 36: 123–143.

Nassar, J., S. Evans, and A. Geliebter. 2009. Use of an operant task to estimate food reinforcement in adult humans with and without BED. *Obesity* 16: 1816–20.

O'Neill, G. and R. Gardner. 1983. *Behavioral principles in medical rehabilitation: A practical guide*. Springfield, IL: Charles C. Thomas.

Pi-Sunyer, X. 2003. A clinical view of the obesity problem. *Science* 299: 859–860.

Rapps, N., S. Becker, M. Teufel, and S. Zipfel. 2009. Binge eating disorder—A comorbid eating disorder in obesity. *Dtsch Med Wochenschr,* 134: 38–47.

Raymond, N., M. deZwaan, J. Mitchell, D. Ackerd, and P. Thuras. 2002. Effects of a very low calorie diet on the diagnostic category of individuals with binge eating disorder. *Int J Eat Disord* 31: 49–56.

Reed, P. 1989. Influence of inter-response time reinforcement on signaled-reward effect. *J Exp Psychol: Animal Behav Processes* 15: 224–231.

Reid, D., M. Parsons, and C. Green. 1989. *Staff management in human services: Behavioral research and application*. Springfield, IL: Charles C. Thomas.

Rieger, E., D. Wilfley, R. Stein, V. Marino, and S. Crow. 2005. A comparison of quality of life in obese individuals with and without binge eating disorder. *Int J Eat Disord* 37: 234–240.

Rincover, A. 1978. Sensory Extinction: A procedure for eliminating self-stimulatory behavior in developmentally disabled children. *J Abnormal Ch Psychol* 6: 299–310.

Skinner, B. 1938. *The behavior of organisms: An experimental analysis*. New York: Appleton-Century-Crofts.

Skinner, B. 1966. What is the experimental analysis of behavior? *J Exp Anal of Behav* 9: 213.

Skinner, B. 1969. *Contingencies of reinforcement: A theoretical analysis*. New York: Appleton-Century-Crofts.

Skinner, B. 1974. *About behaviorism*. New York: Alfred Knopf.

Sulzer-Azaroff, B. 1988. *Behavior analysis in education 1967–1987:* Reprint series, vol. 3. 25–47.

Tate, D., R. Wing, and R. Winnet. 2001. Using internet technology to deliver a behavioral weight loss program. *JAMA* 285: 1172–1177.

Telch, C., and E. Stice. 1998. Psychiatric comorbidity in women with binge eating disorder: Prevalence rates from a non-treatment seeking sample. *J Consult Clin Psychol* 66: 768–776.

Watson, D., and R. Tharp. 1993. *Self-directed behavior: Self-modification for personal adjustment* (6th ed.). Pacific Grove, CA: Brooks-Cole.

Wilfley, D., M. Friedman, J. Dounchis, R. Stein, R. Welch, and S. Ball. 2000. Comorbid psychopathology in binge eating disorder: Relation to eating disorder severity at baseline and following treatment. *J Consult Clin Psychol* 68: 641–649.

Wolpe, J. 1990. *The practice of behavior therapy* (4th ed.). Elmsford, NY: Pergamon Press.

Wylie-Rosett, J., C. Swencionis, and M. Ginsberg. 2001. Computerized weight loss intervention optimizes staff time. *J Am Dietic Assoc* 101: 1155–1162.

Yanovski, S. 2002. Binge eating in obese persons. In *Eating disorders and obesity: A comprehensive handbook*, ed. C. Fairburn & K. Browenell. New York: The Guilford Press.

Yates, B. T. 1986. *Applications in self-management*. Pacific Grove, CA: Brooks-Cole.

Yon, B., R. Johnson, and J. Harvey-Borino. 2007. Personal digital assistants are comparable to traditional diaries for dietary self-monitoring during a weight loss program. *J Behav Modif* 30: 165–175.

15 Social-Emotional Learning, Interpersonal Skills, and Resilience

Marilyn Massey-Stokes and Sean B. Stokes

CONTENTS

15.1 LEARNING OBJECTIVES

After completing this chapter, the reader will be able to

- Examine the connection between emotional vulnerabilities and eating disorders
- Examine the roles of emotional intelligence and social-emotional learning in eating disorder prevention and intervention
- Discuss how the inability to healthfully express emotions can contribute to eating disorders
- Explain how a practitioner can help a female with eating disturbances learn to express her emotions in appropriate, health-promoting ways
- Discuss how unhealthy communication patterns can contribute to eating disorders

- Examine how emotion management, adaptive coping strategies, and effective communication and conflict-resolution skills all work together to prevent eating disorders
- Examine how a practitioner can help females with eating disturbances learn to communicate more effectively
- Discuss protective factors for eating disorders
- Create strategies for developing resilience among girls

15.2 BACKGROUND AND SIGNIFICANCE

15.2.1 Emotional Vulnerabilities and Eating Disorders

According to the World Health Organization (WHO 2007, 1), mental health is defined as "a state of well-being in which the individual realizes his or her own abilities, can cope with the normal stresses of life, can work productively and fruitfully, and is able to make a contribution to his or her community." Thus, mental health provides "the foundation for well-being and effective functioning for an individual and for a community" (WHO 2007, 1). As part of the broad spectrum of mental health, it is essential that individuals learn how to identify and acknowledge their feelings and learn how to express their feelings appropriately. When negative emotions are blocked and not acknowledged, a person can experience anger, anxiety, frustration, and increased levels of perceived stress, thereby creating a negative mood. Furthermore, negative mood appears to interact with stress to increase preoccupation with food (Lingswiler et al. 1989). To try to avoid or cope with negative emotions and the perceived stress, young people may engage in self-destructive behaviors, including harmful dietary practices, such as self-starvation (Fox 2009; Nordbo et al. 2006), bingeing and purging, and binge eating (Eldredge and Agras 1996; Lingswiler et al. 1989; Masheb and Grilo 2006). Moreover, women with bulimia who have higher levels of perceived stress experience an increased urge to binge eat (Tuschen-Caffier and Vogele 1999). In addition, researchers have demonstrated that body dissatisfaction is inversely related to emotional expression (Geller et al. 2000, Hayaki et al. 2002, Ioannou and Fox 2009). Negative body image and body dissatisfaction have been linked to emotional distress, and studies have suggested that emotional vulnerabilities are among the salient predictors of eating disturbances (Connors 1996; Doll et al. 2005; Fox and Power 2009; Littleton and Ollendick 2003; Phares et al. 2004; Stice 2001).

Because eating disorders often present with comorbidities, such as depression and anxiety disorders, the exact relationship between eating disorders and emotions is unclear (Fox and Froom 2009). Nevertheless, researchers have investigated a wide array of psychological variables that appear to be linked with negative body image, body dissatisfaction, and the development of eating disturbances and clinical eating disorders. These variables include the following: (1) negative emotionality (Binford et al. 2004; Martin et al. 2000; Stice 2002); (2) emotional vulnerability and deficits in affect regulation (Corstorphine 2006; Fox 2009; Geller et al. 2000; Gilboa-Schechtman et al. 2006; Ioannou and Fox 2009); (3) avoidance of negative emotions (Nordbo et al. 2006; Schmidt and Treasure 2006); (4) lack of emotional awareness or poor emotional expression (Attie and Brooks-Gunn 1995; Gilboa-Schechtman et al. 2006; Ioannou and Fox 2009); (5) rigidity, compulsivity, and perfectionism (Schmidt and Treasure 2006; Treasure et al. 2008; Wonderlich 2002); (6) low self-esteem (Attie and Brooks-Gunn 1995; Geller et al. 2000; Shisslak and Crago 2001); (7) low self-efficacy (Attie and Brooks-Gunn 1995; Gilboa-Schechtman et al. 2006); (8) depression (Wall et al. 2008); (9) negative emotions, such as anger (Engel et al. 2007; Fox 2009; Fox and Froom 2009; Waller et al. 2003), fear (Fox and Power 2009; Harvey et al. 2002), anxiety (Pallister and Waller 2008; Schmidt and Treasure 2006; Waller 2008), disgust (Harvey et al. 2002), sadness (Fox and Froom 2009), and guilt, shame, and pride (Goss and Allan 2009; Goss and Gilbert 2002; Perkins et al. 2005); (10) rumination (Gilboa-Schechtman et al. 2006); (11) narcissism (Lawson et al. 2008); (12) impulsivity (Fernandiz-Aranda et al. 2008); and (13) poor coping styles (Beaumont 2002; Freeman and Gil 2004; García-Grau et al 2004).

Constricted or blocked expression of emotions can arise from one or more factors, including maladaptive coping styles, ineffective communication skills, insufficient emotional expression, and underdeveloped critical-thinking and creative problem-solving skills (Bowen 1976). For example, research has shown that fathers' psychological control was significantly associated with adolescents' poor emotional regulation and eating disorder symptoms (McEwen and Flouri 2009). Psychological control characterizes fathers "who are intrusive and overprotective, and who create a sense of dependency in children by constraining, invalidating, and manipulating children psychologically and emotionally" (Barber 1996, as cited in McEwen and Flouri 2009, 207). In another study involving patients with anorexia in an inpatient setting, some of the patients indicated that their fathers could not discuss anything emotional (Fox 2009). In addition, Fox (2009, 287) found that participants came from families exhibiting "poverty of emotional environments" where either low levels of emotion were expressed or emotional expression was denied. Interestingly, some participants had difficulty describing the emotional environment they experienced growing up, which is illustrated by the following comment:

> I don't think that emotions weren't something what we talked about really, they're not, it was just like, it was something we didn't talk about really, we don't talk things through we just, if you've got any problems just keep them to yourself kind of thing.

15.2.2 Emotion Management and Coping

Difficulties in emotional processing have been identified as particularly challenging for individuals with eating disorders (Fox 2009; Fox and Power 2009; Geller et al. 2000; Gilboa-Schechtman et al. 2006; Ioannou and Fox 2009). Some research has indicated that eating disorders develop, in part, as an escape from emotional distress, for instance, through maladaptive stress management and skewed self-awareness (Corstorphine 2006; Fox and Power 2009; Gilboa-Schechtman et al. 2006). In a study involving structured interviews with women diagnosed with anorexia nervosa, participants revealed deficits in meta-emotional skills, characterized by a lack of skill in managing their own emotions, particularly anger and sadness. They also tended to avoid conflict, even if it required suppressing their own views and needs (Fox 2009). Other studies have shown that women with eating disorders possess low self-efficacy in their ability to regulate their emotions and improve their mood (Gilboa-Schechtman et al. 2006; Ioannou and Fox 2009). There also appears to be a link between eating disorders, narcissism, and poor emotional awareness, including a lack of empathy (Lawson et al. 2008).

Within families where eating disorders are present, studies have revealed that parental support, empathy, and nurturance are often lacking, and expression of feelings is rarely encouraged (Connors 1996; Loth et al. 2009; Minuchin et al. 1978). Lack of emotion skills within an individual appears to be related to a lack of familial modeling of good emotion skills, thereby creating "emotional confusion, overcontrol of emotions and the use of eating disorder to express emotions" (Fox 2009, 294). This finding corresponds with research suggesting that invalidating family environments that squelch the expression of negative emotions (e.g., anger and sadness) and encourage the expression of positive emotions (e.g., happiness) can create an emotional disconnect (Corstorphine 2006).

In conjunction with emotional disconnect, body dissatisfaction appears to be inversely related to emotional expression (Fox and Power 2009; Ioannou and Fox 2009). According to Geller et al. (2000), unexpressed and particularly negative emotions can be displaced onto the body, resulting in body dissatisfaction and disordered eating behaviors, both of which an individual perceives to have control. For example, research has shown that emotional overeating is connected to the frequency of binge episodes and disinhibition among individuals with binge-eating disorder (Arnow et al. 1995; Lingswiler et al. 1989; Masheb and Grilo 2006). Binge eating also appears to be used to regulate negative emotions (Wright and Blanks 2008). Additionally, in a study of young women who were being treated for anorexia nervosa in a treatment facility, the participants said they did not know how to articulate their problems to family and friends, nor did they feel understood by people around them. They emphasized the desire to change their interpersonal relationships so that their friends and family members could better understand their personal difficulties (Nordbo et al. 2006). In another study of individuals receiving treatment for eating disorders (Loth et al. 2009), patients emphasized the importance of encouraging the discussion and expression of emotions within the family, as well as the importance of teaching children constructive coping skills to handle strong emotions. They also emphasized the importance of parental support, particularly during difficult life transitions, and teaching children how to appropriately love and support themselves when the parents were absent (Loth et al. 2009).

15.2.2.1 Coping Styles

Coinciding with emotion management is the ability to adopt healthy coping styles. Studies have suggested that women with anorexia or bulimia as well as those with eating disorder symptoms tend to use maladaptive coping strategies, such as avoiding problems or using ineffective emotional coping (García-Grau et al. 2004). Ineffective emotional coping is displayed in a variety of ways, including engaging in self-harm (e.g., cutting), bingeing and purging, hoarding food but not eating it, bottling up emotions, and engaging in substance abuse. In addition, eating disorder patients who exhibit more stress tend to have poorer outcomes (Miller et al. 2003). For example, eating-disordered patients with higher cortisol levels had poorer outcomes on 1- and 2-year follow-up assessments of body weight and psychological functioning when compared to patients with lower cortisol levels (Steiner and Levine 1985, as cited in Miller et al. 2003). However, there is very little research analyzing the relationships between coping styles and eating disorders among younger girls (García-Grau et al. 2004). The coping response is important because "how individuals experience and cope with stress affects whether and how they will seek medical care and social support, and how well they adhere to health professionals' advice" (Glanz and Schwartz 2008, 212).

15.3 CURRENT FINDINGS

15.3.1 COPING WITH EMOTIONS

Although there is much to understand about the relationships among emotions, emotion management, coping styles, and eating disorder symptoms, those struggling with eating disorders can learn how to cope with their emotions and reduce their perceived stress. Cook-Cottone and Beck (2008) asserted that an eating disorder treatment program should include an interpersonal component to address interpersonal difficulties, such as articulating emotions, emotional regulation, being assertive, and setting appropriate boundaries within relationships. For example, Bjork and Ahlstrom's (2008, 937) study of eating disorder patients who were in recovery revealed that these individuals had learned how to recognize and accept different emotions and were able to find ways to handle difficult feelings without blaming themselves or engaging in self-harm. As one participant stated, "I allow myself to be sad. I cry, and there's nothing dangerous about being sad anymore. There's that strong emotion and it's not dangerous because it doesn't have to be my fault. There doesn't have to be anything wrong with me because I feel sad." In addition, participants learned how to accept and value themselves for their individuality. Plus, they developed "a positive emotional relationship to themselves [that] diminished the stress of trying to please others as well as achievement anxiety" (Bjork and Ahlstrom 2008, 940). They also learned how to set healthy boundaries, which, in turn, promoted their self-respect and helped them develop assertiveness and resilience.

15.3.2   Emotional Intelligence and Social-Emotional Learning

Emotional intelligence and social-emotional learning are foundational for emotion management and coping and therefore play a significant role in the prevention and management of eating disturbances and clinical eating disorders.

15.3.2.1   Emotional Intelligence

Emotional intelligence is a unique and essential intelligence that encompasses a set of social-emotional competencies that is critically important to health and quality of life. Emotional intelligence can play a salient role in individual resilience and prevention of eating disorders. Salovey et al. (1999) articulated emotional intelligence as involving the ability to monitor one's own feelings and emotions as well as other people's feelings and emotions. Additionally, emotional intelligence involves the ability to regulate these feelings and emotions, and use emotion-based information to guide thinking and action. The competencies involved in emotional intelligence include the following: (1) appraising and expressing emotions in self and others, (2) assimilating emotion and thought, (3) understanding and analyzing emotions, and (4) regulating emotions to promote emotional and intellectual growth (Salovey et al. 1999). Goleman (1995) asserted that fostering emotional intelligence begins in the early years, and opportunities for further development of these competencies should continue throughout the school years. He also viewed emotional intelligence and emotional literacy as preventative and called for schools to become caring communities that teach essential social-emotional skills to youth.

15.3.2.2   Social-Emotional Learning

The Collaborative for Academic, Social, and Emotional Learning (CASEL 2010a) was established to promote social and emotional learning as an essential aspect of success in school and lifelong learning. CASEL (2010b) has identified five core categories of social and emotional competencies that comprise social-emotional learning:

- **Self-awareness**—accurately assessing one's feelings, interests, values, and strengths; maintaining a well-grounded sense of self-confidence.
- **Self-management**—regulating one's emotions to handle stress, control impulses, and persevere in overcoming obstacles; setting and monitoring progress toward personal and academic goals; expressing emotions appropriately.
- **Social awareness**—being able to take the perspective of and empathize with others; recognizing and appreciating individual and group similarities and differences; recognizing and using family, school, and community resources.
- **Relationship skills**—establishing and maintaining healthy and rewarding relationships based on cooperation; resisting inappropriate social pressure; preventing, managing, and resolving interpersonal conflict; seeking help when needed.
- **Responsible decision-making**—making decisions based on consideration of ethical standards, safety concerns, appropriate social norms, respect for others, and likely consequences of various actions; applying decision-making skills to academic and social situations; contributing to the well-being of one's school and community.

Studies have demonstrated that social-emotional learning competencies are essential for life effectiveness and that social-emotional learning has a positive effect on emotional health as well as interpersonal relationships (Durlak and Weissberg 2010; Magee and Perkins 2010). In addition, social-emotional interventions have been shown to decrease health and social development risks and foster protective competencies among youth (CASEL 2003; Durlak and Wells 1998). According to Durlak and Weissberg (2010), young people's social-emotional development is related to their academic development; therefore, promoting social-emotional development can lead to positive outcomes, such as increased positive behaviors and academic performance as well as decreased negative behaviors and emotional distress. Although social-emotional learning studies have not specifically addressed body image and eating disorders, Massey-Stokes (2008, 71) asserted that positive youth development, which promotes multiple health-enhancing competencies, including social-emotional learning, "can be considered a viable framework for promoting healthy body image and preventing eating disturbances among children and adolescents."

15.3.2.3 Self-Awareness and Self-Management of Emotions

As part of the spectrum of emotional intelligence and social-emotional learning, it is important to help preadolescent and adolescent females learn to identify and accept their full range of feelings and learn how to deal with self-defeating, perfectionistic tendencies. In doing so, they can begin to develop a sense of personal power that is conducive to psychological health (Geller et al. 2000). Becvar and Becvar (1997, 123–126) suggested the following guidelines for more effectively managing feelings:

- There are no good feelings and no bad feelings. Feelings just "are." For example, a driver may become angry if she is cut off by another driver in rush-hour traffic. A typical response would be, "That makes me so angry, but I need to try to settle down and not let my anger get the best of me." Or, a person who has experienced abuse feels anger, which is a natural response that is expected and encouraged. For the same emotion (anger), one expression is labeled "bad" and one is labeled "good." In reality, a person simply feels what she feels in reaction to the circumstances.
- Whatever a person is feeling, it is appropriate for her to feel as she does given her experience and her interpretation of this experience. How a person views the world based on her experiences and interpretation of those experiences will influence how she feels. For one person, a particular situation may mean one thing; whereas for another person, the same or similar situation may mean something different based on life experiences, beliefs, etc.
- Feelings can and do change if the interpretation of events changes. In order for a change in interpretation to occur, a person must consciously choose to suspend her interpretation of an event and open herself up to another person's view of the event. In doing so, a person is able to potentially see events from another frame of reference, thereby opening up additional interpretations of an event. Consequently, when a person is able to see multiple possible interpretations of an event, her feelings about the event will change.
- While feelings are not subject to conscious control, a person still has a choice about what she **does** [emphasis added] with those feelings. There will be times when a person acts as if she feels a certain way even when she does not. For example, a person cleans the kitchen even when she does not "feel like" cleaning the kitchen. Another example is that many college students make the choice to study even when they do not "feel like" studying, which pays off in better grades and higher performance than peers who simply let the feeling of "not wanting to study" dictate their actions. An additional way of viewing this guideline is that even though an individual may feel angry, that person has a choice about what to do with that anger (e.g., suppress it or express it in a healthy, appropriate way).

15.3.2.4 Ecological Approach to Address Emotion Management and Coping

Self-awareness and self-management of emotions can be addressed through an ecological approach that recognizes how various factors influence health behaviors, such as intrapersonal experiences, interpersonal interactions, organizational factors, community influences, and public policies (Sallis et al. 2008). In this context, at the intrapersonal or individual level, girls can learn how to recognize their emotions and express these emotions in ways that are health-promoting and not self-defeating. They also can learn a variety of coping skills, including effective ways to cope with negative and often overwhelming emotions, by using a variety of techniques, such as journal writing, relaxation training, and prayer or meditation. In addition, at the interpersonal level, licensed professional counselors or therapists can work with families to strengthen parenting and communication skills and foster stress management and coping skills. At the institutional or organizational level, schools can implement skills-based training, prevention programs, and support groups. They also can provide positive psychosocial influences by promoting prosocial behaviors; creating a culture of caring, acceptance, and belonging; and firmly enforcing zero-tolerance policies regarding teasing and other bullying behaviors. Other factors that influence mental and physical health within the context of eating disorder prevention are discussed in more detail in the following sections of this chapter.

15.3.3 INTERPERSONAL SKILLS

Healthy interpersonal relationships are foundational to health and well-being, and effective interpersonal skills are necessary to establish and maintain quality interpersonal relationships. Research has suggested that individuals "who maintain strong social relationships are healthier and live longer" (Heaney and Israel 2008, 207). Conversely, underdeveloped or poor interpersonal skills can prevent the development of quality interpersonal relationships, which, in turn, can negatively affect a person's quality of life.

According to Johnson (2006), interpersonal skills are measured by one's ability to effectively interact with others and encompass the following abilities and actions:

- Building trust between self and others—Friendships and other significant relationships require a high level of trust. Trust is increased when a person takes a risk to act in a trusting way, and the other person responds in a trustworthy manner.
- Effectively communicating thoughts, ideas, and feelings—Interpersonal communication involves both sending and receiving messages. Effective communication occurs when the receiver of the message (listener) interprets the message the way the sender (speaker) intended.
- Effectively communicating both verbally and nonverbally—It is important to ensure that verbal and nonverbal messages match. Nonverbal messages are more powerful, yet they also are more difficult to interpret. Examples of nonverbal communication include posture, body tension, facial expression, degree of eye contact, hand and body movements, tone of voice, spatial distance, and touch.
- Listening actively and empathically—It is important to listen with undivided attention and strive to understand the message. An active and empathic listener should be able to accurately paraphrase the speaker's message.
- Providing appropriate self-disclosure—Revealing thoughts and perceptions as well as information about oneself requires self-awareness, self-acceptance, and trust in the other person.
- Resolving conflicts constructively—Negotiation is the most important and most difficult strategy for effectively resolving conflict. Negotiation is a process by which people work together to arrive at a mutually acceptable solution to a problem.
- Constructively managing stress and anger—Stress is unavoidable; therefore, it is essential to have a variety of stress management strategies to employ, particularly garncring social support. Anger needs to be dealt with in a constructive manner, such as describing the other person's actions and the angry feelings that resulted from those actions. It also is important engage in self-management strategies in order to stay calm.
- Valuing diversity in people—It is important to recognize diversity and build cooperative relationships with diverse individuals based upon mutual respect.

For more information about interpersonal effectiveness, see Johnson (2006).

15.3.3.1 Communication Skills

Communication is a dynamic process in which "individuals create, send, receive, and interpret messages simultaneously" (Johnson 2006, 124). Communication is a learned skill—a process by which one develops the ability to clearly express thoughts, ideas, feelings, beliefs, opinions, reactions, values, hopes, and dreams. Strong communication skills are a requisite to psychosocial health and are essential for interpersonal-relationship growth and resilience. Communication skills can also serve as a protective factor against body dissatisfaction, low self-esteem, and depression (Ackard et al. 2006). Effective communication encompasses multiple competencies for both sending and receiving messages. According to Johnson (2006), effectively sending messages includes the following steps:

- Clearly "own" your message by using personal pronouns (e.g., *I, me, my*) and expressing your thoughts and feelings to the receiver (i.e., use "I" statements). This entails speaking for oneself, and avoiding the use of generalities. Saying, "I feel ..." is much more direct and effective than saying, "Some people feel ..." or "A lot of people feel ... ." For example, it is more effective to say, "I feel disrespected when you interrupt me" rather than to say, "You know, a lot of people might feel disrespected if you interrupted them."
- Describe the receiver's behavior without using judgmental or evaluative terms. When a person uses judgmental or evaluative terms, it is possible that the receiver will feel invalidated. It is much more effective to say, "You keep ignoring me" rather than "You never listen to anyone because all you care about is yourself. You are so selfish."
- Make the message relevant to the receiver's frame of reference.
- Ask for feedback regarding how the receiver is interpreting your message. One of the easiest means of accomplishing this is to ask the receiver to paraphrase back what she heard. Once the receiver paraphrases what she has heard, the speaker has the opportunity to either confirm that the receiver heard correctly or to correct any misinterpretations.
- Describe your feelings by name, action, or figure of speech (e.g., *I feel angry*, *I feel like screaming*, or *I feel like pounding my fist into the wall*).
- Use appropriate nonverbal messages to help communicate your feelings.
- Ensure that your verbal and nonverbal messages are congruent. The receiver of a message will have a hard time discerning the actual message if the sender's words say one thing, but the nonverbal language says something different. For example, saying, "I get so angry when that happens" while smiling or chuckling creates an incongruent message.
- The process of receiving a message is of utmost importance as well—how a person listens and responds to another person is foundational to the communication process and the formation of a quality relationship (Gordon 2000; Johnson 2006). Markman et al. (1994) posited that everybody has "filters" that influence both what and how they hear a message. These filters influence whether a person will negatively internalize a message or positively internalize a message. The poorer one's self-image, the more likely it is that she will internalize a negative message, even if the sender did not intend to send a negative message.

15.3.3.1.1 Active Listening

The ability to effectively listen and respond appropriately is a buffer against eating disorders as well as an essential factor in the recovery process for those who have an eating disorder (Loth et al. 2009; Nordbo et al. 2006). One of the most effective "receiving" communication techniques is active listening, which requires the receiver of the message to truly seek to understand the perspective of the sender. Using her own words, the receiver relays the message back to the sender without evaluation, opinion, or advice. Phrased a different way, the receiver "feeds back *only what he feels the sender's message meant*—nothing more, nothing less" (Gordon 2000, 62).

15.3.3.1.2 Empathic Listening

A related concept is empathic listening, which is a critically important principle of effective interpersonal communication. Covey (1989, 240–241) described empathic listening as a unique paradigm that involves "listening with intent to *understand*." He explained that most of us listen at one of four levels: (1) we may ignore the person and not listen at all; (2) we may pretend to listen; (3) we may engage in selective listening by hearing only certain aspects of the conversation; or (4) we may practice attentive listening and pay attention to what is said by focusing on the speaker's words. However, few people practice the fifth level, which is empathic listening:

> Empathic (from empathy) listening gets inside another person's frame of reference. You look out through it, you see the world the way they see the world, you understand their paradigm, you understand how they feel. … The essence of empathic listening is not that you agree with someone; it's that you fully, deeply, understand that person, emotionally as well as intellectually … . Next to physiological survival, the greatest need of a human being is psychological survival—to be understood, to be affirmed, to be validated, to be appreciated … . When you listen with empathy to another person, you give that person psychological air. And after that vital need is met, you can then focus on influencing or problem solving. This need for psychological air impacts communication in every area of life.

Individuals with eating disorders can benefit from empathic listening because they often feel the need for permission to express their emotions. They also highly value having someone they can trust and with whom they can discuss their feelings (Fox 2009). Therefore, empathic listening can be an effective component for individual and family approaches to eating disorder prevention and intervention.

15.3.3.1.3 Nonverbal Communication

An estimated 65% to 93% of the social meaning of conversations is transferred through nonverbal messages (Ketrow 1999). Nonverbal communication encompasses a variety of factors, including body posture, body tension, facial expression, eye contact, hand and body movements, tone of voice, spatial distance, touch, and even mode of dress (Johnson 2006). According to Wertheim (2010), nonverbal communication cues can play five roles: (1) repetition—they may repeat a verbal message; (2) contradiction—they may contradict a verbal message; (3) substitution—they may substitute for a verbal message; (4) complementing—they may add to or complement a verbal message; and (5) accenting—they may emphasize a verbal message. In addition, nonverbal communication plays an instrumental role in interpersonal relationships. For example, in using nonverbal messages, a woman communicates how she feels about another person, how she feels about herself, and how she feels about the relationship (Johnson 2006). Therefore, in order to interact more effectively with others, it is important to learn how to interpret nonverbal communication. This excerpt from a U.S. Federal Emergency Management Agency (FEMA) training resource helps to illustrate this point: "By reading your listener, you can gather real-time feedback that tells you whether or not you are communicating successfully. If your message is not getting through, maybe you need to adjust *your* nonverbal broadcast" (FEMA 2010).

For effective communication to occur, the sender of the message needs to ensure that there is congruence between verbal and nonverbal messages (Gordon 2000; Johnson 2006; Markman et al. 1994). Otherwise, a mixed message is sent, which can create confusion, frustration, and anxiety for the receiver. Therefore, a person must be cognizant of the nonverbal messages that she is sending and also have the ability to decode the nonverbal messages that she is receiving in order to effectively communicate with others. Furthermore, it is important to keep in mind that nonverbal communication cues can substantially differ across cultures (FEMA 2005; Johnson 2006; Wertheim 2010). Direct eye contact, touching while speaking, and personal space have meanings that are culture specific (FEMA 2005); thus, it is important to remain culturally relevant so that clear communication can take place.

15.3.3.2 Communication Barriers

Just as effective communication enhances interpersonal relationships, communication barriers often interfere with the transference of a message, and as a result, can hinder the communication process and damage interpersonal relationships. Examples of common communication roadblocks (Markman et al. 1994; Wertheim 2010) include the following:

- Mental-emotional state of people communicating
- Different perceptions concerning the language and words that are used
- Cultural differences
- Personal biases
- Defensiveness and/or distorted perceptions
- Misinterpreting nonverbal cues
- Power struggles
- Assumptions
- Insufficient time set aside for discussing an issue
- The use of "you" statements (as opposed to "I" statements)
- The use of broad generalizations (e.g., *You always ...* or *You never ...*)
- Failure to actively listen

For more information, see Markman et al. 1994.

15.3.3.3 Conflict Resolution

Although conflict is a normal aspect of family relationships, when it is not effectively resolved, conflict tends to escalate and contribute to family dysfunction. Conflict is often heightened when a family member does not communicate effectively or when that person grows up in a family that is invalidating and constricting, and subsequently ignores the communication of emotion or reacts negatively to expressed emotion (Corstorphine 2006). Research has shown that lack of open communication and effective conflict resolution between father and daughter can lead to increased eating-disordered behaviors. For example, increased conflict and inadequate communication skills to resolve conflict may result in bulimic behaviors, such as binge eating and purging cycles, whereas a sense of lack of control over conflict may lead to lack of eating among those with anorexia. In addition, those with anorexia may react differently to conflict than those with bulimia, and these reactions may be totally different from the reactions of those without eating disorders (Botta and Dumlao 2002).

Effective conflict resolution requires a plethora of skills, including direct expression of feelings, effective communication, empathy (including empathic listening), anger management, problem solving, and negotiation (Becvar and Becvar 1997; Covey 1989; Johnson 2006; Markman et al. 1994). Johnson (2006) emphasized the importance of "problem-solving negotiations" and "integrative solutions" in order to maximize joint benefits, strengthen the relationship between parties, and improve the ability of both parties to constructively resolve future conflicts. Furthermore, possessing conflict-resolution skills may prevent young women with a strong drive for thinness from engaging in more frequent bulimic behaviors (Botta and Dumlao 2002).

The ability to effectively communicate and engage in skillful conflict resolution are important skills that link with the development of positive self-esteem, which is considered to be a buffer against poor body image, eating disturbances, and eating disorders (O'Dea 2007). One helpful activity is the Speaker-Listener Technique (Markman et al. 1994), which offers an alternative mode of communication when issues are hot or sensitive and therefore can be useful for resolving conflict. This technique allows two people to work through conflict by allowing each person the opportunity to be the speaker and the listener. There are rules to follow so that each person has a fair turn at speaking. For example, when the person is the speaker, she keeps statements brief and then stops to let the listener paraphrase. The listener focuses on the speaker's message without forming a rebuttal, and then paraphrases what she hears back to the speaker. For more information about this effective communication technique, see Markman et al. (1994). For additional exercises to help an individual develop more effective conflict-resolution skills, refer to Becvar and Becvar (1997), Gordon (2000), and Johnson (2006).

15.3.3.4 Familial Interaction and Communication

The biopsychosocial perspective posits that there are multiple pathways for the development and maintenance of eating disorders that include complex interactions among biological, psychological, sociocultural, and familial factors (Lemmons and Josephson 2001). In line with the biopsychosocial perspective, family factors, such as enmeshment, closed communication, low emotional expression, high levels of stress and conflict, and poor coping skills, can play a role in the onset and maintenance of eating disorders (Le Grange et al. 2009; Minuchin et al. 1978; Polivy and Herman 2002; Tantillo 2006; Vidović et al. 2005); however, the evidence is clear that family factors interact with other important factors, such as individual characteristics and environmental and sociocultural factors, to create vulnerability to eating disorders (Polivy and Herman 2002). An important component of family functioning is communication, which includes the capacity to listen, show mutual respect, and clearly articulate thoughts and feelings (Vidović et al. 2005). In a healthy family system, expression of boundaries, feelings, and needs are encouraged. Additionally, communication is open, and individual growth is fostered. In contrast, within a dysfunctional family system, rules are rigid, communication is closed or strained, and individual growth is stifled (Minuchin et al. 1978).

Adolescents who perceive low levels of family communication, parental expectations, and parental caring and support appear to be at heightened risk for experiencing body dissatisfaction, low self-esteem, and depression (Ackard et al. 2006) and developing eating disorders (Haudek et al. 1999; Lemmons and Josephson 2001; Wade et al. 2006). Research has shown that individuals with eating disturbances often come from families with less open family communication (Miller-Day and Marks 2006; Minuchin et al. 1978). Minuchin et al. (1978) described anorexia nervosa as a disorder reflecting familial dysfunction, particularly characterized by enmeshment, rigidity, overprotection, conflict avoidance, and lack of problem-solving abilities. Within families where anorexia nervosa is present, direct communication is often blocked and conflict is avoided. As a result, problems usually are left unresolved and continue to resurface (Minuchin et al. 1978). In addition, bulimic patients and patients with the bulimic form of anorexia reported more communication difficulties and less cohesion and adaptability within their families than did patients with the restricted form of anorexia (Vidović et al. 2005). Additionally, there is evidence that families of individuals with eating disorders have higher rates of alcoholism, affective disorders, and controlling, conflictual relationships (McGrane and Carr 2002; Vandereycken 2002).

Communication patterns that are learned and practiced within the family are often carried forward into other relationships (Becvar and Becvar 1994; Bowen 1976; Minuchin et al. 1978). In the context of family-of-origin relational processes, Miller-Day and Marks (2006) identified two basic family communication patterns—*conformity* orientation (*closed* communication) and *conversation* orientation (*open* communication). Conformity orientation or closed communication occurs when the flow of information and opinions among family members is tightly controlled, and parental power and control are emphasized. In contrast, conversation orientation or open communication is characterized by a supportive family atmosphere where there is open flow of the exchange of information and opinions, parental beliefs can be challenged, and children can seek out solutions to issues (Booth-Butterfield and Sidelinger 1998; Ritchie 1991, as cited in Miller-Day and Marks 2006). In a large sample of college students, Miller-Day and Marks (2006, 159) found a significant association between father–offspring communication and maladaptive eating. More specifically, "perceptions of fathers as having a conformity orientation was positively associated with maladaptive eating, whereas perceptions of fathers as having a conversation orientation was negatively associated." Botta and Dumlao (2002) reported similar findings, while other studies have also pointed to poor communication with the mother as contributing to eating disturbances (Moreno et al. 2000; Casper and Troiani 2001).

Lemmons and Josephson (2001) summarized the key factors that are generally involved in impaired interactions and deficient communication within families where an eating disorder exists:

- Enmeshment and triangulation
- Overindulgence and overprotectiveness
- Distrust among family members
- Independence/dependence conflict
- Inadequate affective expressions
- Lack of emotional support
- Undefined boundaries
- Rigidity
- Chaotic family environment
- Lack of parental consistency in expectations and consequences
- Poor conflict resolution
- Confusion about family members' roles and responsibilities

Despite agreement that familial factors contribute to the development and maintenance of eating disorders, there is disagreement regarding the exact role of the family in the development and maintenance of eating disorders. Although the Academy for Eating Disorders (Le Grange et al. 2009, 1) acknowledges that family factors can play a role in the development and maintenance of eating disorders, it "stands firmly against any etiologic model of eating disorders in which family influences are seen as the primary cause of anorexia nervosa or bulimia nervosa, and condemns generalizing statements that imply families are to blame for their child's illness." In addition, prospective studies that tested the role of dysfunctional family systems and the lack of parental affection failed to show a relationship between these factors and the onset of eating pathology (Stice 2002). Nevertheless, it is important to point out that reciprocity exists between family function and eating disorders. Maladaptive family dynamics and communication may be a response to the eating disorder rather than a contributor of the problem (Lemmon and Josephson 2001; Stern et al. 1989; Ward et al. 2000, as cited in Polivy and Herman 2002). Then, too, family dysfunction and communication difficulties may intensify eating disorders, but an individual's recovery from an eating disorder may decrease family dysfunction (Steinberg and Phares 2001). Treasure et al. (2008) pointed out that a family's emotional reactions to eating disorder symptoms may play a role in maintaining the problem because the family may forget about their assets and strengths, especially as they become embroiled in interpersonal conflict. Conversely, families who recognize their unique assets and work together to improve familial communication and enhance their relationships can learn to function in a healthier manner. Moreover, as part of a comprehensive approach for treating an eating disorder, a variety of strategies can be employed, including enhancing communication skills and strengthening problem-solving and coping skills in both the individual and in the family (Freeman and Gil 2004; Lemmon and Josephson 2001; Sokol et al. 2005; Tantillo 2006; Treasure et al. 2007; Uehara et al. 2001).

15.3.4 RESILIENCE

Resilience is the "capacity to bounce back, to withstand hardship and repair yourself" (Wolin and Wolin 1993, 5). It also has been described is as a "process of self-righting and growth" (Higgins 1994, 1). Brooks and Goldstein (2001, 1) asserted that "resilience embraces the ability of a child to deal more effectively with stress and pressure, to cope with everyday challenges, to bounce back from disappointments, adversity, and trauma, to develop clear and realistic goals, to solve problems, to relate comfortably with others, and to treat oneself and others with respect." Resilience varies from person to person and can grow and diminish over time, depending upon the balance between risk and protective factors (Henderson and Milstein 1996) and growth and development (Shisslak and Crago 2001). It is important to note that resilience is not a particular character trait that only a select group of children possess. Rather, "resilience is itself normative" (Benard 2004, 9). Therefore, all children have the capacity to be resilient, even those who are faced with difficult challenges, such as eating disorders. As Masten (1994, 9) articulated: "What began as a quest to understand the extraordinary has revealed the power of the ordinary. Resilience does not come from rare and special qualities, but from the everyday magic of ordinary, normative human resources in the minds, brains, and bodies of children, in their families and relationships, and in the communities."

According to Brown and Gilligan (1992, 2), the "edge of adolescence has been identified as a time of heightened psychological risk for girls." Some of the behavioral and psychological health threats that girls face include depression, sexual abuse, suicide, tobacco use, alcohol and other drug use, injury and violence, sexually transmitted diseases and pregnancy, and eating disturbances and eating disorders (Ackard and Neumark-Sztainer 2001; Centers for Disease Control and Prevention 2010; Marcotte et al. 2002). Beginning with this developmental period, girls sometimes lose their resilience and sense of self, which also can make them more likely to experience disconnection from others (Brown and Gilligan 1992). Furthermore, the stress and illness arising out of eating disorders can put family members at increased risk for disconnection, which can involve low self-worth, disempowerment, increased isolation, an inability to tolerate differences, and feelings of tension, doubt, and confusion (Tantillo 2006). Therefore, increasing resilience among girls is important in preventing eating disorders and other problems and promoting wellness and quality of life.

15.3.4.1 Protective Factors

Despite vast research on risk factors associated with eating disorders (see Chapters 1 and 2 of this book), there is little research regarding protective factors and how they may buffer individuals against developing eating disturbances and clinical eating disorders (Cordero and Israel 2009; Shisslak and Crago 2001; Steiner et al. 2003). The primary protective factor that has received the most empirical support is positive family relationships (Ackard et al. 2006; Littleton and Ollendick 2003; Miller-Day and Marks 2006). Other *familial* protective factors that have been considered include: positive comments from parents and parental restraint in referring to children's physical appearance (Connors 1996; Cordero and Israel 2009; Rodgers and Chabrol 2009; Rodgers et al. 2009; Rodin et al. 1990), adaptive problem solving (Drummond et al. 2005), effective communication (Botta and Dumlao 2002; Drummond et al. 2005; Miller-Day and Marks 2006), familial modeling of health-promoting behavioral patterns (Loth et al. 2009), living in a family where parents do not misuse alcohol (Chandy et al. 1995), and social support from the family (Berndt and Hestenes 1996; Stice 2002).

With regard to *individual* factors, research has suggested that the following help protect against the development of eating disorders: self-acceptance (Wertheim et al. 1997), self-directedness and assertiveness (Rodin et al. 1990), the ability to effectively cope with life stressors (Rodin at al. 1990; Striegel-Moore and Cachelin 1999), high self-esteem (Kater 2005; O'Dea 2007; Shisslak and Crago 2001), self-efficacy (Wiser and Telch 1999), and knowledge about the hazards of dieting (Kater 2005; O'Dea 2007; Wertheim et al. 1997). Parents, teachers, and practitioners can help inoculate girls against eating disorders by valuing them for who they are on the inside, teaching them to assume self-responsibility and exert assertiveness, teaching and modeling healthy coping skills, fostering self-esteem and self-efficacy, and talking with them about the negative health effects of dieting.

15.3.4.1.1 Self-Esteem

Within the spectrum of plausible individual protective factors related to eating disorders, self-esteem has been the subject of several studies (e.g., Kater 2005; O'Dea 2007; Shisslak and Crago 2001). Self-esteem encompasses how the individual perceives the self. If individuals have high self-esteem, they experience positive emotions about themselves; conversely, if they have low self-esteem, they experience negative emotions about themselves (Drench et al. 2007). Low self-esteem has been shown to be a contributing factor to body image and eating problems (Kater 2005; O'Dea 2007; Shisslak and Crago 2001; Stice 2002) as well as other problems in adolescence, such as depression, anxiety, and substance abuse (Kelly et al. 2005; Killen et al. 1987). Therefore, the development of positive self-esteem and self-acceptance has been the focus of numerous interventions targeting eating disorder prevention (Kater et al. 2005; McVey et al. 2003, 2004; Neumark-Sztainer et al. 2000; O'Dea 2007; O'Dea and Abraham 2000). However, the exact relationship between self-esteem and eating problems remains complex (Cordero and Israel 2009). For a more complete discussion of both risk and protective factors that affect the development of eating disorders, see Shisslak and Crago (2001) and Stice (2002).

15.3.4.1.2 Growth-Fostering Relationships

Growth-fostering relationships are another critical aspect of fostering resilience and helping girls navigate through preadolescence and adolescence. Resilience research has consistently shown that children and adolescents who have supportive and caring relationships with at least one adult in the community deal more effectively with life events, including severe hardship (Benard 2004). Benard (2004, 109) described the power that accompanies the responsibility of adults who act as "turn-around people for youth":

> In our relationships with young people, we have the power and responsibility to provide the critical supports and opportunities that build resilience strengths. At the same time, we have the power to undermine those inner characteristics. At our best, we can honor the incredible developmental wisdom that propels a young person to seek love and belonging, respect, mastery, challenge, and meaning. We can nurture a youth's innate potential for social competence, problem-solving autonomy, and hope—as models ourselves and by guiding a young person to experience these inner qualities within her own self. Conversely, we can squander the power of our relationship with a young person. We don't have to be perfect, but we do have to be mindful of our immense power, for good or ill.

Similarly, Relational-Cultural Theory (RCT) posits that growth-fostering relationships are critical in promoting the psychological and social-relational health of girls (Jordan et al. 1991, Jordan and Hartling 2002). RCT asserts that individuals need to be in connection with others to transform, heal, and grow (Jordan and Hartling 2002). According to Steese et al. (2006, 56) the "essential mechanisms of healthy connections include the capacity to voice experience honestly and to receive attentive, empathic listening." When empathic interaction is reciprocal, perceived social support increases, which in turn strengthens connections with others (Steese et al. 2006). These relationships and opportunities for communication and connection can occur on different levels, such as individual, interpersonal (e.g., family and peers), community, and even the broader sociocultural level (Jordan and Hartling 2002; Miller-Day and Marks 2006). Within this ecological perspective, it is important to identify "points of tension and disconnection related to the eating disorder and recovery and developing ways to move into better connection with one another" (Tantillo 2006, 94).

15.3.4.2 School- and Community-Based Programs

Schools and other community settings provide other avenues for growth-fostering relationships and empathic interactions. Research has shown that programs designed to foster resilience and build healthy relationships among girls can have a positive effect on body image. For example, an intervention called Girls Circle (Girls Circle 2010) is a unique program that is based on RCT and addresses key relational needs of girls by increasing opportunities for social connection, building empathic skills, and fostering resilience (Steese et al. 2006). An evaluation study of Girls Circle found that the program significantly increased perceived social support, self-efficacy, and perceived body image (Steese et al. 2006). Furthermore, findings from the Girls Circle National Research Project revealed statistically significant gains in self-efficacy, positive body image, and attachment to school as well as statistically significant decreases in self-harming behavior and alcohol use (Roa et al. 2007).

Girls in Motion® (Golman 2009) is another primary prevention program that employs concepts from RCT and Social Cognitive Theory (Bandura 1986). Golman (2009) reported that Girls in Motion® succeeded in reducing body dissatisfaction and drive for thinness among the preadolescent participants, which paralleled findings from other studies (O'Dea and Abraham 2000; Paxton 2002; Scime et al. 2006; Steiner-Adair et al. 2002). In addition, *Inside/Outside Self-Discovery for Teens* (Feinberg-Walker et al. 2009, 11) is a theoretically based prevention program "designed to enhance self-esteem, strengthen protective factors that promote resiliency, and facilitate mutually supportive peer relationships in early adolescent girls." The curriculum also contains suggestions regarding how to modify the lessons for use in mixed-gender settings, such as public schools. See Appendix 15.A for an *Inside/Outside* lesson that focuses on managing feelings, which is a central theme of the curriculum (Feinberg-Walker et al. 2009).

15.3.4.3 The Dynamic Process of Resilience

Resilience plays an essential role in the lives of *all* children and adolescents as well as their families. Additionally, resilience can significantly help those with eating disturbances or eating disorders overcome eating difficulties and negative body image. It is important to emphasize that resilience is a dynamic process, not a program (Benard 2004); and adolescent risk taking and resilience "clearly interface with the concept of responsibility" (Ponton 1997, 269). Developing self-responsibility is a lifelong process that involves a great deal of courage and determined effort by children, adolescents, and families (Ponton 1997). While there is power in a single relationship, "wraparound support" from families, schools, and communities can be even more potent (Benard 2004). Through growth-fostering relationships and empathic interactions, parents, educators, health care providers, and other caring adults can intentionally instill protective factors to mitigate risks, reduce stress, and shift the balance toward overall resilience and quality of life. Moreover, Brooks and Goldstein (2001, 293) asserted that intentionally enhancing resilience in youth has meaningful, long-lasting implications:

> The future lies not in technology but in our children, children instilled by their parents, teachers, and other adults with the resilient qualities necessary to help them shape a future with satisfaction and confidence. We can all serve as the charismatic adults in children's lives—believing in them and providing them with opportunities that reinforce their islands of competence and feelings of self-worth. This is not only a wonderful gift to our children but also an essential ingredient for the future. It is part of our legacy to the next generation.

15.4 SUMMARY AND CONCLUSIONS

Poor emotional processing, maladaptive coping strategies, communication difficulties, and a variety of other risk factors contribute to the complexity of eating disorders. Therefore, social-emotional learning, interpersonal skills, and resilience are essential assets for overcoming these risks. It is important to note that these realms of competence are intertwined and reciprocally influence each other. For example, social-emotional skills, such as self-awareness and emotion management, serve to enhance the ability to cope with stress and also add to the arsenal of important interpersonal skills, including effective communication and conflict resolution. In turn, all of these competencies positively affect individuals' and families' overall resilience. Furthermore, resilience plays a crucial role in the healthy development of individuals and families at every stage of life; and it is foundational in the prevention of body image difficulties, eating disturbances, and eating disorders.

APPENDIX 15.A

Lesson 3: Owning, Accepting, and Managing Feelings

Facilitator's Note

This lesson provides the groundwork for a central theme of the *Inside/Outside Self-Discovery Program*—that we have the ability to influence and shift our own feelings. We can learn how to pause and review the circumstances that generated our feelings and re-examine the interpretation on which our emotional response is based. Often, we discover that we were shortsighted or unaware of the other person's point of view, that we were making different assumptions, or that we have misinterpreted the other's intent. This lesson helps participants develop skills for understanding the complexities of human behavior and increases their capacity for empathy.

Exploring the mind–body relationship allows students to understand how feelings come about and how we can influence our feelings in more constructive ways. It helps students understand why shifting interpretations about the intentions of people's behavior, using a relaxation exercise, going for a walk or run, doing some creative problem-solving, or seeking connection with someone can all contribute to improving their feelings and promote a greater sense of well-being.

This lesson serves as a building block for future lessons on the nature of stress (including how it manifests and affects the mind and body). It teaches about how stress and tension can lead to irritability of mood and negative thinking, and how those factors affect relationships. By helping students understand the basis for misunderstandings and miscommunication, this lesson guides them to examine options for responding to difficult situations and to consider ways to communicate more effectively.

Troubleshooting

In the recommended warm-up for this lesson, we introduce some simple meditation exercises. Students can sit in chairs or on the floor for these exercises. You may want to provide mats if they will be sitting on the floor.

Lesson 3: Owning, Accepting, and Managing Feelings

Goals

Students will

- Increase their awareness of and appreciation for their body
- Understand the interplay between mind, body sensations, and the resulting emotions that they feel
- Learn where feelings come from
- Understand how feelings can change and how changing their thoughts can help change how they feel

Objectives

Students will be able to

- Demonstrate how to tune into or notice their senses/sensations
- Explain how we interpret, and sometimes misinterpret, others' words or behaviors, and how that affects feelings
- Explain the connection between thinking and emotions

Materials and Preparation

Materials Needed

- Rubber cement, markers, and scissors (for continued work on boxes)

Copy one for each student

- **Lesson 3 Vocabulary**

Review

- **Lesson 3 Vocabulary** terms and definitions

Warm-Up

5 minutes

For this lesson, we recommend either the Noticing Your Self or Learning to Notice Sensations warm-up. Both of these exercises encourage students to tune in and become more aware of what they feel in their bodies. Noticing Your Self is a good preliminary exercise for the relaxation exercise done in a later lesson. Learning to Notice Sensations is a slightly different approach to the same end.

See Warm-up Activities section for complete directions.

Brief Presentation

15 minutes

How Do We Get Our Feelings/Where Do They Originate?

Say to students

Today our brief talk is about feelings—where they come from, what we do with them, and where they go. Feelings, also known as emotions, have three parts.

1. Physical sensations: We get information about our sensations by tuning in to our senses of hearing, seeing, smelling, touching, etc. When we direct our attention to noticing what sensations are going on in our bodies (such as sweaty palms, jittery stomach, heat rising in our face), we can become much more aware of what we are feeling.
2. Thinking and interpreting: We interpret our body sensations and the situations that trigger them, give the feeling a name, and describe how the situation affects us. For example: You feel upset and interpret that the other person's actions were disrespectful of you.
3. What we do with our feelings: When we feel something we often react in a particular way. Our reactions are often spontaneous and seem to be automatic. When we slow down and think things through, we can become more deliberate in how we react.

Ask students:
- **What are senses?**
- **What is the value of our senses?**
- **Does everyone experience their senses in the same way? For instance, if we brought in a bunch of fragrant flowers, would everyone smell the flowers in the same way? If you have allergies and flowers make you sneeze, will that influence how you experience the flowers? If we brought a big furry dog in here, might some people who are scared of dogs respond differently from those who are not scared of dogs?**
- **Can you think of some other examples of how we might have different experiences with our senses?** (*Some people like snow/cold weather, while others don't. What about loud music, the sounds of sports on television?*)

Say:
Think for a moment about how you use your senses.
- **How are your senses helpful to you?**
- **Are there times you wish your senses were less aware of your surroundings or more aware of your surroundings (for example, noise)?**
- **How would you function if your senses were extraordinarily keen or extraordinarily weak?**

Say:
Our senses allow us to know what is going on in and around us. They are crucial to helping us know what we need to do in order to adapt, cope, and survive. For example: The sound of a car coming alerts us not to cross the street; seeing our mother put her fingers to the temple portion of her head helps us figure out that she has a headache; feeling jittery in our stomach lets us know that we are worried about a test.

The example of feeling jittery in our bodies before or after a test is a good example of how our senses give us clues about our feelings. When we have a feeling (like being nervous before a test), we feel physical changes in our bodies. These physical sensations, such as heart fluttering, sweaty palms, or tight stomach, help us know what emotion we are feeling.

Many of us have learned to disregard these physical signals. Sometimes, that might be useful, such as when we have a cold and don't feel well but need

to concentrate on the teacher's explanation of a math concept. At other times, it can be really important to notice these physical signals (for example, when we aren't feeling safe in a situation), so we can ask ourselves questions to help figure out why we are feeling that way. Using our body signals and the feelings that go along with them can help us to decode a message that our body–mind system is trying to give us.

How do we get our feelings and where do they originate? They always have a "because" that helps us to decode why we are feeling the way we are. For example, "This is happening because I am responding to ... ." When we understand why we feel the ways that we do, we can learn how to cope with our more challenging feelings. We can learn how to decode the messages sent to us from our body signals and how to work with them so that we are not controlled by them.

Draw the following diagram (Anderson 1981) on the board and explain it to students.

Situation	We Think	We Feel
Your teacher didn't call on you.	She doesn't like me.	Angry/sorry for self
Your teacher calls on Ted.	That's not fair; Ted always gets to answer.	Jealous
Your teacher calls on another student.	Thank goodness she didn't pick me; I didn't know the answer.	Happy/relieved
Your teacher calls on another student.	She thinks I don't know anything.	Feel bad about self/ depressed/defeated
Your teacher calls on another student.	She never calls on me.	Frustrated

Situation/What Happened → We Think → We Feel

(The explanation we give for a situation causes us to end up feeling the way that we feel.)

Say to students:

Step 1: Something happens.

Step 2: We notice sensations in our body and make an interpretation of what these sensations mean. We explain the physical changes that go along with the emotions by considering the context or situation (such as who the other people involved are and what events are going on). Misinterpretation often occurs because we see the situation through the filter of our automatic feelings, not from a more neutral perspective that looks at the bigger picture.

Step 3: This produces a feeling. We name or label what we are feeling and that leads to a reaction. Sometimes, we react impulsively, and other times, we can slow ourselves down and give consideration to how we might prefer to react. When we practice holding back from expressing our automatic responses, we then have more opportunity to react constructively.

Step 4: The response we make/our reaction.

We all tend to have particular ways that we respond to situations. We might be pleased with these ways of reacting, or we might wish we could react differently. When we practice slowing down and experiment with reacting in new and different ways, we get to see how that might help us handle our feelings in a more effective way and how it might help strengthen our relationships. Many of us feel the need to explode in order to get relief, but when we do that our friends or family members get mad at us because they feel like they just got hit in the face by our screaming, harsh words. We have to learn how to speak about our feelings in ways that invite others to listen. That takes practice, just like learning our multiplication tables and learning to ride a bike.

Many of us don't want to speak up because we are afraid that others will get mad at us; we fear that they won't like us if we say anything. If we give in to this way of thinking and feeling, we don't get to practice the skills we need to stand up to our fears and to give others feedback. When we react in this way, we aren't usually thinking about how we are also shortchanging the other person. Think about this: If you were doing something that caused your friend to feel hurt or offended and you didn't know that your actions were causing her to feel that way, would you want her to tell you so that you could stop doing it? When we don't develop the courage to talk to our friends about how they are affecting us, we both lose out. Often people don't know that they affect others in the ways they do.

For example: Your friend tells something private about you to another friend. What might you think about this? How would this make you feel? Are there other ways you might feel? Do different explanations for what happened make a difference in how you might react to your friend?

Ask students:

- **What do you typically do when you feel angry? Why?**
- **Do you "take after" anyone else in your family? In other words, does anyone else in your family tend to do the same thing when he or she feels angry?**

Give some examples from your own experience and then ask students for other examples. Possible examples include the following:

- When I feel angry, I want to run away before I say something mean.
- Some people hold a grudge for a very long time, not realizing that everyone in middle school will make mistakes and that we all learn, grow, and change as we experience life's circumstances. Someone you are mad at this year may well turn out to be a good friend in high school.

Ask students:

- **Why do you think some people tend to hold grudges?** (*They have a hard time letting go of being hurt or angry; they have a hard time being forgiving; they hold unrealistic expectations of others and think that others are supposed to act in ways that are meant to please them; they often care more about feeling "right" than they do about building a connection with another person; they get locked in to their own way of seeing things and don't have much ability to see things from a different perspective.*)
- **Sometimes we get the idea that we're not supposed to get angry at our parents. Do you ever feel like that? How do we get this idea?**
- **Can you think of a time when you were able to explain that you were feeling upset or angry because of something a friend did and you got a good response from your friend?**

Review the following points with students:

- A situation occurs. Something happens and we feel stirred up.
- We have a thought about what happened and that produces feelings.
- We label and describe the feeling to ourselves.

Beliefs Systems Influence Our Feelings

Say to students:

When we think about a situation, our belief systems will influence the way we feel. For example: If we believe that honesty is important in friendship and then we find out that a friend has told a lie about us, how might we feel? If we believe that friends should always be nice to each other, then how might we feel when our friend slights us?

Sometimes, the ideas that we hold are framed in the ideal—meaning that we hold onto the belief that the world could be a perfect place where people never make mistakes. But real life isn't that way. In real life, people are imperfect and do make mistakes. The key is to notice whether people (including ourselves) are willing to learn from the mistakes they make. In order to do this, we have to be willing to look at ourselves in a realistic and honest way and to be forgiving.

An example of an unrealistic idea is that someone should only be our friend and not be friends with someone else, or the idea that friends should never hurt our feelings. These kinds of beliefs are irrational because they aren't the way things actually work in the real world. Good friends, just like family members, can hurt each other's feelings at times. The key to determining whether someone can be a good friend is by seeing if she or he cares about having hurt you and if they try to do things differently the next time.

Ask students:

- **What are some of your most uncomfortable feelings?** *(Examples: jealousy, anger, resentment, anxiety, stress, embarrassment, shame, pride)*
- **What are some of your favorite feelings?**
- **What situations can get you nervous? happy? sad?**
- **What helps you feel good about yourself? Who has helped you feel good about yourself and how?**
- **Do you think it would help to remind yourself of your strong areas (your strengths) and your successes when you feel disappointed?**
- **Do you think it would help to remind yourself that the person you are upset with might not have acted that way intentionally?**
- **What about when you feel jealous? Would either of these reminders – that the person is not trying to make you feel jealous or that you have your own things that you're good at doing – help change your interpretation—and the thoughts you are telling yourself?**
- **Can you think of a time when a friend was upset and you helped your friend feel better? How did you help?**

Activity

15 minutes

(Continued from Lesson 3.)

Allow students time to continue to work on the Inside/Outside boxes. Ask them to consider including their inside feelings, something that other people don't know. For example, what gets them scared, worried, happy, jealous, or sad?

Wrap-Up

5 minutes

Ask students:
Were you surprised by anything you learned today? Did you learn anything you hadn't thought about before?

Thoughts/Self-Discoveries for the Week

2 minutes

Students can take boxes home to finish them and to add any small objects that are meaningful to them, or represent some aspect of themselves. Let them know that they will be sharing parts of their boxes in the next lesson, and that they can decide what they share and if they would like to share. Remind students to bring their boxes to the next lesson. You might offer to loan students materials if they need to continue their work at home.

Lesson 3 Vocabulary

Feeling or Emotion: We are born with the biological readiness to feel basic, primary-level emotions: anger, sadness, joy, surprise, fear, disgust, guilt/shame, and interest. Emotions come and go like waves in the ocean, and they become associated with events and people. Emotions involve body changes, such as tensing or relaxing of muscles and heart rate or temperature changes, and they involve changes in our brains' production of chemicals.

We label particular patterns of physical response as being a particular feeling. For example: We feel our face getting warm (physical change) when the teacher calls on us and we're uncertain of the answer (situation); we recognize (interpret) that we feel embarrassment. We feel heavy and sluggish, even tearful, and realize that we feel sad and discouraged because we miss our parent who is traveling for work.

Sensations: Noticeable physical changes in our bodies. These changes can signal an emotion, depending on a given situation or context. We all experience different sensations in our bodies for each given situation—we are wired to do so. For example, some people feel nervous in their stomachs, sometimes described as "butterflies;" other people may feel nervous in their legs and find themselves holding their foot in a stiff or tense position or constantly jiggling their foot. Then, there are other people who jiggle their foot when they feel impatient or bored.

Thought: What we say to ourselves, often in response to a situation. These statements often help us understand or interpret the sensations that we are feeling and then name the feeling or emotion. For example, when I started to jiggle my leg in math lesson, I made the interpretation that I was feeling tense and impatient because I wasn't following the teacher's explanation.

Mind–Body Connection: What our mind thinks affects what our body feels. What our body feels also influences the emotion we experience. For example: If my friend doesn't wait for me, I can make an interpretation that my friend didn't wait for me on purpose. If that's what I think, then I am more likely to feel rejected. Another person in that same situation may wonder if her friend is annoyed with her, and she might feel less hungry for lunch because her stomach reacts with pain.

Fact: Known to be true, can be proven, and is accepted by almost everyone. For example: Ice cream is a food.

Belief: A belief is an idea that some people may think is true, but to which not all agree. It is like an opinion. Usually, you can insert "I think" before the statement. For example: (I think) Chocolate ice cream is great.

Rational Beliefs: Rational beliefs make sense. Although they may not be true for everyone, they are true for many people.

Irrational Beliefs: Irrational beliefs don't make sense, and they are not true; they are based in feelings. (I feel it therefore it is true.) For example: The teacher wanted all of us to fail her lesson. When you wear the color purple, your school team will win the game.

Naming or labeling the feeling: We tell ourselves what we are feeling when we tell ourselves a story of what happened; that is, when we make an interpretation. For example: I feel upset and angry because my friend didn't sit with me at lunch and that means she must not want to be my friend.

Pause and think it over: To help ourselves, we can ask ourselves if we can think of another explanation or interpretation for a given situation. We can choose to check it out before we assume that our hurtful explanation is accurate.

Sources

Feeling Diagram and Example: From Jill Anderson, *Thinking, Changing, Rearranging: Improving Self Esteem in Young People* (Eugene, OR: Timberline Press, 1981) p. 7.

REFERENCES

Ackard, D. M., and D. Neumark-Sztainer. 2001. Family mealtime while growing up: Associations with symptoms of bulimia nervosa. *Eat Disord* 9: 239–249.

Ackard, D. M., D. Neumark-Sztainer, M. Story, and C. Perry. 2006. Parent-child connectedness and behavioral and emotional health among adolescents. *Am J Prev Med* 30: 59–66.

Arnow, B., J. Kenardy, and W. S. Agras. 1995. The emotional eating scale: The development of a measure to assess coping with negative affect by eating. *Int J Eat Disord* 18: 79–90.

Attie, I., and J. Brooks-Gunn. 1995. The development of eating regulation across the life span. In *Developmental psychopathology*, ed. C. Dante and D. J. Cohen, 332-368. New York: Wiley.

Bandura, A. 1986. *Social foundations of thought and action*. Englewood Cliffs, NJ: Prentice Hall.

Beaumont, P. J. V. 2002. Clinical presentation of anorexia nervosa and bulimia nervosa. In *Eating disorders and obesity*, ed. C. G. Fairburn and K. D. Brownell, 162–170. New York: Guilford Press.

Becvar, D. J., and R. S. Becvar. 1994. *Hot chocolate for a cold winter night: Exercises for relationship enhancement*. Denver, CO: Love.

Becvar, D. J., and R. S. Becvar. 1997. *Pragmatics of human relationships*. Galena, IL: Geist and Russell.

Benard, B. 2004. *Resiliency: What we have learned*. San Francisco: WestEd.

Berndt, T. J., and S. L. Hestenes. 1996. The developmental course of social support: Family and peers. In *The developmental psychopathology of eating disorders*, ed. L. Smolak, M. P. Levine, and R. Striegel-Moore, 77–106. Mahwah, NJ: Erlbaum.

Binford, R. B., M. Mussell, C. B. Peterson, and S. J. Crow. 2004. Relation of binge eating age of onset to functional aspects of binge eating in binge eating disorder. *Int J Eat Disord* 25: 286–292.

Bjork, T., and G. Ahlstrom. 2008. The patient's perception of having recovered from an eating disorder. *Health Care Women Int* 29: 926–944.

Booth-Butterfield, M., and R. Sidelinger. 1998. The influence of family communication on the college-aged child: Openness, attitudes and actions about sex and alcohol. *Commun Q* 46: 295–308.

Botta, R. A., and R. Dumlao. 2002. How do conflict and communication patterns between fathers and daughters contribute to or offset eating disorders? *Health Commun* 14:   199–219.

Bowen, M. 1976. Theory in the practice of psychotherapy. In *Family therapy: Theory and practice,* ed. P. J. Guerin, Jr., 42–90. New York: Gardner Press.

Brooks, R., and S. Goldstein. 2001. *Raising resilient children*. Chicago, IL: McGraw-Hill/Contemporary Books.

Brown, L. M., and C. Gilligan. 1992. *Meeting at the crossroads*. New York: Ballantine Books.

Casper, R. C., and M. Troiani. 2001. Family functioning in anorexia nervosa differs by subtype. *Int J Eat Disord* 30: 338–342.

Centers for Disease Control and Prevention. 2010. *Healthy youth!* http://www.cdc.gov/HealthyYouth/ (accessed May 20, 2010).

Chandy, J. M., L. Harris, R. W. Blum, and M. D. Resnick. 1995. Female adolescents of alcohol misusers: Disordered eating features. *Int J Eat Disord* 17: 283–289.

Collaborative for Academic, Social, and Emotional Learning (CASEL). 2010a. *Welcome to CASEL*. http://www.casel.org/ (accessed March 24, 2010).

Collaborative for Academic, Social, and Emotional Learning (CASEL). 2010b. *What is SEL: Skills & competencies*. http://www.casel.org/basics/skills.php (accessed March 24, 2010).

Collaborative for Academic, Social, and Emotional Learning (CASEL). (2003). *Safe and sound: An educational leaders' guide to evidence-based social and emotional learning (SEL) programs*. Chicago: Collaborative for Academic, Social, and Emotional Learning.

Connors, M. E. 1996. Developmental vulnerabilities for eating disorders. In *The developmental psychopathology of eating disorders: Implications for research, prevention, and treatment*, ed. L. Smolak, M. P. Levine, and R. Striegel-Moore, 285–310. Mahwah, NJ: Lawrence Erlbaum Associates.

Cook-Cottone, C., and M. Beck. 2008. Manualized-group treatment of eating disorders: Attunement in mind, body, and relationship (AMBR). *J Spec Group Work* 33: 61–83.

Cordero, E. D., and T. Israel. 2009. Parents as protective factors in eating problems of college women. *Eat Disord* 17: 146–161.

Corstorphine, E. 2006. Cognitive-emotional-behavioural therapy for the eating disorders: Working with beliefs about emotions. *Eur Eat Disord Rev* 14: 448–461.

Covey, S. R. 1989. *The seven habits of highly effective people: Restoring the character ethic*. New York: Simon & Schuster/Fireside.

Doll, H. A., S. E. Petersen, and S. L. Stewart-Brown. 2005. Eating disorders and emotional and physical well-being: Associations between student self-reports of eating disorders and quality of life as measured by the SF-36. *Qual Life Res* 14: 705–717.

Drench, M. E., A. C. Noonan, N. Sharby, and S. H. Ventura. 2007. *Psychosocial aspects of health care* (2nd ed.). Upper Saddle River, NJ: Prentice Hall (Pearson).

Drummond, J., D. Fleming, L. McDonald, and G. M. Kysela. 2005. Randomized controlled trial of a family problem-solving intervention. *Clin Nurs Res* 14: 57–80.

Durlak, J., and R. Weissberg. 2010. Social and emotional learning programmes that work. *Better Evid Based Educ* 2: 4–5. http://casel.org/downloads/BETTER_Evidence_based_Education_Social_Emotional_Learning.pdf. (accessed June 3, 2010).

Durlak, J. A., and A. M. Wells. 1998. Evaluation of indicated preventive intervention (secondary prevention) mental health programs for children and adolescents. *Am J Community Psychol* 26: 775–802.

Eldredge, K. L., and W. S. Agras. 1996. Weight and shape overconcern and emotional eating in binge eating disorder. *Int J Eat Disord* 19: 73–82.

Engle, S. G., J. J. Boseck, R. D. Crosby, S. A. Wonderlich, J. E. Mitchell, J. Smyth, R. Miltenberger, and H. Steiger. 2007. The relationship of momentary anger and impulsivity to bulimic behavior. *Behav Res Ther* 45: 437–447.

Feinberg-Walker, H., S. Barrett, and J. Shure. 2009. *Inside/outside self-discovery for teens: Strategies to promote resilience, relationships, and positive body image.* The Miles Family Foundation.

FEMA. 2010. Effective communication: Independent study 242.a. http://training.fema.gov/EMIWeb/IS/IS242A.pdf (accessed June 9, 2011).

Fernandiz-Aranda, F., A. P. Pinheiro, L. M. Thornton, W. H. Berrettini, S. Crow, M. M. Fichter, K. A. Halmi et al. 2008. Impulse control disorders in women with eating disorders. *Psychiatry Res* 157: 147–157.

Fox, R. E. 2009. A qualitative exploration of the perception of emotions in anorexia nervosa: A basic emotion and developmental perspective. *Clin Psychol Psychother* 16: 276–302.

Fox, R. E., and K. Froom. 2009. Eating disorders: A basic emotion perspective. *Clin Psychol Psychother* 16: 328–335.

Fox, R. E., and M. J. Power. 2009. Eating disorders and multi-level models of emotion: An integrated model. *Clin Psychol Psychother* 16: 240–267.

Freeman, L. M. Y., and K. M. Gil. 2004. Daily stress, coping, and dietary restraint in binge eating. *Int J Eat Disord* 36: 204–212.

García-Grau, G., A. Fusté, A. Miró, C. Saldaña, and A. Bados 2004. Coping style and vulnerability to eating disorders in adolescent boys. *Eur Eat Disord Rev* 12: 61–67.

Geller, J., S. J. Cockell, P. L. Hewitt, E. M. Goldner, and G. L Flett. 2000. Inhibited expression of negative emotions and interpersonal orientation in anorexia nervosa. *Int J Eat Disord* 28: 8–19.

Gilboa-Schechtman, E., L. Avnon, E. Zubery, and P. Jeczmien. 2006. Emotional processing in eating disorders: Specific impairment or general distress related deficiency? *Depress Anxiety* 23: 331–339.

Girls Circle. 2010. http://www.girlscircle.com/Default.aspx (accessed December 6, 2010).

Glanz, K., and M. D. Schwartz. 2008. Stress, coping, and health behavior. In *Health behavior and health education: Theory, research, and practice* (4th ed.), ed. K. Glanz, B. K. Rimer, and K. Viswanath, 211–236. San Francisco: Jossey-Bass.

Goleman, D. 1995. *Emotional intelligence: Why it can matter more than IQ.* New York: Bantam.

Golman, M. 2009. A study to evaluate the effectiveness of the Girls in Motion® program in improving body satisfaction in preadolescent girls. PhD diss., Texas Woman's Univ.

Gordon, T. (2000). *Parent effectiveness training: The proven program for raising responsible children.* New York: Three Rivers Press.

Goss, K. P., and S. Allan. 2009. Shame, pride, and eating disorders. *Clin Psychol Psychother* 16: 303–316.

Goss, K. P., and P. Gilbert. 2002. Eating disorders, shame and pride: A cognitive-behavioral functional analysis. In *Body shame: Conceptualization, research, and treatment*, ed. P. Gilbert, and J. Miles, 219–255. Hove, UK: Brunner-Routledge.

Harvey, T., N. A. Troop, J. L. Treasure, and T. Murphy 2002. Fear, disgust, and abnormal eating attitudes: A preliminary study. *Int J Eat Disord* 32: 213–218.

Haudek, C., M. Rorty, and B. Henker. 1999. The role of ethnicity and parental bonding in the eating and weight concerns of Asian–American and Caucasian college women. *Int J Eat Disord* 25: 425–433.

Hayaki, J., M. A. Friedman, and K. D. Brownell. 2002. Emotional expression and body dissatisfaction. *Int J Eat Disord* 31: 57–62.

Heaney, C. A., and Israel, B. A. 2008. Social networks and social support. In *Health behavior and health education: Theory, research, and practice* (4th ed.), ed. K. Glanz, B. K. Rimer, and K. Viswanath, 189–210. San Francisco: Jossey-Bass.

Henderson, N., and M. M. Milstein. 1996. *Resiliency in schools: Making it happen for students and educators.* Thousand Oaks, CA: Sage/Corwin Press.

Higgins, G. O. 1994. *Resilient adults: Overcoming a cruel past.* San Francisco: Jossey-Bass.

Ioannou, K., and J. R. E. Fox. 2009. Perception of threat from emotions and its role in poor emotional expression within eating pathology. *Clin Psychol Psychother* 16: 336–347.

Johnson, D. W. 2006. *Reaching out: Interpersonal effectiveness and self-actualization* (9th ed.). Boston, MA: Pearson.

Jordan, J. V., and L. M. Hartling. 2002. New developments in relational-cultural theory. In *Rethinking mental health and disorders: Feminist perspectives*, ed. M. Ballou, and L. S. Brown, 48–70. New York: Guilford.

Jordan, J. V., A. G. Kaplan, J. B. Miller, I. P. Stiver, and J. L. Surrey. 1991. *Women's growth in connection: Writings from the Stone Center.* New York: Guilford.

Kater, K. 2005. *Healthy body image: Teaching kids to eat and love their bodies too!* (2nd ed.). Seattle, WA: National Eating Disorders Association.

Kelly, A. M., M. Wall, M. E. Eisenberg, M. Story, and D. Neumark-Sztainer. 2005. Adolescent girls with high body satisfaction: Who are they and what can they teach us? *J Adolesc Health* 37: 391–396.

Ketrow S. 1999. Nonverbal aspects of group communication. In *Handbook of group communication theory and research*, ed. L. Frey, 251–287. Thousand Oaks, CA: Sage.

Killen J. D., C. B. Taylor, M. J. Telch, T. N. Robinson, D. J. Maron, and K. E. Saylor. 1987. Depressive symptoms and substance use among adolescent binge eaters and purgers: A defined population study. *Amer J Pub Health* 77: 1539–1541.

Lawson, R., G. Waller, J. Sines, and C. Meyer. 2008. Emotional awareness among eating-disordered patients: The role of narcissistic traits. *Eur Eat Disord Rev* 16: 44–48.

Le Grange, D., J. Lock, K. Loeb, and D. Nicholls. 2009. *Academy for Eating Disorders position paper: The role of the family in eating disorders.* http://www.aedweb.org/policy/documents/RoleofFamily.pdf (accessed May 10, 2010).

Lemmon, C. R., and A. M. Josephson. 2001. Family therapy for eating disorders. *Child Adolesc Psychiatr Clin N Am* 10: 519–542.

Lingswiler, V. M., J. H. Crowther, and M. A. P. Stephens. 1989. Affective and cognitive antecedents to eating episodes in bulimia and binge eating. *Int J Eat Disord* 8: 533–539.

Littleton, H. L., and T. Ollendick. 2003. Negative body image and disordered eating behavior in children and adolescents: What places youth at risk and how can these problems be prevented? *Clin Child Fam Psychol* 6: 51–66.

Loth, K. A., D. Neumark-Sztainer, and J. K. Croll. 2009. Informing family approaches to eating disorder prevention: Perspectives of those who have been there. *Int J Eat Disord* 42: 146–152.

Magee, N., and P. Perkins. 2010. Implementing a SEL programme. *Better Evidence-based Education* 2: 10–11. http://casel.org/downloads/BETTER_Evidence_based_Education_Social_Emotional_Learning.pdf (accessed June 3, 2010).

Marcotte, D., L. Forton, P. Potvin and M. Papillon. 2002. Gender differences in depressive symptoms during adolescence: Role of gender-typed characteristics, self-esteem, body image, stressful life events, and pubertal status. *J Emot Behav Disord* 10: 29–42.

Markman, H., S. Stanley, and S. L. Blumberg. 1994. *Fighting for your marriage: Positive steps for preventing divorce and preserving a lasting love.* San Francisco, CA: Jossey-Bass.

Martin, G. C., E. H. Wertheim, M. Prior, D. Smart, A. Sanson, and F. Oberklaid. 2000. A longitudinal study of the role of childhood temperament in the later development of eating concerns. *Int J Eat Disord* 27: 150–162.

Masheb, R. M., and C. M. Grilo. 2006. Emotional overeating and its associations with eating disorder psychopathology among overweight patients with binge eating disorder. *Int J Eat Disord* 39: 141–146.

Massey-Stokes, M. 2008. Body image and eating disturbances in children and adolescents. In *The active female: Health issues throughout the lifespan,* ed. J. McComb, R. Norman, and J. Slauterbeck, 57–79. Totowa, NJ: Humana.

Masten, A. 1994. Resilience in individual development: Successful adaptation despite risk and adversity. In *Educational resilience in inner-city America*, ed. M. Wang and E. Gorden, 2–35. Hillsdale, NJ: Lawrence Erlbaum.

McEwen, C., and E. Flouri. 2009. Fathers' parenting, adverse life events, and adolescents' emotional and eating disorder symptoms: The role of emotion regulation. *Eur Child Adolesc Psychiatry* 18: 206–216.

McGrane, D., and A. Carr. 2002. Young women at risk for eating disorders: Perceived family dysfunction and parental psychological problems. *Contemp Fam Ther* 24: 385–398.

McVey G. L., R. Davis, S. Tweed, and F. Shaw. 2004. Evaluation of a school-based program designed to improve body image satisfaction, global self-esteem and eating attitudes and behaviours. A replication study. *Int J Eat Disord* 36: 1–11.

McVey G. L., M. Lieberman, N. Voorberg, D. Wardrope, and E. Blackmore. 2003. School-based peer support groups: A new approach to the prevention of disordered eating. *Eat Disord* 11: 169–185.

Miller, S. P., A. D. Redlich, and H. Steiner. 2003. The stress response in anorexia nervosa. *Child Psychiatry Hum Dev* 33: 295–306.

Miller-Day, M., and J. D. Marks. 2006. Perceptions of parental communication orientation, perfectionism, and disordered eating behaviors of sons and daughters. *Health Commun* 19: 153–163.

Minuchin, S., B. L. Rosman, and L. Baker. 1978. *Psychosomatic families: Anorexia nervosa in context.* Cambridge, MA: Harvard Univ. Press.

Moreno, J. K., M. J. Selby, K. Aved, and C. Besse. 2000. Differences in family dynamics among anorexic, bulimic, obese and normal women. *J Psychother Indep Pract* 1: 75–87.

Neumark-Sztainer, D., N. E. Sherwood, T. Coller, and P. J. Hannan. 2000. Primary prevention of disordered eating among preadolescent girls: Feasibility and short-term effect of a community-based intervention. *J Am Diet Assoc* 100: 1466–1473.

Nordbo, R. H. S., E M. S. Espeset, K. S. Gulliksen, F. Skårderud, and A. Holte. 2006. The meaning of self-starvation: Qualitative study of patients' perception of anorexia nervosa. *Int J Eat Disord* 39: 556–564.

O'Dea, J. 2007. *Everybody's Different: A Positive Approach to Teaching about Health, Puberty, Body Image, Nutrition, Self-Esteem and Obesity Prevention.* Camberwell, Victoria, Australia: ACER Press.

O'Dea, J., and S. Abraham. 2000. Improving the body image, eating attitudes and behaviours of young male and female adolescents: A new educational approach that focuses on self-esteem. *Eat Disord* 28: 43–57.

Pallister, E., and G. Waller. 2008. Anxiety and eating disorders: Understanding the overlap. *Clin Psychol Rev* 28: 366–386.

Paxton, S. J. 2002. *Research review of body image programs: An overview of body image dissatisfaction prevention interventions.* Body Image and Health, Inc., and Psychology Department, University of Melbourne, Prepared for the Victorian Government Department of Human Services, Melbourne, Victoria.

Perkins, S., U. Schmidt, I. Eisler, J. Treasure, I. Yi, S. Winn, P. Robinson, R. Murphy et al. 2005. Why do adolescents with bulimia nervosa choose not to involve their parents in treatment? *Eur Child Adolesc Psychiatry* 14: 376–385.

Polivy, J., and C. P. Herman. 2002. Causes of eating disorders. *Annu Rev Psychol* 53: 187–213.

Ponton, L. E. 1997. *The romance of risk: Why teenagers do the things they do.* New York: Basic Books.

Roa, J., A. Irvine, and K. Cervantez. 2007. *Girls Circle national research project.* http://www.girlscircle.com/docs/Final_Report_2007.pdf (accessed October 29, 2010).

Rodgers, R., and H. Chabrol. 2009. Parental attitudes, body image disturbance and disordered eating amongst adolescents and young adults: A review. *Eur Eat Disord Rev* 17: 137–151.

Rodgers, R. F., S. J. Paxton, and H. Chabrol. 2009. Effects of parental comments on body dissatisfaction and eating disturbance in young adults: A sociocultural model. *Body Image* 6: 171–177.

Rodin, J., R. H. Streigel-Moore, and L. R. Silberstein. 1990. Vulnerability and resilience in the age of eating disorders: Risk and protective factors for bulimia nervosa. In *Risk and protective factors in the development of psychopathology*, ed. J. Rolf, A. S. Masten, D. Cicchetti, K. H. Neuchterlein, and S. Weintraub, 361-383. Cambridge: Cambridge Univ. Press.

Salovey, P., B. T. Bedell, J. B. Detweiler, and J. D. Mayer. 1999. Coping intelligently: Emotional intelligence and the coping process. In *Coping: The psychology of what works*, ed. C. R. Snyder, 141–164. New York: Oxford Univ. Press.

Sallis, J. F., N. Owen, and E. B. Fisher. 2008. Ecological models of health behavior. In *Health behavior and health education: Theory, research, and practice* (4th ed.), ed. K. Glanz, B. K. Rimer, and K. Viswanath, 465–485. San Francisco, CA: Jossey-Bass.

Schmidt, U., and J. Treasure. 2006. Anorexia nervosa: Valued and visible. A cognitive-interpersonal maintenance model and its implications for research and practice. *Brit J Clin Psychol* 45: 343–366.

Scime, M., C. Cook-Cottone, L. Kane, and T. Watson. 2006. Group prevention of eating disorders with fifth-grade females: Impact on body dissatisfaction, drive for thinness, and media influence. *Eat Disord* 14: 143–155.

Shisslak, C. M., and M. Crago. 2001. Risk and protective factors in the development of eating disorders. In *Body image, eating disorders, and obesity in youth*, ed. J. K. Thompson and L. Smolak, 103–125. Washington, DC: American Psychological Association.

Sokol, M. S., T. K. Jackson, C. T. Selser, H. A. Nice, N. D. Christiansen, and A. K. Carroll. 2005. Review of clinical research in child and adolescent eating disorders. *Prim Psychiatry* 12: 52–58.

Steese, S., M. Dollette, W. Phillips, E. Hossfeld, G. Matthews, and G. Taormina. 2006. Understanding Girls' Circle as an intervention on perceived social support, body image, self-efficacy, locus of control, and self-esteem. *Adolesc* 41: 55–74.

Steinberg, A. B., and V. Phares. 2001. Family functioning, body image, and eating disturbances. In *Body image, eating disorders, and obesity in youth*, ed. J. K. Thompson and L. Smolak, 127–147. Washington, DC: American Psychological Association.

Steiner, H., W. Kwan, T. G. Shaffer, S. Walker, S. Miller, A. Sagar, and J. Lock. 2003. Risk and protective factors for juvenile eating disorders. *Eur Child Adolesc Psychiatry* 12: 38–46.

Steiner-Adair, C., L. Sjostrom, D. Franko, S. Pai, R. Tucker, A. E. Becker, and D. B. Herzog. 2002. Primary prevention of risk factors for eating disorders in adolescent girls: Learning from practice. *Eat Disord* 32: 401–411.

Stern, S. L., K. N. Dixon, D. Jones, M. Lake, E. Nemzer, and R. Sansone. 1989. Family environment in anorexia nervosa and bulimia. *Int J Eat Disord* 8: 25–31.

Stice, E. 2001. A prospective test of the dual pathway model of bulimic pathology: Mediating effects of dieting and negative affect. *J Abnorm Psychol* 110: 123–135.

Streigel-Moore, R. H., and F. M. Cachelin. 1999. Body image concerns and disordered eating in adolescent girls: Risk and protective factors. In *Beyond appearance: A new look at adolescent girls*, ed. N. G. Johnson and M. C. Roberts, 85–108. Washington, DC: American Psychological Association.

Tantillo, M. 2006. A relational approach to eating disorders multifamily therapy group: Moving from difference and disconnection to mutual connection. *Fam Syst Health* 24: 82–102.

Treasure, J., A. R. Sepulveda, P. MacDonald, W. Whitaker, C. Lopez, M. Zabala, O. Kyriacou, and G. Todd. 2008. The assessment of the family of people with eating disorders. *Eur Eat Disord Rev* 16: 247–255.

Treasure, J., A. R. Sepulveda, W. Whitaker, C. Lopez, and J. Whitney. 2007. Collaborative care between professionals and non-professionals in the management of eating disorders: A description of workshops focused on interpersonal maintaining factors. *Eur Eat Disorders Rev* 15: 24–34.

Tuschen-Caffier, B., and C. Vogele. 1999. Psychological and physiological reactivity to stress: An experimental study on bulimic patients, restrained eaters, and controls. *Psychother Psychosom* 68: 333–340.

Uehara, T., Y. Kawashima, M. Goto, S. Tasaki, and T. Someya. 2001. Psychoeducation for the families of patients with eating disorders and changes in expressed emotion: A preliminary study. *Comp Psychiatry* 42: 132–138.

Vandereycken, W. 2002. Families of patients with eating disorders. In *Eating disorders and obesity: A comprehensive handbook* (2nd ed.), ed. C. G. Fairburn and K. D. Brownell, 215–220. New York: Guilford Press.

Vidović, V., V. Jureša, I. Begovac, M. Mahnik, and G. Tocilj. 2005. Perceived family cohesion, adaptability and communication in eating disorders. *Eur Eat Disord Rev* 13: 19–28.

Wade, T. J., J. L. Bergin, N. G. Martin, N. A. Gillespie, and C. G. Fairburn. 2006. A transdiagnostic approach to understanding eating disorders. *J Nerv Ment Dis* 194: 510–517.

Wall, A. D., E. J. Cumella, and J. L. O'Connor. 2008. Depression and eating disorders. In *Eating disorders: A handbook of Christian treatment*, ed. E. J. Cumella, M. C. Eberly, and A. D. Wall, 319–340. Carlsbad, CA: Gürze Books.

Waller, G. 2008. A trans-transdiagnostic model of the eating disorders: A new way to open the egg? *Eur Eat Disord Rev* 16: 165–172.

Waller, G., M. Babbs, R. J. Milligan, C. Meyer, V. Obanian, and N. Leung. 2003. Anger and core beliefs in the eating disorders. *Int J Eat Disord* 34: 118–124.

Wertheim, E. G. 2010. *The importance of effective communication.* http://helpguide.org/mental/eq6_nonverbal_communication.htm (accessed May 19, 2010).

Wertheim, E. H., S. J. Paxton, H. K. Schutz, and S. L. Muir. 1997. Why do adolescent girls watch their weight? An interview study examining sociocultural pressures to be thin. *J Psychosom Res* 42: 345–355.

Wiser, S., and C. F. Telch. 1999. Dialectical behavior therapy for binge-eating disorder. *J Clin Psychol* 55: 755–768.

Wolin, S. J., and S. Wolin. 1993. *The resilient self: How survivors of troubled families rise above adversity.* New York: Villard Books.

Wonderlich, S. A. 2002. Personality and eating disorders. In *Eating disorders and obesity: A comprehensive handbook* (2nd ed.), ed. C. G. Fairburn and K. D. Brownell, 204–209. New York: Guilford Press.

World Health Organization. 2007. *Mental health: Strengthening mental health promotion* (fact sheet #220). http://www.who.int/mediacentre/factsheets/fs220/en/print.html (accessed March 18, 2010).

Wright, K., and E. E. Blanks. 2008. The secret and all-consuming obsessions: Eating disorders. In *Youth at risk: A prevention resource for counselors, teachers, and parents* (5th ed.), ed. D. Capuzzi and D. R. Gross, 203–247. Alexandria, VA: American Counseling Association.

16 Exercise Guidelines: Specific Recommendations for Women and Children with Eating Disorders

Jacalyn J. Robert-McComb and Vanessa Bayer

CONTENTS

16.1 LEARNING OBJECTIVES

After reading this chapter, you should be able to
- Describe the evaluation criteria for safe exercise participation
- Describe the components of physical fitness
- Identify normative values for the components of physical fitness for girls and women
- Prescribe and assess a safe exercise program for both women and girls
- Discuss the importance of a balanced exercise program
- Discuss the use of exercise in the treatment of eating disorders

16.2 BACKGROUND AND SIGNIFICANCE

16.2.1 INTRODUCTION

Many people do not fully understand what is meant by the term physical activity. Physical activity is a broad term that encompasses both activities of daily living (such as climbing the stairs at work or doing house work) and structured exercise sessions (such as attending a fitness class). Both types of activities are important for maintaining a healthy lifestyle. The beginning of this chapter will focus on exercise assessment and prescription for the general population, with specific recommendations for women and children. The culmination of the chapter will be exercise recommendations for individuals who are exercise dependent or are being treated for eating disorders (ED). Types of physical activity covered will include cardiorespiratory, muscular strength and endurance, flexibility, and yoga exercises. The assessment and attainment of a healthy body composition (e.g. weight and percent body fat [BF]) will also be covered. We hope you enjoy your reading and gain a better understanding of the physical activity needs for health throughout the lifespan for women and children.

16.2.2 PHYSICAL ACTIVITY LEVELS

Research shows that physical activity levels decline with age. Individuals are more likely to be active during childhood when they engage in more spontaneous and active play, whereas physical activity levels often begin to decline in adolescence as other interests and behaviors take precedence over active play time (Biddle et al. 2004). In their 2009 national Youth Risk Behavior Survey (YRBS), the U.S. Department of Health and Human Services (HSS) found that (1) only 18.4% of students surveyed engaged in the recommended 60 minutes (min) per day, seven days per week, of physical activity; (2) roughly twenty-three percent (23.1%) did not participate in 60 min of physical activity any day of the week; (3) roughly twenty-five percent (24.9%) played video or computer games or used the computer for reasons other than doing school work for 3 or more hours on an average school day; and (4) thirty-three percent (32.8%) watched television for an average of 3 h on an average school day. These prevalence rates have shown little to no change over the last several years (U.S. Department of Health and Human Services [HSS], 2010).

At the other end of the healthy physical activity spectrum, some women and adolescents engage in excessive or pathological amounts of physical activity. Garman et al. (2004) defined exercise as problematic when an individual rigidly pursues a structured physical activity program for 360 or more min of physical activity each week that is continued despite negative physical, emotional, or social consequences. In a study of college students, 21.8% of them engaged in this sort of physical activity. This group of individuals (referred to as exercise dependent) exercised for an average of 735.6 min each week, whereas the nondependent group exercised for an average of 102.9 min per week, a finding that was consistent with other research in college populations. One important point is that defining excessive physical activity is difficult because high amounts of physical activity for some individuals, such as elite athletes, may not be harmful.

16.2.3 BENEFITS AND RISKS ASSOCIATED WITH PHYSICAL ACTIVITY

Physical activity has many physical and psychological benefits. Weight-bearing physical activity is beneficial for children because it aids in the growth and maintenance of a healthy musculoskeletal system (through increased deposit of bone mineral), helps regulate weight and BF levels (Hills et al. 2007), helps to prevent and reduce high blood pressure, contributes to mental and social development, builds motor skills, and improves self-esteem, energy levels, sleep quality, and the ability to concentrate (Faigenbaum et al. 2009).

As one ages, regular participation in physical activity can decrease one's risk for premature death, colon and breast cancers, type 2 diabetes (decreased insulin needs, increased glucose tolerance), cardiovascular and coronary artery disease (reduced resting systolic/diastolic pressure, increased HDL-cholesterol, decreased triglyceride levels), strokes, gallbladder disease, osteoporosis, anxiety, depression, and obesity (American College of Sports Medicine [ACSM] 2010a; HHS 2008).

16.2.4 SCREENING FOR RISK

Overall, physical activity is safe; however, there are some risks: (1) It can increase the risk of orthopedic injury, particularly in overweight and obese individuals or those with weak bone structures (e.g. individuals with osteoporosis [ACSM 2006]). (2) Inadequate caloric consumption in an ED population may contribute to hypoglycemia during exercise. (3) Binge eating and purging may result in electrolyte imbalances (see Chapters 3 and 4) that could contribute to arrhythmias during exercise. (4) Engagement in vigorous physical activity can also increase the risk of having a heart attack, and individuals with heart disease may be more vulnerable for sudden cardiac death (ACSM 2010a). Table 16.1 lists risk factors for cardiovascular disease. Signs and symptoms for cardiovascular disease include but are not limited to the following: (1) a rapid or racing heart rate (HR); (2) dizziness; (3) aches or discomfort in the chest, neck, jaw, or arms; (4) shortness of breath at rest; (5) sudden weakness or numbness of the face, arm, or leg on one side of the body; (6) sudden dimness or loss of vision; and (7) sudden difficulty speaking (ACSM 2010a).

In order to provide a safe physical activity program, individuals should be screened before participation in exercise. A screening should include a health history questionnaire, which includes questions about eating habits and binge/purge behaviors, lab reports (cholesterol, blood glucose, and triglyceride levels), and a blood pressure assessment. Appendix 16.A contains a sample health history questionnaire. An individual could also determine his or her readiness for exercise participation by filling out the Physical Activity Readiness Questionnaire (PAR-Q). The PAR-Q is a simple screening device that indicates when individuals should consult their physician before beginning an exercise program (ACSM 2010a). The PAR-Q can be found in Appendix 16.B.

Based on the information gathered from the initial screening, an individual may be placed in one of three risk categories (see Table 16.2). A medical exam, an exercise test, or a physician's supervision of the physical activity program is not required for low-risk individuals, but is required for moderate-risk individuals who participate in vigorous physical activity and high-risk individuals who participate in moderate or vigorous physical activity (ACSM 2010a).

16.3 CURRENT FINDINGS

Cardiorespiratory endurance, muscular strength and endurance, flexibility, and body composition are health-related components of physical fitness. The most up-to-date guidelines for achieving these health-related components are presented in this chapter. Attention is also given to yoga because it has been found to be beneficial for those who have an ED.

TABLE 16.1
Coronary Artery Disease Risk Factors

Primary Modifiable Risk Factors	Defining Criteria
Prediabetes	Impaired fasting glucose (IFG) = fasting plasma glucose ≥ 100 mg·dL^{-1} but <126 mg·dL^{-1}
Cigarette smoking	Current smoker, quit within past 6 months, or exposed to environmental tobacco smoke
Hypertension (or using antihypertensive medication)	Blood pressure $> 140/90$ mmHg or taking antihypertensive medication confirmed on 2 separate occasions
Dyslipidemia	Low density lipoprotein cholesterol ≥ 130 mg/dL, high density lipoprotein cholesterol <40 mg/dL, total serum cholesterol > 200 mg/dL, or taking medication to lower cholesterol levels
Sedentary lifestyle	Not participating in at least 30 min of moderate-intensity physical activity on at least three days of the week for at least 3 months
Secondary Nonmodifiable Risk Factors	Defining Criteria
Age	Men > 45 years; women > 55
Family history	MI or sudden death before 55 years of age in father or before 65 years of age in mother
Secondary Modifiable Risk Factors	
Obesity	Body mass index ≥ 30 kg·m^2 *or* waist girth >102 cm (40 in) for men and >88 cm (35 in) for women

Source: Adapted from *JAMA*, 269: 3015–3023, 1993 and the American College of Sport Medicine (ACSM). 2010. *ACSM guidelines for exercise testing and prescription.* Philadelphia, PA: Lippincott, Williams, & Wilkins.

TABLE 16.2
Risk Stratification

Low risk	Individuals who are asymptomatic and apparently healthy with no more than one primary coronary risk factor either modifiable or nonmodifiable (see Table 16.1)
Moderate risk	Individuals who are asymptomatic and apparently healthy and have two or more primary or secondary coronary risk factors either modifiable or nonmodifiable
High risk or have disease	Individuals with known disease (cardiovascular, pulmonary, or metabolic) or who exhibit one or more signs and symptoms suggestive of cardiovascular disease

Source: Adapted from the American College of Sport Medicine (ACSM). 2010. *ACSM guidelines for exercise testing and prescription.* Philadelphia, PA: Lippincott, Williams, & Wilkins.

16.3.1 CARDIORESPIRATORY ENDURANCE

Cardiorespiratory endurance is related to the development of the cardiovascular, respiratory, and muscular systems. Aerobic activities, such as bike riding, running, and brisk walking, involve prolonged, rhythmical movements of the body's large muscle groups and increased respiration. As one's rate of respiration increases, greater amounts of oxygen are taken in and transported through the blood to the body's muscles to be used for energy production. Cardiorespiratory endurance is a measure of cardiorespiratory output as well as oxygen uptake by the muscles. The maximum amount of blood containing oxygen that the heart can pump and the muscles can use for energy production is known as VO_{2max}. Improvements in cardiorespiratory endurance lead to increases in VO_{2max}.

16.3.1.1   Assessment of Cardiorespiratory Endurance

Cardiorespiratory standards for girls are most easily calculated by a 1-mile walk/run test. To perform the test, a 1-mile course is marked off. A circular track is helpful and should be used if available. A girl is asked to complete the mile in the quickest time possible and is allowed to walk or run at her discretion.

Standards for the 1-mile walk/run are set so that at the age of 5, girls should complete the course in 14 min. Time will then decrease 1 min per year for the next 2 years (age 6–13 min; age 7–12 min). After 8 years of age, however, the standard is 11.5 min, the standard only decreases by 30 seconds (s). Girls ages 9 through 12 should be able to complete the course in 11 min. Girls aged 13 or more should complete the course in 10.5 min or less (McSwegin et al. 1989).

Other options include the .5-mile, suggested for girls aged 5 through 9, and the 1.5-mile run, suggested for girls aged 13 through 18. Standards for the .5-mile run are as follows: (1) a 5-year-old girl should complete the course under 6.33 min, (2) a 6-year-old, under 5.66 min, (3) a 7-year-old, less than 5.33 min, (4) an 8-year-old, under 5 min, and (5) a 9-year-old, under 4.75 min (McSwegin et al. 1989). There are only two time standards in the 1.5-mile course. Girls 13 and 14 years old should complete the course under 17 min, whereas, any girl over the age of 14 should complete the course under 16.5 min (McSwegin et al. 1989).

Cardiorespiratory standards for women are similarly assessed (Hoegar and Hoegar 1999, 2011). Before beginning, two items will be needed: a stopwatch; and a 1.5-mile walking course (preferably on a track). Cardiorespiratory endurance for women is expressed in VO_{2max} in ml kg^{-1} min^{-1} and is estimated using a regression equation. In order to use the regression equation to estimate VO_{2max}, running time is expressed in min and s should be changed to a decimal figure (i.e., 14 min and 25 s would be 14 + 25/60 or 14.4 min). The formula to estimate VO_{2max} ml kg^{-1} min^{-1} = (483 divided by run time in min) + 3.5.

Women younger than 30 years of age should have a VO_{2max} of 38 ml kg^{-1} min^{-1} or greater. After age 30, this figure will drop two points per decade (↓2 points for every 10 years after age 30; so someone age 40 would have a VO_{2max} of 36). After the age of 50, a woman's VO_{2max} will decrease by only one point per decade.

The 1-mile walk test is another option, particularly for individuals at risk for orthopedic injury or cardiovascular difficulties, or who find running uncomfortable. Before beginning, three items will be needed to make calculations: one's weight, a stopwatch, and a 1-mile walking course (preferably on a track). An individual should walk briskly for 1 mile at a pace that elevates the HR above 120 beats per min (bpm). At the completion of the walk, the pulse is counted for 10 s and multiplied by 6 to convert it to bpm. The next step is to convert the time from min and s into min and fractions of a min (as explained above). The final step is to insert the information into an equation to obtain VO_{2max}. The equation is: $VO_{2max} = 88.768 - (0.0957 \times \text{weight in pounds}) - (1.4537 \times \text{time in min}) - (0.1194 \times HR)$.

16.3.1.2   Guidelines for Cardiorespiratory Endurance Training

16.3.1.2.1   Determining Exercise Intensity

There are different ways to determine the intensity of aerobic physical activity. Some use a percentage of either a person's maximal HR (MHR) or HR reserve (HRR) when engaging in activity. Recently, a new formula for women has been proposed (Parker-Pope 2010). To estimate target heart rate using the MHR formula, please see Table 16.3. To estimate target heart rate using the HHR formula, please see Table 16.4.

During exercise, HR can be measured using a HR monitor or by palpating the carotid (in the neck, below the jaw, next to the Adam's apple) or the radial artery (on same side of the wrist as the thumb) with the index and middle fingers for 6 s, 10 s, or 15 s. This count would then have to be converted to bpm. If counting for 6 s, simply add a 0 (zero), for 10 s multiply by 6, and for 15 s multiply by 4 to get bpm. The longer the time the HR is counted, the more accurate the count. If the HR is above 100 bpm before the individual begins exercising and stays elevated after 15 min of rest, he or she should not exercise and should be seen by a physician.

Resting HR is best measured in the morning before rising by palpitating the carotid or radial artery and counting the pulse for 1 min. Resting HR could also be measured at other times while the individual is seated and relaxed, but may not be as accurate because the true resting HR may be altered by a variety of variables, such as food intake and emotional status that change throughout the day.

For improvements in cardiovascular fitness, the ACSM (2010a) suggests cardiovascular activities of moderate or vigorous intensities. The intensity and duration of these activities depend on one's fitness level and needs. According to ACSM (ACSM 2010b), moderate-intensity activities are activities that fall between 40% and 60% of HRR (or 64% and 77% of MHR), and vigorous-intensity activities are activities that fall above 60% of HRR (or above 77% of MHR). The recommended intensity varies based on the duration of the exercise session, with shorter durations

TABLE 16.3
Adjusted Maximum Heart Rate Formula to Determine Exercise Intensity[a] for Women

Steps	Procedure
1	206 − (age × .88) = estimated maximum heart rate (MHR)
2	MHR × desired % (i.e., 64% lower limit)[a]
3	HRR × desired % (i.e., 777% upper limit)
4	Target heart rate would then range from lower limit to upper limit

[a] Training zone ranges from 64% to 77%.

Source: Adapted from the American College of Sport Medicine (ACSM). 2010. *ACSM guidelines for exercise testing and prescription.* Philadelphia, PA: Lippincott, Williams, & Wilkins.

TABLE 16.4
Karvonen's Formula to Determine Exercise Intensity Using Heart Rate Reserve

Steps	Procedure
1	220 − age = estimated maximum heart rate (MHR)
2	MHR − resting heart rate = heart rate reserve (HRR)
3	HRR × desired % (i.e., 50%)
4	Add resting heart rate to answer in step 3; this is lower limit
5	HRR × desired % (i.e., 85%)
6	Add resting heart rate to answer in step 5; this is upper limit
7	Target heart rate would then range from lower limit to upper

Source: Adapted from the American College of Sport Medicine (ACSM). 2010. *ACSM guidelines for exercise testing and prescription.* Philadelphia, PA: Lippincott, Williams, & Wilkins.

recommended for higher intensity activities (e.g., running, high-impact aerobics, heavy yard work, swimming continuous laps) and longer durations recommended for lower intensity activities (e.g., brisk walking, recreational swimming, nonstrenuous yard work). Nonfit or deconditioned individuals may see benefits with lower intensities, whereas individuals who are more physically fit will need to exercise in the higher part of the % HHR or % MHR ranges to see benefits in cardiovascular fitness. However, higher intensities involve greater risk for cardiovascular and orthopedic injury (ACSM 2010a).

Another way to determine intensity is to use one of the Borg Scales: (1) the Rating of Perceived Exertion (RPE); or (2) the Rating of Perceived Breathlessness (RPB) scale (Borg 1982). These scales are illustrated in Table 16.5. On the RPE scale, the individual rates his or her overall exertion and fatigue while exercising. A rating from moderate (3) to very strong (6 to 9) has been shown to correlate with an intensity level of 50% to 85% of HRR or 60% to 90% of MHR (Pollock and Wilmore 1990). If individuals have moderate to severe respiratory diseases, such as asthma, they may want to use the perceived breathlessness scale to choose an appropriate conditioning level (see Table 16.5). The target range for breathlessness is 3 for exercise intensity at 50% and 6 for training at an intensity of 85% (Wilson and Jones 1989).

16.3.1.2.2 Recommended Duration and Frequency of Cardiovascular Activities

The development of cardiovascular endurance for children is more related to play than to structured exercise. The HHS recommends that children accumulate at least 60 min of moderate- to vigorous-intensity physical activity each day. The ACSM (2010a) suggests that 30 min of this daily activity be of a moderate intensity and 30 min be of a vigorous intensity. Many children, particularly younger, may not need a structured activity program because they acquire the recommended amounts of physical activity through intermittent bouts of free play and games (HHS 2008). As children grow older, they are able to engage in longer periods of physical activity and more likely to engage in structured physical activity, such as sports or fitness programs.

TABLE 16.5

Borg Scales[a]

Rating of Perceived Exertion (RPE)		Rating of Perceived Breathlessness (RPB)
0	None	0
0.5	Very, very weak	0.5
1	Very weak	1
2	Weak	2
3	Moderate	3
4	Somewhat strong	4
5	Strong	5
6		6
7	Very severe	7
8		8
9	Very, very strong	9
10	Maximal	10

[a] Use only one of these scales as a monitoring device during exercise. If fatigue tends to limit you during aerobic workouts, use the exertion scale on the left.

Source: Adapted from Borg, G. A. V. 1982. Psychophysical basis of perceived exertion. *Med. Sci. Sports Exercise* 14: 377–381 and Wilson, R. C., and P. W. Jones. 1989. A comparison of the visual analogue scale and modified Borg scale for the measurement of dyspnea during exercise. *Clin. Sci.* 76: 277–282.

The current recommendation for cardiovascular exercise for adults is 150 min of moderate-intensity (e.g., brisk walking) or 75 min of vigorous-intensity physical activity (e.g., running) each week (HHS 2008, ACSM 2010a). The ACSM (2010a) also defines the recommended amounts of activity in daily values, suggesting that individuals engage in at least 30 min of moderate-intensity activity 5 days per week or at least 20 min of vigorous activity 3 days per week. Individuals can vary how the recommended amount of activity is accumulated. For example, a person who engages in 30 min of moderate-intensity aerobic activity 5 days per week, a person who engages in 25 min of vigorous-intensity aerobic physical activity 3 days per week, and a person who engages in 10 min periods of moderate-intensity activity 3 times a day, 5 days per week would all meet the recommended amount. Whether an individual should exercise at moderate or high intensity depends on his or her current health status, fitness level, goals, and preferences.

For even greater health benefits (i.e., prevention of weight gain and lower risk of colon cancer, breast cancers, diabetes, and heart disease), a person who has reached the recommended 150 min of moderate-intensity activity each week can work towards obtaining 300 min of moderate-intensity activity, 150 min of vigorous-intensity activity, or an equivalent combination of moderate- and vigorous-intensity aerobic activity each week (HHS 2008). For most individuals, 250 to 300 min of moderate-intensity or 150 min of vigorous-intensity aerobic activity per week would be needed for weight loss or maintenance (ACSM 2010a). It is important to note that some health benefits can be seen if the individual accumulates at least 60 min of physical activity each week (HHS 2008).

Individuals who are sedentary or unfit should first work towards the goal of 150 min of exercise per week with a focus on increasing the number of min per week before increasing the intensity. Programs of vigorous-intensity exercise will allow for the needed amount of activity to be obtained from a shorter duration of activity; however, vigorous-intensity exercise is not required. Individuals who are obese may be at increased risk for orthopedic or cardiovascular injury; therefore, the intensity of the activity prescribed may need to be lowered to avoid potential injury. Furthermore, some individuals may find vigorous-intensity activity undesirable and should exercise at a lower intensity to keep themselves motivated (ACSM 2010a). Individuals who cannot tolerate long duration of exercise can engage in several shorter periods of activity (e.g., three 10-min periods each day; Jakicic and Otto 2005).

16.3.2 Muscular Strength and Endurance

Muscular strength is the maximal force that can be generated during a single voluntary muscle contraction (known as 1 Repetition Max—RM). Muscular endurance involves the repetition of submaximal contractions for a sustained amount of time (e.g., lifting and lowering a 10 lb weight for 15 repetitions). Exercises that improve muscular strength and endurance can involve isotonic, isometric, or isokinetic muscle contractions.

Isotonic contractions involve movement of the joint where the muscle shortens while a set amount of resistance or weight is lifted (concentric movement) and lengthens while the weight is lowered (eccentric movement). Isometric contractions involve static contractions of the muscle where there is no movement around the joint or the resistance is unmovable (such as pushing against a static object or holding a 5-s contraction at maximum intensity without moving the joint angle). Isokinetic contractions involve muscle contractions that occur at a constant rate through the full range of motion. The speed of contraction is controlled mechanically so that the limb moves through the full range at a set speed, as on a Cybex machine. Training can involve any of these types of muscle contractions.

Important components of a resistance training program include the amount of weight lifted (also referred to as load), the number of repetitions (or number of times the weight is lifted), the number of sets (composed of a certain number of consecutive repetitions), the speed that the weight is lifted and lowered, the range of motion through which the weight is lifted and lowered, and the number of min and days per week the individual trains. It is also important to know one's repetition max (RM), or the greatest amount of weight that can be lifted for a certain number of repetitions, the maximal voluntary contraction, or the maximal resistance that can be held in a 6-s static contraction, and the amount of time needed to sustain the static contraction for strength or endurance gains.

16.3.2.1 Assessment of Muscular Strength and Endurance

Commonly used methods to assess childhood muscular strength and endurance capabilities are sit-up and pull-up exercises. The maximum repetitions a child can perform in 1 min are counted. Typically the standard is 20 sit-up repetitions for a 5-year-old girl with the standard progressing by one sit-up per year as the child ages. The standard for the pull-up exercise is 1 pull-up regardless of the age of the girl (McSwegin et al. 1989).

The assessment for muscular strength and endurance for women is slightly more complex. Rather than performing only two exercises, the adult must perform five exercises: (1) latissimus dorsi pull-down, (2) leg extension, (3) bench press, (4) leg curl, and (5) arm curl. Familiarization with the individual exercises and the proper techniques must precede testing. The weight required for testing must be calculated. The leg extension exercise is tested first, using 50% of body weight (BW). This is followed by bench press and latissimus dorsi pull-downs at 45% of BW, and the leg curl at 25%. The last exercise is the arm curl using 18% of BW. For example, a woman weighing 120 pounds would multiply her weight by the percentage necessary for testing procedures. Thus, the leg extension calculation would be $120 \times 0.5 = 60$ pounds; bench press and pull-downs would be $120 \times .45 = 54$ pounds; leg curl would be $120 \times .25 = 30$ pounds; the arm curl would be $120 \times .18 = 21.6$ pounds. During the assessment, a woman performs as many repetitions as possible of each exercise. The number of repetitions performed is then compared with set standards. Standards are as follows: (1) leg extension—10 repetitions; (2) bench press and pull-downs—11 repetitions; (3) leg curl—7 repetitions; and (4) arm curl—12 repetitions (Hoeger and Hoeger 2011). This is the minimal suggested number of repetitions. Higher repetitions reflect greater muscular strength and endurance capabilities.

16.3.2.2 Guidelines for Muscular Strength and Endurance Training

Individuals should engage in an appropriate warm-up before engaging in a resistance training session. The warm-up should include 5 to 10 min of cardiovascular exercise and 5 to 10 min of dynamic stretching along with initial sets of the exercises to be performed using a light load (ACSM 2010b). After lifting weights, a cool-down session lasting at least 10–15 min is recommended. The cool-down should include general calisthenics and static stretches with the aim of relaxing the body and improving flexibility (Faigenbaum et al. 2009; Grossmann 2004).

Many children improve their muscle strength and endurance through free-play exercises involving weight-bearing activities or movements that act against resistance (e.g., climbing trees, playing on playground equipment [HHS 2008]). Children who are able to engage in play that involves high-impact forces should be ready to participate in resistance training, usually occurring around the age of 7 or 8 years when they show improved balanced and postural control (Council on Sports Medicine and Fitness 2008; Faigenbaum et al. 2009; Wallace and Wallace 2008).

Children should be gradually introduced to resistance training. Children younger than 7 years old should begin training with calisthenics (e.g., push-ups) before beginning light-resistance exercises. It is important for beginners to learn how to perform simple weight-bearing exercises (e.g., biceps curls) with no or little weight before they begin to train with heavier weights (Faigenbaum et al. 2009; Grossmann 2004).

Guidelines for resistance training for children emphasize muscular endurance rather than muscular strength; hence, there is an emphasis on more repetitions rather than heavier weight. Due to their inexperience with resistance training, beginners should start training by doing one set of each exercise until they have learned the proper technique (Vehrs 2005), and they should not train more than 2 days per week (ACSM 2010b). For children, 1 to 3 sets of 8 to 15 repetitions per set of each exercise at a moderate intensity (60%–80% 1 RM) are recommended. For prepubescent children, the amount of weight lifted should be decreased if the child is unable to lift the weight for at least

8 repetitions. Once 15 repetitions can be performed with proper form, the child can increase the amount of weight lifted by 1 to 3 pounds. When children have reached late adolescence, they can begin tailoring the guidelines for resistance training so that muscular strength rather than endurance is emphasized (load is high, repetitions are low). For example, older adolescents may perform sets with higher loads but with fewer repetitions when they show maturity. At 16 years of age, adolescents may progress to entry-level adult programs. However, progression in training should be gradual, avoiding training that is too intense or demanding (ACSM 2010a). Appendices 16.C and 16.D highlight resistance training recommendations for children.

Children, as well as individuals with hypertension, diabetes, or those at risk for a stroke or other problems resulting from an increase in blood pressure, should train at a lower intensity and not work their muscles to exhaustion through maximal or near-maximal lifts (Council on Sports Medicine and Fitness 2008; Grossmann 2004). Children should not do spine loading, power lifting, or body building exercise because of risks to the spine and growth plates (Ashmore 2003). These activities should be done after the individual has reached skeletal maturity (Council on Sports Medicine and Fitness 2008). Many weight machines were designed to fit an adult's body; therefore, they may be too large for children to use them correctly. Care should be taken to ensure that a child will be able to use a weight machine with proper technique and range of motion (ACSM 2010b).

Most healthy adults should be able to engage in regular strength training, whereas individuals with health problems will need to modify their resistance training program. The guidelines for muscular strength and endurance training for children and adults are similar. However, there should be increased emphasis on form and proper technique during repetitive lifts for children and also an emphasis on motor-skill development.

The recommended frequency of resistance training is 2–3 days per week with a 48-h period between training sessions when working the same muscle groups (ASCM 2010a). Greater than 4 days of training per week is not recommended due to an increased risk of injury due to overtraining (Council on Sports Medicine and Fitness 2008). Gains in strength and endurance should be seen after at least 8 weeks, with initial increases in strength coming from enhanced neural control (Council on Sports Medicine and Fitness 2008; Grossman 2004; Wescott and Faigenbaum 2003). In order to maintain strength gains, a person must continue to engage in at least one weekly resistance training session. The resistance lifted should be the same as the weight needed to see the improvements in strength at the completion of the 8 weeks of training sessions.

High-intensity resistance is achieved when momentary muscle fatigue (being unable to lift the weight for another repetition while maintaining proper form) occurs. A lower number of repetitions (i.e., 3–6) will be required to reach muscle fatigue when a heavy weight is used, whereas a higher number of repetitions (i.e., 8–12) will be required when using a lighter resistance (ACSM 2010a).

For healthy adults to see improvements in muscle strength and endurance, ACSM (2010a) recommends 2 to 4 sets of 8 to 12 repetitions done in the full range of motion at an intensity of about 60%–80% of 1 RM. The individual should rest 2 to 3 min between sets of exercises working the same muscle groups. The intensity of the lift (i.e., % RM) should vary depending on the number of sets that will be performed. For example, if you perform one set of the exercise, for maximum benefits you should perform the set at 90%–100% of RM after your warm-up. If you are performing 2–3 sets, use the first set as a warm-up by only doing 40%–50% RM. The second set could be done at 60%–75% RM, and the third set at 90%–100% RM.

Several multijoint (involving muscles surrounding multiple joints such as squats) and single-joint (involving muscles surrounding only one joint such as biceps curls) exercises that work all of the major muscle groups (e.g., gluteal muscles, quadriceps, hamstrings, abdominals, spinal erectors, pectoralis major, latissmus dorsi, upper trapezius, deltoids, biceps, and triceps) should be included in a training regimen. The individual should start with the large muscle groups (e.g., quadriceps, gluteal, pectoralis major) and end with the smaller muscle groups (e.g., biceps, triceps), as well as do multijoint exercises before single-joint exercises (ACSM 2010a; Grossmann 2004; Wescott and Faigenbaum 2003). For example, squats and chest presses (multijoint exercises involving larger muscles groups) should be done before biceps curls and heel raises (single-joint exercises involving smaller muscle groups). Additionally, training should include a balance between opposing muscle groups (e.g., the biceps and the triceps, the quadriceps and the hamstrings; ACSM 2010a; Faigenbaum et al. 2009; Grossmann 2004).

Individuals should rest long enough between sets of exercises so that they can perform the next set using proper technique (ACSM 2010a). The duration of the rest period is dependent upon how intense their training load is, how many repetitions and sets they are doing, the types of exercises they are doing, and their fitness level. A general rule is that rest between sets should be greater (about 2 min) when the load is high and the number of repetitions per set is low (e.g., doing 4 sets of 6 repetitions) and can decrease (about 30–45 s) as the load becomes lighter and repetitions increase (e.g., doing 3 sets of 15 repetitions; Faigenbaum et al. 2009; Wescott and Faigenbaum 2003).

To obtain maximal benefits from a resistance training program and reduce the risk of injury and boredom, the intensity, volume, rest interval, and types of exercises should be varied (Faigenbaum et al. 2009; Grossmann 2004). To vary the types of exercises being done, exercises that work the same muscle groups can be substituted for each other, such as by doing the chest press in place of push-ups. Another idea would be to change the exercise equipment being used (e.g., use resistance bands rather than dumbbells). Intensity and volume can be varied by progressively increasing load, the number of sets completed, the number of repetitions completed, or the number of days per week the individual trains (ACSM 2010a). An overview of the ACSM position on progression models in resistance training for healthy adults can be found in Appendix 16.E.

Appropriate weightlifting technique is important to avoid being injured. The concentric (toward the body) and eccentric (away from the body) movements involved in resistance training exercises should be done in a slow and controlled manner, exhaling during the concentric movement and inhaling during the eccentric movement. One strategy to ensure that the exercise is being done in a slow and controlled manner is to count to two or three during the concentric movement, then to count to two or three for the eccentric movement. For most exercises, an individual should stand or sit tall, shoulders down and back, torso erect, and hips level with the shoulders. This will allow for proper technique and easier breathing, as it is important that normal breathing be maintained. Twisting, turning, and squirming should be avoided during exercises that do not require those movements; it often signals that the weight being lifted is too heavy or that the muscles are getting close to being exhausted. It is more important to use correct form than to lift a heavier weight or do more repetitions. Lifting a heavy weight incorrectly will increase one's risk of injury (ACSM 2010; Ashmore 2003; Grossman 2004; Wescott and Faigenbaum 2003).

16.3.3 HEALTHY BODY COMPOSITION

Body composition can be divided into fat and fat-free weight (FFW). FFW includes all of the tissues of the body—muscle, bone, skin, blood, and organs minus the amount of fat. Chemically, FFW is composed of water, proteins, and bone mineral. The fat component of the body includes both storage and essential fat. Storage fat includes subcutaneous adipose tissues and the fat surrounding the internal organs. Essential fat includes the fat in the bone marrow, central nervous system, cell membranes, heart, lungs, liver, spleen, kidneys, intestines, and muscles. In the female, essential fat includes sex-specific or sex-characteristic fat. This component of essential fat is important for childbearing and other hormone-related functions. Many times, the terms lean body mass (LBM) and FFW are used interchangeably, but technically, they are not identical. LBM includes essential fat and FFW does not.

16.3.3.1 Assessment of Body Composition

A detailed explanation of the methods for assessing body composition is beyond the scope of this chapter. However, for children, skinfold data estimating body composition seems to be the most accurate method. Research has shown a systematic increase in skinfold thickness among 6- to

9-year-old girls from the 1960s to the 1980s. Body composition values in the 6- to 11-year-old age group increased from 17.6% between 1963 and 1965 to 27.1% between 1976 and 1980 (Gortmaker et al. 987). Healthy scores for percent BF for girls ages 5 through 17 range from 17% to 32% according to the Prudential FITNESSGRAM standards (Meredith 1987).

When using skinfold data to estimate BF, it is imperative to use equations that have been developed for a particular population or a similar population. Equations that have been developed for eumenorrheic females (normal menstruating females) may overestimate the percentage of BF for females with anorexia nervosa (AN) because the bone mineral content levels of eumenorrheic females may be higher than those of amenorrheic females (Barrow and Saha 1988; Drinkwater et al. 1984).

One simple way to determine one's health risk due to BF is the calculation of the body mass index (BMI), using an individual's height and weight. The BMI score should not be confused with an actual BF percentage score. It simply enables one to assess level of risk for diseases that are based on excessive BW. A higher score is associated with a high prevalence of mortality from heart disease, diabetics, and cancer. To calculate your BMI multiply your weight in pounds by 705 and divide this number by the square of your height in inches. For example, if a person weighed 120 pounds and was 63 in tall, her BMI would be calculated as follows: (1) $120 \times 705 = 84,600$; (2) $63 \times 63 = 3,969$; and (3) $84,600/3,969 = 21.32$. A BMI in the 18.5–24.9 range is considered acceptable. Those individuals with a BMI in the 25.0–29.9 range are classified as overweight and are at increased risk for heart disease, high cholesterol, hypertension, diabetes, and cancer, and those individuals with a BMI that is 30 or above are classified as obese and are at an even greater risk for those health problems. Additionally, individuals with a BMI less than 18.5 are classified as underweight and are at a greater risk for cardiovascular disease (ACSM 2010a).

Norms for children are based on age- and sex-specific percentiles because the amount of BF changes with age and differs for boys and girls. The following website provides information on evaluating a child's BMI: http://www.cdc.gov/healthyweight/assessing/bmi/childrens_bmi/about_childrens_bmi.html.

For adult women, standards for desirable body composition depend on health goals, athletic performance goals, and aesthetic goals. Standard values for % BF are presented in Table 16.6. However, these values must be interpreted with consideration of a person's goals. For example, if the goal is athletic prowess in a specific sport, a lower percentage of acceptable BF may be the standard. If the objective is health rather than fitness (e.g., the resumption of normal menstrual cycles), values in the average category are acceptable and should be promoted. Educators must make recommendations for acceptable levels of BF depending on the needs and goals of their clients. For the average adult woman, a healthy level of BF is 18% to 22% (Williams 1988).

TABLE 16.6
Standard Values for Percent Body Fat for Women

Rating	Age				
	18–29	30–39	40–49	50–59	60+
Excellent	<16	<17	<18	<19	<20
Good	16–19	17–20	18–21	19–22	20–23
Average	20–28	21–29	22–30	23–31	24–32
Fair	29–31	30–32	31–33	32–34	33–35
Poor	>31	>32	>33	>34	>35

Source: Adapted from Jackson, A.S. et al. 1978. *Br. J. Nutr.* 40: 497; and Jackson, A.S. et al. 1980. *Med. Sci. Sports Exercise* 12: 175.

For women with AN, especially, it is important to emphasize the importance of a healthy body composition. Low BF is associated with alteration in estrogen metabolism (Fishman et al. 1975; Petterson et al. 1973). It has been suggested that individuals with AN use internal fat as a means of providing calories, possibly decreasing the role it plays in converting androgen to estrogen because fat tissue is a site for estrogen formation and storage (Bale et al. 1996). In the human female, adipose tissue of the breasts, abdomen, omentum, and fatty marrow of the long bones convert androgen to estrogen; therefore, adipose tissue is a significant extragonadal source of estrogen (Frisch et al. 1981). Additionally, being below a critical level of BF has also been emphasized as a potential contributor to menstrual irregularity (Brooks-Gunn et al. 1987; Myerson et al. 1991; Walberg and Johnston 1991). The theory that low BF is related to menstrual irregularity is based on Frisch's findings (Frisch and MacArthur 1974). Frisch contended that both the onset and maintenance of regular menstrual function are dependent on a critical weight for the person's height, representing a critical lean-to-fat ratio or percent BF. Frisch also stated that the minimal amount of BF needed to begin menarche is approximately 17%, and after age 16, at least 22% BF is needed to maintain normal menstruating cycles. Because a characteristic of AN is the absence of menstruation for at least 3 months, normal levels of BF must be emphasized in the recovery process.

16.3.3.2 Guidelines for Improving Body Composition

The premises or bases for healthy body composition are similar for children and women. While body composition is determined by a complex set of genetic and behavioral factors, healthy values of body composition for women and children can be maintained by balancing energy intake with energy expenditure. If energy intake exceeds expenditure, BW will increase. Conversely, weight is lost when the opposite situation occurs. Energy intake consists of the food that is consumed, and energy expenditure is composed of the amount of calories used while at rest (known as the Basal Metabolic Rate or BMR) and through physical activity.

To lose one pound of fat, an individual would need a deficit of about 3,500 kcal of energy. A weight loss of 1–2 pounds per week, equating to a deficit of 500 to 1,000 calories per day, respectively, is recommended as a healthy rate of weight loss. This small caloric deficit is recommended in order to promote loss of BF while maintaining lean body tissue (ASCM 2010b). It can be attained through healthy dietary changes (e.g. 250–500 kcal less consumed per day) and an increase in physical activity (e.g. expending 250–500 kcal through exercise each day ACSM 2010a, 2010b). Various websites allow individuals to determine the energy costs of their activities. Two are listed below:

http://www.primusweb.com/fitnesspartner/calculat.htm. A calculator at this website estimates the number of calories burned for over 200 activities. http://www.coolrunning.com/engine/4/4_1/94.shtml. A calculator at this website estimates the number of calories burned after swimming, biking, or running various distances.

As mentioned previously, the ACSM (2010a) recommends 300 min of moderate-intensity or 150 min of vigorous-intensity aerobic activity each week for weight loss. In their review of the literature on exercise treatment for obesity, Atlantis et al. (2006) found 155–180 min of moderate- to high-intensity physical activity each week to be effective at decreasing BF in overweight children and adolescents.

Resistance training is also important for weight loss. The effectiveness of a combined aerobic/strength training program in aiding weight loss was demonstrated by Wescott's (1991) comparison of two groups of exercisers. One group performed aerobic exercises for 30 min 3 days a week. The other performed 15 min of aerobic exercises and 15 min of strength training exercises 3 days a week. Both groups spent the same amount of time exercising. The group that combined aerobic exercise with resistance exercises lost more fat than the group who performed only aerobic exercise, and also gained more lean muscle mass. Each additional pound of muscle tissue can raise the BMR 30 to 50 kcal a day (Hafen and Hoeger 1994).

The American Council on Exercise (ACE) and ACSM provide specific guidelines for caloric restriction for weight loss purposes (American Council on Exercise [ACE] 1991, ACSM 1993, 1995,

2006). The intention of these guidelines is to enhance the loss of BF rather than lean body tissue. Normal adults should consume at least 1200 kcal per day; however, this requirement may not be appropriate for athletes or older individuals. If caloric intake is less than 1200 kcal per day, the BMR can drop as low as 20%. This drop is caused by the loss of lean tissue and the body's efforts to conserve energy by slowing the BMR. Negative caloric balance should not exceed 500 to 1000 kcal per day. For example, if an individual is expending 2,000 kcal per day in energy expenditure, they should not take in less than 1,500 kcal or 1,000 kcal in energy intake (i.e., food sources). The minimal amount of energy consumption needed to maintain normal physiological functioning is estimated to be somewhere around 1,000 kcal for adults. This is an extremely rough estimation and simply serves as a rule of thumb. Therefore, the rule is that caloric intake should not be less than 1,000 kcal per day. To get an estimation of energy needs, use the worksheet in Appendix 16.F.

The diet should consist of foods that are acceptable to the dieter in terms of sociocultural background and usual eating habits, provided that the nutrient intake is adequate. These habits should be sustainable for life. A dietary fat intake of less than 30% of total energy intake and an emphasis on eating whole grains, lean protein, fruits, and vegetables are recommended (ACSM 2010a). Yo-yo diets with severe calorie restriction only make it harder in the long run for you to lose weight and keep it off because your resting metabolic rate decreases because of severe food restriction. When you begin eating normally again, you may gain weight. Be sensible and choose a balanced approach to weight loss.

16.3.4 Flexibility

Static flexibility is the total range of motion (ROM) at the joint. Dynamic flexibility is a measure of the torque or resistance to movement. Flexibility is related to age, sex, and physical activity. However, the major limitation to both static and dynamic flexibility is the tightness of soft tissue structures. The relative contribution of soft tissues to the total resistance encountered by a joint during movement is estimated to be: (1) joint capsule—47%; (2) muscle and its fascia—41%; (3) tendons and ligaments—10%; and (4) skin—2% (Johns and Wright 1962). Inactivity is a major cause of inflexibility but it can also be associated with the aging process as well. Flexibility increases with age until puberty and thereafter begins to decline through the teenage and adult years (Cooper et al. 1995).

16.3.4.1 Assessment of Flexibility

Flexibility is a joint-specific attribute of fitness. In order to achieve a total flexibility score, one should perform a battery of flexibility tests. However, time and resources often are limited. Thus, the sit-and-reach test has become widely accepted as a general test for flexibility. This test primarily measures flexibility of two main groups of muscles—the hamstrings and lower back muscle—and one joint—the hip. To perform the sit-and-reach test, one should sit on the floor with the back against a wall, legs straight, and arms and feet extended directly in front. A box is placed in front of the extended legs with the bottom of the feet resting on the end of the box. A ruler is placed on top of the box parallel to the length of the box and to the extended arms and legs. The end of the ruler nearest the extended fingertips should read 0 cm. A partner holds the ruler in place and reads the measurement as the participant leans forward and reaches as far as possible down the length of the ruler without bouncing. The final position reached and held for 2 s is the score.

Individuals 18 and younger should be able to reach 40.6 cm (Hoeger and Hoeger 2011). In earlier publications, Hoeger and Hoeger (1999) stated that girls between the ages of 5 and 17 should be able to reach a minimum of 25 cm with a progression of 1 cm for every year after age 5. Women between the ages of 19 and 35 should be able to reach 40.1 cm; between 36 and 49, 36.8 cm; and over 50, 31.2 cm. Reaching further indicates greater flexibility (Hoeger and Hoeger 2011).

16.3.4.2 Guidelines for Flexibility Exercises

The general principles for flexibility apply to individuals of all ages. Flexibility exercises should be performed in a slow, controlled manner with gradual progression to a full range of motion. Static stretches should be performed for at least 10 min at least 2 to 3 days per week. Stretches should include all major muscle tendon groups (hips, legs, pelvis, upper and lower back, shoulders, and neck) with four or more repetitions of stretches for each group. Static stretches should be held for 15 to 60 s to a point of mild tightness without discomfort (ACSM 2010a).

Children have much shorter attention spans and may not be able to hold stretches for as long, or do as many stretches in one session, as an adult. For this reason, stretching routines should be made fun and lively. Activities that more closely resemble games are preferred by children and will be better accepted and have higher participation rates. Another point to remember is that when children learn new skills, the concepts need to be taught in a way that they understand. For instance, instead of telling a child to stretch to a position of mild discomfort, it is better to have the child stretch to a point where she can feel the muscle pull in a certain area.

16.3.5 YOGA AND EATING DISORDERS

Yoga involves the combination of asanas (body postures emphasizing physical awareness) and pranayamas (awareness of breathing) and may include dharana and dhyama, or meditation involving a nonjudgmental focus on inner processes (Dale et al. 2009, McIver et al. 2009). The Mayo Clinic recommends that individuals with the following conditions be medically cleared to participate in yoga: high blood pressure that is difficult to control, a risk of blood clots, eye conditions (e.g., glaucoma), osteoporosis, pregnancy, and artificial joints (see http://www.mayoclinic.com/health/yoga/CM00004).

Yoga helps improve balance and flexibility and strengthens the muscles and bones of the body because it involves weight-bearing exercises. This is true for adults as well as children. A great resource for yoga for children is Bersma and Visscher's (2003) book. The authors provide guidelines for developing yoga programs for children of different ages as well as examples of child-focused yoga games and postures.

The cardiovascular benefits of yoga depend on the intensity of the exercises. Beginner's yoga is reported as being metabolically similar to walking at a slow pace while more vigorous forms of yoga, such as Ashtanga Yoga, performed for at least 10 min could improve cardiovascular fitness for unfit or sedentary individuals (Hagins et al. 2007). Studies have shown that the practice of yoga can improve cardiopulmonary endurance in healthy individuals, with greater benefits arising from regular, long-term participation. The improvement in cardiopulmonary endurance results from an increase in lung capacity and the delivery of oxygen to the working muscles brought about from yoga's emphasis on breathing during the postures (Raub 2002). Regular practice of yoga may aid in weight loss and maintenance through improved physical fitness, particularly the more active forms of yoga (e.g., Ashtanga Yoga). Research has also found yoga to be related to decreases in depression, anxiety, and stress and improvements in body image, mental focus, and attention (Brown and Gerbarg 2005; Granath et al. 2006; Jhansi Rani and Krishna Rao 2005). It can also promote skills in emotion regulation, cooperation, and concentration for children (Bersma 2003; McGonigal 2006).

Numerous studies support the use of yoga in the prevention and treatment of EDs. Including yoga as a component of an ED prevention program has led to decreases in body dissatisfaction, drive for thinness, and thinking about and engaging in uncontrollable eating (Scime and Cook-Cottone 2008; Scime et al. 2006). Research has also found including yoga in ED treatment to improve awareness of and responsiveness to internal bodily states, body acceptance, body satisfaction, and the ability to identify emotional states and self-soothe (Dale et al. 2009; Daubenmeir 2005; Douglass 2009; Jhansi Rani and Krishna Rao 1994). Decreases in feelings of anxiety and fear about eating, guilt and shame after eating, self-objectification, mood disturbances, food preoccupation, and other ED attitudes and symptoms have also been observed (Carei et al. 2009; Daubermeir 2005).

Individuals with EDs have been found to be disconnected from physical sensations and emotional states (Spoor et al. 2005) and to view their bodies as objects that are evaluated within the cultural ideal of a thin body (known as self-objectification [Daubenmeir 2005]). Yoga focuses on developing a connection between the mind and body. Attention is paid to the subtle cues provided by the body while breathing and holding poses and during meditation. A nonjudgmental awareness of physical states within the body is developed, and focus is taken off of the body's outer appearance and onto bodily sensations and the movements and positioning of the body. Thus, an appreciation of what the body is able to do, rather than its outer appearance, and acceptance of its limitations, rather than a need to control it or push it beyond its limitations, can be gained from practicing yoga (Dale et al. 2009). Yoga can also help a person become better able to recognize and cope with emotional states, such as being able to recognize and release tension through breathing and relaxation (Close 2007; Dale et al. 2009).

Individuals with EDs lose their natural ability to regulate food intake by eating when the body sends signals of hunger and stopping when the body feels satiated. Individuals who are restrictive eaters ignore bodily cues of hunger, whereas binge eaters start eating due to emotional cues (i.e., eating to distract themselves from disturbing emotions or thoughts) or external cues (e.g., seeing commercials about food, social events). An awareness of bodily cues can help these individuals reconnect to and trust the body's natural cues of hunger and satiation, so that they begin to eat when physically hungry and stop when the body is satiated. It can also help them differentiate these natural cues from external cues (Benavides and Caballero 2009; Dale et al. 2009; Daubenmeir 2005; McIver et al. 2009). A reconnection to the body's natural hunger and satiation cues may also be beneficial to non-eating disordered individuals who overeat and are trying to lose or maintain their weight (Kristal et al. 2005).

16.3.6 EXCESSIVE EXERCISE

Exercise can become problematic when an individual exercises too intensely, too frequently, or at too high of a volume without allowing the body time to recover (Faigenbaum 2009). Exercising in this way will lead to physical and psychological symptoms—a state often referred to as the overtraining syndrome (Morgan et al. 1987). Signs of the overtraining syndrome include soreness, stiffness, fatigue, amenorrhea, decreased VO_{2max}, decreased blood lactate levels, poorer physical performance during workouts, a higher resting HR, decreased HR response to exercise, decreased immune functioning, more frequent injuries, appetite loss, weight loss, insomnia, and mood disturbances (Costin 2007; De Mond 1991). Excessive exercise can lead to osteopenia or osteoporosis (decreased bone mass), increasing one's risk of stress fractures.

Some excessive exercisers have maladaptive attitudes about exercise and exercise behaviors. Excessive physical activity in its pathological state has been referred to as exercise dependence, obligatory exercise, compulsive exercise, or activity disorder (Costin 2007). It can involve either structured exercise sessions that include weight training and cardiovascular exercise or random movement, such as standing instead of sitting (Costin 2007). When an individual feels guilty for not exercising and exercises to improve physical appearance or control weight, he or she is at risk for decreased psychological well-being and ED behaviors (Mond et al. 2004). These factors have been found to best differentiate eating-disordered and noneating-disordered exercisers (Mond and Calogero 2009).

Other characteristics of pathological excessive exercise include (Beaumont et al. 1994; Costin 2007; Powers and Thompson 2008; Shroff et al. 2006):

1. Feeling depressed, irritable, or anxious when not able to engage in physical activity.
2. Keeping detailed records of the amount and intensity of physical activity and the number of calories used for physical activity.
3. Reducing caloric intake when not able to exercise.
4. Using exercise to compensate for an episode of binge eating.
5. Not allowing oneself to miss an exercise session, having a schedule that revolves around physical activity, and neglecting social, vocational, household, and other responsibilities in order to exercise.

6. Engaging in rigid and repetitive exercise routines.
7. Continuing to exercise despite being overtrained.
8. Increasing the amount or intensity of exercise in response to the decreased physical abilities and fatigue resulting from being overtrained.
9. Being secretive about workouts.
10. Engaging in strenuous physical activity for more than 2 h per day. (This amount of activity may not be maladaptive for athletes and other people of a healthy weight.)

16.3.6.1 Excessive Exercise and Eating Disorders

Excessive exercise has frequently been seen in individuals with EDs (Shroff et al. 2006). Davis et al. (1997) found that 81% of their sample of patients with AN, and 57% of those diagnosed with BN, engaged in excessive exercise during the acute phase of their disorder. Bryant-Waugh (2007) suggested that excessive exercise, along with purging and dietary restriction, may be frequently used as a weight-management strategy for young children and adolescents as they are less likely than older adolescents and adults to have access to substances, such as appetite suppressants, diuretics, and amphetamines.

The physical risks of exercise can be greater in individuals with EDs, particularly if the individual is consuming an inadequate number of calories to refuel the body after exercise. This can lead to the breakdown of muscle and increase the risk for cardiovascular problems (e.g., hypotension, bradycardia, and cardiac arrhythmia), particularly if the individual has electrolyte imbalances from purging. Individuals with AN are susceptible to osteopenia and can experience stress fractures and damage to the joints as a result, particularly when engaging in high-impact activities. Excessive exercise can also exacerbate peripheral edema in emaciated individuals (Beaumont et al. 1994).

16.3.6.2 Treatment of Excessive Exercise

Treatment for someone who exercises excessively involves having him or her take time to rest between workouts, decrease the frequency or duration of workouts, include lower intensity workouts on days between intense workouts, incorporate more variety to the workout routine, do flexibility exercises more often, include warm-up and cool-down periods to workouts, and develop realistic goals with regards to abilities and fitness level (De Mond 1991). The difference between healthy and unhealthy exercise behaviors and attitudes should be taught. Individuals who engage in pathologically excessive exercise may also require psychological treatment to address their maladaptive attitudes toward exercise and possible exercise withdrawal symptoms, such as anxiety or depression.

16.4 SUMMARY AND CONCLUSIONS

A variety of treatment approaches targeting exercise in ED patients have been investigated. Most incorporate gradual increases in physical activity, making participation and progress in the program dependent on percent BF, ideal weight, or medical clearance. Programs have included activities such as stretching, yoga, pilates, strength training, balance exercises, low-impact aerobic exercise, recreational games, and group activities (Calogero and Pedrotty 2004; Sungot et al. 2002; Thien et al. 2000; Tokumura et al. 2005).

Strength training, particularly of the large muscle groups, should be included in the exercise routine to improve bone density and to rebuild the muscle mass that was lost due to malnutrition. Exercises should initially be non-weight-bearing, progressing to partial-weight-bearing as the patient regains strength and muscle control. Once BW has been increased to healthy levels (70%–80% of ideal BW), complete weight-bearing exercises as well as low-impact aerobic activity can gradually be included (Close, 2007; Calogero and Pedrotty 2004; Thien et al. 2000).

Some programs also address attitudes toward exercise and educate patients about healthy physical activity. Patients should be educated about: (1) misconceptions about exercise (e.g.,

"If I miss this one exercise session I will get fat" or "No pain, no gain"); (2) exercise safety; (3) avoiding exercise when sick or injured; (4) the need to include variety in exercise routines; (5) the importance of refueling the body after exercise; (6) the negative effects of excessive exercise; and (7) the importance of discontinuing exercise if dizziness, faintness, nausea, muscle cramps, painful shortness of breath, chest pain, or irregular heart beat occur (Powers and Thompson 2008).

Programs should emphasize the health and psychological benefits of regular physical activity rather than the use of exercise to control weight (Calogero and Pedrotty 2004). Participants should be taught the appropriate amount, frequency, and intensity of exercise as well as how to adjust these aspects of their program as they become more physically fit. Gradually giving participants more autonomy in choosing what types of exercise to do is also recommended (Calogero and Pedrotty 2004).

Individuals who binge eat without engaging in compensatory behaviors, such as purging, can also benefit from physical activity. A decrease in or abstinence from binge eating behaviors has been seen in individuals with binge eating disorders (BED) who increased their physical activity levels. Levine et al. (1996) found that 81.4% of 44 obese women participating in treatment for BED who also participated in an additional exercise program increased their weekly physical activity levels from an average of .4 days per week to an average of 2.9 days per week after treatment and were abstinent from binge eating after treatment. The women being treated for BED who did not change their exercise frequency continued to binge eat, although many had decreased the amount of their binge eating.

One concern might be that including physical activity in the treatment of AN may interfere with weight gain. Several studies have shown that that does not happen, that including physical activity in the treatment of individuals with AN may even lead to weight gain, and physical activity can be beneficial to the individual's recovery in several other ways (Calogero and Pedrotty 2004; Touyz et al. 1993). Benefits seen in research include the following: (1) increased compliance with treatment; (2) improved exercise capacity; (3) a greater increase in BMI than individuals who do not participate in an exercise program; and (4) reductions in emotional distress, exercise abuse, emotional commitment to and rigidity in their exercise routines, and ED symptoms (Beaumont et al. 1994; Calogero and Pedrotty 2004; Sungot-Borgen et al., 2002; Thien et al. 2000; Tokumura et al. 2005).

Yoga has been found to be therapeutic for women with EDs. Yoga is also becoming more popular for children. Yoga for children should emphasize the concept of fun and play. For the most benefits, Brown and Gerbarg (2005) recommend practicing yoga for 30 min every day; however, any amount of training can be beneficial. When choosing a yoga class, be sure the instructor is knowledgeable about EDs and is properly trained in yoga. Yoga classes that emphasize breathing, relaxation, and meditation rather than perfection of the postures are recommended for individuals with EDs.

APPENDIX 16.A   HEALTH HISTORY QUESTIONNAIRE

Last name _____ First name _____Middle initial _____

Date of birth _____ Sex _____ Home phone _____ Work phone _____

Address _____

City _____ State _____ Zip _____

Dietary habits

1. What is your current weight? _____lb.   height? _____ in.
2. What would you like to weigh? _____ lb.
3. What is the most you ever weighed as an adult? _____ lb.
4. What is the least you ever weighed as an adult? _____ lb.
5. What weight loss methods have you tried?

6. Which do you eat regularly?
   ☐ Breakfast   ☐ Mid-afternoon snack
   ☐ Midmorning snack   ☐ Dinner
   ☐ Lunch   ☐ After-dinner snack
7. Do you occasionally go all day without eating, followed by a
   large dinner later in the evening?   ☐ Yes   ☐ No
8. What size portions do you normally have?
   ☐ Small   ☐ Moderate   ☐ Large
   ☐ Extra large   ☐ Uncertain
9. How often do you eat more than one serving?
   ☐ Always   ☐ Usually
   ☐ Sometimes   ☐ Never
10. Do you usually eat at least 1200 calories a day?   ☐ Yes   ☐ No
11. When you snack, how many times a week do you eat the following?
    Cookies, cake, pie _____ Candy _____ Diet soda
    Soft drinks _____ Doughnuts _____ Fruit
    Milk or milk beverage _____ Potato chips, pretzels, etc.

Medical History

12. When was the last time you had a physical examination?
13. If you are allergic to any medications, food, or other substances, please name them.
14. If you have been told that you have any chronic or serious illnesses, please list them.
15. Give the following information pertaining to your last three hospitalizations. Do not list
    normal pregnancies.
    Hospitalization 1   Hospitalization 2 Hospitalization 3
    Type of operation _____
    Month and year hospitalized _____
    Name of hospital_____
    City and state _____
    During the past 12 months _____
16. Has a physician prescribed any form of medication for you?   Yes ☐   No ☐
17. Has your weight fluctuated more than a few pounds?   Yes ☐   No ☐
18. Did you attempt to bring about this weight change through
    diet or exercise?   Yes ☐   No ☐
19. Have you experienced any faintness, light-headedness,
    or blackouts?   Yes ☐   No ☐
20. Have you occasionally had trouble sleeping?   Yes ☐   No ☐
21. Have you experienced any blurred vision?   Yes ☐   No ☐
22. Have you had any severe headaches?   Yes ☐   No ☐
23. Have you experienced chronic morning cough?   Yes ☐   No ☐
24. Have you experienced any temporary change in your speech
    pattern, such as slurring or loss of speech?   Yes ☐   No ☐
25. Have you felt unusually nervous or anxious for no apparent
    reason?   Yes ☐   No ☐
26. Have you experienced unusual heartbeats such as skipped beats
    or palpitations?   Yes ☐   No ☐
27. Have you experienced periods in which your heart felt as
    though it were racing for no apparent reason?   Yes ☐   No ☐

At present:

28. Do you experience shortness of breath or loss of breath while walking with others your own age?   Yes ☐ No ☐
29. Do you experience sudden tingling, numbness, or loss of feeling in your arms, hands, legs, feet, or face?   Yes ☐ No ☐
30. Have you ever noticed that your hands or feet sometimes feel cooler than other parts of your body?   Yes ☐ No ☐
31. Do you experience swelling of your feet or ankles?   Yes ☐ No ☐
32. Do you get pains or cramps in your legs?   Yes ☐ No ☐
33. Do you experience any pain or discomfort in your chest?   Yes ☐ No ☐
34. Do you experience any pressure or heaviness in your chest?   Yes ☐ No ☐
35. Have you ever been told that your blood pressure was abnormal?   Yes ☐ No ☐
36. Have you ever been told that your serum cholesterol or triglyceride level was high?   Yes ☐ No ☐
37. Do you have diabetes? If yes, how is it controlled?
    ☐ Dietary means   ☐ Insulin injection   ☐ Oral medication   ☐ Uncontrolled
38. How often would you characterize your stress level as being high?
    ☐ Occasionally   ☐ Frequently   ☐ Constantly
39. Have you ever been told that you have any of the following illnesses?
    ☐ Myocardial infarction   ☐ Arteriosclerosis   ☐ Heart disease   ☐ Heart block
    ☐ Coronary thrombosis   ☐ Rheumatic heart   ☐ Heart attack   ☐ Aneurysm
    ☐ Coronary occlusion   ☐ Heart failure   ☐ Heart murmur   ☐ Angina
40. Has any member of your immediate family been treated for or suspected to have had any of these conditions? Please identify their relationship to you (father, mother, sister, brother, etc.).
    ☐ Diabetes   ☐ Heart disease   ☐ Stroke   ☐ High blood pressure
    Relationship   Relationship   Relationship   Relationship
    _____   _____   _____   _____

APPENDIX 16.B   THE PHYSICAL ACTIVITY READINESS QUESTIONNAIRE (PAR-Q)

Becoming more active is very safe for most people, but if you're in doubt, please complete the questionnaire below. Some people should check with their doctor before they start becoming much more physically active. Start by answering the seven questions below. If you are between the ages of 15 and 69, the PAR-Q will tell you if you should check with your doctor before you start. If you are over 69 years of age, and you are not used to being very active, definitely check with your doctor. Common sense if your best guide when you answer these questions. Please read the questions carefully and answer each one honestly: check YES or NO.

YES   NO
☐   ☐   Has your doctor ever said that you have a heart condition and that you should only do physical activity recommended by a doctor?
☐   ☐   Do you feel pain in your chest when you do physical activity?

In the past month, have you had chest pain when you were not doing physical activity?
☐   ☐   Do you lose your balance because of dizziness or do you ever lose consciousness?
☐   ☐   Do you have a bone or joint problem that could be made worse (e.g., back, knee or hip) by a change in your physical activity?
☐   ☐   Is your doctor currently prescribing drugs (e.g., water pills) for your blood pressure or heart condition?

☐   ☐   Do you know of any other reason why you should not do physical activity?

If you answered YES to one or more questions, talk with your doctor before you start becoming much more physically active.

If you answered NO to all questions, you can be reasonably sure that you can start becoming more physically active right now. Be sure to start slowly and progress gradually—this is the safest and easiest way to go.

Delay becoming much more active if:

- You are not feeling well because of a temporary illness such as a cold or a fever—wait until you feel better; or
- You are or may be pregnant—talk to your doctor before you start becoming much more active.

Note: If your health changes so that you then answer YES to any of the above questions, ask for advice from your fitness or health professional.

Source: Physical Activity Readiness Questionnaire (PAR-Q) © 2010. Reprinted with permission from the Canadian Society for Exercise Physiology (see http://www.csep.ca/forms.asp).

APPENDIX 16.C   SPORT MEDICINE GUIDELINES FOR RESISTANCE TRAINING FOR CHILDREN

- ✓ Children should be supervised by a qualified instructor when performing exercises
- ✓ High-intensity exercises such as 1RM should be avoided and progressive loading should be utilized instead.
- ✓ Equipment should be appropriate for the size and skill level of the child.
- ✓ The goals of the resistance program should work to increase motor skill and fitness level.
- ✓ The child should perform each exercise between 8 and 15 repetitions and weight should only be increased when they can perform this number of repetitions with correct form. If eight repetitions cannot be performed, then the resistance weight needs to be lowered so the child can perform the eight repetitions with correct form.
- ✓ Young children should not perform below eight repetitions. A training load of eight or below should be utilized only for older adolescents.
- ✓ The focus should be on developing correct form rather than maximizing weight.

Source: Adapted from American College of Sports Medicine. 2006. *ACSM's guidelines for exercise testing and prescription* (7th ed.). Philadelphia, PA: Lippincott Williams & Wilkins.

APPENDIX 16.D   KRAEMER'S AGE SPECIFIC RESISTANCE TRAINING GUIDELINE

Resistance Training Guidelines by Age Group

7 years or younger
- ✓ Use little or no weight
- ✓ Focus on technique
- ✓ Volume should stay low

8–10 years of age
- ✓ Can increase number of exercises as well as resistance and volume
- ✓ Important to monitor progression and tolerance of increases

11–13 years of age
- ✓ Continue slow progression of resistance and volume
- ✓ Begin to introduce advanced exercises using little or no weight
- ✓ Add sport specific exercises

14–15 years of age	✓ Continue resistance progression
	✓ Advance sport specific components
16 years and older	✓ After demonstrating mastery of proper technique the child should be progressed to entry-level adult programs

Source: Adapted from Kraemer, W. J. and S. J. Fleck. 2005. *Strength training for young athletes* (2nd ed.). Champaign: Human Kinetics.

APPENDIX 16.E GUIDELINES FOR PROGRESSION MODELS THROUGHOUT A RESISTANCE TRAINING PROGRAM

Recommendations should be viewed in context of individual's target goals, physical capacity, and training status. Exercise selection should include concentric and eccentric muscle actions as well as both single- and multiple-joint exercises.

Exercise Sequence
> Exercise large muscle groups before small muscle groups
> Perform multiple-joint exercises before single-joint exercises
> Perform higher intensity exercises before lower intensity exercises

When training at a specific RM load
> A 2%–10% increase in load should be applied when one to two repetitions can be performed over the current workload

Training frequency
> 2–3 days per week for novice and intermediate training
> 4–5 days per week for advanced training

Novice training
> 8–12 repetition maximum (RM)

Intermediate to advanced training
> 1–12 RM in periodized fashion with emphasize on the 6–12 RM zone using 1- to 2-min rest periods between sets at a moderate velocity (1–2 s concentric, 1–2 s eccentric)
> Eventual emphasis on heavy loading (1–6 RM) with at least 3-min rest periods between sets at a moderate contraction velocity (1–2 s concentric, 1–2 s eccentric)

Hypertrophy training
> 1–12 RM in periodized fashion with emphasis on the 6–12 RM zone, 2-min rest periods between sets, moderate contraction velocity (1–2 s concentric, 1–2 s eccentric)
> moderate loading for novice (70%–85% of 1 RM), advanced training (70%–100% for 1–12 reps) higher volume, multiple-set programs result in greater hypertrophy than low volume, single set programs

Power training(novice- and intermediate-trained individuals)
> One to three sets per exercise using light to moderate loads (30%–60% of 1 RM) at a fast contraction velocity for 3–6 repetitions with 2–3 min of rest between sets for multiple sets, emphasize multiple-joint exercises, especially those involving the total body, progression of power enhancement uses various loading strategies in a periodized manner

Local muscular endurance training
> Light to moderate loads, 40%–60% of 1 RM, high repetitions (> 15), short rest periods (< 90 s)

Source: Adapted from American College of Sports Medicine Position Stand. 2002. Progression models in resistance training in healthy adults. *Med Sci Sports Exerc* 34: 364–380.

APPENDIX 16.F ESTIMATING YOUR DAILY ENERGY NEEDS

Your weight in pounds =

Your weight in kilograms = _____ = $\dfrac{wt(lbs)}{2.2}$

1. Calculate your BMR:
   Males: multiply your wt. (kg) × 1 kcal/kg/h × 24 h/day = _____ kcal/day
   Females: multiply your wt (kg) × 0.9 kcal/kg/h × 24 h/day = _____ kcal/day
2. Account for slower metabolism during sleep:
   Subtract from your BMR: .1 kcal/kg/h sleep × your wt (kg) × ?hours of sleep. Adjusted BMR = _____ kcal/day
3. Add the appropriate activity increment:

	Males	Females
Sedentary/light	225 kcal	225 kcal
Moderate	750	500
Heavy	1500	1000
Very heavy	2500	1750

   Energy Expenditure – Adjusted BMR + Activity Increment = _____ kcal/day
4. Add 10% to the value in 3 for the increased metabolism due to digestion. Total expenditure = kcal/day (from 3) _____ + 10% of kcal/day (from 3) _____ = kcal/day.
5. How does this energy expenditure compare with your daily kcal consumption?
6. Please finish the sentence:
   To increase weight I must …
   To decrease weight I must …
   To maintain weight I must …

REFERENCES

American College of Sports Medicine. 1993. *Resource manual for guidelines for exercise Exercise testing and prescription.* Baltimore, MD: Lea & Febiger.

American College of Sports Medicine. 1995. *Guidelines for exercise testing and prescription.* Baltimore, MD: Williams & Wilkins.

American College of Sports Medicine. 2006. *ACSM's guidelines for exercise testing and prescription* (7th ed.), ed. M. H. Whaley, P. H. Brubaker, and R. M. Otto. Baltimore, MD: Williams & Wilkins.

American College of Sports Medicine. 2010a. *ACSM's guidelines for exercise testing and prescription* (8th ed.). Philadelphia: Lippincott, Williams, & Wilkins.

American College of Sports Medicine. 2010b. *ACSM's resource manual for guidelines for exercise testing and prescription* (6th ed.). Philadelphia: Lippincott, Williams, & Wilkins.

American Council on Exercise. 1991. *Personal trainer manual.* Boston, MA: Reebok Univ. Press.

Ashmore, A. 2003. Strength training guidelines for children. *Am Fit* 21: 62.

Atlantis, E., E. H. Barnes, and M. A. Fiatarone-Singh. 2006. Efficacy of exercise for treating overweight in children and adolescents: a systematic review. *Int J Obes* 30: 1027–1040.

Bale, P., D. Doust, and D. Dawson. 1996. Gymnasts, distance runners, anorexics, body composition, and menstrual status. *J Sports Med Phys Fit* 36: 49–53.

Barrow, G., and S. Saha. 1988. Menstrual irregularity and stress factors in collegiate female distance runners. *Am J Sports Med* 16: 209–216.

Beaumont, P. J. V., B. Arthur, J. D. Russell, and S. W. Touyz. 1994. Excessive physical activity in dieting disorder patients: Proposals for a supervised exercise program. *Int J Eat Disord* 15: 21–36.

Benavides, S., and J. Caballero. 2009. Ashtanga yoga for children and adolescents for weight management and psychological well being: An uncontrolled open pilot study. *Complement Ther Clin Pract* 15: 110–11 4.

Bersma, D., and M. Visscher. 2003. *Yoga games for children: Fun and fitness with postures,movements, and breath.* Alameda, CA: Hunter House.

Biddle, S. J. H., T. Gorely, and D. J. Stensel. 2004. Health-enhancing physical activity and sedentary behaviour in children and adolescents. *J Sports Sci* 22: 679–701.

Borg, G. A. V. 1982. Psychophysical basis of perceived exertion. *Med Sci Sports Exercise* 14: 377–381.

Brook-Gunn, J., M. P. Warren, and L. H. Hamilton. 1987. The relation of eating problems and amenorrhea in ballet dancers. *Med Sci Sports Exercise* 19: 41–44.

Brown, R. P., and P. L. Gerbarg. 2005. Sudarshan Kriya yogic breathing in the treatment of stress, anxiety, and depression: Part II—clinical applications and guidelines. *J Altern Complement Med* 11: 711–717.

Bryant-Waugh, R. 2007. Anorexia nervosa in children and adolescents. In *Eating disorders in children and adolescents*, ed. T. Jaffa and B. McDermott, 111–122. New York: Cambridge Univ. Press.

Carei, T. R., A. L. Fyfe-Johnson, C. C. Breuner, and M. A. Brown. 2009. Randomized controlled clinical trial of yoga in the treatment of eating disorders. *J Adolesc Health* 46: 346–351.

Calogero, R. M., and K. N. Pedrotty. 2004. The practice and process of healthy exercise: An investigation of the treatment of exercise abuse in women with eating disorders. *Eat Disord* 12: 273–291.

Carei, T. R., C. C. Breuner, and A. Fyfe-Johnson. 2009. The evaluation of yoga in the treatment of eating disorders. *J Adolesc Health* 40: S31–32.

Close, M. 2007. Physiotherapy and exercise. In *Eating disorders in childhood and adolescence*. 3rd ed., ed. B. Lask, and R. Bryant-Waugh, 294–311. New York: Routledge/Taylor & Francis Group.

Cooper, C., M. Cawley, A. Bhalla, P. Egger, F. Ring, L. Morton, and D. Barker. 1995. Childhood growth, physical activity, and peak bone mass in women. *J Bone Miner Res* 10: 940–947.

Costin, C. 2007. Activity disorder: When a good thing goes bad. In *The eating disorder sourcebook: A comprehensive guide to the causes, treatments, and prevention of eating disorders* (3rd ed.), ed. C. Costin, 45–58. New York: McGraw-Hill.

Council on Sports Medicine and Fitness. 2008. Strength training by children and adolescents. *Pediatrics* 121: 835–839.

Dale, L. P., A. Maher-Mattison, K. Greening, G. Galen, W. P. Neace, and M. L. Matacin. 2009. Yoga workshop impacts psychological functioning and mood of women with self-reported history of eating disorders. *Eat Disord* 17: 422–434.

Daubenmier, J. J. 2005. The relationship of yoga, body awareness, and body responsiveness to self-objectification and disordered eating. *Psychol Women Q* 29: 207–219.

Davis, C., D. K. Katzman, S. Kaptein, C. Kirsh, H. Brewer, K. Kalmbach, M. P. Olmsted, D. B. Woodside, and A. S. Kaplan. 1997. The prevalence of high-level exercise in the eating disorders: Etiological implications. *Compr Psychiatry* 38: 321–326.

De Mond, T. E. 1991. Recognizing overtraining: The young, the old, even fitness pros may be at risk. *Am Fit* 9: 48–59.

Douglass, L. 2009. Yoga as an intervention in the treatment of eating disorders: Does it help? *Eat Disord* 17: 126–139.

Drinkwater, B. L., K. Nilson, C. Chestnut, W. Bremner, S. Shainholtz, and M. Southworth. 1984. Bone mineral content of amenorrheic and eumenorrheic athletes. *New England J Med* 311: 277–281.

Faigenbaum, A. D. 2009. Overtraining in young athletes: How much is too much? *ACSM's Health Fit J* 13: 8–13.

Faigenbaum, A. D., W. J. Kraemer, C. J. R. Blimke, I. Jefferys, L. J. Micheli, M. Nitka, and T. W. Rowland. 2009. Youth resistance training: Updated position statement paper from the National Strength and Conditioning Association. *J Strength Cond Res* 23: S60– S79.

Fishman, J., R. M. Boyar, and L. Hellman. 1975. Influence of body weight on estradiol metabolism in young women. *J Clin Endocrinol Metabol* 41: 989–991.

Frisch, E. R., A. V. Gotz-Welbergen, J. W. McArthur, T. Albright, J. Witschi, B. Bullen, J. Binholz, R. B. Reed, and H. Herman. 1981. Delayed menarche and amenorrhea of college athletes in relation to age of onset of training. *JAMA* 246: 1559–1563.

Frisch, E. R., and J. MacArthur. 1974. Menstrual cycles: Fatness as a determinant of minimum weight for height necessary for their maintenance or onset. *Science* 185: 949–951.

Garman, J. F., D. M. Hayduk, D. A. Crider, and M. M. Hodel. 2004. Occurrence of exercise dependence in a college-aged population. *J Am Coll Health* 52: 221–228.

Gortmaker, S. L., W. H. Dietz, A. M. Sobol, and C. A. Wehler. 1987. Increasing pediatric obesity in the United States. *Am J Dis Child* 141: 535–540.

Granath, J., S. Ingvarsson, U. von Thiele, and U. Lundberg. 2006. Stress management: A randomized study of cognitive behavioral therapy and yoga. *Cogn Behav Ther* 35: 3–10.

Grossman, K. M. 2004. Safe and effective strength training for grades 3–8. *Teach Elem Phys Educ* 15: 13–16.

Hafen, B., and W. Hoeger. 1994. *Wellness guidelines for a healthy lifestyle*. Englewood, CO: Morton.

Hagins, M., W. Moore, and A. Rundle. 2007. Does practicing hatha yoga satisfy recommendations for intensity of physical activity which improves and maintains health and cardiovascular fitness. *BMC Complement Altern Med* 7, http://www.biomedcentral.com/1472-6882/7/40 (accessed September 19, 2010).

Hills, A. P., N. A. King, and T. P. Armstrong. 2007. The contribution of physical activity and sedentary behaviors to the growth and development of children and adolescents: Implications for obesity and overweight. *Sports Med* 37: 533–545.

Hoeger, W. K., and S. A. Hoeger. 1999. *Principles and labs for physical fitness.* Englewood, CO: Morton.

Hoeger, W. K., and S. A. Hoeger. 2011. *Lifetime physical fitness & wellness: A personalized program.* 11th ed. Belmont, CA: Wadsworth.

Kristal, A. R., A. J. Littman, D. Benitez, and E. White. 2005. Yoga practice is associated with attenuated weight gain in healthy middle-aged men and women. *Altern Ther Health Med* 11: 28–33.

Jhansi Rani, N., and P. V. Krishna Rao. 2005. Impact of yoga training on body image and depression. *Psychol Stud* 50: 98–100.

Jakicic, J. M., and A. D. Otto. 2005. Physical activity recommendations in the treatment of obesity. *Psychiatr Clin N Am* 28: 141–150.

Johns, R. J., and V. Wright. 1962. Relative importance of various tissues in joint stiffness. *J Appl Physiol* 17: 824–828.

Levine, M. D., M. D. Marcus, and P. Moulton. 1996. Exercise in the treatment of binge eating disorder. *Int J Eat Disord* 19: 171–177.

McGonigal, K. 2006. Yoga for kids. *IDEA Fit J* 3: 91–93.

McIver, S, M. Gartland, and P. O'Halloran. 2009. Overeating is not about the food: Women describe their experience of a Yoga treatment program for binge eating. *Qual Health Res* 19: 1234–1245.

McSwegin, P., C. Pemberton, C. Petray, and S. Going. 1989. *Physical best.* Reston, VA: AAPHERD.

Meredith, M. D. 1987. *FITNESSGRAM User's manual.* Dallas, TX: Institute for Aerobics Research.

Mond, J. M., and R. M. Calogero. 2009. Excessive exercise in eating disorder patients and in healthy women. *Aust N Z J Psychiatry* 43: 227–234.

Mond, J. M., P. J. Hay, B. Rodgers, C. Owen, and P. J. V. Beumont. 2004. Relationships between exercise behavior, eating-disordered behavior, and quality of life in a community sample of women: When is exercise 'excessive'? *Eur Eat Disorders Rev* 12: 265–272.

Morgan, W. P., D. R. Brown, J. S. Raglin, P. J. O'Connor, and K. A. Ellickson. 1987. Psychological monitoring of overtraining and staleness. *Br J Sports Med* 21: 107–114.

Myerson, M., B. Gutin, M. Warren, M. May, I. Contento, M. Lee, F. Pi-Sunyer, R. Pierson, and J. Brooks-Gunn. 1991. Resting metabolic rate and energy balance in amenorrheic and eumenorrheic runners. *Med Sci Sports Exercise* 23: 15–22.

Parker-Pope, T. 2010. Recalibrated formula eases women's workouts. New York Times Health Update, http://well.blogs.nytimes.com/2010/07/05/recalibrated-formula-eases-womens-workouts (accessed September 19, 2010).

Petterson, F., H. Fries, and S. Nillius. 1973. Epidemiology of secondary amenorrhea: Incidence and prevalence rates. *Am J Obstetr Gynecol* 117: 80–86.

Pollock, M. L., and J. H. Wilmore. 1990. *Exercise in health and disease: Evaluation and prescription for prevention and rehabilitation.* Philadelphia: W.B. Saunders.

Powers, P., and R. Thompson. 2008. *Exercise balance: What's too much, what's too little, and what's just right for you!* Carlsbad, CA: Gürze Books.

Raub, J. A. 2002. Psychophysiologic effects of Hatha Yoga on musculoskeletal and cardiopulmonary function: A literature review. *J Altern Complement Med* 8, no. 2: 797–812.

Scime, M., and C. Cook-Cottone. 2008. Primary prevention of eating disorders: A constructivist integration of mind and body strategies. *Int J Eat Disord* 41: 134–142.

Scime, M., C. Cook-Cottone, L. Kane, and T. Watson. 2006. Group prevention of eating disorders with fifth-grade females: Impact on body dissatisfaction, drive for thinness, and media influence. *Eat Disord* 14: 143–155.

Shroff, H., L. Reba, L. M. Thornton, F. Tozzi, K. L. Klump, W. H. Berrettini, H. Brandt, et al. 2006. Features associated with excessive exercise in women with eating disorders. *Int J Eat Disord* 39: 454–461.

Spoor, S. T. P, M. H. J. Bekker, G. L. Van Heck, M. A. Croon, and T. Van Strien. 2005. Inner body and outward appearance: The relationships between appearance, orientation, eating disorder symptoms, and internal body awareness. *Eat Disord* 13: 479–490.

Sungot-Borgen, J., J. H. Rosenvinge, R. Bahr, and L. Sundgot Schneider. 2002. The effect of exercise, cognitive therapy, and nutritional counseling in treating bulimia nervosa. *Med Sci Sports Exercise* 34: 190–195.

Thien, V., A. Thomas, D. Markin, and C. L. Birmingham. 2000. Pilot study of a graded exercise program for the treatment of anorexia nervosa. *Int J Eat Disord* 28: 101–106.

Tokumura, M., T. Tanaka, S. Nanri, and H. Watanabe. 2005. Prescribed exercise training for convalescent children and adolescents with anorexia nervosa: Reduced heart rate response to exercise is an important parameter for the early recurrence diagnosis of anorexia nervosa. In *Adolescent eating disorders*, ed. P. I. Swain, 69–83. New York: Nova Science Publishers.

Touyz, S. W., W. Lennerts, B. Arthur, and P. J. V. Beumont. 1993. Anaerobic exercise as an adjunct to refeeding patients with anorexia nervosa: Does it compromise weight gain? *Eur Eat Disorders Rev* 1: 177–181.

U. S. Department of Health and Human Services (HHS). 2008. Physical activity guidelines for Americans: Be active, healthy, and happy, http://www.health.gov/PAguidelines/pdf/paguide.pdf (accessed September 19, 2010).

U. S. Department of Health and Human Services (HHS). 2010. Trends in the prevalence of physical activity. National YRBS: 1991–2009, http://www.cdc.gov/HealthyYouth/yrbs/pdf/us_physical_trend_yrbs.pdf (accessed October 18, 2010).

Vehrs, P. R. 2005. Strength training in children and teens: Implementing safe, effective, and fun programs—Part two. *ACSM's Health Fit J* 9: 13–18.

Walberg, J., and C. Johnston. 1991. Menstrual function and eating behavior in female international weight lifters and competitive body builders. *Med Sci Sports Exercise* 23: 30–36.

Wallace, K. L., and B. J. Wallace. 2008. Raising the bar: Pushing away the misconceptions and pulling out new ideas regarding youth strength training. *Phys Health Ed J* 75: 16–22.

Wescott, W. L. 1991. You can sell exercise for weight loss. *Fit Manage,* 7: 33.

Wescott, W. L., and A.D. Faigenbaum. 2003. Strength training (for kids). *IDEA Health Fit Source* 21: 36–43.

Williams, M., 1988. *Nutrition for fitness and sport.* Dubuque, IA: William C. Brown.

Wilson, R. C., and P. W. Jones. 1989. A comparison of the visual analogue scale and modified Borg scale for the measurement of dyspnea during exercise. *Clin Sci* 76: 277– 282.

17 Nutritional Evaluation and Treatment of Eating Disorders

Ann A. Thompson and Amanda J. Danielson

CONTENTS

17.1 LEARNING OBJECTIVES

After completing this chapter, you should be able to do the following:

- Describe the importance of the role of the registered dietitian in the treatment of eating disorders
- Identify the major nutritional problems of individuals with anorexia nervosa, bulimia nervosa, and binge eating disorder
- Identify the key steps in nutritional evaluation and therapy for individuals with eating disorders
- Explain the similarities and differences between the work of the registered dietitian and the work of other professionals in treating an individual with an eating disorder

17.2 CONSEQUENCES OF INHIBITING FOOD INTAKE

Inhibiting food intake has consequences that may not have been anticipated by those attempting such restriction. Starvation and self-imposed dieting can lead to eating binges and can also result in psychological manifestations, such as preoccupation with food, increased emotional responsiveness, dysphoria, and distractibility (Polivy 1996).

17.2.1 DISORDERED EATING BEHAVIORS

Disordered eating can be distinguished from occasional, maladaptive eating changes by looking at the purpose behind the behavior and the consistency of the behavior. Behaviors associated with disordered eating can include compulsive dieting, excessively skipping meals, or avoiding specific food groups in order to lose weight. Individuals who later develop eating disorders are more likely to have had abnormal eating patterns, such as skipping breakfast or eating excessive amounts of unhealthy foods, even before the age of 12 (Fernandez-Aranda et al. 2007).

17.2.2 NUTRITIONAL STATUS

The psychopathologies of all eating disorders overlap. Disordered food behaviors adversely affect one's nutritional status and medical status. Food-related complications are most evident in anorexia nervosa (AN) and bulimia nervosa (BN); however, they also occur in binge eating disorder (BED; Mitchell and Peterson 2005). Nutritional and health status changes are observed as an eating disorder progresses. Impaired nutritional status can cause future medical complications including cardiac and blood pressure problems, diabetes and insulin complications, osteoporosis, gastrointestinal disorders, and dental problems. Chapters 3 and 4 provide detailed information regarding these changes.

17.3 THE REGISTERED DIETITIAN

The registered dietitian is uniquely qualified to provide medical nutritional therapy for the normalization of eating patterns and nutritional status. This professional term is a legally protected term regulated by the American Dietetic Association (ADA 2010; Henry and Ozier 2006). An individual with this professional credential is registered with the Commission on Dietetic Registration (the certifying agency of the ADA) and is able to use the title "registered dietitian" only when specific educational and professional prerequisites are completed and a national registration exam has been passed (Emerson et al. 2006).

17.3.1 IMPORTANCE OF THE REGISTERED DIETITIAN

It is the position of the ADA that registered dietitians are an important part of the treatment team for individuals with AN, BN, or BED. Registered dietitians have unique qualifications and training in dealing with clinical problems related to food and eating that arise when treating eating disorders (Henry and Ozier 2006). Registered dietitians are especially important in treating eating disorders, because interventions, whether inpatient or outpatient, almost always include changes in diet (Spear et al. 2007). Registered dietitians have been trained in conducting nutritional evaluations, which can include both food records and biochemical measurements. They are also trained in providing a nutritional treatment plan and nutritional therapy that is safe and suitable for the eating-disordered individual. Registered dietitians working with eating disorders should have additional skills and training in counseling and psychology.

To be effective, a registered dietitian should be comfortable working with a multidisciplinary treatment team that includes physicians, psychologists, and psychiatrists. A registered dietitian who is treating an individual with an eating disorder should know and provide referrals to a physician, a psychologist, and a psychiatrist who specialize in the treatment of eating disorders. Diagnosing an eating disorder is always the responsibility of the physician or the licensed clinical psychologist. The registered dietitian must stay in regular contact with other members of the treatment team (Whisenant and Smith 1995).

The standard protocol followed by registered dietitians when treating individuals with eating disorders has four steps: nutritional assessment, nutritional diagnosis, nutritional intervention, and nutritional support, monitoring, and evaluation. Registered dietitians have many tools available to them through the ADA that help them perform these tasks, including the Nutrition Care Process, the American Dietetic Evidence Analysis Library, and the Nutrition Care Manual® (Eat Right 2010). The Nutrition Care Process is a standardized model intended to guide registered dietitians in providing high-quality nutritional care. Likewise, the ADA Evidence-Based Guidelines assist the registered dietitian in applying up-to-date, synthesized research into practice. ADA's Nutrition Care Manual® is useful as a comprehensive online resource that covers all aspects of nutritional management.

17.3.2 THE ROLE OF THE REGISTERED DIETITIAN

Food behaviors and thoughts must be addressed at the beginning of the treatment of an individual with an eating disorder. The registered dietitian's role in an interdisciplinary treatment team is to help accomplish this. The registered dietitian provides nutritional therapy, assists the medical team in assessing the physiological effects of the eating disorder, and helps in monitoring laboratory values, vital signs, and physical symptoms. The registered dietitian should also provide nutritional rehabilitation to help restore normal eating patterns and appropriate nutritional requirements (Henry and Ozier 2006).

It is important for the family and friends of an individual with an eating disorder, as well as the individual herself, to understand what to expect from the registered dietitian. The intake appointment for nutritional therapy usually occurs within a week of initial therapy interviews. It includes a discussion of food and eating patterns and difficulties. Although some of the topics covered in nutritional therapy may be covered by other members of the treatment team, the registered dietitian will approach these topics from a different perspective and will focus almost exclusively on the nutritional aspects of the eating disorder. The topics discussed can include, but are not limited to, the effect of inadequate nutrition on the body, food fears, inaccurate beliefs about nutrition, and information about nutritional terms such as body mass index (BMI) and metabolic rate. A registered dietitian tries to correct inaccurate beliefs and creates an individualized meal plan to help restore adequate nutritional status. Nutritional therapy also includes a maintenance plan for long-term full recovery (Kolodny 2004).

Establishing a trusting relationship between the registered dietitian and the patient is crucial in order to achieve maximal progression toward recovery. Actions by the eating disorder patient that can help promote this trust include being reliable with appointment schedules, being honest, being consistent, admitting uncertainties and mistakes, and following rules established in the treatment plan. The registered dietitian should promote trust by being knowledgeable about the evaluation and treatment of eating disorders, maintaining confidentiality, engaging in active listening, and being patient (Kronberg 2002).

17.4 NUTRITIONAL ASSESSMENT

The nutritional assessment will include physical observations, the individual's history, diagnostic tests, a food history, and calculations for nutritional assessment. The assessment should also include the individual's nutritional status, motivation for change, current eating and behavioral status, and goals for recovery. All eating disorders have a variety of biochemical, nutritional, and physical complications (Kovacs and Winston 2003).

17.4.1 PHYSICAL OBSERVATIONS

Physical complications are those that can be discovered during a physical examination and do not require a blood analysis. These can include complications that can be visually detected by the registered dietitian such as facial hair, "chipmunk checks," callused knuckles, or dental problems. Further physical examination and nutritional interviews may provide observations such as gastrointestinal, sleep, or cardiac complications.

17.4.2 HISTORY

Obtaining the patient's history allows the registered dietitian a view of what has happened and what is happening. The history may include information about the patient's eating disorder symptoms, weight, dieting, and exercise. Curry and Jaffe (1998) provide an example of a nutritional assessment for individuals with eating disorders that includes this information.

An individual's medical history is pertinent to nutritional assessment and treatment. This history includes any chronic medical conditions, the frequency of medical appointments, past hospitalizations or surgical procedures, pregnancies, allergies, and significant medical problems of the individual's family members. Special attention should be paid to incidences of hyperthyroidism or hypothyroidism, diabetes, malabsorption syndrome, inflammatory bowel disease, chronic pancreatitis, and past psychiatric disorders associated with weight loss or gain. Diagnoses of any of these conditions will affect the nutritional treatment plan and food recommendations. A family medical history can also reveal information that is crucial to planning treatment (see case study in Chapter 8). Research shows that a family history of eating disorders increases a child's risk of developing an eating disorder (Strober et al. 1985).

A registered dietitian should obtain a list of the individual's current or recent medications. Common medications taken by individuals with eating disorders include antidepressants, antianxiety medications, hormones, vitamins, minerals, herbs, and nutritional supplements (see Chapter 22). Many prescribed medications influence weight changes. Reviewing these medications and their potential effects on weight change will be important in nutritional planning and in the education of the patient (Vanina et al. 2002). Abuse of weight-losing medications, such as laxatives, diuretics, diet pills, Ipecac, or thyroid medication, may first be recognized during this phase of a nutritional assessment (Mitchell et al. 1988).

17.4.3 LABORATORY TESTS

The registered dietitian working with the patient's physician will review a number of medical tests including: analysis of vital signs, laboratory values for electrolytes, complete blood count, thyroid function tests, hormonal work up, mineral levels, erythrocyte sedimentation rates, and gastrointestinal work-ups if necessary (Halmi 2002; Seidenfeld et al. 2004). Whether there are biochemical and nutrient problems depends on the stage and severity of the eating disorder. Many of the values from laboratory tests may remain in the normal range until the eating disorder is in its advanced stages (Whitney and Rolfes 1999). In the advanced stages of an eating disorder, various biochemical and nutrient levels should be closely evaluated. Table 17.1 shows abnormal values for laboratory tests that are frequently found in eating disorders. As nutritional intake improves, so should these abnormal values (Altern 2002).

Severe biochemical and nutrient deficiencies are especially prevalent in individuals with AN; these abnormalities are secondary to starvation. Misra et al. (2004) evaluated the nutritional, hormonal, and bone-density status of a sample of outpatient adolescent girls with AN and compared them to measures from a comparison group. Adolescents with AN had lower BMI, fat mass, and lean body mass, and they also had significantly lower blood pressure, heart rate, body temperature, red blood cell count, and white blood cell count. Girls with AN also had lower serum estradiol

TABLE 17.1

Common Patterns of Abnormal Physiological Functioning among Individuals with Eating Disorders that are Detected by Laboratory Tests

AN	BN	BED
Hypokalemia	Hypokalemia	Elevated lipids
Plasma albumin < 3.6 g/dL	Hypocholermia	Elevated glucose
Hypomagnesmia	Hypomagnesmia	
Low zinc	Low sodium	
Low vitamin B_{12}	Low potassium	
Alkalosis	Metabolic alkalosis	
Elevated bicarbonate	Elevated uric acid	
Elevated cholesterol	Abnormal serum lipase	
Hypophosphatemia (in refeeding)	Hypophosphatemia	
Elevated beta-carotene	Elevated nitrogen in urine	
Leukopenia	Blunted thyroid-stimulating hormone response	
Lymphocytosis	Elevated prolactin	
Low fasting blood glucose		
Low T-4; low or blunted T-3		
Low insulin		

Source: Data from Mehler and Andersen (1999) and Schebendach and Carlson (1999).
Note: AN = anorexia nervosa; BN = bulimia nervosa; BED = binge eating disorder.

values, luteinizing hormone values, insulin-like growth factor I, and bone mineral density. These severe nutritional and hormonal deficits suggest a strong need for close monitoring of hormone and nutrient values throughout the treatment of an individual with AN.

Individuals with AN have numerous problems associated with bone growth. Specifically, bone resorption (bone breakdown), bone formation, and bone mineral density levels are all adversely affected. These abnormalities eventually result in osteoporosis and bone fractures in many individuals with AN. Premenopausal osteoporosis occurs in some individuals with calcium deficiencies and accelerated bone loss, complications commonly found in individuals with AN. Nutrient deficiencies in individuals with premenopausal osteoporosis may also limit their peak bone mass because calcium accumulation and bone consolidation occur before the age of 30 years, which is when women are at greatest risk for the development for AN. Amenorrhea (cessation of menstrual cycle) and the resulting low estrogen levels can lead to significant bone loss, both of which are symptoms of AN. Amenorrhea results from the severe caloric restriction associated with this disorder (Seidenfeld et al. 2004).

Gourlay and Brown (2004) described specific factors leading to bone loss that are associated with AN. Women with amenorrhea have lower spinal bone mineral density compared to other women, and they also have a higher incidence of fractures. Women with AN also have significantly lower bone mineral content compared to women who do not restrain their eating. Most individuals with AN meet the criteria for osteopenia (reduced bone mineral density), and many of them also meet the criteria for osteoporosis (thinning of bone tissue and loss of bone density). Two key factors in obtaining a healthy bone mineral density are sufficient calcium and vitamin D consumption (Taylor et al. 2009). Therefore, identifying individuals with AN who are deficient in these nutrients is very important for treatment. Individuals with a lower BMI have higher rates of bone resorption and lower rates of bone formation (Weinbrenner et al. 2003).

Abnormalities for BN are secondary to the complications associated with vomiting and with other compensatory behaviors, such as the abuse of Ipecac, laxatives, or diuretics. Although the deficiencies in BN are not usually as severe as they are for AN, past research shows that individuals with BN who diet excessively can have severe energy deprivation leading to other serious biological consequences (Alpers and Tuschen-Caffier 2004). Experts suggest that a full blood count and serum electrolyte levels be measured in patients with BN. Electrolyte imbalance and damage to the heart muscle are often associated with the vomiting and laxative use associated with this disorder (Henry and Ozier 2006). Hypokalemia (low potassium) is often a symptom of BN, partially as a result of hypomagnesaemia (low magnesium) and hypocalcaemia (low calcium). These deficiencies can result in abnormally rapid heart rhythms that originate in the lower chambers of the heart called the ventricles, also known as ventricular arrhythmias. Therefore, it is recommended that serum potassium be routinely measured in the nutritional assessment of individuals with BN. Magnesium and potassium should also be measured regularly to detect imbalances in these important electrolytes (Kovacs and Winston 2003).

BED is often associated with complications linked to obesity. Past research on individuals with BED has shown that these individuals have significantly larger stomach capacity and higher insulin levels than other individuals (Geliebter et al. 2004). These differences can account for the increased appetite associated with BED. In addition, research has shown that peripheral neuropeptide abnormalities exist in individuals with BED. Specifically, individuals with this disorder have decreased levels of ghrelin and PYY (Peptide YY 3–36) compared to healthy individuals (Munsch et al. 2009). Ghrelin is a gastrointestinal hormone that acts on the hypothalamus to stimulate feeding, and PYY is a gastrointestinal hormone that serves as a potent feeding inhibitor. These neuropeptides help regulate hunger and satiety, so their imbalance can lead to an increase in appetite, perpetuating BED, obesity, or both. In the treatment of BED, these measurements and their relationship to appetite should be considered. Individuals with BED are at an increased risk for chronic diseases such as Type 2 diabetes, so it is recommended that glucose and insulin be measured as well (Henry and Ozier 2006).

17.4.4 ANTHROPOMETRICS

Anthropometrics are physical measurements that reflect body composition and development. Anthropometric measures such as height and weight measurements are important in the beginning of eating disorder treatment, especially in individuals with AN. The registered dietitian can perform these objective measurements, which are part of a total nutritional assessment, in determining whether the person is underweight or overweight. A combination of BMI, total body fat, and ideal body weight is important in anthropometric measurement (Mitchell and Peterson 2005).

BMI is a basic measurement of whether the individual's weight is healthy for her. It does not consider the individual's gender or body frame, but it is a fast and effective way to determine whether further evaluation is necessary. Tools to calculate the BMI are available to the registered dietitian in the ADA Nutrition Care Manual. After computing an individual's BMI, the following ranges can be used to determine whether that person is underweight, overweight, or of normal weight: a BMI that is less than 18.5 indicates that the person is underweight; a BMI between 18.5 and 24.9 represents a normal weight for the person's height; a BMI between 25 and 29.9 indicates that the person is overweight; and a BMI greater than 30 indicates that the person is obese.

Body composition measurements compare adipose tissue and lean body mass. An individual's percentage of body fat is the weight of that person's fat divided by her total weight. Methods to measure this include near-infrared interactance (Conway et al. 1984), dual-energy X-ray absorptiometry (DEXA; Kohrt 1998), bioelectrical impedance analysis (Kyle et al. 2004), skin-fold measurements (Durnin and Rahaman 1967), hydrodensitometry measurement by under-water weighing (Probst et al. 2001), and hip-to-waist ratio (Dobbelsteyn et al. 2001). Of these alternatives, skin-fold measurements are used most frequently by the registered dietitian.

Ideal body weight is an estimate of an individual's healthy body weight, taking into account one's frame size, height, and current weight. Measuring elbow breadth appears to be the most practical way to determine frame size (Novascone and Smith 1989). Once the individual's frame size is measured, ideal body weight can be determined by using the Metropolitan Life Insurance height and weight tables. Calculations for frame size and Metropolitan Life Insurance height and weight charts are available in *Understanding Nutrition* (Whitney and Rolfes 1999) and from many health-related web sites (National Center for Health Statistics 2010).

Height determination is especially important in patients with AN, because growth retardation is a common symptom of individuals with this disorder. Up to 75% of adolescents with AN will not reach their full growth potential, even after recovery. Some height gain is associated with weight gain in these individuals (Modan-Moses et al. 2003).

The Resting Energy Expenditure (REE) was developed using a multiple-regression analysis to determine how many calories a person needs to consume for optimal functioning based on that person's weight, height, age, and sex (Mifflin et al. 1990). The formulas are: REE (males) = $10 \times$ weight (kg) + $6.25 \times$ height (cm) − $5 \times$ age (years) + 5; REE (females) = $10 \times$ weight (kg) + $6.25 \times$ height (cm) − $5 \times$ age (years) − 161 (Mifflin et al. 1990). These formulas are based on normal, healthy adults and can be used as a basis for determining kcal needs of individual patients with eating disorders.

17.4.5 FOOD RECALL

Asking individuals to recall the food that they have eaten will provide insight into their current eating behavior. Asking what is eaten on a "good" day and on a "bad" day is especially helpful when working with individuals with eating disorders. A registered dietitian is needed to accomplish this task because self-reported data about food consumption are rarely accurate. Usually, energy intake is underreported (Mitchell and Peterson 2005). The registered dietitian will compare the collected data regarding an individual's food intake to scientifically based recommendations, such as dietary reference intakes (DRIs; Food and Nutrition Information Center: Dietary Reference Intakes 2010). Appropriate food intake can also be assessed using the Food Guide Pyramid or Dietary Guidelines for Americans (Dietary Guidelines for Americans 2010, MyPyramid 2010). Evaluating reported energy intake compared to healthy recommendations in individuals with eating disorders is important because it will help determine the goal for energy consumption in treatment (Mitchell and Peterson 2005).

17.5 NUTRITIONAL DIAGNOSIS

The nutritional diagnosis provides a concise representation of problems associated with an eating disorder, and it can also provide a blueprint for needed nutritional interventions (Eat Right 2010). The nutritional diagnosis is never meant to diagnose an eating disorder; this is the responsibility of the physician or psychologist. Instead, it describes the nutritional deficiencies and abnormalities that need clinical attention. The nutritional diagnosis contains three parts (Snetselaar 2008):

1. Problem (diagnostic label): alterations in one's nutritional status;
2. Etiology: factors that cause or contribute to the existence of the problem; and
3. Signs and symptoms (defining characteristics): data identified during the assessment phase that provide evidence for the problem, its etiology, and its consequences

17.6 NUTRITIONAL INTERVENTION AND PRESCRIPTION

During nutritional intervention, the registered dietitian sets goals and prioritizes them, defines the basic plan for nutritional prescription, makes connections with other professionals, and matches intervention strategies both with the patient's needs and nutritional diagnosis, and with current reference standards and dietary guidelines. Critical thinking is needed in those tasks and in choosing from among alternatives to determine a course of action and specify the time and frequency of care (The American Dietetic Association Quality Management Committee 2008). Nutritional intervention focuses on changing an individual's behaviors and thoughts related to eating to more normal, healthy patterns. Registered dietitians use intervention techniques to help the individual with an eating disorder make behavior changes that will over time reflect a new understanding and relationship to food (Herrin 2003). Nutritional intervention helps the patient to consume an appropriate amount of nutrients, to dispel food myths, to end ritualistic food behaviors, to develop regular meal schedules, to plan reasonable menus, and to deal effectively with gastrointestinal complaints. For patients with AN, nutritional intervention also includes providing information about metabolism and the physiological changes that will occur as weight is regained (Seidenfeld et al. 2004).

17.7 NUTRITIONAL THERAPY AND EDUCATION

Gaining weight is an essential and immediate goal in the treatment of a patient with AN. A severely malnourished individual may be unable to respond to psychological therapy (Lucas 2004). The first step is to persuade the patient to participate in treatment. The second major step is weight restoration and refeeding, which often require inpatient treatment and a dietitian. Several studies have indicated that tube feeding for weight restoration can be beneficial in severe cases of AN (Grilo 2006). However, some specialists in the treatment of AN have offered cautions about this intervention (Lucas 2004).

Recovery of neurological and other medical systems requires balanced nutrition, often at higher calorie levels than usual, with a wide variety of foods containing abundant fats, calories, and nutrients. The foods needed during recovery can temporarily increase the physical discomfort and the anxiety of the individual with an eating disorder, which makes refeeding difficult. Dramatic reversal of eating disorder symptoms and personality changes are generally seen once weight is restored to an appropriate level and maintained for several months. Nutritional intervention and weight restoration can occur prior to or concurrent with other therapeutic interventions. Psychotherapy may not be fully effective without full nutritional restoration (Agras et al. 2004).

Complications, such as hypophosphatemia (low level of phosphorous in the blood caused by starvation), can arise in response to refeeding due to severe changes in electrolyte and fluid levels. One strategy for avoiding these complications is to gradually increase the caloric intake of patients undergoing refeeding in the first week and closely monitor electrolytes. A refeeding schedule for an AN patient below 70% target weight would include 1,200 kcals, no added salt, low fat, and low lactose for 4 days. The kcal should then be increased by 500 kcal daily, every 4 days, up to an average of 3,500 kcal (Mehler and Andersen 1999). The registered dietitian will modify this as clinically indicated. Oral phosphate treatment in the first week can help to maintain proper electrolyte balance (Birmingham et al. 1996). Various cardiovascular complications should be considered during treatment of patients with AN, so it is important to monitor the patient's electrolytes, protein breakdown measured by blood urea nitrogen, blood pressure, EKG, creatinine, magnesium, and phosphorus. These are especially important because of the high mortality rates associated with bradycardia and hypertension among individuals with AN (McCallum et al. 2006). These levels should be monitored at the beginning of treatment, and patients who are chronically malnourished may be monitored every other day for the first 7 to 10 days of refeeding (Mehler and Andersen 1999).

Malnourished patients will also need additional medical monitoring. Twenty-four-hour monitoring is suggested in especially severe cases (McCallum et al. 2006). This can consist of close monitoring of blood glucose, nutrient tolerance, hydration status including fluid retention, and vital signs, such as pulse and blood pressure. Patients may need bathroom monitoring to prevent purging or falling due to muscle weakness. Patients should be predominately on bed rest, and their activity should be limited. Exercise should also be monitored, and a low amount of exercise is recommended.

Patients with BN frequently have difficulty when they resume eating a normal, healthy amount of food because of their damaged gastric functioning. This difficulty is especially prevalent in patients who have developed a conditioned vomiting response to eating after having used excessive purging as a primary compensatory behavior. In these severe situations, a slow drip of isotonic formula is suggested to initiate gastric motility, as well as total parenteral nutrition (intravenous feeding) until the gastrointestinal system is at least partially normalized (Mitchell et al. 1997).

Nutritional education is a major component of nutritional intervention during recovery from an eating disorder because it provides the individual with the necessary tools for maintaining recovery. Nutritional education can include the following information: adequate nutrition and its role in reversing physical symptoms of eating disorders, the functions of nutrients, those nutrients important to brain functioning, metabolic processes, set point theory, and establishing and maintaining a healthy weight range. It is also important to include information about the physical complications of purging behaviors and the adverse effects of starvation. Educating the patient about disordered eating patterns can help the patient realize how her beliefs and attitudes perpetuate the eating disorder. For example, it may be useful to discuss self-imposed food rules, feared foods, food that the patient has labeled as "good" or "bad," the difference between emotional eating and physical hunger, the causes of restriction or overeating, and ritualistic eating behaviors. After the disordered eating patterns have been highlighted, the registered dietitian focuses on educating the individual about healthy food and eating behaviors. This education can include foods that will help the patient meet nutritional needs, meal planning, grocery shopping, portion control, social eating, eliminating dieting, and simply enjoying food. If necessary, this education may also include appropriate amounts of exercise. When hospitalized patients with AN evaluate their own physical activity, their assessments are often inaccurate (Van Elburg et al. 2007). Therefore, the amount of exercise should be closely monitored in patients with AN, and these patients should be helped to accurately evaluate their physical activity.

Registered dietitians will use a variety of counseling methods during the nutritional intervention process. These techniques provide the registered dietitian with the proficiency and confidence to handle the complex issues of eating disorders. Psychological treatment approaches also facilitate teamwork with other members of the health care team (Herrin 2003). The psychological techniques helpful in nutritional counseling for eating disorders may include behavioral counseling, cognitive-behavioral therapy, dialectical behavioral therapy, and intuitive eating. Behavioral counseling allows the patient's eating disorder to be redefined as a food, exercising, or weight management problem for which there is an effective management system (Herrin 2003). Cognitive-behavioral therapy for a registered dietitian includes educational components, the prescription of a meal plan, weight monitoring, and written self-observation (Fairburn, Marcus, and Wilson 1993). Dialectical behavioral therapy is helpful in recognizing trigger foods and situations, in stopping unwanted food thoughts, and in getting back on track with healthy food patterns. Intuitive eating allows the registered dietitian to teach the client how to create a healthy relationship with food (Tribole and Resch 2003). When a registered dietitian is considering using psychological treatment methods within nutritional therapy, it is especially important to work closely with the other members of the treatment team to make sure that the different components of the treatment are appropriately coordinated, and that the psychological components of the nutritional therapy are being conducted properly (McCallum et al. 2006).

17.8 NUTRITIONAL GOALS: ESTABLISHING NORMAL EATING PATTERNS

The registered dietitian will work with the individual with an eating disorder to identify nutritional goals. These goals consist of defining desired nutritional behaviors, determining appropriate conditions or circumstances for performing these behaviors, and establishing the extent or level of the desired behaviors (Snetselaar 2008). Goals should be specific, detailed, and relevant to the needs of the individual with an eating disorder. The registered dietitian, working with other treatment team members, will determine the psychological, educational, and behavioral change models that will work best for each individual. There will be variations in the nutritional therapy goals for AN, BN, and BED.

The major goals of nutritional therapy for AN are achieving and maintaining medical stability, adequate body weight for height, and normalized eating behaviors. The goals of nutritional therapy for BN include obtaining a healthy weight and focusing on lifelong healthy nutrition and exercise. The goals for BED include normalizing eating behaviors, emphasizing a nondiet approach to weight loss, and focusing on lifelong eating and exercise habits (Kotler et al. 2003).

17.9 FOOD AND FEEDING DIFFICULTIES

Developing normal eating patterns is essential for all types of eating disorders. One of the most important aspects of normal eating is eating three planned meals each day, plus two or three planned snacks (Fairburn, Jones et al. 1993). Patients should choose what they eat in their planned meals and snacks. Vomiting, spitting, laxative misuse, or any other form of compensatory behavior must not be allowed to follow the meals and snacks. Changing disordered eating patterns may be a slow process, with progress made in small increments. Many individuals with eating disorders have difficulty recognizing hunger and satiety cues (Canals and Arija 2009). This difficulty may be due to imbalances in leptin (a satiety-signaling hormone) and ghrelin (a hunger-signaling hormone; Stoving et al. 2009). When treating these individuals, it is crucial to develop their appetite in an appropriate way in order to see long-term changes in eating behaviors. It may be useful to include assistance in the detection of hunger and satiety in nutritional intervention.

A registered dietitian should not recommend a diet of less than 1,200 calories and should not agree with a patient that certain foods are fattening and should be avoided. A registered dietitian should recommend foods that are rich in vitamins and minerals, especially those vitamins and minerals that the patient may have a deficiency in. Table 17.2 provides initial meal plans for individuals with either AN or BN. However, a meal plan should be individualized according to the patient's needs and deficiencies. Registered dietitians should also be aware that individuals with BN are very susceptible to food deprivation (Hetherington et al. 2000). Inadequate nutritional intake may lead

---

TABLE 17.2

Food Plans for Initial Nutritional Intervention (Minimum Kcal) for Individuals with Anorexia Nervosa and Bulimia Nervosa

	Anorexia nervosa	Bulimia nervosa
Breakfast	1 Bread, ½ 1% Milk, 1 Fruit	3 Bread, 1 Fat, 2 Fruit
First snack	1 Bread	2 Bread, 1 Fat
Lunch	2 Bread, 2 Very lean protein, 1 Fruit, 1 Vegetable	2 Bread, 2 Lean protein, 1 Fruit, 1 Vegetable, 1 Fat
Second snack	1 Fruit	2 Bread, 1 Fat
Dinner	2 Bread, 2 Very lean protein, 1 1% Milk, 1 Vegetable	3 Bread, 3 Lean protein, 1 1% Milk, 2 Vegetable, 1 Fat
Third snack	1 Bread	2 Bread
Carbohydrate %	64%	60%
Protein %	22%	20%
Fat %	14%	20%
Calorie total	1,200 kcal	1,900 kcal

Source: Keddy (2002).

Note: Numbers are for dietary exchange values (Mayo Clinic 2010).

to a reoccurrence of unwanted eating patterns, such as binges, in these individuals. It is important to ensure adequate intake when developing healthy eating patterns. Research on AN shows that patients who reach higher levels of weight gain during treatment and avoid immediate weight loss following intense treatment are more likely to be successful in proper long-term weight management (Kaplan et al. 2009). Therefore, nutritional intake at treatment time for AN should focus on obtaining a higher BMI to prevent future weight loss. Adequate nutritional intake helps to restore a healthy body and mind. Table 17.3 lists important nutrients for a healthy nervous system, as well as dietary sources that are high in these nutrients.

TABLE 17.3
Essential Nutrients for Health Brain Functioning

Function	Nutrients	DRIs	Food sources
CNS development and structural maintenance	Folic acid	400 mcg	Dark greens, dried legumes, kidneys, and liver
	Omega-3 fatty acid	***	Salmon, mackerel, tuna, sardines, flaxseed, and canola, soy, and walnut oils
Neurotransmitter production and maintenance	Tryptophan	***	Cheese, eggs, meat, milk, nuts, seeds, and yogurt
	Phenylalanine	***	Cheese, eggs, meat, milk, nuts, seeds, and yogurt
	Choline	***	Egg yolks, legumes, and organ meats
	Folic acid	400 mcg	Dark greens, dried legumes, kidneys, and liver
Nerve impulse transition	Iron	15 mg	Dark greens, dried apricots, dried legumes, egg yolks, enriched and wholegrain cereals, kidneys, liver, molasses, potatoes, prunes, raisins, and red meats
	Calcium	1,000 mg	Canned salmon or sardines with bones, fortified citrus juice, corn tortillas, dairy products, dark greens, and dried lentils
	Magnesium	310 mg	Almonds, cashews, raw leafy green vegetables, seeds, soybeans, and whole grains
	Zinc	12 mg	Eggs, liver, meat, milk, poultry, seafood, and whole grains
	Manganese	***	Fruit, instant coffee, nuts, tea, vegetables, and whole grains
Antioxidants	Beta-carotene	800 mg RE	Dark greens and orange or yellow fruits and vegetables
	Vitamin C	60 mg	Citrus fruits, strawberries, green pepper, dark greens, melon, potatoes, and tomatoes
	Vitamin E	8 mg	Dried legumes, leafy green vegetables, liver, margarine, vegetables oils, wheat germ, and whole grains
	Selenium	55 mcg	Brazil nuts, chicken, egg yolks, garlic, meat, milk, and whole grains
	Glutathione	***	Avocados, asparagus, grapefruit, okra, oranges, peaches, strawberries, watermelon, and white potatoes

Sources: Woolsey (2002).
Notes: DRI = dietary reference intake. The DRIs are for women who are 19 to 30 years old. RE = retinal equivalent.
*** = no established DRI.

Developing normal eating patterns for individuals with BED should be comparable to developing an effective eating plan for individuals with obesity. Caloric restriction does lead to weight loss, but there are other nutritional treatments and dietary behaviors that should be considered when treating patients with obesity (Taylor et al. 2004). Other options can include encouraging the individual to follow regular, healthy eating patterns and to consume specified amounts of dietary fat, carbohydrates, fiber, and glycemic load (a ranking system for carbohydrate content in food servings). Eating plans for these individuals should also discourage passive overconsumption (Taylor et al. 2004). One study examined self-monitoring by parents and their children with morbid obesity. Research has shown that children who are morbidly obese are more likely to lose weight when their food intake is self-monitored and also monitored by their parents (Germann et al. 2006). Therefore, self-monitoring should be included in weight-control treatments for obese children. Self-monitoring of food intake is also important for future meal planning and for increasing awareness of thoughts and behaviors related to food (Grilo 2006).

17.10   NUTRITIONAL SUPPORT, MONITORING, AND EVALUATION

Nutritional support in the form of supplements may be required in some special instances, such as when a patient engages in chronic vomiting, refuses to eat or consumes an inadequate amount of food, or has a condition such as pancreatitis or gastrointestinal dysfunction. When providing nutritional support for patients with these problems, the registered dietitian should refer to the Nutrition Care Manual available from the American Dietetic Association (2010).

During nutritional monitoring and evaluation, the registered dietitian and the individual being treated for an eating disorder identify outcomes relevant to the nutritional diagnosis and to the intervention plan and goals. Data sources and tools for nutritional monitoring and evaluation can include self-monitoring food records, food records made by medical professionals, anthropometric measurements, biochemical data, questionnaires (pre- and post-treatment), and mail or telephone follow-up. The registered dietitian or appropriately trained and supervised support personnel monitor food and nutrient intake and other physical outcomes.

Nutritional monitoring and evaluation can be separated into three interrelated steps. The first step is monitoring progress. The registered dietitian should evaluate the patient's understanding and compliance with the treatment plan and should also determine if the intervention is being implemented as prescribed. This step may include determining if the patient's eating behavior or nutritional status has changed, identifying other positive or negative nutritional or psychological outcomes of the intervention, and considering possible reasons for any lack of progress. Conclusions need to be supported with specific evidence. The second step is measuring outcomes. In this step, the registered dietitian selects outcome indicators that are relevant to the nutritional diagnosis and the treatment goals. These indicators may include biochemical or anthropometric measurements, or physical signs and symptoms, and may be based on medical or psychological diagnoses and outcomes. The third and final step is evaluating outcomes. This is simply comparing current findings with the previously established outcome indicators. A positive or negative evaluation can be based on the patient's meeting intervention goals or the patient's physical state. The latter can be evaluated based on how close the current state matches biochemical, anthropometric, and physical reference standards.

The registered dietitian may actively continue care, or the patient may be discharged if nutritional care is complete or no further change is expected. If nutritional care is to be continued, reassessment may result in refinements to the diagnosis and to the intervention plan. If care does not continue, the patient may still be monitored for a change in status and for possible reentry to nutritional care at a later date (The American Dietetic Association Quality Management Committee 2008).

Evaluating the effectiveness of the nutritional care plan provides a basis for determining the need for continued nutritional care and support during recovery. Sessions for nutritional intervention will become less frequent as an individual reports and shows evidence of having fewer thoughts and behaviors characteristic of disordered eating behaviors. The road to a healthy recovery is unpredictable and often involves frustrations, as times of success alternate with relapses or times when the patient is uncooperative.

A healthy weight should be reached before an individual with an eating disorder is discharged, no matter what the eating disorder. Apart from achieving this goal, there are additional criteria for AN, BN, and BED that should be met before a patient is discharged from treatment. Individuals with AN should be able to sustain their goal weight for at least 2 months, should eat a variety of foods, and should have tried any previously feared foods. Individuals with BN should be maintaining a healthy weight, should be abstinent from bingeing and compensatory behaviors for at least 3 months, and should be able to eat any fear foods. Individuals with BED usually need long-term nutritional therapy, often for approximately 1 year. These individuals will be able to end their nutritional therapy when they are able to maintain a healthy eating pattern and their relationship with food has returned to normal (Keddy 2002).

When a relapse occurs during treatment and recovery, it is important to help the individual return as quickly as possible to a regular pattern of healthy eating. There are several warning signs that may indicate a relapse. These can include unwanted eating patterns such as skipped meals, decreased social eating, planned ways to compensate for eating, or an increased focus on calories or fat intake. Warning signs can also include unwanted behaviors such as over-exercising or frequent weighing (Hall and Ostroff 1999). When an individual notices any of these signs, it is important to talk to members of the treatment team.

17.11 SUMMARY

Nutritional evaluation and treatment are essential components of the overall treatment of an eating disorder. Nutritional therapy is best provided by a registered dietitian who possesses knowledge and expertise in nutrition, physiology, and skills for promoting change in eating behavior (Rieter and Graves 2010). The Nutrition Care Process follows a standard protocol that includes a nutritional assessment, nutritional intervention, and nutritional monitoring and evaluation. Through this process the registered dietitian will assist the patient in recovering from the physical and mental problems associated with inadequate or poor nutrition. The ultimate goal is to help the patient create a healthy relationship with their food, mind, and body (Mathieu 2009). Additional research is needed to identify the most effective strategies for nutritional therapy in the treatment of eating disorders (Rieter and Graves 2010) along with effective prevention strategies (Berkman et al. 2006).

REFERENCES

Agras, W. S., H. A. Brandt, C. M. Bulik, R. Dolan-Sewell, C. G. Fairburn, K. A. Halmi, D. B. Herzog, et al. 2004. Report of the National Institutes of Health workshop on overcoming barriers to treatment research in anorexia nervosa. *Int J Eat Disord* 35: 509–521.

Alpers, G. W., and B. Tuschen-Caffier. 2004. Energy and macronutrient intake in bulimia nervosa. *Eat Behav* 5: 241–249.

Altern, P. 2002. Eating disorders: A review of the literature with emphasis on medical complication and clinical nutrition. *Med Rev* 7: 184–202.

The American Dietetic Association. 2010. Nutrition care manual. http://nutritioncaremanual.org (accessed November 1, 2010).

The American Dietetic Association Quality Management Committee. 2008. American Dietetic Association Revised 2008 Standards of Practice for Registered Dietitians in Nutrition Care; Standards of Professional Performance for Registered Dietitians: Standards of Practice for Dietetic Technicians, Registered, in Nutrition Care. *J Am Diet Assoc* 108: 1538–1542.

Berkman, N. D., C. M. Bulik, K. A. Brownley, K. N. Lohr, J. A. Sedway, A. Rooks, and G. Gartlehner. 2006. *Management of eating disorders*. Rockville, MD: Agency for Healthcare Research and Quality (Publication No. 06-E010).

Birmingham, C. L., A. F. Alothman, and A. M. Goldner. 1996. Anorexia nervosa: Refeeding and hypophospha-temia. *Int J Eat Disord* 20: 211–223.

Canals, J., and M. V. Arija. 2009. Influence of parents' eating attitudes on eating disorder in school adolescents. *Eur Child Adolesc Psychiatry* 18: 353–359.

Conway, J. M., K. H. Norris, and C. E. Bodwell. 1984. A new approach for the estimation of body composition: Infrared interactance. *Am J Clin Nutr* 40: 1123–1130.

Curry, K. A., and A. Jaffe. 1998. *Nutrition counseling & communication skills.* Philadelphia, PA: W. B. Saunders.

Dietary Guidelines for Americans. 2010. http://www.cnpp.usda.gov/dietaryguidelines.htm (accessed October 18, 2010).

Dobbelsteyn, C. J., M. R. Joffres, D. R. MacLean, and G. Flowerdew. 2001. A comparative evaluation of waist circumference, waist-to-hip ratio and body mass index as indicators of cardiovascular risk factors: The Canadian Heart Health Surveys. *Int J Obes Relat Metab Disord* 25: 652–661.

Durnin, J. V. G. A., and M. M. Rahaman. 1967. The assessment of the amount of fat in the human body from measurements of skinfold thickness. *Br J Nutr* 21: 681–689.

Eat Right. 2010. http://www.eatright.org (accessed October 18, 2010).

Emerson, M., P. Kerr, M. D. C. Soler, T. A. Girard, R. Hoffinger, E. Pritchett, and M. Otto. 2006. American Dietetic Association: Standards of practice and standards of professional performance for registered dietitians (generalist, specialty and advanced) in behavioral health care. *J Am Diet Assoc* 106: 608–613.

Fairburn, C. G., R. Jones, R. C. Peveler, R. A. Hope, and M. O'Connor. 1993. Psychotherapy and bulimia ner-vosa: The longer-term effects of interpersonal psychotherapy, behavior therapy and cognitive behavior therapy. *Arch Gen Psychiatry* 50: 419–428.

Fairburn, C. G., M. D. Marcus, and G. T. Wilson. 1993. Cognitive-behavioral therapy for binge eating and buli-mia nervosa: A comprehensive treatment manual. In *Binge eating: Nature, assessment, and treatment,* ed. C. G. Fairburn and G. T. Wilson, chapter 16. New York, NY: Guilford Press.

Fernandez-Aranda, F., I. Krug, R. Granero, J. M. Ramon, A. Badia, L. Gimenez, R. Solano, D. Collier, A. Karwautz, and J. Treasure. 2007. Individual and family eating patterns during childhood and early ado-lescence: An analysis of associated eating disorder factors. *Appetite* 49: 476–485.

Food and Nutrition Information Center: Dietary Reference Intakes. 2010. http://fnic.nal.usda.gov/nal_display/index.php?info_center=4&tax_level=1&tax_subject=620 (accessed October 18, 2010).

Geliebter, A., E. K. Yahav, M. E. Gluck, and S. A. Hashim. 2004. Gastric capacity, test meal intake and appeti-tive hormones in binge eating disorder. *Physiol Behav* 81: 735–740.

Germann, J. N., D. S. Kirschenbaum, and B. H. Rich. 2006. Child and parental self-monitoring as determinants of success in the treatment of morbid obesity in low-income minority children. *J Pediatr Psychol* 32: 111–121.

Gourlay, M., and S. Brown. 2004. Clinical consideration is premenopausal osteoporosis. *Arch Intern Med* 167: 603–614.

Grilo, C. M. 2006. *Eating and weight disorders.* New York, NY: Psychology Press.

Hall, L., and M. Ostroff. 1999. *Anorexia nervosa: A guide to recovery.* Carlsbad, CA: Gurze Books.

Halmi, K. A. 2002. Eating disorders in females: Genetics, pathophysiology, and treatment. *J Pediatr Endocrinol Metab* 15: 1379–1386.

Henry, B. W., and A. D. Ozier. 2006. Position of the American Dietetic Association: Nutrition intervention in the treatment of anorexia nervosa, bulimia nervosa, and other eating disorders. *J Am Diet Assoc* 106: 2072–2082.

Herrin, M. 2003. *Nutrition counseling in the treatment of eating disorders.* New York, NY: Routledge.

Hetherington, M. M., A. E. Stoner, A. E. Andersen, and B. J. Rolls. 2000. Effects of acute food deprivation on eating behavior in eating disorders. *Int J Eat Disord* 28: 155–161.

Kaplan, A. S., B. T. Walsh, M. Olmsted, E. Attia, J. C. Carter, M. J. Devlin, K. M. Pike, et al. 2009. The slippery slope: Prediction of successful weight maintenance in anorexia nervosa. *Psychol Med* 39: 1037–1045.

Keddy, D. 2002. Outpatient nutrition therapy for eating disorders. In *Eating disorders: A clinical guide to counseling and treatment,* ed. M. M. Woolsey, 286–311. Chicago, IL: American Dietetic Association.

Kohrt, W. M. 1998. Preliminary evidence that DEXA provides an accurate assessment of body composition. *J Appl Physiol* 84: 372–377.

Kolodny, N. J. 2004. *The beginner's guide to eating disorder recovery.* Carlsbad, CA: Gurze Books.

Kotler, L. A., G. S. Boudreau, and M. J. Devlin. 2003. Emerging psychotherapies for eating disorders. *J Psychiatr Pract* 9: 431–441.

Kovacs, D., and A. P. Winston. 2003. Physical assessment of patients with anorexia nervosa and bulimia ner-vosa: An international comparison. *Eur Eat Disord Rev* 11: 456–464.

Kronberg, S. 2002. Development of psychotherapeutic techniques to facilitate successful change. In *Eating disorders: A clinical guide to counseling and treatment*, ed. M. M. Woolsley, 312–334. Chicago: American Dietetic Association.

Kyle, U. G., I. Bosaeus, A. D. De Lorenzo, P. Deurenberg, M. Elia, J. M Gomez, B. L. Heitmann, et al. 2004. Bioelectrical impedance analysis—part II: Utilization in clinical practice. *Clin Nutr* 23: 1430–1453.

Lucas, A. R. 2004. *Demystifying anorexia nervosa: An optimistic guide to understanding and healing*. New York, NY: Oxford University Press.

Mathieu, J. 2009. What should you know about mindful and intuitive eating? *J Am Diet Assoc* 109: 1982–1987.

Mayo Clinic. 2010. Your diabetes diet: Exchange lists. http://www.mayoclinic.com/health/diabetes-diet/DA00077 (accessed October 30, 2010).

McCallum, K., O. Bermudez, C. Ohlemeyer, E. Tyson, M. Portilla, and B. Ferdman. 2006. How should the clinician evaluate and manage cardiovascular complications of anorexia nervosa? *Eat Disord* 14: 73–80.

Mehler, P. S., and A. E. Andersen. 1999. *Eating disorders: Guide to medical care and complications*. Baltimore, MD: Johns Hopkins University Press.

Mifflin, H. D., S. T. St Jeor, L. A. Hill, B. J. Scott, S. A. Daugherty, and Y. O. Koh. 1990. A new predictive equation for resting energy expenditure in healthy individuals. *Am J Clin Nutr* 51: 241–247.

Misra, M., A. Aggarwal, K. K. Miller, C. Almazan, M. Worley, L. A. Soyka, D. B. Herzog, and A. Klibanski. 2004. Effects of anorexia nervosa on clinical, hematologic, biochemical, and bone density parameters in community-dwelling adolescent girls. *Pediatrics* 114: 1574–1583.

Mitchell, J. E., and C. B. Peterson. 2005. *Assessment of eating disorders*. New York, NY: Guilford Press.

Mitchell, J. E., C. Pomeroy, and D. E. Adson. 1997. Managing medical complications. In *Handbook for treatment of eating disorders*, ed. D. M. Garner and P. E. Garfinkel, 383–393. New York, NY: Guilford Press.

Mitchell, J. E., C. Pomeroy, and M. Huber. 1988. A clinician's guide to the eating disorders medicine cabinet. *Int J Eat Disord* 7: 211–223.

Modan-Moses, D., A. Yaroslavsky, I. Novikov, S. Segev, A. Toledano, E. Miterany, and D. Stein. 2003. Stunting of growth as a major feature of anorexia nervosa in male adolescents. *Pediatrics* 111: 270–276.

Munsch, S., E. Biedert, A. H. Meyer, S. Herpertz, and C. Beglinger. 2009. CCK, ghrelin, and PYY responses in individuals with binge eating disorder before and after a cognitive behavioral treatment (CBT). *Physiol Behav* 97: 14–20.

MyPyramid. 2010. http://www.mypyramid.gov (accessed October 19, 2010).

National Center for Health Statistics. 2010. *Height weight charts*. http://www.heightweightchart.org/ (accessed November 1, 2010).

Novascone, M. A., and E. P. Smith. 1989. Frame size estimation: A comparative analysis of methods based on height, wrist circumference, and elbow breadth. *J Am Diet Assoc* 89: 964–966.

Polivy, J. 1996. Psychological consequences of food restriction. *J Am Diet Assoc* 96: 589–592.

Probst, M., M. Goris, W. Vandereycken, and H. Van Coppenolle. 2001. Body composition of anorexia nervosa patients assessed by underwater weighing and skinfold-thickness measurements before and after weight gain. *Am J Clin Nutr* 73: 190–197.

Rieter, C. S., and L. Graves. 2010. Nutrition therapy for eating disorders. *Nutr Clin Pract* 25: 122–136.

Schebendach, J., and A. T. H. Carlson. 1999. Laboratory data in nutrition assessment. In *Karause's food, nutrition and diet therapy* (10th ed.), ed. L. K. Mahan and S. Escott-Stump, 380–390. Philadelphia, PA: W. B. Saunders.

Seidenfeld, M. E., E. Sosin, and V. I. Rickert. 2004. Nutrition and eating disorders in adolescents. *Mt Sinai J Med* 71: 155–161.

Snetselaar, L. G. 2008. *Nutrition counseling skills for the nutrition care process* (4th ed.). Sudbury, MA: Jones and Bartlett Publishers.

Spear, B. A., S. E. Barlow, C. Ervin, D. S. Ludwig, B. E. Saelens, K. E. Schetzina, and E. M. Taveras. 2007. Recommendations for treatment of child and adolescent overweight and obesity. *Pediatrics* 120: S254–S288.

Stoving, R. K., A. Andries, K. Brixen, A. Flyvbjerg, K. Horder, and J. Frystyk. 2009. Leptin, ghrelin, and endocannabinoids: Potential therapeutic targets in anorexia nervosa. *J Psychiatr Res* 43: 671–679.

Strober, M., W. Morrell, J. Burroughs, B. Salkin, and C. Jacobs. 1985. A controlled family study of anorexia nervosa. *J Psychiatr Res* 19: 239–246.

Taylor, C., B. Lamparello, K. Kruczek, E. Anderson, J. Hubbard, and M. Misra. 2009. Validation of a food frequency questionnaire for determining calcium and vitamin D intake in adolescent girls with anorexia nervosa. *J Am Diet Assoc* 109: 479–485.

Taylor, E., E. Missik, R. Hurley, S. Hudak, and E. Logue. 2004. Obesity treatment: Broadening our perspective. *Am J Health Behav* 28: 242–249.

Tribole, E., and E. Resch. 2003. *Intuitive eating*. New York, NY: St. Martin's Press.

Van Elburg, A. A., H. W. Hoek, M. J. H. Kas, and H. Van Engeland. 2007. Nurse evaluation of hyperactivity in anorexia nervosa: A comparative study. *Eur Eat Disord Rev* 15: 425–429.

Vanina, Y., A. Podolskaya, K. Sedky, H. Shahab, A. Siddiqui, F. Munshi, and S. Lippmann. 2002. Body weight changes associated with psychopharmacology. *Psychiatr Serv* 53: 842–847.

Weinbrenner, T., A. Zitterman, I. Gouni-Berthold, P. Stehle, and H. K. Berthold. 2003. Body mass index and disease duration are predictors of disturbed bone turnover in anorexia nervosa: A case–control study. *Eur J Clin Nutr* 57: 1262–1267.

Whisenant, S. L., and B. A. Smith. 1995. Eating disorders: Current nutrition therapy and perceived needs in dietetics education and research. *J Am Diet Assoc* 95: 1109–1112.

Whitney, E. N., and S. R. Rolfes. 1999. *Understanding Nutrition* (8th ed.). Belmont, MA: Wadsworth, 1999.

Woolsey, M. M. 2002. Nutrition and nervous system function. In *Eating disorders: A clinical guide to counseling and treatment*, ed. M. M. Woolsey, 269–285. Chicago, IL: American Dietetic Association.

18 Nutrition Needs for Special Populations with Eating Disorders

Stephanie Rushing

CONTENTS

18.1 LEARNING OBJECTIVES

After reading this chapter you should be able to do the following:

- Identify groups of people who are particularly vulnerable to developing eating disorders
- Understand the prevalence and risk factors contributing to eating disorders in children, adolescents, female athletes, and pregnant women

- Recognize health consequences associated with eating disorders in children, adolescents, female athletes, and pregnant women
- Determine appropriate nutrition goals and therapies for eating disorders in children, adolescents, female athletes, and pregnant women
- Appreciate special nutrition needs that exist for children, adolescents, female athletes, and pregnant women

18.2   BACKGROUND AND SIGNIFICANCE

Long before Mary Lou Retton or Kerri Strug, Cathy Rigby was an elite, young Olympian gymnast who won a medal in 1968. She forever changed the course of gymnastics for the United States, but what America did not know was the struggle inside of a developing eating disorder. The same attributes that pushed her to success, including a strong work ethic, the quest for perfection, and a desire for absolute control, were also the attributes that posed a risk for the development of an eating disorder. She found herself in a sport that emphasized weight control and physical appearance, which also encouraged the development of an eating disorder. Add increasing tension at home because her father lost his job and became an alcoholic, and Cathy had brewing family dynamics that would lend itself to an emerging eating disorder.

Initially, Cathy was just under 5 ft and weighed 92 pounds. However, after a weight gain to 104 pounds following puberty, she panicked but discovered that she could control her weight by starving herself and by vomiting after eating. Fighting dizziness and exhaustion from starvation, binge eating, and self-induced vomiting, Cathy was unable to perform at a competitive level, and her career as a world-class gymnast slowly melted away. Unfortunately, her eating disorder did not.

After the Olympics and in the midst of her failing gymnastics career, Cathy retired from the sport and married another former athlete. However, she continued to obsess about thinness. Throughout her pregnancies, Cathy continued to engage in eating disorder behaviors and purged up to six times per day. Eventually, Cathy sought treatment, but her eating disorder persisted and jeopardized her health and negatively affected her personal relationships. For instance, she was rushed to the emergency room twice due to electrolyte imbalances, and her first marriage ended in divorce (Pendergast and Pendergast 2000).

Nutrition education and recommendations for special populations, such as young athletes, did not exist during Cathy's time. Coaches and parents would tell athletes what they should eat and what they should weigh, and these recommendations were somewhat arbitrary. Since then, research and science have developed to address the special nutritional needs for young people, athletes, and pregnant women. Beyond the basic nutrient needs for the average person, people with eating disorders have special needs. Specific guidelines for children and adolescents, female athletes, and pregnant women with current or prior eating disorder behaviors are included in this chapter.

18.2.1   EATING DISORDERS IN CHILDREN AND ADOLESCENTS

18.2.1.1   Prevalence

The prevalence of eating disorders in children and young adolescents has increased, and children are developing eating disorders at ever-earlier ages (Lask and Bryant-Waugh 2000). Like eating disorders in general, various factors contribute to the development of eating disorders in children and adolescents, including significant genetic, biological, psychological, and sociocultural risk factors. The exact contribution of each of these factors remains unclear, but biological predisposition, comorbid psychopathology, and family factors have all been suggested to be especially influential in the development of eating disorders in young children (Rosen 2003).

18.2.1.2   Risk Factors

Weight and body image concerns develop early in childhood and are well established prior to puberty (Rosen 2003). One of the first studies to examine these factors was conducted by Maloney and colleagues (1989), who studied over 300 girls in the third through sixth grades (age 7–13 years) from two randomly selected, middle-income elementary schools. Results of this study showed significant body and weight dissatisfaction in this population of girls, with 55% of girls wanting to be thinner and 41% of the girls reporting some weight loss activities. As grade in school increased, both desire for thinness and weight-control behavior increased. In fact, among sixth-grade girls, 70% wished to be thinner and 60% had tried to lose weight. Skipping meals, fasting, vomiting, and the use of diet pills were all reported. Nearly 10% of the girls in this study scored in the anorexia nervosa range of the Children's Eating Attitudes Test (Maloney et al. 1989).

The onset of puberty itself has also been recognized as a critical period for the development of disordered eating in girls. Killen and colleagues (1992) studied a nonclinical, community-based sample of over 900 sixth- and seventh-grade girls (11 and 12 years old) in California. More than 4% of the sample engaged in disordered eating behaviors. Girls who were more physically mature were more likely to be symptomatic, independent of age. For each advance in the Tanner Sexual Maturity Rating, a scale used to measure stages and onset of puberty, girls in the study doubled their risk of disordered eating. Girls who indicated any symptom of disordered eating reported fear of weight gain, a sense of ineffectiveness or worthlessness, and depressive symptoms (Killen et al. 1992).

Family dysfunction has been implicated frequently in the development of eating disorders. Specifically, anorexia nervosa may emerge in enmeshed families with rigid styles of interactions and difficulty managing conflict (Steiner and Lock 1998). Similarly, sexual abuse is also frequently identified in patients with disordered eating and at rates higher than those in the general population (Wonderlich et al. 2001). Sexual victimization is especially seen in patients with binge–purge behaviors (Rosen 2003).

18.2.1.3 Assessment and Classification

Eating disorders in children and young adolescents are often not suspected by health care providers until the disturbance has existed for an extended time or until dramatic physical consequences have appeared (Rosen 2003). Part of the delay in diagnosis is related to the atypical presentation of eating disorders in younger patients. Eating disorders in young girls are more likely to appear in the context of stressful family life events and are often present with comorbid psychiatric symptoms, especially obsessive thinking and symptoms of depression (Lask and Bryant-Waugh 2000). Compared to older adolescents and adult women, girls and younger adolescents are less likely to report disturbances in body image, are more likely to describe themselves as thin, may seem more willing to entertain some changes in their eating habits, and generally have a smaller repertoire of weight loss behaviors (Rosen 2003). Some patients report being motivated solely by a focus on "health" rather than concerns about weight. For example, a patient may be concerned about prevention efforts for heart health and increase her exercise level and change her eating habits. However, as the patient continues to pursue a healthy lifestyle, she might be unsure how to balance these efforts, so her changes become extreme and lead to too much weight loss. Many times, the parent of a child pursuing these changes has experienced some type of health problem.

These atypical eating disorders, not fully meeting diagnostic criteria for anorexia nervosa or bulimia nervosa, are especially prevalent in children and adolescents and are often diagnosed as "eating disorder not otherwise specified." There is wide agreement that unspecified eating disorders represent an ambiguous category of patients with disordered eating that creates clinical confusion and may impede access to treatment (Rosen 2003). For example, in a large sample of children with eating disorders (ages 6–16 years), half of the participants were diagnosed with unspecified eating disorders using the *DSM* classification system (Fisher et al. 2001), reiterating that eating problems in children can be overlooked.

In addition to anorexia nervosa, bulimia nervosa, and unspecified eating disorders, the Great Ormond Street criteria for childhood and early adolescence includes food avoidance emotional disorder, selective eating disorder, pervasive refusal, and functional dysphagia. Table 18.1 briefly summarizes each of these disorders.

TABLE 18.1

The Great Ormond Street Criteria for Eating Disorders

Disorder	Criteria
Anorexia nervosa	Determined weight loss
	Abnormal cognitions of weight and/or shape
	Morbid preoccupation with weight and/or shape
Bulimia nervosa	Recurrent binges and purges
	Lack of control
	Morbid preoccupation with weight and/or shape
Food avoidance emotional disorder	Food avoidance
	Weight loss
	Mood disturbances (but not primary affective disorder)
	No abnormal cognitions of reoccupation regarding weight or shape
	No organic brain disease or psychosis
Selective eating disorder	Narrow food choices for at least 2 years
	Unwillingness to try new foods
	No abnormal cognitions regarding weight or shape
	No fear of choking or vomiting
Functional dysphagia	Food avoidance
	Fear of swallowing, choking, or vomiting
	No abnormal cognitions or preoccupation regarding weight or shape
	No organic brain disease or psychosis
Pervasive refusal syndrome	Refusal to eat, drink, walk, talk, or care for self
	Determined resistance to efforts to help

Source: Adapted from Nicholls, D., R. Chater, and B. Lask. 2000. Children into DSM don't go: Comparison of classification systems for eating disorders in childhood and early adolescence. *Int J Eat Disord* 28: 317–324.

Anorexia nervosa is characterized by determined attempts to lose weight or avoid weight gain through fasting, self-induced vomiting, laxative abuse, or excessive exercise. Weight drops to a level below what is necessary to allow appropriate growth and development for the child. The weight loss is often associated with abnormal cognitions about weight, shape, and size (Lask and Bryant-Waugh 2000).

Bulimia nervosa is characterized by episodes of overeating in which the child experiences a loss of control and seeks compensatory behaviors to avoid weight gain. Children and adolescents with bulimia nervosa share the same weight and shape concerns as those with anorexia nervosa but maintain an appropriate weight for their age and level of development. Other forms of self-harm and other risky behaviors, such as wrist scratching, skin burning, and drug abuse, can also be present in children with bulimia nervosa (Lask and Bryant-Waugh 2000).

Food avoidance emotional disorder is manifested by determined food avoidance, as is seen in anorexia nervosa, as well as mood disturbance in the form of mild depression and anxiety. Phobias and obsessions, especially for specific foods, might also be present. However, the child does not experience abnormal cognitions about weight or shape that are characteristic of anorexia nervosa or bulimia nervosa. Food avoidance emotional disorder is commonly seen as part of an emotional response to physical ill health, although it may not be the primary symptom of the child's illness (Lask and Bryant-Waugh 2000).

Selective eating describes the behavior of children who limit their food intake to a very narrow range of preferred foods, such as breads, cereals, crackers, and other foods that are high in carbohydrates. Selective eating often begins during the preschool years and appears to be an extension of food jags. Food jags are often characteristic of preschool children who will only eat the same foods every day, prepared in the same way, and possibly even the same brand of food. Attempts to increase the variety of foods that the child consumes are usually met with extreme resistance and distress. Despite the narrow range of foods, most children do not manifest impaired growth or low weight, and there is no preoccupation with weight, shape, or size (Lask and Bryant-Waugh 2000).

Functional dysphagia characterizes children who have a marked fear of swallowing. Thus, they tend to avoid food, particularly solid foods and those foods of a certain type or texture. In many cases, there is a traumatic event that contributes to the fear, such as choking on a piece of food or witnessing someone else choking on food. Sometimes, the traumatic event could be related to abuse, such as taping the child's mouth shut after stuffing the child's mouth with food. There are no abnormal weight or shape concerns associated with this problem. Instead, anxiety associated with eating and swallowing is the key feature (Lask and Bryant-Waugh 2000).

Pervasive refusal syndrome describes a potentially life-threatening condition in a small group of children who refuse to eat, drink, talk, or care for themselves in any way over a period of several months. Children with this condition are underweight and are often dehydrated because they adamantly refuse food and drink. Often, the condition is misdiagnosed as anorexia nervosa, even though children with this syndrome have a much wider range of symptoms. It has been suggested that this condition is an extreme form of post-traumatic stress disorder or learned helplessness (Lask and Bryant-Waugh 2000).

18.2.1.4 Health Consequences

The nutritional impact of disordered eating on younger patients may be unusual or misleading. Younger people typically do not lose a large amount of weight like some adults with eating disorders. However, any amount of weight loss in children and adolescents is concerning because they should be growing and gaining weight. Furthermore, children and young adolescents have less body fat than older patients, so they exhaust their nutritional stores more quickly. Thus, the nutritional consequences of weight loss in children and young adolescents are quite severe.

When a young person engages in disordered eating behavior, every organ system can be affected. The most obvious signs and symptoms of malnutrition involve the cardiovascular system and gastrointestinal system. Electrolyte disturbances are most often seen in patients who purge by vomiting or by using laxatives. When growth and development are impaired, interruption of hormonal processes may lead to irreversible stunting of growth or damage to the reproductive system. Magnetic resonance imaging studies of the brain have shown loss of brain volume in patients with anorexia nervosa that may persist even after weight recovery (Katzman et al. 2001). Finally, younger patients with eating disorders are susceptible to osteopenia and osteoporosis as a result of bone loss and a failure to accrue bone mass during the critical developmental periods of childhood and adolescence. Osteopenia is described as thin, soft bones and the beginning stage of osteoporosis. Osteoporosis is a "skeletal disorder characterized by compromised bone strength predisposing a person to an increased risk of fracture" that develops not only through bone loss during adulthood, but also through the failure to accumulate sufficient bone mass during adolescence (National Institute of Health 2001).

18.2.1.5 Nutrition Goals

Nutrition therapy for children is based on classic principles of nutritional rehabilitation for starving humans. Renourishment should begin with a gradual increase in energy intake. Typically, calorie intake begins at 1,000–1,200 cal per day and is increased by 50–150 cal per day. This gradual increase in caloric intake allows for slow weight change with minimal anxiety. Calorie amounts for children and adolescents should be adjusted based on the desired rate of weight gain, with the goal of one pound per week for those in outpatient treatment and 3 pounds per week for those in inpatient treatment. Sometimes, it is necessary to increase calories to an elevated level of 3,000–4,000 cal per day in order to reverse the body's catabolic state and move it into an anabolic state. Once the child achieves a healthy weight, caloric intake is gradually decreased in order to maintain weight.

In addition to improving energy intake, the nutrition therapist should prescribe adequate protein and fat to meet basic needs. Sodium and sugars should be moderated, as they may enhance fluid retention, resulting in artificial weight gain. High-fiber foods should also be included to achieve bowel regularity, but only after gastrointestinal complications related to starvation, binge eating, and purging have been considered.

If a child or an adolescent refuses to eat normal, solid food, a nutritionally complete liquid formula may be used to meet the prescribed meal plan. Nourishment by mouth is the preferred route and is almost always possible. However, if oral feedings are refused, it may be necessary to use nasogastric methods, or in rare cases, parenteral nutrition. When invasive methods are used, they will be presented to the patient and to the family as life-saving procedures, not as punishment for refusing to eat.

The nutrition therapist should involve the entire family during the nutrition intervention, not only to provide support for the child or adolescent, but also to educate family members about food, nutrition, and health. For example, the nutrition therapist is responsible for educating a parent who is trying to lose weight using an unhealthy fad diet about the health consequences that may occur if the parent continues the diet. The nutrition therapist can also discuss the parent's potential to be a role model for the child and the possible sabotage to the child's recovery from an eating disorder if the parent continues to diet. The nutrition therapist should also review basic nutrition principles and metabolic changes that can occur in response to eating disorder behaviors. Often, nutrition sessions can provide a forum for discussion of difficulties and myths about food. Guided experiences, such as cooking, eating out, grocery shopping, and introducing new foods, prepare the child and the family to manage food in multiple environments.

18.2.2 Eating Disorders in Athletes

18.2.2.1 Prevalence

The reported prevalence of disordered eating and eating disorders among female athletes has ranged from as low as 2% and to as high as 62% (Beals and Manore 1994; Petrie 1996; Hulley and Hill 2001; Sundgot-Borgen 2004). Prevalence varied since different studies used varying methods to assess the occurrence of eating disorders. Some studies used criteria derived from the strict diagnostic definitions of eating disorders, whereas other studies estimated prevalence using instruments that screened for eating disordered behaviors and attitudes. In addition, the type of athlete varied greatly, and several studies examined 10–15 different sports within the same study.

18.2.2.2 Risk Factors

Disordered eating in athletes is characterized by a wide spectrum of maladaptive eating patterns as well as various weight-control behaviors and attitudes. These disordered eating patterns include concerns about body weight and shape; poor nutrition or inadequate caloric intake; binge eating; misuse of laxatives, diuretics, and diet pills; and extreme weight-control behaviors, such as fasting, vomiting, and excessive exercise (Shisslak et al. 1995).

Sundgot-Borgen and Torstveit (2004) studied the risk for developing eating disorders in female athletes. Results of this study indicated that athletes are at a greater risk than nonathletes for developing eating disorders due to a heightened emphasis on appearance in their sport as well as pressure in some sports to have a low weight, low percentage of body fat, and low body mass in order to enhance performance. Additionally, these authors found that female athletes competing in aesthetic sports, such as dance, gymnastics, and figure skating, were found to be at the highest risk for eating disorders, and athletes competing in weight class and endurance sports, such as powerlifting, wrestling, and running, were also at elevated risk for eating disorders.

Many athletes also share psychological qualities similar to individuals with eating disorders. These characteristics include perfectionism (Halmi et al. 2000; Chang 2004; Hopkinson and Lock

2004), obsessive personality traits and high achievement expectations (Yates 1989), and feelings of personal ineffectiveness, guilt, and distrust (Klemchuk et al. 1990). Other characteristics seen specifically in athletes who develop bulimia nervosa include impulsiveness, narcissism, and intolerance to hunger or psychological distress (Petrie 1996). Athletes who develop anorexia nervosa tend to be sensitive, obsessive, perfectionistic, and avoidant (Petrie 1996). Unfortunately, many of the characteristics that are helpful to become a successful athlete might also contribute to the development of an eating disorder.

18.2.2.3 Health Consequences

Disordered eating of any degree can lead to adverse health consequences, with risk of impaired athletic performance or even death, and the effects of these consequences increase as the severity of the eating disorder increases. Weight loss, food restriction, and purging practices associated with eating disorders have powerful physiological and psychological effects for athletes specifically. These effects can include decreased exercise capacity, increased risk of injury, and potentially fatal medical complications, such as nutrient deficiencies, fluid and electrolyte imbalances, and adverse changes in the cardiovascular, digestive, endocrine, skeletal, and thermoregulatory systems.

This section will briefly describe the special problems that have come to be identified as the female athlete triad. In 1992, the American College of Sports Medicine coined the term "the female athlete triad" to represent the set of associations between disordered eating behaviors, menstrual cycle abnormalities, and bone loss. Alone, each problem is of medical concern, but when all three components of the triad are present, there is potential for more serious consequences for health and a greater risk of death (American College of Sports Medicine 2008).

Dietary energy is used in basic physiological processes, such as cellular maintenance, thermogenesis, immune functioning, growth, reproduction, and locomotion. Energy that is used in any one of these areas limits the amount of energy that is available in another area. Low-energy intake coupled with high-energy expenditure during training and athletic competitions results in an inadequate amount of energy available to the body. This lack of available energy impairs body functions in many areas, including suppressing reproductive function and compromising the menstrual cycle.

Menstrual abnormalities include oligomenorrhea (menstrual cycles exceeding 35 days), primary amenorrhea (delayed menarche when menstruation has not begun by 16 years of age), and secondary amenorrhea (absence of menstrual cycle for more than 90 days). Amenorrhea is related to dysfunction of the hypothalamic-pituitary-ovarian axis. Evidence suggests that a dysfunctional pattern exists between luteinizing hormone (LH) and follicle stimulating hormone (FSH) in which LH is suppressed more than FSH (Loucks and Thuma 2003). LH suppression leads to ovarian suppression with subsequent low levels of estrogen and progesterone. In the past, it was proposed that a critical level of body fat was needed to achieve and maintain reproductive function. This idea was based on clinical observations rather than empirical studies, and no specific percentage of body fat has been shown to cause an athlete to cease regular menses. Instead, low energy availability resulting in an energy deficit has been correlated with low LH (Loucks et al. 1998; Loucks and Thuma, 2003), and amenorrhea has been shown to be reversed with appropriate caloric supplementation (Williams et al. 2001). The prevalence of amenorrhea in athletes varies widely with sport, age, training, and body weight. It is a common misconception among some athletes, coaches, and trainers that amenorrhea is a consequence of strenuous exercise and is an indicator that training is at an optimal level for a sport. In fact, the altered hormonal environment is a risk factor for the development of impaired bone health and osteoporosis.

Bone development is influenced by genetics, nutrition, exercise, and overall hormone status. Imbalances in any of these factors can lead to insufficient deposition of calcium in the bone and increased loss of calcium from the bone. In particular, estrogen increases intestinal absorption of calcium, reduces renal excretion of calcium, and regulates calcium homeostasis in the blood. Thus, a low estrogen level in an athlete with an eating disorder who also has menstrual dysfunction is one etiological factor in the development of osteopenia or osteoporosis. Bone strength and the risk of fracture depend on the density and internal structure of bone mineral and on the quality of bone protein. Osteoporosis is diagnosed in terms of a bone mineral density (BMD); however, data are lacking for premenopausal women and children, including female athletes. Currently, it is recommended that BMD in these populations be expressed as Z-scores to compare individuals to age- and sex-matched controls. Generally, Z-scores that are below −2.0 define low bone density (International Society for Clinical Densitometry 2004). An athlete's BMD reflects her cumulative history of energy availability and menstrual status, as well as genetic endowment and exposure to other nutritional, behavioral, and environmental factors.

All athletes would benefit from a comprehensive assessment as a means of screening for disordered eating patterns and behaviors. If an athlete is identified to have any psychological, behavioral, or physical characteristics of an eating disorder, appropriate interventions should be implemented from knowledgeable health care professionals, including a nutrition therapist who specializes in eating disorders.

18.2.2.4 Nutrition Goals

Initially, a nutrition assessment should be conducted to evaluate the athlete's food intake, metabolic status, and readiness to make changes. Habits and general lifestyle choices, such as drinking and smoking, should also be assessed. The primary goal of nutrition counseling and management is to help athletes maintain adequate energy availability. Athletes need to consume adequate energy during periods of high-intensity training and during long-duration training to maintain health, body weight, and to maximize training effects. In fact, improving an eating disordered athlete's overall energy availability may be the key to reversing menstrual dysfunction and reducing fracture risk. Athletes should try to maintain energy availability between 30 and 45 cal per kg per day for weight maintenance and more than 45 cal per kg per day for weight gain and growth (Manore et al. 2007). Increasing energy intake in moderate increments, such as 100–200 cal per day, will be the most acceptable approach for an athlete with an eating disorder. If the athlete has suffered from marked weight loss, reestablishment of a healthy weight is also a primary focus. According to the International Olympic Committee (IOC), a goal of at least 90% of ideal body weight is recommended in order for the athlete to return to participation in the athlete's sport. Body weight and body mass index have been shown to be closely associated with BMD and resumption of the menstrual cycle (Manore 2002). Therefore, appropriate weight status, in addition to dietary intake, is important for the athlete with eating disordered behaviors.

Although limited data are available regarding the protein requirements of female athletes, it is recommended that they consume more protein (1.2–1.5 g of protein per kg) than the Recommended Dietary Allowance (0.8 g of protein per kg; American Institute of Medicine 2009). Top sport endurance athletes, such as elite cyclists or marathon runners, may have protein requirements as high as 1.7 g of protein per kg (Tarnopolsky 2004). In addition, recent research has suggested that high quality protein consumed immediately after exercise may improve overall net protein balance (Koopman et al. 2004). Generally, recommended protein intake can be met through diet alone without the use of protein or amino acid supplements.

Consuming enough calories to maintain body weight is necessary for optimal protein use and performance. The athlete should help to develop the meal plan, and the plan should include a variety of food options and encourage her to eat regularly and to consume enough food to meet her energy needs. Athletes who restrict energy intake or eliminate food groups from their diet can have low micronutrient intakes, especially nutrients that build energy (B-complex vitamins), blood (folate, vitamin B_{12}, iron), and bones (calcium, magnesium, and vitamin D; Manore 2000, 2002). The nutrition therapist should consider calcium and vitamin D supplementation to achieve and maintain the recommended dietary intakes of 1,000–1,500 mg per day of calcium and 400–600 IU per day of vitamin D. High doses of both supplements are necessary to prevent or treat osteoporosis and minimize fracture risk.

18.2.3 Eating Disorders in Pregnancy

18.2.3.1 Prevalence

The prevalence of eating disorders among women of childbearing potential has been estimated at approximately 4% (Mitchell-Gieleghem et al. 2002). The prevalence in pregnancy, however, appears to be lower (Blais et al. 2000). The only population-based study on the prevalence and course of eating disorders in pregnant women reported a variable course (Bulik et al. 2007). The Norwegian Mother and Child Cohort Study assessed the presence of eating disorders in 41,157 pregnant women at approximately 18 weeks of gestation using self-administered questionnaires. Broad criteria were used to define eating disorders, instead of formal *DSM-IV* criteria. Before pregnancy, 0.1% of the women were diagnosed with anorexia nervosa, 0.7% were diagnosed with bulimia nervosa, and 3.6% were diagnosed with eating disorder not otherwise specified (EDNOS), which included binge eating disorder and self-induced purging without binge eating. At 18 weeks of gestation, the prevalence of bulimia nervosa fell to 0.2%, but the proportion of women with EDNOS increased to 4.9%. Although some women with bulimia nervosa or EDNOS had partial or complete remission, those with binge eating disorder did not. In fact, binge eating disorder was more likely than other eating disorders to develop during pregnancy. Specifically, in this study, there were 711 new cases of binge eating disorder that developed during pregnancy (Bulik et al. 2007).

18.2.3.2 Risk Factors

Predisposing factors for eating disorders during pregnancy are generally the same as for other eating disorders: genetics, family dynamics, certain personality traits, and different psychiatric disorders. Predisposed individuals may be triggered into active eating disorders at times of profound body changes, such as puberty or pregnancy. "Pregorexia" has become a common term used to describe pregnant women who reduce their caloric intake and increase the amount that they exercise in order to control weight gain, and individuals who are pregnant and suffer from these problems need to be considered high risk (American Dietetic Association 2009).

18.2.3.3 Health Consequences

There are several significant health consequences for a woman with an eating disorder who is pregnant or is trying to get pregnant, including amenorrhea or oligomenorrhea. Individuals with eating disorders may also experience low libido, sexual dysfunction, infertility, and inadequate weight gain during pregnancy, and they may give birth to preterm children or children with low birth weights (Andersen and Ryan 2009).

Research has examined potential complications for both the baby and the mother in relationship to the eating disorder. For the baby, findings suggest that both anorexic and bulimic behavior may negatively affect fetal outcomes (Kouba et al. 2005). Although disordered eating behaviors tend to subside during pregnancy, preterm delivery, intrauterine growth restriction, and low birth weight have been associated with past or current eating disorder behaviors. Franko and colleagues (2001) reported that women experiencing eating disorder symptoms reported more fetal and neonatal complications and a higher rate of complicated deliveries than women who were nonsymptomatic. In addition, this study suggested that women with bulimia nervosa have an increased risk of miscarriage and fetal deaths (Franko et al. 2001).

For the mother, existing research shows that some women with eating disorders experience a reduction in the severity of their symptoms during pregnancy. However, the late postpartum period has been shown to be a high-risk time for the recurrence or exacerbation of eating disorder symptoms (Blais et al. 2000). Among individuals with bulimia nervosa, purging frequency and binge eating frequency both decreased during pregnancy and remained reduced for 9 months postpartum. Individuals with anorexia nervosa showed a similar pattern of symptom reduction, as both anorexic and bulimic symptoms decreased during the course of the pregnancy. However, 9 months after the birth, eating disorder symptoms returned to prepregnancy levels for all of the women in the study

(Blais et al. 2000). Since pregnant women with eating disorders are considered high-risk pregnancies, close monitoring by the nutrition therapist and the treatment team is essential.

18.2.3.4 Nutrition Goals

Most pregnant women receive very little formal nutrition counseling during pregnancy. Most obstetricians do not have the time to provide in-depth nutritional counseling, so they rely on booklets or pamphlets to provide information about detailed dietary changes that are needed during pregnancy. Although information in nutritional booklets or pamphlets might be adequate for most women, pregnant women with eating disorders need more attention. Weekly nutrition sessions are recommended for pregnant women with eating disorders in order to determine energy needs for appropriate weight gain and lactation, to design an individualized food plan, and to discuss hydration shifts and rebound edema.

The body needs additional energy during pregnancy because of added maternal tissues and the growth of the fetus and placenta. Adequate maternal weight gain, including some maternal fat storage, is needed to ensure that the size of the newborn is optimal for survival. Thus, storage of energy is included as part of the energy requirement for pregnancy. According to the National Research Council (1989), it is recommended that a pregnant woman should increase her daily intake by 300 cal and sustain this increase throughout the remainder of the pregnancy. However, if a woman with an eating disorder becomes pregnant with depleted body reserves, it might be necessary for her to increase her daily caloric intake by 500 cal per day. During lactation, the additional caloric intake needed is proportional to the quantity of milk produced. Since most women have some fat stores that remain after birth and help to meet energy needs during lactation, 500 additional calories per day is the standard recommendation. However, if a woman's weight gain during pregnancy was below normal or if her weight falls below a healthy level, an additional 650 cal per day is recommended during the first 6 months (National Research Council 1989).

The nutrition therapist needs to work closely with the pregnant woman to determine her emotional tolerance for increased caloric intake and subsequent weight gain. An optimal range of weight gain during pregnancy should be determined. According to the guidelines set by the Institute of Medicine (2009), new recommendations for total weight gain and rate of weight gain during pregnancy have been established and are based on prepregnancy body mass index. Table 18.2 summarizes these recommendations.

It is important to promote slow, gradual weight gain and to monitor weight status throughout the pregnancy. To ensure appropriate and adequate weight gain, pregnant women with eating disorders typically need a detailed and practical meal plan. The meal plan should include the total amount of daily calories, protein, carbohydrate, and fat required to achieve healthy weight gain during the pregnancy. Because food consumption patterns vary among people with eating disorders, the nutrition therapist should respect food choices to avoid additional stressors during the pregnancy. When

TABLE 18.2

American Institute of Medicine's (2009) Recommended Weight Gain Guidelines for Pregnant Women

Prepregnancy Body Mass Index	Body Mass Index	Recommended Weight Gain	Rate of Weight Gain
Underweight	<18.5	28 to 40 lbs.	1 to 1.3 lbs/week
Normal Weight	18.5 to 24.9	25 to 35 lbs.	.8 to 1 lbs/week
Overweight	25 to 29.9	15 to 25 lbs.	.5 to .7 lbs/week
Obese	>30	11 to 20 lbs.	.4 to .6 lbs/week

Source: Adapted from Mathieu, J. 2009. What is pregorexia? *J Am Diet Assoc* 109: 976–979 with permission.

developing the meal plan, high-calorie, high-protein, and low-volume foods should be encouraged, such as peanut butter, eggs, milk, cheese, and dried fruit. High-quality protein sources are often the least threatening inclusion to the meal plan, because these foods cause very few hydration shifts.

Weight shifts can occur due to fluid changes, and these shifts may evoke fear in a person with an eating disorder. Hormonal changes might also affect fluid balance and water retention, and both are a normal part of childbirth. If a woman with an eating disorder restricts fluid in an attempt to lose weight, the nutrition therapist should discuss rebound edema with her. She should be informed that her restriction does not promote temporary or permanent weight loss and may even cause additional water retention and increased body weight. It may be helpful to discuss a specific goal for consumption of fluids in addition to the individualized food plan created for a pregnant woman to ensure that she is consuming an appropriate amount of liquid as well as an appropriate amount of calories.

18.3 CASE STUDIES

18.3.1 CASE STUDY 1

Please read this scenario and answer the questions in the *Your Response* section of this Chapter.

KT is a 15-year-old, female, high school track star. She was asked to leave the track team for a semester because of malnutrition and was referred to a student health center for evaluation. Her history revealed severe restriction of food intake and more than 50 pounds of weight loss in a 6- to 9-month period. Her training regimen consisted of running 6–9 miles each day and occasional biking and swimming in addition to running. She reported no vomiting or laxative use, but she admitted to using diet pills. Menstrual history revealed secondary amenorrhea for 1 year. She stated that she was seen by her internal medicine doctor during the previous summer and was cleared to return to school and track. She was also told to "eat better." Her physical exam indicated that she was 5 ft, 10 in tall and weighed 109 pounds. Her pulse was 32 bpm, and her blood pressure was 88/56. Lab values revealed hyponatremia, hypokalemia, hypophosphatemia, abnormal liver function tests, and abnormal renal function tests. She had an abnormal electrocardiogram with heart block and prolonged QT wave signifying irregular heart beat. Her echocardiogram showed a dilated right ventricle, left ventricle, and mitral valve regurgitation. Her bone scan revealed osteoporosis by Z score.

18.3.1.1 Your Response

1. Should this individual be allowed to return to school? If so, should she be allowed to rejoin the track team? Why or why not? If she needs treatment, at what level of care should she receive this treatment?
2. What are the health consequences of her current condition, and are they more serious because of her age?
3. What are your recommendations for food intake, activity level, and weight range?

18.3.1.2 Appropriate Response

1. This individual has lost an excessive amount of weight and is at high nutrition risk. She should be admitted to inpatient treatment based on her medical complications and compromised health status. Once she has received appropriate nutrition therapy to increase her weight to 90% of her ideal body weight (at least 135 pounds, as recommended by the IOC) and is consistently following an adequate meal plan, then she may incorporate some physical activity into her life and may resume participation in track.
2. This individual is suffering from several serious health consequences and medical complications. Her cardiovascular, hepatic, renal, skeletal, and reproductive systems have all been compromised due to malnutrition. Because she is an adolescent, these health consequences are critical because of disruption of growth and development. Examples might include permanent heart damage and failure to maximize bone mass density.

3. Food intake recommendations may be initiated at ~1,000–1,200 kcal per day. It is important to increase her food intake to 100 kcal per day to a goal of ~3,000 kcal per day (45 kcal per kg ideal body weight) and to reevaluate periodically based on weight changes to promote slow and steady weight gain. An appropriate healthy weight range goal is 135–145 pounds (61.3–65.9 kg). Activity should be limited during the weight gaining process and once the individual reaches her minimum healthy weight, she may be able to incorporate physical activity into her routine. In addition, calories will need to be adjusted to a level of maintenance which should be ~2,000–2,400 kcal per day to manage basic metabolic needs plus additional intake to compensate for exercise expenditure.

18.3.2 Case Study 2

Please read this scenario and answer the questions in the *Your Response* section of this Chapter.

CR is a 24-year-old, pregnant female with a history of bulimia nervosa since age 18. Prior to conception, CR was restricting daily, binge eating and vomiting two to three times per week, and compulsively exercising for 2 h per day. In addition, she weighed herself at home one to four times per day. CR weighed 137 pounds when she conceived and is 5 ft, 4 in tall. Her doctor advised her to gain 25 pounds, but she decided that she would only allow herself to gain a total of 20 pounds. Her doctor became concerned because during the fifth month, CR did not gain any weight and during the sixth month, she lost 2 pounds. CR reported "eating healthfully" during her pregnancy and told her doctor that she was confused by the weight loss. Upon further prompting, however, CR admitted that she continued to exercise compulsively and returned to binge eating followed by vomiting one to three times per week starting in the second trimester. After engaging in these behaviors, CR reported feelings of fear, self-hatred, and guilt.

18.3.2.1 Your Response

1. Does this individual need to be referred on by her doctor? If so, what type of professional(s) should this individual be referred to?
2. What type of meal plan and/or meal practices would you incorporate for this individual? How would you approach this individual about her eating disorder behaviors during pregnancy?
3. How much weight is appropriate for this individual to gain? Would it be helpful to focus on weight status and changes throughout the pregnancy? Why or Why not?

18.3.2.2 Appropriate Response

1. Because this individual is pregnant with a history of an eating disorder as well as active in her eating disorder behaviors, she needs to work with other specialized professionals besides her doctor. A registered dietitian specializing in eating disorders can help her with her fear of weight changes and can help her plan her diet and activity to promote adequate weight gain upon the doctor's recommendation. A mental health professional may also be necessary if the pregnancy is triggering or causing mental health problems that are interfering with the patient's functioning and care of herself and the baby.
2. A meal plan that is adequate in caloric intake to support her pregnancy should be recommended. This patient needs approximately 2,200 cal based on her age, weight, and height. However, due to pregnancy, the patient must consume an additional 300 cal. Therefore, a total of 2,500 cal per day should be recommended. These additional cal can easily be added by consuming 2 cups (16 oz) of whole milk per day. By adding a high protein, high calories source, fluid changes affecting weight status is less likely. Also, the addition is small in volume, which reduces the likelihood that the patient will feel overwhelmed. Addressing eating disorder behaviors can be very tricky. Rather than expecting immediate cessation of the restriction/binge/purge cycle, emphasize small, specific changes, such as

increasing calorie and/or protein intake or other positive self-care behaviors. Repetitive discussions about the high-risk aspects of the pregnancy and statements regarding harm of the child and the possible death of the fetus are not advised.

3. Appropriate weight gain is based on prepregnancy body mass index. The patient's body mass index is 23.5 kg/m², which is calculated from her height and weight at conception. According to the Institute of Medicine, an individual with a body mass index between 18.5 and 24.9 is considered normal weight and should gain between 25–35 pounds. Therefore, a minimum of 25 pounds of weight gain is recommended, which is consistent with the doctor's initial recommendation. It is also important to emphasize that the rate of weight gain in the second and third trimesters should be an average of 1 pound per week. Although the individual's weight should be monitored, it is important to focus on positive outcomes and de-emphasize weight gains and losses. The overall weight trend can be tracked and plotted on a weight graph to demonstrate and ensure slow but steady weight gain.

REFERENCES

American College of Sports Medicine. 2008. Position Stand: The female athlete triad. *Med Sci Sport Exerc* 1867–1882.

American Dietetic Association. 2009. What is pregorexia? *J Am Diet Assoc* 109: 976–979.

American Institute of Medicine. 2009. *Weight gain during pregnancy: Reexamining the guidelines.* Washington, DC: National Academies Press.

Andersen, A. E., and G. L. Ryan. 2009. Eating disorders in the obstetric and gynecologic patient population. *Obstet Gynecol* 114: 1353–1367.

Beals, K. A., and M. M. Manore. 1994. The prevalence and consequences of subclinical eating disorders in female athletes. *Int J Sport Nutr* 4: 175–195.

Blais, M. A., A. E. Becker, R. A. Burwell, A. T. Flores, K. M. Nussbaum, D. N. Greenwood, E. R. Ekeblad, and D. B. Herzog. 2000. Pregnancy: Outcome and impact on symptomatology in a cohort of eating-disordered women. *Int J Eat Disord* 27: 140–149.

Bulik, C. M., A. Von Holle, R. Hamer, C. K. Berg, L. Torgersen, P. Magnus, C. Stoltenberg, A. M. Siega-Riz, P. Sullivan, and T. Reichborn-Kjennerud. 2007. Patterns of remission, continuation and incidence of broadly defined eating disorders during early pregnancy in the Norwegian Mother and Child Cohort Study (MoBa). *Psychol Med* 37: 1109–1118.

Chang, E. C. 2004. Perfectionism as a predictor of positive and negative psychological outcomes: Examining a mediation model in younger and older adults. *J Couns Psychol* 47: 8–26.

Fisher, M., M. Schneider, J. Burns, H. Symons, and F. Mandel. 2001. Differences between adolescents and young adults at presentation to an eating disorders program. *J Adolesc Health* 28: 222–227.

Franko, D. L., M. A. Blais, A. E. Becker, S. S. Delinsky, D. N. Greenwood, A. T. Flores, E. R. Ekeblad, K. T. Eddy, and D. B. Herzog. 2001. Pregnancy complications and neonatal outcomes in women with eating disorders. *Am J Psychiatry* 158: 1461–1466.

Halmi, K. A., S. R. Sunday, M. Strober, A. Kaplan, D. B. Woodside, M. Fichter, J. Treasure, W. H. Berrettini, and W. H. Kaye. 2000. Perfectionism in anorexia nervosa: variation by clinical subtype, obsessionality, and pathological eating behavior. *Am J Psychiatry* 157: 1799–1805.

Hopkinson, R. A., and J. Lock. 2004. Athletics, perfectionism, and disordered eating. *Eat Weight Disord* 9: 99–106.

Hulley, A. J., and A. J. Hill. 2001. Eating disorders and health in elite women distance runners. *Int J Eat Disord* 30: 312–317.

International Society for Clinical Densitometry Writing Group for the ISCD Position Development Conference. 2004. Diagnosis of osteoporosis in men, women, and children. *J Clin Densitom* 7: 17–26.

Katzman, D. K., B. Christensen, and A. R. Young. 2001. Starving the brain: Structural abnormalities and cognitive impairment in adolescents with anorexia nervosa. *Sem Clin Neuropsychiatry* 6: 146–152.

Killen, J. D., C. Hayward, I. Litt, L. D. Hammer, D. M. Wilson, B. Miner, C. B. Taylor, A. Varady, and C. Shisslak. 1992. Is puberty a risk factor for eating disorders? *Am J Did Child* 146: 323–235.

Klemchuk, H. P., C. B. Hutchinson, and R. I. Frank. 1990. Body dissatisfaction and eating-related problems on the college campus: Usefulness of the Eating Disorder Inventory with a nonclinical population. *J Counsel Psychol* 37: 297–305.

Koopman, R., D. L. Pannemans, A. E. Jeukendrup, A. P. Gijsen, J. M. Senden, and D. Halliday. 2004. Combined ingestion of protein and carbohydrate improves protein balance during ultra-endurance exercise. *Am J Physiol Endocrinol Metabol* 287: 712–720.

Kouba, S., T. Hallstrom, C. Lindholm, and A. L. Hirschberg. 2005. Pregnancy and neonatal outcomes in women with eating disorders. *J Obstet Gynecol* 105: 255–260.

Lask, B., and R. Bryant-Waugh. 2000. *Anorexia nervosa and related eating disorders in childhood and adolescence.* Hove, UK: Psychology Press.

Loucks, A. B., and J. R. Thuma. 2003. Luteinizing hormone pulsatility is disrupted at a threshold of energy availability in regularly menstruating women. *J Clin Endocrinol Metab* 88: 297–311.

Loucks, A. B., M. Verdun, and E. M. Heath. 1998. Low energy availability, not stress of exercise, alters LH pulsatility in exercising women. *J Appl Physiol* 84: 37–46.

Maloney, M. J., J. McGuire, S. R. Daniels, and B. Specker. 1989. Dieting behavior and eating attitudes in children. *Pediatrics* 84: 482–489.

Manore, M. M. 2000. Effect of physical activity on thiamin, riboflavin, and vitamin B-6 requirements. *Am J Clin Nutr* 72: 598S–606S.

Manore, M. M. 2002. Dietary recommendations and athletic menstrual dysfunction. *Sports Med* 32: 887–901.

Manore, M. M., L. C. Kam, and A. B. Loucks; International Association of Athletics Federations. 2007. The Female Athlete Triad: Components, Nutrition Issues, and Health Consequences. *J Sports Sci* 25: S61–S71.

Mathieu, J. 2009. What is pregorexia? *J Am Diet Assoc* 109: 976–979.

Mitchell-Gieleghem, A., M. E. Mittelstaedt, and C. M. Bulik. 2002. Eating disorders and childbearing: Concealment and consequences. *Birth* 29: 182.

National Institutes of Health Consensus Development Panel. 2001. Osteoporosis prevention, diagnosis, and therapy. *JAMA* 285: 785–795.

National Research Council. 1989. *Recommended daily allowances* (10th ed.). Washington DC: National Academy Press.

Nicholls, D., R. Chater, and B. Lask. 2000. Children into DSM don't go: Comparison of classification systems for eating disorders in childhood and early adolescence. *Int J Eat Disord* 28: 317–324.

Pendergast, T. and S. Pendergast. 2000. *St. James encyclopedia of popular culture.* Detroit, MI: St. James Press.

Petrie, T. A. 1996. Differences between male and female college lean sport athletes, nonlean sport athletes, and nonathletes on behavioral and psychological indices of eating disorders. *J Sport Exerc Physiol* 8: 218–230.

Rosen, D. S. 2003. Eating disorders in children and young adolescents: Etiology, classification, clinical features, and treatment. *Adolescent Med* 14: 49–59.

Shisslak, C. M., M. Crago, and L. S. Estes. 1995. The spectrum of eating disturbances. *Int J Eat Disord* 18: 209–219.

Steiner, H., and L. Lock. 1998. Anorexia nervosa and bulimia nervosa in children and adolescents: Review of the past 10 years. *J Am Acad Child Adolesc Psychiatry* 37: 352–359.

Sundgot-Borgen, J. 1994. Risk and trigger factors for the development of eating disorders in female elite athletes. *Med Sci Sports Exerc* 26: 403–425.

Sundgot-Borgen, J., and M. K. Torstveit. 2004. Prevalence of eating disorders in elite athletes is higher than in the general population. *Clin J Sport Med* 14: 25–32.

Tarnopolsky, M. 2004. Protein requirements for endurance athletes. *Nutrition* 20: 662–668.

Williams, N. I., A. L. Caston-Balderrama, D. L. Helmreich, D. B. Parfitt, C. Nosbisch, and J. L. Cameron. 2001. Longitudinal changes in reproductive hormones and menstrual cyclicity in cynomolgus monkeys during strenuous exercise training: Abrupt transition to exercise-induced amenorrhea. *Endocrinol* 142: 2381–2389.

Wonderlich, S., R. Crosby, J. Mitchell, K. Thompson, J. Redlin, G. Demuth, and J. Smyth. 2001. Pathways mediating sexual abuse and eating disturbances in children. *Int J Eat Disord* 29: 270–279.

Yates, A. 1989. Current perspectives on the eating disorders: I. History, psychological, and biological aspects. *J Am Acad Child Adolesc* 6: 813–828.

Part VI

Therapeutic Approaches to the
Treatment of Eating Disorders

19 Cognitive Behavioral Approaches for Treating Eating Disorders

Marcia M. Abbott and Kristin L. Goodheart

CONTENTS

19.1 LEARNING OBJECTIVES

After completing this chapter, you should be able to do the following:

- Describe cognitive processes and their relevance to treating people with eating disorders
- Generate examples of common cognitive distortions among people with eating disorders
- Describe methods to help change distorted thought patterns in people with eating disorders

- Explain the process of therapy, including the referral, the initial interview, and the treatment stages of therapy
- Describe when and how to refer people who need professional assistance

19.2 INTRODUCTION

Working with women with eating disorders can be extremely challenging because maladaptive knowledge structures or schemata are acquired early in childhood. Aaron Beck (1976) explained that these schemata are ways of perceiving the world that are made up of attitudes, beliefs, and concepts that individuals use when they interpret their experiences. When some women experience stressful events in childhood, they become vulnerable to making dysfunctional interpretations that lead to emotional disorders, such as anorexia nervosa and bulimia nervosa. In addition to maladaptive cognitions, external factors, such as societal pressure, can contribute to the maintenance of these disorders. Therefore, the treatment of eating disorders is complicated and requires much patience of the therapist. The purpose of this chapter is to provide an overview of cognitive behavioral strategies that we have found to be clinically useful. In addition, specific examples for establishing rapport, making appropriate referrals, and engaging the client and her family in the therapeutic process are discussed.

19.3 RESEARCH BACKGROUND AND SIGNIFICANCE

19.3.1 Cognitive Behavioral Model

In his classic Cognitive Therapy of Depression, Beck (1976) explained that irrational and distorted patterns of thinking lead to negative emotions and self-defeating behaviors. He theorized that learning how to recognize specific thoughts and beliefs that precede negative emotional reactions and behaviors could provide the chance to change unhealthy thinking patterns. Many irrational patterns are acquired from early childhood and lead to emotions and behaviors that are so automatic that they feel as though they occur spontaneously. In people with eating disorders, cognitive distortions can lead to feelings of low self-esteem; mistaken attributions of problems in life due to weight, shape, and appearance; and maintenance of eating disorders as ways to manage weight and emotions. For example, a woman who restricts her diet believes that she is able to control her environment as long as she maintains a low weight. She may believe that she cannot be successful or liked by others unless she is thin. The thinner she becomes, the more weight she wants to lose because her perception of perfection becomes distorted, as does her image of her body. A person who binges and purges believes she cannot lose weight without engaging in unhealthy behaviors, such as self-induced vomiting, laxative abuse, or excessive exercise. This belief is maintained even though the client may remain at an average weight for her height. One reason this belief is maintained is because the mechanism of bingeing and purging can cause swelling in the face and neck, which can contribute to body image distortion and provides "proof" to the client that she is, indeed, fat.

19.3.2 Restructuring Cognitive Distortions

In practice, clinicians often observe that a client's concern with her body shape and weight has become a preoccupation by the time she enters puberty. She may recall criticism of her size and weight by a parent, teacher, coach, or other authority figure. She incorporates what she hears as part of her self-esteem and body image and develops distorted beliefs at a preconscious level. Her self-defeating behaviors with food stem from her irrational beliefs. The fears and tensions that are alleviated through the use of these unhealthy behaviors reflect deficient coping abilities in several areas, including maturity fears, developmental transition from childhood to puberty, dysfunctional family relationships, and separating from parents and going away from home. Her preoccupation with food and weight becomes consuming, and the preoccupation distracts her from overwhelming feelings of anxiety, fear, and depression triggered by developmental or family events. She, therefore, mistakenly feels in control of herself and those around her, although her eating behaviors are out of control. As she becomes more and more ill, she views negative comments about her thinness as compliments.

Culture has a strong influence on beliefs and expectations, particularly in those cultures where thinness is highly valued (Garner and Garfinkel 1985). For example, in American culture, the media constantly glorify the virtues of dieting and thinness. Young girls are bombarded by images of ultra-thin models, actresses, and entertainers, and incorporate these images into their beliefs about their own body images. Even when a celebrity comes forward to reveal problems with an eating disorder, an adolescent's distorted body image rarely changes. A young person begins to develop the irrational belief from these media examples that being thin equals beauty, happiness, and success. These values are reinforced by influential people, such as friends or family members who praise weight loss.

Irrational eating behaviors become patterns that persist independent of emotional situations that occur. What begins as a desire to lose a few pounds becomes an obsession. The more weight that the client loses, the more she restricts her diet, and the more fearful she becomes about food. She begins to limit her food choices based on irrational beliefs. For example, she may believe that any fat intake will result in an instant weight gain, so she will cut out fat entirely. If she is unable to successfully restrict her diet, she might engage in unhealthy behaviors, like self-induced vomiting or excessive exercise, to attempt to compensate for the food consumption and regain control.

Cognitive distortions occur in the areas of personality functioning, self-esteem, self-efficacy, and competence. They influence the client's perception of food and the effects that particular foods and eating patterns have on weight loss. Therefore, the cognitive behavioral model is best used in the context of a multidisciplinary setting in which cognitive distortions are addressed by both a psychotherapist and a registered dietician.

19.3.3 COMMON COGNITIVE DISTORTIONS OF EATING DISORDER CLIENTS

Based on Beck's (1976) model of thinking errors, various types of cognitive distortions have been linked to the difficulties that are often present in eating disorder clients (Garner and Garfinkel 1985).

19.3.3.1 Dichotomous Reasoning

Dichotomous reasoning involves thinking in extreme and absolute terms, commonly referred to as "all or nothing" thinking. For example, a client may divide food into "good" and "bad" categories. She might believe that all foods containing fat are "bad" and all foods that belong to a certain food group, like fruits or vegetables, are "good," not realizing that some fat is essential to good nutrition and that some fruits and vegetables, like avocados and coconuts, contain some fat. Therefore, if a woman who characterizes foods as "good" or "bad" eats something from her list of "bad" foods, she might view herself as a failure and as losing total control of her willpower. As a result, she might engage in an episode of binge eating, purging, or both.

This type of thinking can also extend to personality functioning and personal relationships. For example, a young woman might expect perfection in grades, sports, and other extra-curricular activities. She might expect herself to always be happy, in control, and accepted by others. If she finds herself lacking in even one area, she feels she is a total failure. Additionally, she might think that if she is not in complete control of every aspect of her life that she will lose control of everything. By viewing the world in a dichotomous way, she is setting herself up to either remain successful in all areas of her life or to be a total failure.

19.3.3.2 Overgeneralizing, Labeling, and Mislabeling

A client's pattern of drawing a general conclusion about her ability, performance, and worth on the basis of a single incident is called overgeneralization (Beck 1976). Because of the emphasis on appearance, people with eating disorders often draw conclusions about themselves based on their weight, shape, or food consumption. For example, a woman might think that if she gains one pound, she will not be attractive to anyone. Similarly, she might view herself as a bad person after eating something she does not think she should eat, such as a cookie or a piece of chocolate. Not all overgeneralizations, however, are specific to weight or food. For example, a young woman might view herself as a complete failure if she earns a B on an exam.

Related to overgeneralizing, sometimes clients will label or mislabel behaviors or events. More specifically, they will attempt to explain behaviors or events simply by assigning an absolute and emotionally loaded word or name to them. For example, a young woman with an eating disorder might mislabel herself as "fat, stupid, and ugly" after failing an exam or getting into a fight with a friend or family member.

19.3.3.3 Catastrophizing

Catastrophizing is magnification of the negative consequences of a particular event. When people catastrophize, it can seem as though they are acting or speaking in an overly dramatic way because they focus on the worst possible outcome, even if that outcome is unlikely. However, to the person who is catastrophizing, there is a lack of awareness that this magnification is nonsensical. For example, a young woman who thinks that she must be thin in order to be happy might believe that no one will ever love her if she gains weight. Similarly, a woman might attribute all of her problems to her appearance. Therefore, if she is not thin and does not always look perfect, she might think that she will never be successful and will never have the life that she wants. Yet, by catastrophizing, she experiences tremendous anxiety and precludes herself from experiencing happiness.

19.3.3.4 Mental Filtering and Disqualifying the Positive

Mental filtering refers to a biased, incomplete way of viewing life, such as focusing one's attention almost exclusively on negative aspects of an event while ignoring positive aspects. When a person filters information in such a way that she overlooks all positive feedback, even the slightest piece of constructive criticism can be difficult for her to digest. For example, even after earning an "A" on an assignment, a young woman might focus on the problems that she did not answer correctly, and she might view herself as inadequate because she did not earn a perfect score.

Similar to mental filtering, disqualifying the positive refers to continually disregarding positive experiences for arbitrary reasons. When a person disqualifies positive experiences, she recognizes that there might be positive aspects to a situation, but she thinks about them in ways that diminish their importance. Using the same example as just mentioned, the young woman might continue to focus on the problems that she missed on the assignment to remind herself that she is "stupid," or she might rob her success of any special significance by focusing on the high grades obtained by other students on the same assignment.

19.3.3.5 Jumping to Conclusions

In clinical practice, it is often observed that eating disorder clients will form conclusions hastily and with little supporting evidence. They might assume that they know what other people are thinking (mind reading), or they might be certain about the outcome of a particular event before it actually occurs (fortune telling). For example, after gaining a pound or eating a cookie, a young woman assumes that her boyfriend thinks she is fat. As a consequence, she convinces herself that he intends to break up with her. Therefore, she avoids his attempts to contact her and eventually ends the relationship herself.

19.3.3.6 Should Statements

Should statements refer to patterns of thinking that are indicative of the way a person believes things "ought to be" rather than the reality of a given situation. Should statements are often linked to rigid rules that a person endorses and often reflect unrealistic expectations for oneself. For example, women with eating disorders often think that they "should always" be in control, "should never" gain weight, "should never" eat "bad" foods, and "should never" be less than perfect.

19.3.3.7 Emotional Reasoning

When a person relies on visceral reactions rather than rational thinking to make decisions or build arguments, she is engaging in emotional reasoning. For example, women with eating disorders often suggest that they "feel fat," and, as a consequence, base behavior on this "feeling." For example, a woman with an eating disorder might think that because she "feels fat," she is fat, even if she is severely underweight. In addition to identifying this cognitive distortion in individuals with eating disorders, it can be advantageous to encourage clients to use other words to describe their feelings since "fat" is not an emotion like shame, anger, or sadness.

19.3.3.8 Personalization

Sometimes, a client will take personal responsibility for an event that is completely out of her control. For example, a young girl might blame herself for her parents' divorce. An adolescent female might blame herself for the normal physical body changes she is experiencing. A young woman might blame herself for her husband's infidelity. Irrational thoughts related to personalization might make a woman feel that she has lost control of her life, so she might focus her energy on over-controlling one area of her life, such as her diet.

Any number of cognitive distortions can be present in clients with eating disorders, and the distortions are often related. For example, a woman who thinks she should never consume foods that contain fat (should statement) labels herself as a complete failure after eating a cookie (mislabeling), and concludes that she will gain 10 pounds and be completely unattractive to her partner because she ate one cookie (castastrophizing). In working with eating disorder clients, it is important for clinicians to make clients aware of their irrational thoughts and to challenge these cognitive distortions by asking for evidence, further explanation, or alternative solutions. Additional strategies for clinicians working with eating disorder clients are included later in this chapter.

19.3.4 Cognitive Behavioral Therapy, Enhanced: A Transdiagnostic Approach to Treatment

Fairburn (2008) developed a modified and "enhanced" version of cognitive behavioral therapy (CBT) to work specifically with people with eating disorders. CBT-Enhanced (CBT-E) is a transdiagnostic approach to treating individuals with eating disorders, so this approach can be used with any person with an eating disorder regardless of the specific diagnosis. The assumption is that underlying psychological processes that contribute to the development and maintenance of dysfunctional relationships with food are similar even though the presentation of observable symptoms, such as food restriction or purging behaviors, is different (Fairburn 2008). A broad, flexible, encompassing approach to treating eating disorders is important because 80% of eating disorder cases change within 3 years (Fairburn 2009), and the majority of clinical eating disorder clients are diagnosed with unspecified eating disorders rather than specific eating disorders, like anorexia nervosa or bulimia nervosa (Fairburn et al. 2003; Machado et al. 2007). To date, CBT-E is the only treatment that has been shown to be effective for unspecified eating disorders and is the only effective treatment for significantly underweight clients (Fairburn 2009).

There are two forms of CBT-E. One approach focuses specifically on eating disorder psychopathology, and the other approach incorporates obstacles to change, such as perfectionism, low self-esteem, interpersonal problems, and emotional intolerance, into the treatment. Anticipated length of treatment is determined by the client's weight. For those who are not significantly underweight, Fairburn recommends 20 weeks. For those who are significantly underweight, 40 weeks are recommended since a significant portion of the treatment process will be devoted to weight restoration.

Four stages comprise CBT-E. In the first stage, the therapist focuses on establishing therapeutic rapport, engaging the client in therapy, and increasing her awareness that change is necessary. The client is educated about her illness, the necessity of regular eating, and the consequences associated with her eating disorder symptoms. Of great importance during Stage 1 is to shift the client's perspective from a need to lose weight to an admitted need for professional help. Once her perspective has shifted, the deceit associated with the maintenance of eating disorder symptoms is minimized (Fairburn 2009). The second stage includes evaluation and preparation. Specifically, the therapist and client analyze therapeutic progress and identify obstacles to change, such as media and peer influence or poor treatment compliance. Additionally, they discuss their future work together. In the third stage, the focus of therapy is to identify and explore key factors that contribute to the maintenance of the eating disorder. For example, the extreme value that the client places on her weight and shape would be addressed during this stage. The deep issues that are addressed during Stage 3 make it a key component of CBT-E, so Stage 3 requires the most time of all the stages. Finally, Stage 4 prepares the client to function independently and to cope with future obstacles. During this stage, the client and therapist discuss ways that the client will maintain the changes that she had made throughout the therapeutic process and therefore minimize her risk of relapsing. Additionally, it is important to discuss her options if the client does relapse. Reflection on the client's progress can be incorporated into this phase as well. A follow-up session 20 weeks after the termination of therapy is also recommended (Fairburn 2008).

Although CBT-E was originally developed for use with adults in outpatient settings, adaptations of this therapy allow for its use with inpatient (Dalle Grave et al. 2008) and adolescent clients (Cooper and Stewart 2008). Fairburn's (2008) treatment manual provides guidelines and more detailed information regarding the application and individualization of this approach for eating disorder clients.

CBT is only one approach to treating clients with eating disorders. Other effective approaches to individual treatment include interpersonal therapy, constructivist therapy, and narrative therapy (see Chapters 20 and 21). Sometimes, psychotropic medication is used in conjunction with therapy to treat eating disorder clients (see Chapter 22). Most often, clinicians use individual therapy to treat eating disorders (Haas and Clopton 2003). However, group therapy and family approaches can be used exclusively or in addition to individual therapy (Lock and de Grange 2005, McGilley 2006).

19.4   APPLICATION OF RESEARCH AND ENHANCING TREATMENT WITH EATING DISORDER CLIENTS

The value of research knowledge contained in this chapter is in helping a client recognize and reform cognitive distortions. Modifications of Beck's model of CBT, including Fairburn's (2009) CBT-E, have been researched and the procedures have been recommended for use when counseling eating-disordered clients. Cognitive approaches have been shown to be more effective or at least as effective as any other psychological or pharmacological treatments for eating disorders (Ricca et al. 2000). Sessions are semi-structured, problem-oriented, and mainly concerned with the client's present and future rather than the past. The following pages include a thorough discussion of the outpatient treatment process, and the views presented in this section are based upon clinical experiences and therapeutic strategies that this chapter's authors have found to be most effective in working with eating disorder clients.

19.4.1   INITIAL CONSULTATION

19.4.1.1   Referral

Since it is most common for eating disorders of both the restricting and binge/purge types to begin during mid- to late adolescence, when the client is still dependent on her family (Polivy et al. 2003), the referral will almost always be made by someone other than the client herself. Often, the client's teacher or a friend will be the first to identify the problem and notify the client's parents. They will then seek help from a pediatrician, family physician, or clinical psychologist. If the client is a college student, she may be self-referred at the recommendation of a counselor, friend, or professor.

Based on clinical experience, the most effective treatment for eating disorders includes the use of a multidisciplinary team. Eating disorders are complex, so several professionals are often needed to effectively treat the disorder. These professionals can include a clinical psychologist, physician, registered dietitian, exercise physiologist, family therapist, and other professionals, including an addiction specialist, if applicable. Most often, the professional who accepts the referral assumes the leadership role since the first person contacted most usually has the trust of the family.

Because both physical and emotional problems are evident in people with eating disorders (see Chapters 2, 3, and 4 of this book), the multidisciplinary team must include at least one professional who can address the medical problems and at least one professional to address the psychological problems associated with the disorder. Therefore, the therapist or professional who assumes the leadership role should make a referral for the physical exam at the end of the initial interview and should have the client and her parents sign a release for the therapist to talk to the physician. If the client has been evaluated prior to the initial interview, the therapist should request access to these records in the first interview. If the client has not had a physical examination, the therapist should make a referral for a complete physical evaluation, including blood work. Stressing the need for this evaluation to the patient and her parents reinforces the seriousness of the illness and helps the family recognize the need to follow through with treatment.

19.4.1.2 Initial Interview

This section of the chapter provides information about the initial interview with the client and her parents, which is a crucial aspect of the therapeutic process. During the first meeting, the therapist can convey support and instill hope in the client and her parents, which can improve attendance, assist in establishing rapport, and set the stage for future work together. Although the suggestions within this section fit well with a cognitive behavioral approach, these suggestions are not specific to CBT and are appropriate to use with other treatment approaches.

When the parent calls to set up the first appointment, it is important to obtain as much information as possible prior to the first visit. One way to accomplish this is to mail various forms to the client and her family. These forms should include an explanation of office practices, limits of confidentiality, and financial information for the parents. Forms requesting identifying information and a personal history of the problem should also be included. Finally, an eating disorder questionnaire should be completed by the client. It is important to obtain these documents prior to the first visit so that the therapist can prepare for the initial interview.

If the client is younger than 18 or living at home, the practitioner should request that a parent accompany the client to the first visit. At the initial visit, the parent and client are invited into the office, and the parent is asked to provide information about the nature of the problem and the reason for seeking therapy. This explanation is given in the presence of the client so that all understand the reason for the intervention and hear the same information. The client is then asked to provide both the therapist and the parent with her version of the problem.

Next is a thorough discussion of confidentiality issues. Because enmeshment or control issues often exist between the client and her parents, the therapist explains that the policy is not to discuss the client with her parents unless they are all present in the office. However, the client is informed that she can invite her parents to attend a session any time she wishes. Additionally, parents are invited to call the office manager to request a meeting with the therapist and the client when important issues arise. Parents are also instructed to speak to the office manager regarding any scheduling or financial issues. The agreement of the client and the family to these policies is essential in establishing rapport and trust with the client.

In addition to the information described previously, a detailed explanation about office practices and HIPPA guidelines are given to the client and her parents during the initial session. It is especially important to discuss the ethical guidelines regarding a professional's duty to warn in case of suicidal or homicidal thoughts. Additionally, the practitioner should make the client and her parents aware of how to contact the therapist outside of business hours, who will be on call if the therapist should be out of town, and the need for written release forms in order to request records or to contact another treating professional, such as the physician.

After completing the discussions mentioned previously, the parents are asked to leave the room and the initial interview begins. Detailed questions about the development of the eating disorder are asked using the self-report questionnaire completed by the client. The questionnaire should be comprehensive and should include her weight history and the client's perception of her weight both in childhood and adolescence. The questionnaire should also contain questions about body image, dieting behaviors, binge eating behaviors, purging behaviors, exercise, substance use, sexual history, medical history, psychological history, social history, quality of family and peer relationships, and any medical or psychological problems of family members. Depending on the age of the client, the parents might be asked for medical history information before they leave the room.

Next, the practitioner reviews the history form with the client, starting with her earliest memories. Questions included in the history form involve her memories and perceptions of (1) the quality of life in her family, (2) relationships with the family, friends and teachers, and (3) school and social issues. Special attention should be paid to her perception of the authority figures in her life. It is important to ask the client if any sexual, physical, emotional, or other type of abuse has occurred. These questions should be asked in a candid manner, and the therapist should never suggest or assume that abuse has definitely occurred, as clients are susceptible to the development of false memories. Questions about trauma should also be included, because any childhood trauma may be important to the development of the eating disorder. These traumas may include physical illness or accidents, loss of a parent through death or divorce, relocation of the family at a sensitive time in the client's life, or other issues that have been particularly upsetting to the client. Because the client may not understand the meaning of words like trauma or abuse, the therapist should ask specific questions about her experiences. For example, rather than asking the client if she has a history of childhood trauma, she should be asked specific questions about accidents, physical illness, and family challenges. Additionally, the therapist should inquire about traumatic experiences specific to weight or shape. For example, many eating disorder clients have early memories of their weight or shape being criticized by an authority figure (Ghaderi 2001).

It is vital to the case formulation and to the treatment plan that a careful history is taken so that the therapist will begin to understand the origin and content of the cognitive distortions that drive the eating disorder. The presence of any concurrent illness, such as depression, anxiety, or a personality disorder, might also be discovered at this time. If the case appears to be very complicated or unclear, there are other assessment instruments that can be helpful with the diagnosis (for specific measures, refer to Chapters 2 and 5 of this book).

At the end of the interview, the therapist will ask the client's permission to share general impressions with her parents, stressing that no private information will be shared. She will also be asked if she would feel comfortable working with the therapist. If the client admits that she will not be comfortable working with the therapist, the therapist should offer to make referral to another professional after sharing the diagnostic impressions with her parents.

When the initial interview is completed, the therapist will have an impression of the diagnosis and can begin generating ideas about a treatment plan. Although the type of eating disorder is discussed with the client and her parents, the therapist makes them aware that deciding on a specific diagnosis requires further inquiry. The parents and client are invited to ask questions about the impressions that the therapist has presented. Based on the provisional diagnosis, a general treatment plan is discussed with the client and her parents. The components of this plan can include individual psychotherapy, a comprehensive physical examination, and referrals to a registered dietitian, an exercise physiologist, and a support group. Most commonly, weekly psychotherapy sessions are recommended with the goal of completing the detailed history and case formulation within

3 weeks. Referral to a medical professional for a complete physical examination is also made at this time. Additional referrals to the dietitian and other members of the team can be made when the formal diagnosis and treatment plan is completed. If a dual diagnosis is suspected, such as alcohol or substance abuse, a referral to an adjunct treatment program such as Alcoholics Anonymous or Narcotics Anonymous can be made after rapport with the client and family is firmly established. Medication should not be suggested in the first session, since it will not yet be clear whether it will be helpful.

If the client is a college student living away from home, the diagnostic impression and preliminary treatment plan are given to her individually. If appropriate, she is asked to invite her parents to attend at least one session so that they can support her and participate in her treatment. However, there are times that the therapist may choose not to include the family of a client over 18, especially if there is a history of abuse or neglect that might cause the family to be unsupportive of treatment. If the client is an adult with a family of her own or a support system that is not her biological family, it will be up to her to decide who to include in her treatment plan.

Recommendations for treatment are based on the nature and severity of the eating disorder and any accompanying problem, such as a mood disorder, personality disorder, suicidal ideations, or substance abuse. It is most commonly recommended for eating disorder clients to be treated for 20 weeks (Garner and Garfinkel 1985; Halmi 1992; Fairburn, 2008). However, some eating disorder clients are in therapy for a longer amount of time. A dual diagnosis of severe depression, anxiety, or a personality disorder, such as obsessive-compulsive personality disorder, may require longer treatment. If clients are significantly underweight, hospitalization may be necessary before outpatient eating disorder treatment can begin. In addition, if clients are seriously dependent on illegal drugs, alcohol, or prescription medications, treatment for substance dependence must be addressed before eating disorder treatment can be successful.

19.4.1.3 Treatment

As the therapist continues to obtain a detailed history from the client, the therapist must also work to establish rapport and trust. The therapist should refrain from being judgmental or confrontational during this phase of treatment. As the development of the eating disorder is discussed, a psychoeducational approach is used to make the client aware of triggers for the dysfunctional eating behavior (Weiss et al. 1985). These triggers can be emotional in nature and can be related to certain "trigger foods," such as pizza, cake, or other high-fat, high-carbohydrate foods. Other psychoeducational issues may include educating the client about body image distortion, the influence of the media and other pressures, and the physical effects of the eating disorder, including, osteoporosis, fatigue, infertility, tooth erosion, thinning hair, loss of muscle mass, difficulty with concentration and attention, and vitamin and electrolyte deficiency (American Psychiatric Association 2000).

When the client begins to understand that there is a connection between her emotions and her eating behaviors, she should be encouraged to begin a journal. The client can complete the journal using a computer spreadsheet or a handwritten record. The journal should include the types and amount of food consumed, the times and place food is eaten, and any emotional triggers or unusual or stressful feelings that the client notices. Clients who binge and purge are asked to place an asterisk beside any food or meal that is purged. If exercise is problematic for the client, the clinician might also request that the client include information about the time, place, amount, and type of exercise completed. The client is advised to bring her journal to each session of psychotherapy. As the therapist reviews the record during each session, patterns of restricting or bingeing and purging emerge that are previously unnoticed by the client. Eating behaviors and choices may improve because the client is now paying more attention to what she is eating and when she is eating. Journaling might also help her to cope with automatic thoughts and behaviors, particularly those that occur as a result of anxiety. A common example of automatic behavior occurs when the client is anxious about deadlines at school. At these times, her carbohydrate intake may increase, and more bingeing and purging will result. Discussing these patterns with the client eventually helps her to separate coping with her feelings from the eating disorder behaviors. Once the pattern of reviewing the journal is established, the therapist should be careful not to forget to ask about it, as forgetting will send a message that completing the journal is not important. The client may forget to bring the journal during times of acute stress, which may indicate resistance to becoming aware of her problems.

Early in treatment, the CBT process is introduced to the client. Many therapists use a published, self-help manual, such as *Overcoming Binge Eating* (Fairburn 1995), to help explain the process. A modification of Beck's model of CBT for depression has also been used for both restricting clients and clients who binge and purge (see Section 19.2.1; Beck et al. 1979). The therapist will help the client look for schemas, or underlying ways of organizing one's thoughts and experiences, that explain irrational beliefs about body image, self-efficacy, self-worth, and self-esteem. These beliefs also affect how the client thinks about food. For example, a client's father often went on a diet that prohibited all bread, butter, potatoes, and dessert. The client, therefore, grew up believing that any amount of these foods would make her fat and should be forbidden. As she became more ill, she removed even more types of food from her diet. By the time that treatment began, she would only consume cereal with a small amount of skim milk. Because cognitive therapy helped her realize that her beliefs were irrational, she was able to slowly incorporate more types of food into her meal plan.

Another common example of irrational thoughts is the fear of gaining weight and being fat. For example, a client's father told her that her legs were "chunky" when she was in junior high school. As a result, she worried severely about the size of her legs and measured them with a tape measure every morning. As she lost more weight, her thoughts became more irrational and her body image became more distorted. As the client learned to examine and dispute her irrational thoughts, she was able to change her body image, her eating behaviors, and her beliefs about food.

Generalized anxiety can also be a trigger for eating-disordered behaviors. Stress management tools can help the client reduce the anxiety that often contributes to binge eating, purging, or restricting. When clients are highly anxious, they frequently begin eating automatically to calm themselves. In fact, it has been shown that carbohydrates increase brain serotonin temporarily (Fernstrom 1988; Wurtman and Wurtman 1989). Learning simple deep breathing techniques and other methods of relaxation, such as progressive muscle relaxation, can help the client decrease her anxiety so that she can stop and analyze her thoughts and change her dysfunctional eating behaviors (Benson and Klipper 2000).

Anxiety, depression, and low self-esteem are sometimes fueled by learned passive or aggressive communication styles. These styles often invite rejection from others, and this rejection is misinterpreted by the client as being associated with her appearance. Cognitive restructuring of this belief along with assertiveness training can help the client communicate more effectively (Beck and Emery 1985). Practicing assertive behaviors in group settings can be especially useful in challenging a client's fears about standing up for herself.

A very helpful adjunct to treatment, especially for younger patients, can be family therapy. The therapist can establish a safe place for the client to explore her fears and other feelings with her family members, and they can learn to better understand her eating behaviors and what they can do to help. Frequently, parents will say, "Just eat and you'll be okay." With the help of family therapy, parents can learn to refrain from mentioning the client's food intake and can learn the importance of avoiding comments about the client's weight or body. Family members are often surprised by how difficult it is to have a meal without discussing food. In addition to educating parents about inappropriate comments, it is also important for issues of control and enmeshment to be addressed in family therapy. A high level of dependence is frequently fostered in these families, and they often require the assistance of a professional to become comfortable letting go of the need for control. An excellent reference for parents is *Surviving an Eating Disorder* (Siegel et al. 2009). This book provides guidelines for communicating about food and also explains how parents can be helpful as treatment progresses.

Because clients are often very isolated and secretive about their eating disorder, it can be advantageous to include group psychotherapy as part of the multidisciplinary approach. The group should be led by a therapist who is well-versed in the treatment of eating disorders and who is trained in the cognitive behavioral approach. Group therapy can help clients see that they are not alone in their struggles and can help them to be more open in their communication about their problems. The goal of group therapy is similar to that of individual therapy in that clients learn to identify, separate, and deal with their emotions and learn to stop using food as a way of preoccupying themselves or numbing their emotions. Despite potential benefits of participating in group therapy, leaders should be aware of the competitive nature of eating disorder clients. In some instances, individuals might strive to exercise more or eat less than others in the group. Additionally, discussion of specific behaviors might provide group members with information about additional maladaptive strategies. Leaders must be proactive in minimizing these problems, and conversations about food behaviors should be discouraged in group therapy.

19.4.2 Summary of the Therapeutic Process

- Because eating disorder clients are, in general, resistant to treatment and secretive about their thoughts and behaviors, plenty of time should be taken to establish a therapeutic, trusting relationship with them. In order to establish a strong working relationship with the client, the therapist should convey a supportive attitude and a desire to help the client. The therapist should be careful not to challenge the client too soon and should refrain from making statements that might be perceived as judgmental and critical until a strong, trusting relationship is established. Additionally, the client and therapist should work together to generate goals for therapy so that both have a personal investment in the process. In establishing goals for therapy, it is important for the therapist and client to identify the problem and devise a plan to address the problem, which can include identifying thoughts and feelings contributing to the problem and using strategies, such as relaxation techniques, to reduce anxiety or other emotions that are associated with the problem. Repeatedly using healthy strategies, like relaxation techniques, to cope with uncomfortable thoughts or feelings, like anxiety, can help the client to eventually develop healthy and positive behavior changes. Establishing clear goals is important because meeting one's goals becomes the focus of therapy.
- The client is taught to monitor her own thoughts and discover irrational perceptions or beliefs. Education about body weight regulation, the adverse effects of dieting, and the physical consequences of behaviors like self-induced vomiting, laxative misuse, and excessive exercise is introduced to challenge the common cognitive distortion that these behaviors do not have negative or long-term consequences. A journal that is structured to help the client to monitor her thoughts and behaviors is recommended. It works best to give the patient a form for each day or each week that includes details about food intake, such as portion sizes and times food is eaten. Feelings and behaviors that may have influenced the food choices or that follow after the food is ingested are also recorded. Exercise can also be included in this chart. It is useful to have this information because it helps the client to separate food behaviors from the client's emotions. Examining the feelings and behaviors recorded on this chart in the therapy session can help the patient discover irrational thoughts.
- The client should learn to recognize the connection between distorted perceptions and irrational behaviors. For example, through the use of a daily journal, the client might notice that her hours of exercise increase as she contemplates going to the senior prom. This connection might indicate an increase of anxiety based on her irrational belief that she must be thin to get a date. As her fear of failure increases, her level of exercising, incidence of binge and purge episodes, and restriction of food intake might also increase.
- The client and therapist should examine the validity of the client's beliefs. The therapist should question the beliefs in a kind, nonthreatening manner and should communicate to

the client that she is accepted no matter what her beliefs are. The therapist asks questions to confront the irrational beliefs, such as:

- How do you know you can't get a date if you weigh what you do now?
- How do you know that people think you are fat and don't like you?
- How many calories per week do you have to overeat to gain one pound?

- The client is taught to substitute healthy and positive thoughts, which are more realistic and logical, for her earlier irrational beliefs. She should be encouraged to verbalize her thoughts to trusted friends so that she can gain a more realistic view. She should confront her irrational thoughts by making a list of advantages and disadvantages for maintaining these irrational thoughts. She should ask herself what objective data support her thoughts. Are there data that cast doubt on her thoughts? She should also ask herself what other people would think under similar circumstances.

- After learning to use the information she has gathered to change her beliefs and substitute healthy and positive thoughts, she should practice by verbalizing the new thoughts to her therapist.

- The new thoughts should be used to guide behavior, even if the client does not fully believe them. For example, if she is studying for a test and her anxiety level is increasing, she may find herself obsessing about carbohydrates and constantly wanting to eat. If she has changed her belief that she is hungry to a belief that she is anxious, she can use a relaxation technique, such as deep breathing, to calm herself instead of rushing off to binge. That will give her time to analyze her thoughts. A common problem for a person who severely restricts her diet is the irrational belief that if she eats anything, she will gain weight. She practices new beliefs by forcing herself to stay on her meal plan even though she is afraid to do so. To accomplish this monumental change, she needs to trust her therapist and get positive support from those around her.

- Some clients are quite resistant to the cognitive behavioral process. They feel that exploring their thoughts and attitudes is too intrusive, especially since some of their thoughts and attitudes are learned from their family members. They often feel guilty revealing their family histories to therapists because they feel they are betraying family secrets. This is almost always the case if a family history includes serious problems with abuse or addiction. Other clients are unable to engage in cognitive restructuring because of limited intelligence or a tendency to be concrete thinkers. These clients can sometime benefit from a group approach. This allows them to relate to other eating disorder clients who share their problems.

- If eating-disordered behavior accompanies another diagnosis, such as addiction, depression, anxiety, borderline personality disorder, or obsessive-compulsive disorder, the patient should be referred for therapy to a well-trained expert. Additionally, a physician should evaluate the client for prescription of medication. This is particularly important if suicidal or homicidal ideation or tendency to self-injury is present (Beck et al. 1979).

19.5 CONCLUSION

The purpose of this chapter was to illustrate the usefulness of cognitive behavioral strategies in working with eating disorder clients. Vulnerability to the development of eating disorders begins in childhood with stressful events and with development of maladaptive patterns of thinking that lead to dysfunctional behaviors. The cognitive behavioral perspective suggests that changes in thinking result in significant changes in maladaptive behavior. Thus, successful treatment includes the use of CBT to help the patient identify and change irrational perceptions of herself and irrational perceptions of her world that contribute to disordered eating behaviors. An attempt has been made in this chapter to describe not only what is done in CBT, but also specific ways to enhance the effectiveness of those treatment strategies.

REFERENCES

American Psychiatric Association. 2000. *Diagnostic and statistical manual of mental disorders* (4th ed., text revision). Washington, DC: American Psychiatric Association.

Beck, A. T. 1976. *Cognitive therapy and the emotional disorders.* New York: International Press.

Beck, A. T., and G. Emery. 1985. *Anxiety disorders and phobias: A cognitive perspective.* New York: Basic Books.

Beck, A. T., J. Rush, B. Shaw, and G. Emery. 1979. *Cognitive therapy of depression.* New York: Guilford Press.

Benson, H., and M. Z. Klipper. 2000. *The relaxation response.* London, UK: HarperCollins.

Cooper, Z., and A. Stewart. 2008. CBT-E for Adolescents. In *Cognitive behavior therapy and eating disorders,* ed. C. G. Fairburn, 221–230. New York: Guilford Press.

Dalle Grave, R., K. Bohn, D. M. Hawker, and C. G. Fairburn. 2008. Inpatient CBT-E. In *Cognitive behavior therapy and eating disorders,* ed. C. G. Fairburn, 231–244. New York: Guilford Press.

Fairburn, C. G. 1995. *Overcoming binge eating.* New York: Guilford Press.

Fairburn, C. G. (ed.) 2008. *Cognitive behavior therapy and eating disorders.* New York: Guilford Press.

Fairburn, C. G. 2009. Transdiagnostic cognitive behavioral therapy for eating disorders. Presentation at the annual meeting of the Association for Behavioral and Cognitive Therapies (ABCT) annual convention, New York.

Fairburn, C. G., Z. Cooper, and R. Shafran. 2003. Cognitive behavior therapy for eating disorders: A transdiagnostic theory and treatment. *Behav Res Ther* 41: 509–528.

Fernstrom, J. D. 1998. Carbohydrate ingestion and brain serotonin synthesis: Relevance to a putative control loop for regulating carbohydrate ingestion, and effects of aspartame consumption. *Appetite* 11: 35–41.

Garner, D. M., and P. E. Garfinkel. 1985. *Handbook of psychotherapy for anorexia nervosa and bulimia.* New York: Guilford Press.

Ghaderi, A. 2001. Review of risk factors for eating disorders: Implications for primary prevention and cognitive behavioral therapy. *Scand J Behav Ther* 30: 57–74.

Haas, H. L., and J. R. Clopton. 2003. Comparing clinical research treatments for eating disorders. *Int J Eat Disord* 33: 412–420.

Halmi, K. A. 1992. *Psychobiology and treatment of anorexia nervosa and bulimia nervosa.* Washington, DC: American Psychiatric Press.

Lock, J., and de Grange. 2005. Family-Based Treatment of Eating Disorders. *Int J Eat Disord* 37: S64–S67.

Machado, P. P., B. C. Machado, S. Goncalves, and H. W. Hoek. 2007. The prevalence of eating disorders not otherwise specified. *Int J Eat Disord* 40: 212–217.

McGilley, B. 2006. Group therapy for adolescents with eating disorders. *Group* 30: 321–336.

Polivy, J., C. Herman, J. Mills, and H. Wheeler. 2003. Eating disorders in adolescence. In *Blackwell handbook of adolescence,* ed. G. R. Adams and M. D. Berzonsky, 523–549. Malden, MA: Blackwell Publishing.

Ricca, V., E. Mannucci, T. Zucchi, C. M. Rotella, and C. Faravelli. 2000. Cognitive-behavioral therapy for bulimia nervosa and binge eating disorder: A review. *PsychotherPsychosom* 69: 287–295.

Siegel, M., J. Brisman, and M. Weinshel. 2009. *Surviving an eating disorder: strategies for family and friends* (3rd ed.). London, UK: Harper Collins.

Weiss, L., M. Katzman, and S. Wolchik. 1985. *Treating bulimia. A psychoeducational approach.* New York: Pergamon Press.

Wurtman, R. J., and J. J. Wurtman. 1989. Carbohydrates and depression. *Sci Am* 260: 68–75.

20 Interpersonal Approaches for Treating Eating Disorders

Kristin L. Goodheart, Marcia M. Abbott, and James R. Clopton

CONTENTS

20.1 LEARNING OBJECTIVES

After completing this chapter, you should be able to do the following:

- Explain the theory behind interpersonal therapy and its potential for treating people with eating disorders
- Generate examples of interpersonal problems that could contribute to the development or the maintenance of eating disorders
- Understand methods to help change problematic interpersonal patterns in people with eating disorders
- Explain the interpersonal process and identify times when it may be appropriate to use this strategy in the therapeutic setting

20.2 INTRODUCTION

This chapter presents a way of conducting psychotherapy with clients with eating disorders that focuses on their interpersonal relationships. Such a focus seems developmentally appropriate, because eating disorders begin at a time when a girl or young woman is highly concerned about finding a way to relate well to family members, peers, and other people in her life. Clinicians commonly find that clients with eating disorders have problems relating to other people, and these interpersonal problems can lead to stress, increase the severity of the eating disorder, and make treatment more complicated. Interpersonal therapy can be viewed either as a method—an approach to doing therapy comparable to cognitive behavioral therapy (Klerman et al. 1984, Fairburn 1997, Apple 1999, Wilfley et al. 2000), or it can be viewed as a more general orientation—a way of developing a therapeutic relationship between the therapist and the client that will enhance the effectiveness of the techniques and strategies of any other approach used to help a client with an eating disorder (Teyber 2006).

Interpersonal therapy can be a natural complement to cognitive behavioral therapy (see Chapter 19 in this book). Both approaches to therapy were originally developed for the treatment of other problems but have been recognized as being empirically supported treatments for eating disorders for the past 20 years (Wilson and Pike 1993). Although both can be highly effective, they achieve their effectiveness in contrasting ways. In cognitive behavioral therapy, the therapist often uses specific treatment techniques that directly address the eating problems of the client. Interpersonal therapy is an indirect approach that is often based on the assumption that maladaptive eating patterns will no longer occur once the client has better interpersonal skills and experiences less stress in her relationships with other people. In some forms of interpersonal therapy, the focus is less on specific treatment techniques than on broad strategies for promoting greater self-understanding and interpersonal effectiveness in clients (Teyber 2006).

20.3   RESEARCH BACKGROUND AND SIGNIFICANCE

Interpersonal therapy was initially developed to treat depression (Klerman et al. 1984), as it was suggested that disturbances in social functioning were related to the onset and maintenance of depressive symptoms. More generally, interpersonal dysfunction is considered a salient component of most any type of psychological maladjustment or psychological distress (Wilfley et al. 2000). Thus, the focus of interpersonal therapy is to resolve the social problems that contribute to the development and maintenance of psychological dysfunction. Specifically, interpersonal therapy focuses on problems that typically develop within four social areas: dealing with abnormal grief, alleviating interpersonal role disputes, coping with role transitions, and overcoming interpersonal deficits (Klerman et al. 1984).

With regard to eating disorders, the theory behind interpersonal therapy suggests that, over time, underlying interpersonal dysfunction has contributed to the development or maintenance of eating disorder symptoms. Thus, interpersonal therapy has been adapted to treat people with some types of eating disorders, including bulimia nervosa (Fairburn et al. 1991) and binge eating disorder (Wilfley et al. 1993, 1998). There is also evidence to suggest that interpersonal therapy might be effective in treating people with anorexia nervosa (McIntosh et al. 2000).

The focus of interpersonal therapy is to treat problematic eating behaviors, such as binge eating and purging, by linking these problematic eating behaviors to current social problems (Fairburn et al. 1991, Wilfley et al. 1998). However, the theory behind interpersonal therapy does not necessarily suggest that interpersonal dysfunction causes dysfunctional eating behaviors; rather, eating problems might be viewed by some individuals as a way to alleviate or solve interpersonal problems (Wilfley et al. 1998). For example, a person might binge to alleviate uncomfortable feelings like anger or boredom. Therefore, when using an interpersonal approach to treat an eating disorder, one focus of therapy might be to change the interpersonal context in which a specific eating problem has been developed or maintained. (Section 20.4 of this chapter provides specific examples of interpersonal problems that can contribute to eating problems and strategies to achieve needed interpersonal changes.)

Because the focus of interpersonal therapy is on interpersonal relationships and difficulties within these relationships, maladaptive eating patterns are rarely discussed in the therapeutic setting. Instead, the client and the therapist focus on goals to improve interpersonal interactions that will, in turn, alleviate the maladaptive eating patterns (Fairburn 1997; Apple 1999; Wilfley et al. 2000). Because specific eating patterns are not targeted directly, as they are when using other therapeutic approaches like cognitive behavioral therapy (see Chapter 19 of this book), interpersonal therapy often requires more time before a change in eating behavior is evident (McFarlane et al. 2005; Carr and McNulty 2006). However, studies have shown that interpersonal therapy is as effective as cognitive behavioral therapy in generating lasting effects and abstinence from behaviors like binge eating and purging (Fairburn 1997). Additionally, because approximately one-third of all women with eating disorders relapse (Keel et al. 2005), interventions that target the factors that maintain eating disorder symptoms, such as interpersonal therapy, might help to prevent relapse in some women with eating disorders more than interventions that target the symptoms directly.

20.4 CURRENT FINDINGS

There is some research evidence indicating that interpersonal therapy is more effective for some women with eating disorders than other treatments, such as cognitive behavioral therapy (e.g., Wei et al. 2005; Chui et al. 2007; Tasca et al. 2007; Schembri and Evans 2008). Thus, research studies have attempted to identify certain characteristics in women with eating disorders who will benefit most from interpersonal therapy. For example, interpersonal therapy might be especially effective for people who have problems with emotion regulation, as emotion regulation has been associated with interpersonal problems (Wei et al. 2005), as well as for people who respond well to gentle encouragement and for people who will benefit from semi-structured sessions that are not specifically guided by behavioral instruction (Apple 1999). Additionally, research suggests that interpersonal therapy might be especially beneficial for women with eating disorders who are anxious about losing their relationships, who have a high need for approval, or who rely on others to validate their sense of self-worth (Tasca et al. 2007; Schembri and Evans 2008).

In a study that examined changes in attachment security (i.e., how secure women felt about their significant relationships) and changes in binge eating for women who received interpersonal therapy compared to women who received cognitive behavioral therapy, Tasca et al. (2007) found that both types of therapy contributed to improvements in attachment insecurity. For women who received interpersonal therapy, improvements in attachment anxiety were related to improvements in depression; however, this relationship was not found for women who received cognitive behavioral therapy. Therefore, interpersonal therapy might be especially advantageous for women who are anxious about their interpersonal relationships and who have a high need for approval from others, since interpersonal therapy would address these specific issues. In a different study, Schembri and Evans (2008) studied the intimate relationships of a large sample of women who experienced symptoms of bulimia nervosa and found that many of these women tried to change themselves and their bodies to accommodate their perceptions of their partners' desires. Thus, interpersonal therapy would be particularly beneficial for these women since the symptoms of the disorder are likely maintained by misperceptions about their partners' expectations and hypothesized consequences if they do not meet these expectations. Finally, Chui et al. (2007) found that a small sample of African–American women with bulimia nervosa responded better to interpersonal therapy than to cognitive behavioral therapy, perhaps because of the strong emphasis on familial relationships within the African–American culture.

Some research has suggested that interpersonal therapy or interpersonal strategies might be an effective supplement with other treatment approaches, like cognitive behavioral therapy (McFarlane et al. 2005; Teyber 2006). Yet, other studies have suggested that adding interpersonal therapy to the treatment plan does not enhance the overall effectiveness of the treatment or may not be effective for patients who do not respond to other treatments (Agras et al. 1995). Additionally, as is true with other therapeutic approaches, interpersonal therapy will likely be an ineffective therapeutic approach when the client and the therapist are not able to form a strong therapeutic alliance (Constantino et al. 2005). Although few studies have examined the use of interpersonal therapy with children with eating disorders, the limited research does suggest that interpersonal therapy might be an effective approach for children or adolescents who have symptoms of bulimia nervosa (Gleaves and Latner 2008).

20.5 APPLICATION OF RESEARCH AND ENHANCING TREATMENT WITH EATING DISORDER CLIENTS

Interpersonal therapy targets relational problems that cause or maintain eating disorder symptoms, and once the interpersonal problems are resolved, eating disorder symptoms should also stop (Fairburn 1997; Apple 1999; Wilfley et al. 2000; Carr and McNulty 2006). Because of the emphasis on interpersonal relationships, the therapeutic relationship is a vital component of interpersonal therapy. Throughout the course of treatment, the therapist maintains a warm, empathic, and respectful attitude toward the client. Additionally, the therapist serves as an advocate for the client and remains optimistic about her ability to recover (Wilfley et al. 2000). The therapist also empowers the client and encourages her to take responsibility for the content and direction of therapy, but redirects her when conversations are not directly related to the established goals for treatment (Fairburn 1997; Wilfley et al. 2000). Both the client and the therapist must agree on the goals of therapy, and both must understand the relationship between the client's eating problems and her interpersonal dysfunction.

20.5.1 STAGES OF INTERPERSONAL THERAPY

The amount of time that is needed to work with a client with an eating disorder varies based on individual factors, such as the complexity of the problem and the client's motivation to change. It is estimated that many clients can complete interpersonal therapy in 15 to 20 sessions (Fairburn 1997) but might need as many as 24 to 36 sessions (Apple 1999).

Interpersonal therapy consists of three phases. In the first phase, the therapist works to engage the client in treatment, and current interpersonal problems are identified so that an appropriate treatment plan can be formed. This phase typically requires three to five sessions. In the middle phase, the identified interpersonal problems are addressed. This phase is the longest and typically requires 12 to 24 sessions. In the final phase, the therapist and the client review their work together and prepare for termination. This phase typically requires three to five sessions, and at this point in therapy, sessions can be held every 2 weeks rather than every week. The following section of the chapter provides more detailed information about these specific phases.

20.5.1.1 Phase 1: Collecting Information, Identifying the Interpersonal Problem, and Establishing Rapport

In the first phase of therapy, the therapist conducts a full psychological evaluation and collects a thorough history, focusing specifically on current relationships and past interpersonal patterns. Although therapists who use interpersonal therapy focus more on a client's current social interactions than on analyzing past relationships, therapists do collect information about past experiences and relational patterns during the initial therapy sessions to develop a better understanding of the client's current social functioning (Wilfley et al. 2000). Gathering a thorough history allows both the client and the therapist to gain a better understanding of the eating disorder and other factors, specifically interpersonal factors, that are contributing to the disorder. The therapist should ask the client about significant life events, shifts in her mood and self-esteem, past and current interpersonal relationships, and changes in her weight throughout the course of her life (Fairburn 1997; Apple 1999; Carr and McNulty 2006). One way to organize this data is to record a timeline for each area individually and then to compare the timelines to each other so that the client and therapist can see connections among mood changes, important life events, interpersonal relationships, and eating disorder symptoms. To gain specific information about the client's interpersonal functioning, the therapist should ask about frequency and duration of interactions in addition to the types of activities or conversations that the client has with each person. The therapist should also inquire about aspects of the relationship that are satisfying as well as aspects of the relationship that the client would like to change (Carr and McNulty 2006). Finally, the therapist should ask specifically when eating disorder symptoms like binge eating and purging are most likely to occur (Fairburn 1997), as these specific interactions become an important focus of treatment in Phase 2.

After this information has been collected, the therapist and the client discuss the diagnosis and contributing factors, especially current interpersonal patterns that are contributing to the eating disorder (i.e., grief, role dispute, role transition, social skills deficit, or a combination of these difficulties). The therapist and the client also work together to generate goals that will alleviate these difficulties. When the interpersonal difficulties are related to grief, goals should include mourning the loss and reestablishing relationships. If the problem is related to interpersonal role disputes, goals of therapy might include identifying the dispute and modifying one's communication with others or her expectations of others. When the identified problem area is related to role transitions, goals should be centered around mourning the loss of the old role, accepting the new role, and restoring one's self-esteem. If the problem is connected to interpersonal deficits, goals can include reducing isolation, increasing socialization, and forming close relationships with other people. Goals do not focus on changing specific eating behaviors, such as not binge eating or not restricting one's food intake. Rather, goals should focus on improving interpersonal relationships and improving one's overall health (Wilfley et al. 2000).

In addition to discussing problems that contribute to the eating disorder and goals for treating these problems, the client and the therapist discuss potential obstacles to treatment. If, for example, the client has a tendency to neglect herself and put the needs of others first, the therapist and the client might need to discuss the importance of focusing on herself and on recovering from the eating disorder rather than worrying about other people's needs (Carr and McNulty 2006).

20.5.1.2   Phase 2: Working through the Identified Interpersonal Problem

In the second phase of therapy, the client and the therapist work toward achieving the goals that were established in the first phase of treatment, or more specifically, work toward resolving the interpersonal problems (e.g., grief, role transition, role dispute, interpersonal deficit) that are maintaining the eating disorder symptoms. Specific techniques used to achieve the therapeutic goals and to improve interpersonal interactions might include role playing, open-ended questioning, examining advantages and disadvantages of change, and encouraging expression of feelings (Apple 1999). In each session, the therapist and the client discuss progress toward the agreed-upon goals as well as specific improvements in the client's interpersonal interactions. By addressing these problematic interactions and alleviating the strained interpersonal relations that are related to the eating disorder, the symptoms of the eating disorder eventually subside. However, the client and the therapist do not specifically discuss changes in eating disorder symptoms until they reflect upon their work together in the final stage of therapy (Fairburn 1997). Specific interpersonal difficulties that could contribute to eating disorders and the strategies that can be used to alleviate these interpersonal difficulties are included in the following sections of the chapter.

20.5.1.2.1   Grief

After experiencing a significant loss, such as the death of a loved one or the break-up of an important relationship, some people might cope with the loss by developing maladaptive behaviors rather than experiencing the difficult emotions and coping with the loss in a healthier way. For example, a person might begin to severely restrict her diet or might begin to engage in episodes of binge eating and purging to avoid or to suppress the uncomfortable emotions that she is experiencing. Results of two research studies that were conducted by Fairburn and his colleagues showed that grief was the primary problem that was identified for 6% of women with anorexia nervosa and 12% of women with bulimia nervosa (Fairburn et al. 1991, 1993).

When the primary problem area is related to grief or an inability to tolerate the painful emotions associated with a loss, the therapist's role is to facilitate the mourning process. After the client and therapist have identified this underlying problem area, they work together to identify ways to deal with the grief. For some clients, acknowledging the difficult emotions associated with the loss and receiving validation for the experience of these emotions might be enough. Other times, clients might need the therapist's help to work through unresolved issues. Eventually, the therapist might need to encourage the client to seek out other relationships to replace the relationship that has been lost and help the client identify healthy, enjoyable activities that help compensate for the loss. After the interpersonal issue has been resolved (e.g., the uncomfortable emotions become easier to tolerate, the client works through the unfinished business, or the client embraces alternate relationships that help compensate for the loss), the eating problems eventually subside as well, even without directly addressing the eating problems, because the underlying problems that contributed to the eating problems have been addressed.

20.5.1.2.2   Interpersonal Role Dispute

Sometimes, psychological problems like eating disorders are related to disputes with significant persons in one's life, including partners, children, parents, siblings, teachers, friends, bosses, and coworkers. The two research studies mentioned earlier found that interpersonal role disputes were the primary presenting problem for 33% of women with anorexia nervosa and for 64% of women with bulimia nervosa (Fairburn et al. 1991, 1993).

When the focus of treatment is resolving a role dispute, such as a conflict with a parent, a romantic partner, or a competitive sibling, the therapist helps the client to identify and understand the dispute and also works with the client to identify strategies to resolve the dispute. For example, an adolescent who believes that her mother is overcontrolling and feels like she has no control of her life might begin restricting her diet because she thinks this is one aspect of her life that she actually can control. In this instance, the therapist would work with the client to identify the problem and her associated emotions. Together, they would develop a plan to address the interpersonal conflict. For example, they might discuss ways to talk with the mother about the adolescent's feeling of being controlled by her mother, and they might practice the conversation with the adolescent's mother by using a role-play strategy in the therapy session. Additionally, the therapist could help mother and daughter improve the way that they communicate with one another by inviting the mother to several therapy sessions and then addressing their troublesome communication. Once the role dispute between mother and daughter has been resolved, the adolescent should feel less compelled to overcontrol her food intake.

Using a different example, a woman who does not feel appreciated or loved by her partner might try to fill this void with food, and thus begin to binge eat in an attempt to find the comfort, love, and support that she is seeking. The therapist might work with this client to identify the reason that she binge eats, and then help her think of ways to communicate to her partner that she does not feel loved. Sometimes, the other person involved in the role dispute might need to attend a few therapy sessions, so that the therapist can work with the couple to improve affection and communication, to facilitate compromise between both parties, or to focus on other problem areas. If the dispute cannot be resolved, the therapist and the client discuss ways to end the relationship or decrease the frequency of interactions and then to mourn the loss of this relationship. When the client feels loved and appreciated by her partner or leaves her partner and finds other loving and appreciating relationships, she should eventually stop binge eating because she no longer feels like she needs to fill her emotional void with food.

20.5.1.2.3   Role Transitions

It is not uncommon for people to experience eating problems during periods of transition or while experiencing stressful life events (Ball and Lee 2000). These changes could include the transition from middle school to high school, high school to college, college to the workforce, or being single to being married. Other changes, such as divorce, becoming a parent, or beginning a new job, can also contribute to eating problems for some people. Two research studies indicated that a role transition was the primary problem that was identified for 17% of women with anorexia nervosa and for 36% of women with bulimia nervosa (Fairburn et al. 1991, 1993).

When working with clients who are experiencing difficulty with a role transition, therapists work with clients to understand the transition, to mourn and accept the loss of the previous role, and to develop a strong sense of self related to the new role. The therapist and the client also discuss the advantages of the new role and skills needed to be successful in this new role. For example, a therapist might work with a new mother to identify all the benefits of being a parent while mourning the loss of independence that new parents often report. The therapist might also help the client explore her fears about being a new parent and work with her to reduce excessive or unrealistic fears. Again, once the underlying, identified problem (i.e., the changing role of the client) is resolved, the symptoms of the eating disorder should also subside.

20.5.1.2.4 Interpersonal Deficits

Problems such as loneliness, social isolation, low self-esteem, or an inability to establish and maintain close relationships are significant "interpersonal deficits." Indeed, research has linked these problems to symptoms of eating disorders (Ball and Lee 2000; Ghaderi 2001), and interpersonal deficits were identified in the two research studies as the primary problem for 33% of women with anorexia nervosa and for 16% of women with bulimia nervosa (Fairburn et al. 1991, 1993).

When a person feels lonely or isolated, she might attempt to compensate for these deficits by using food (e.g., binge eating) to decrease these feelings. A person with low self-esteem or with problems establishing relationships might try to counter these problems by placing strong emphasis on her appearance and on changing the shape of her body, because she might think that being "prettier" or "skinnier" will help her to feel better about herself, to make friends, or to have a boyfriend. As a consequence, she might develop symptoms of an eating disorder, such as purging or severely restricting her food intake, in a desperate attempt to change the way that she looks. In situations like the ones described, the therapist should work with the client to reduce her social isolation, improve her interpersonal skills, form new relationships, and improve current relationships. Again, once these interpersonal deficits are addressed and resolved, her problems with eating should also improve.

20.5.1.2.5 Combination of Identified Interpersonal Problems

The previous examples illustrate how one specific interpersonal problem (i.e., grief, role dispute, role transition, or social skills deficit) could contribute to eating disorder symptoms. However, several different interpersonal problems could contribute to the development of an eating disorder or the maintenance of the symptoms. For example, a woman might experience difficulty coping with the death of her spouse (grief) and also have difficulty accepting her new role as a single parent (role transition). Or, an adolescent might lack the ability to communicate effectively with other people (interpersonal skills deficit), and therefore have difficulty navigating her roles in her relationships with her parents, siblings, and friends (interpersonal role dispute). When more than one interpersonal problem is identified, the therapist and the client need to work together to identify the primary problem or discuss which problem to address first. For example, the woman who lost her husband might need to adequately grieve this loss before she can accept her new role as a single parent. The adolescent who has several chaotic interpersonal relationships might benefit from focusing on learning social skills that will make her interactions less chaotic before attempting to have a conversation with her parents about her role in their relationship. Sometimes, resolving one problem eventually helps resolve the other problem. Other times, both problems might be resolved almost simultaneously.

20.5.1.3 Phase 3: Reflecting, Celebrating, Grieving, and Troubleshooting

In the final phase of interpersonal therapy, the client and the therapist reflect upon their work together and discuss the ways that the client has grown throughout treatment as well as ways to maintain these gains. They also anticipate potential future problems and work together to develop possible solutions for these potential problems, including returning to therapy, if necessary. This phase typically requires three or four sessions, and these sessions can occur at 2-week intervals rather than weekly (Fairburn 1997). The final phase of interpersonal therapy is extremely important for those people who have experienced chaotic interpersonal relationships or those who often experience problems when relationships end. For these clients, this phase can serve as a model for ending relationships in a healthy way.

During this phase of therapy, clients are also asked to reflect upon changes in eating patterns and to explore how these changes are related to positive changes in their interpersonal relations. The client and the therapist also discuss emotions associated with ending the therapeutic relationship. For clients who are told from the beginning of treatment that therapy is time limited and are reminded regularly about the number of sessions remaining, ending therapy is usually less troublesome because they are able to prepare for the termination (Fairburn 1997). Therefore, therapists are encouraged to talk to clients about the anticipated length of treatment at the beginning of therapy.

20.5.2 Using the Interpersonal Process in Therapy

Although the focus of interpersonal therapy is on the client's relationships outside of the therapeutic context (Apple 1999; Wilfley et al. 2000), there are times when it might be appropriate to focus on the interpersonal processes that are occurring between the client and the therapist (Fairburn 1997; Teyber 2006). For instance, if the client has a very limited social support system and few significant relationships, it could be beneficial to focus on the relationship within the therapeutic setting. Additionally, it might be beneficial for clients to get specific feedback from the therapist about how other people might perceive their behaviors and their ways of communicating, and this feedback would be based upon the therapist's observations of the client or interactions with the client. Teyber's (2006, 6) interpersonal process approach focuses specifically on the relationships between clients and therapists and ways that "therapists can use their current interaction to help clients change." When an issue arises between the client and therapist, the therapist addresses the issue so that the client and therapist can work together to resolve the issue in an appropriate way. As the client and therapist work through more interpersonal conflicts, the client is able to apply these positive interactions to her life outside of the therapeutic setting.

The premise of the interpersonal process approach to therapy is that most therapy clients develop maladaptive coping strategies during childhood to combat interpersonal conflicts, such as faulty beliefs or insecurities about relationship attachments. Often, these interpersonal conflicts go unresolved as they progress through later phases of life. As a consequence, people engage in maladaptive behaviors to avoid or manage the anxiety they experience in their interpersonal interactions (Sullivan 1968).

Using this theory, maladaptive strategies, such as symptoms of eating disorders, can develop in different ways. Internalizing familial roles is one way that a person can develop maladaptive eating patterns to compensate for interpersonal difficulty. For example, a person who played the role of "the perfect child" will probably be perfectionistic, will have extremely high expectations for herself, and will tend to avoid conflict, and all of these characteristics have been linked to eating disorders (see Chapter 2 of this book). A girl who has played the role of "the perfect child" might be afraid of becoming fat or might expect herself to maintain a certain weight or eat a "perfectly healthy" diet. As a result, she might restrict her diet in order to meet her own standards and to maintain the role of "the perfect child."

People can also develop maladaptive strategies because they have faulty beliefs. For instance, if a girl grows up hearing her father make disrespectful comments about her mother's body, the girl might develop the belief that she must be thin in order to be loved, and if she is able to maintain a thin figure, she will never displease her partner. The girl has now placed enormous importance on being thin, and as a result, might go to any extreme to achieve thinness, including self-starvation or self-induced vomiting. If she maintains this faulty belief as she progresses through life, she might undermine her other qualities that potential romantic partners might find appealing, such as intelligence, kindness, or humor, and consider herself unworthy of love if she is not at a weight that she deems acceptable. When she enters into a new relationship, she might put pressure on herself to lose weight or to maintain a low weight to gain her partner's affection. However, this overemphasis on weight loss and on the appearance of her body might interfere with the relationship and put distance between the couple rather than achieving a loving relationship like she originally believed. When the relationship ends, this young woman might attribute the break-up to "being too fat" or "not being pretty enough" rather than recognizing that her attempts to lose weight or maintain a low weight interfered with her ability to be authentic and invested in the relationship. As a consequence, she may go through life continuing to believe that the only way to find love is to be thin, and therefore symptoms of the eating disorder persist. Using the interpersonal process, the therapist's challenge is to help the client resolve this problem by providing her with an alternative emotional experience with the therapist. If she can see that the therapist's respect and liking are not dependent on her weight and appearance, then this new learning can later be generalized to other relationships.

Personality, according to Sullivan (1968), develops through interpersonal interactions with parents and other individuals, and therefore reflects the strategies that a person has adopted to avoid or minimize anxiety. For instance, if a child is ridiculed by her parents every time she expresses an emotion like sadness or anger, she will learn that these aspects of herself are inappropriate or unacceptable and therefore will develop coping strategies to avoid the expression of anger or sadness in the presence of her parents, and eventually when she is in the presence of other individuals as well. The child might turn to food, for example, to avoid sad or angry feelings and grow up overeating or binge eating when she is sad or angry rather than learning to appropriately express anger, sadness, and other types of emotions. Throughout her adolescence and adulthood, she may continue using overeating or binge eating as a coping mechanism, rather than expressing emotion in a healthy way. Eventually, she might also develop strategies to compensate for the excessive food that she is consuming (e.g., self-induced vomiting, excessive exercise, or periods of food restriction), especially if she is dissatisfied with the appearance of her body. The therapist's role is to help the client recognize this pattern and the basis for this behavior. Using the interpersonal process, the therapist can ask the client directly how the client thinks the therapist will react if the client expresses sadness or anger in the therapeutic context. The therapist can then help to alleviate the client's concern about being ridiculed, for example, and encourage the appropriate expression of anger and sadness. As the client practices the expression of sadness and anger in the supportive therapeutic environment, she will eventually learn that it is possible to express anger and sadness without being rejected by other people. Therefore, she will be able to express emotions like anger and sadness in the presence of other people rather than avoiding these emotions and turning to food.

Using the interpersonal process, the relationship between the client and therapist is viewed as the foundation of therapy and is considered the most important avenue for change in the client. Specifically, the therapist helps the client identify unhealthy thinking and maladaptive interpersonal patterns that contribute to problems in the client's life. They then explore whether these identified problematic interactions that exist outside of the therapeutic relationship also exist in the therapeutic relationship. For those problems that are present in the therapeutic setting, the client and the therapist collaborate to identify ways to change the problematic interactions. Later, the client and the therapist discuss how to transfer the new insights and skills that were acquired as the client and the therapist worked to resolve the interpersonal problem in their relationship to other relationships where the same problems are occurring.

Understanding the meaning of interpersonal interactions with the client allows the therapist to intervene when change is needed. For example, therapists can work through misunderstandings, inaccurate perceptions, and other interpersonal conflicts that might arise between the client and therapist. If problems are not addressed, the client's relationship with the therapist will mimic her negative interactions outside of therapy. For example, a submissive client who feels like her parents are overcontrolling might view the therapist as being similar to her parents, especially if the therapist tells her what to do rather than working with her to determine appropriate strategies for therapy. Rather than being open to change, she might resent the therapist and be unwilling to fully participate in treatment. Other examples of maladaptive interactions could include the client being overly accommodating, protecting the therapist, playing the role of the "good" client, and working to maintain constant approval from the therapist. Processing these problematic interactions in the moment is effective because clients are invited to actively participate in increasing the effectiveness of an interpersonal interaction rather than simply talking about how to improve an interaction.

Regardless of the problem being addressed in the therapeutic setting, the therapist attempts to challenge the client's beliefs and behavioral strategies, by offering a "corrective emotional experience" and showing the client that sometimes relationships can be different (Teyber 2006, 23–24). Specifically, the therapist tries to be appropriately supportive toward the client who was always discouraged, tries to be "responsive to the client who was always ignored," tries to be "flexible with the client who grew up with rigidity," and tries to be "consistent with a client who grew up without discipline" (Teyber 2006, 13). When a client is able to experience a healthy relationship with her therapist that differs from other dysfunctional relationships in her life, the client learns to trust the therapist and to view her as a competent person who is able to help improve her circumstances. Conversely, when the therapeutic relationship mimics other dysfunctional relationships in the client's life (e.g., the therapist seems critical like the client's parents), the client will have difficulty trusting and respecting the therapist, and therapeutic strategies and techniques will not be effective (Teyber 2006). In order to gain the necessary respect and trust from the client to work in an experiential way, the therapist must be empathic, genuine, and understanding of the client's circumstances. Additionally, the therapist and the client must develop a strong, trusting, collaborative relationship, and both the therapist and client must be invested in the process and committed to the relationship. Because of the importance that is placed on the therapeutic relationship, therapists might need to spend extra time establishing rapport and gaining trust before moving through the issues that need to be addressed in therapy. Specifically, therapists can ask about previous therapeutic experiences and inquire about helpful and unhelpful aspects of previous therapy. Additionally, therapists must empower clients and ask for their ideas about treatment goals and problems to address. Therapists should be cautious, however, to maintain appropriate boundaries with clients, as therapy will be ineffective if the therapist becomes too close to the client (Teyber 2006).

The interpersonal process approach can be used with any type of theoretical orientation, and therapists are encouraged to personalize, integrate, and modify the strategies associated with this process. Incorporating this process into therapy can increase the effectiveness of the treatment, because the client and the therapist focus on developing a collaborative relationship and on establishing a strong rapport (Teyber 2006). By incorporating attention to the interpersonal process into therapy, clients do not simply talk with therapists. Instead, they often recreate maladaptive relational patterns that exist outside of therapy. Therefore, the therapist has the opportunity to confront the maladaptive interaction, and the therapist and client can work together to improve the interaction. In turn, the client becomes more flexible and learns more effective ways to interact with people. The client also learns that people do not always respond in the same expected way (e.g., not everyone is critical, not everyone ignores them, not everyone is competitive), and therefore she is challenged to develop a wider range of expectations, rather than assuming that each person in her life will respond to her in an identical manner.

20.6   CONCLUSION

Interpersonal therapy assumes that the best way to help someone with problematic eating behavior is to focus on that individual's difficulties in dealing with other people. One way of doing that is to help the individual resolve specific interpersonal problems that are contributing to the development and maintenance of disordered eating and other psychological dysfunction. Four specific interpersonal areas that are often linked to disordered eating patterns by interpersonal therapists are grief, role disputes, role transitions, and interpersonal deficits. This chapter has summarized the therapeutic strategies used by interpersonal therapists in each of those areas. For example, if the focus of treatment is alleviating grief, the interpersonal therapist might work with the client to mourn the loss and to find ways to compensate for the loss through other relationships and enjoyable activities. If the focus of treatment is resolving a role dispute, such as a conflict with a parent, the therapist helps the client to identify and understand the dispute and also works with the client to identify strategies to resolve the dispute. If the focus of treatment is to help the client accept her new role in a new phase of life, the therapist helps the client understand the transition, mourn the loss of the old role, and might discuss the advantages of the new role and skills needed to be successful in this new role. If the focus of treatment is on a specific social skill deficit, such as difficulty making new friends or problems keeping a boyfriend, the therapist and the client work together to identify ways that the client can reduce her social isolation, can form new relationships, or can improve current relationships.

An alternative treatment strategy is to focus on the therapeutic relationship, expecting that the problems that a client with an eating disorder has had with other individuals will also occur in her relationship with the therapist. As the client's interpersonal problems are enacted in the therapeutic relationship, the therapist and the client can identify and resolve those problems. Whether the therapist emphasizes the client's relationship with the therapist or her relationship with other individuals, the main focus in therapy is on current relationships. Another key assumption of interpersonal therapy is that the best way to assist an individual with an eating disorder is not to work directly to change that individual's maladaptive eating patterns but to work on interpersonal problems that are linked to her problematic eating patterns.

The use of interpersonal therapy with individuals with eating disorders may take more time than other therapeutic approaches, but there are many aspects of this approach that are appealing to therapists. Interpersonal therapy can be a therapist's main source of ideas for helping clients with eating disorders, or elements of interpersonal therapy can be combined with strategies from other treatment approaches. Previous research indicates that interpersonal therapy is effective in producing lasting benefits for clients and that it might be the best treatment option for particular types of clients (e.g., those who are anxious about interpersonal relationships or who have a high need for approval).

REFERENCES

Agras, W. S., C. F. Telch, B. Arnow, K. Eldredge, M. J. Detzer, J. Henderson, and M. Marnell. 1995. Does interpersonal therapy help patients with binge eating disorder who fail to respond to cognitive behavioral therapy? *J Consult Clin Psychol* 63: 356–360.

Apple, R. F. 1999. Interpersonal therapy for bulimia nervosa. *J Clin Psychol* 55: 715–725.

Ball, K., and C. Lee. 2000. Relationship between psychological stress, coping and disordered eating: A review. *Psychol Health* 14: 1007–1035.

Carr, A., and M. McNulty. 2006. Eating disorders. In *The handbook of adult clinical psychology: An evidence-based practice approach,* eds. A. Carr and M. McNulty, 724–765. New York: Taylor-Francis Group.

Chui, W., D. L. Safer, S. W. Bryson, W. S. Agras, and G. T. Wilson. 2007. A comparison of ethnic groups in the treatment of bulimia nervosa. *Eat Behav* 8: 485–491.

Constantino, M. J., B. A. Arnow, C. Blasey, and W. S. Agras. 2005. The association between patient characteristics and the therapeutic alliance in cognitive behavioral and interpersonal therapy for bulimia nervosa. *J Consult Clin Psychol* 73: 203–211.

Fairburn, C. G. 1997. Interpersonal psychotherapy for bulimia nervosa. In *Handbook of treatment for eating disorders,* eds. D. M. Garner and P. E. Garfinkel, 278–294. New York: Guilford Press.

Fairburn, C. G., R. Jones, R. C. Peveler, R. A. Hope, and M. O'Connor. 1993. Psychotherapy and bulimia nervosa: Longer term effects of interpersonal psychotherapy, behavior therapy, and cognitive behavior therapy. *Archiv Gen Psychiatry* 50: 419–428.

Fairburn, C. G., R. Jones, R. C. Peveler, S. J. Carr, R. A. Solomon, M. E. O'Connor, J., Burton, and R. A. Hope. 1991. Three psychological treatments for bulimia nervosa: A comparative trial. *Archiv Gen Psychiatry* 48: 463–469.

Ghaderi, A. 2001. Review of risk factors for eating disorders: Implications for primary prevention and cognitive behavioural therapy. *Scand J Behav Ther* 30: 57–74.

Gleaves, D. H., and J. D. Latner. 2008. Evidence-based therapies for children and adolescents with eating disorders. In *Handbook of evidence-based therapies for children and adolescents: Bridging Science and Practice,* eds. R. G. Steele, T. D. Elkin, and M. C. Roberts, 335–353. New York: Springer.

Keel, P. K., D. J. Dorer, D. L. Franko, S. C. Jackson, and D. B. Herzog. 2005. Postremission predictors of relapse in women with eating disorders. *Am J Psychiatry* 162: 2263–2268.

Klerman, G. L., M. M. Weissman, B. J. Rounsaville, and E. S. Chevron. 1984. *Interpersonal psychotherapy of depression.* New York: Basic Books.

McFarlane, T., J. Carter, and M. Olmsted. 2005. Eating disorders. In *Improving outcomes and preventing relapse in cognitive behavioral therapy,* eds. M. M. Antony, L. R. Ledley, and R. G. Heimberg, 268–305. New York: Guilford Press.

McIntosh, V. V., C. M. Bulik, J. M. McKenzie, S. E. Luty, and J. Jordan. 2000. Interpersonal psychotherapy for anorexia nervosa. *Int J Eat Disord* 27: 125–139.

Schembri, C., and L. Evans. 2008. Adverse relationship processes: The attempts of women with bulimia nervosa symptoms to fit the perceived ideal of intimate partners. *Eur Eat Disord Rev* 16: 59–66.

Sullivan, H. S. 1968. *The interpersonal theory of psychiatry.* New York: Norton.

Tasca, G., L. Balfour, K. Ritchie, and H. Bissada. 2007. Change in attachment anxiety is associated with improved depression among women with binge eating disorder. *Psychotherapy: Theory, Research, Practice, Training* 44: 423–433.

Teyber, E. 2006. *Interpersonal process in therapy: An interpersonal model.* Belmont, CA: Thomson.

Wei, M., V. L. Vogel, T. Y. Ku, and R. A. Zakalik. 2005. Adult attachment, affect regulation, negative mood, and interpersonal problems: The mediating roles of emotional reactivity and emotional cutoff. *J Counsel Psychol* 52: 14–25.

Wilfley, D. E., W. S. Agras, C. F. Telch, E. M. Rossiter, J. A. Schneider, A. G. Cole, L. A. Sifford, and S. D. Raeburn. 1993. Group cognitive behavioral therapy and group interpersonal psychotherapy for the nonpurging bulimic individual: A controlled comparison. *J Consult Clin Psychol* 61: 296–305.

Wilfley, D. E., J. Z. Dounchis, and R. R. Welch. 2000. Interpersonal psychotherapy. In *Comparative treatments for eating disorders,* eds. K. J. Miller and J. S. Mizes, 128–159. New York: Springer Publishing Company.

Wilfley, D. E., M. A. Frank, R. Welch, E. B. Spurrell, and B. M. Rounsaville. 1998. Adapting interpersonal psychotherapy to a group format (IPT-G) for binge eating disorder: A model for adapting empirically-validated treatments. *Psychother Res* 8: 379–391.

Wilson, G. T., and K. M. Pike. 1993. Eating disorders. In *Clinical handbook of psychological disorders: A step-by-step treatment manual,* ed. D. H. Barlow, 278–317. New York: Guilford Press.

21 Constructivist and Narrative Approaches for Treating Eating Disorders

Kristin L. Goodheart and Stephanie L. Harter

CONTENTS

21.1 LEARNING OBJECTIVES

After completing this chapter, you should be able to do the following:

- Understand the basic assumptions and related practices of constructivist and narrative approaches to treating people with eating disorders
- Engage in practices that validate the client as a construing person separate from his or her eating disorder
- Facilitate a therapeutic relationship in which clients can elaborate new dimensions of meaning and stories about their lives, which offer alternatives to eating disorders and related oppressive self-constructions
- Elaborate questioning practices that foster alternative constructivism, positioning dominant stories as a limited set of potential ways of organizing experience, rather than as taken for granted realities

- Assist clients to collaborate with relationship partners in continued coauthoring of meanings, stories, and conversational practices that are respectful of persons and foster their continued growth

21.2   INTRODUCTION

Constructivist and narrative approaches to therapy (see Kelly 1955; White and Epston 1990; Neimeyer and Mahoney 1995; Freedman and Combs 1996; Smith and Nylund 1997; Mahoney 2006; White 2007) focus on understanding the meaning of life experiences (i.e., meaning making) as a personal process embedded within social contexts that both offer and constrain possible ways of organizing these experiences. Meanings are shaped by the person's engagement in social processes, within which constructions or stories of experiences are enacted, validated or invalidated, and maintained or revised. Healthy personal and social processes involve the ongoing creation of new meanings that are respectful and inclusive of personal experience. Both therapists' and clients' personal meanings, including ways of nurturing the self and being with others, evolve within social and cultural stories. Therapists' and clients' positions within and experiences of these stories may be very different, leading to differing constructions of themselves, each other, their therapeutic relationship, and larger social processes. Within the therapeutic relationship, the therapist and the client collaborate to "deconstruct" or to evaluate and break down stories that limit the client's possibilities for creative elaboration of new meanings, to consider alternative constructions, and to create new possibilities (Harker 1997; Harter 1988, 2004). Disordered eating and related behaviors can be considered to stem from limiting stories of identity, gender, and relationships located within cultural practices (Gremillion 2003; Maisel et al. 2004).

Within a constructivist and narrative framework, we each see the world through the lens of our own experience—within the cultures, relationships, and related roles in which we participate. Thus, both the therapist and the client bring personal "biases" and "knowledges" to their work together. Among other contributions, the therapist brings experience in co-creating therapeutic conversations, and clients bring expert knowledge of their own lives, including experiences of the problems for which they are seeking consultation. Together, the therapist and the client are involved in a therapeutic conversation that inevitably leads them to co-author ways of understanding the client's experience. In this way, therapy is recreated with each client, rather being an application of *a priori* techniques. Each therapy relationship is also embedded within social and cultural processes that include other collaborators, co-authors, or conversational partners (Harter 2004, 2007; White 2007).

Similar processes are involved in the co-authoring of this chapter, which extends beyond the acknowledged academic collaboration to previous authors of constructivist and narrative texts and to our interactions with friends, family, colleagues, and clients who have experienced painful relationships with food and related limiting constructions of themselves, gender, and relationships. Thus, this chapter is multiply authored as one stream within many contributing conversations. As Mahoney (2006, 4) states, "Every life and every act within a life makes a difference."

21.3   RESEARCH BACKGROUND AND SIGNIFICANCE

Disordered eating and distress related to body dissatisfaction encompass the most common of all psychological problems, affecting by some estimates nearly 800 million people worldwide (Malowe 2007). Although specific eating disorders, such as anorexia nervosa and bulimia nervosa are rare, a larger number of people experience some sort of dysfunctional relationship with food (Fairburn and Bohn 2005; Fairburn et al. 2007). A variety of approaches are used to treat eating disorders, including cognitive behavioral therapy, interpersonal therapy, and drug therapy (see Chapters 19, 20, and 22 of this book). Treatment outcome studies for clients with eating disorders, particularly for those diagnosed with anorexia nervosa, remain limited (Berkman et al. 2007; Bulik et al. 2007). Reviews suggest that treatments for eating disorders are effective in helping some clients (Lundgren et al. 2004; Brownley et al. 2007; Bulik et al. 2007; Shapiro et al. 2007), but many clients continue to have limited to poor outcomes. For instance, Clausen's review (2004) of outcome studies of treatment of bulimia nervosa estimated that only about half of the clients obtained a good outcome. Vanderlinden (2008) concluded that, in spite of being one of the most empirically supported and empirically tested treatments for eating disorders, cognitive behavioral therapy is only effective in the longer term for 45% to 50% of clients with bulimia nervosa, and the longer term outcome for clients with anorexia nervosa is unknown. He suggested a need for increasing attention to family and peer influences, emotional experiencing, and underlying implicit emotional messages, versus a dominant focus on cognitions. These suggestions are quite compatible with Kelly's (1955) holistic description of meaning making as including processes that are more traditionally described as physiological, emotional, behavioral, and social, in addition to cognitive. Kelly's (1955) description of meaning making was later elaborated by more contemporary constructivists (e.g., Mahoney 1991).

There is a continued need to create more inclusively effective treatment strategies and to individualize treatment with individual clients. All people differ in their personalities, their life experiences, their genetic make-up, and their individual vulnerabilities. Clients with eating problems are no exception. Within diagnostic categories, clients may differ in their particular constellation of symptoms, in the underlying meanings and functions of the symptoms, and in their experience of the disorder, diagnosis, and related treatment (Harter 1995; Raskin and Lewandowski 2000). After all, "… (therapeutic) techniques are like languages. The more languages one knows, the more people with whom one can communicate" (Mahoney 2006, 58).

21.3.1 OVERVIEW OF CONSTRUCTIVIST THERAPY

Constructivist approaches to therapy emphasize the client's active engagement in the change process, rather than the therapist as the director of change. Constructivists view change as an interpersonal process, not a procedure. Co-construction of a creative therapeutic process allows exploration and experimentation with new meanings. The focus of constructivist psychotherapy is on the ongoing conceptualization of a person's experience, knowledge, and development, rather than on specific techniques, as individuals are expected to differ in their responses to the same technique (Mahoney 2006). Because of this, constructivism can serve as a meta-theory within which practitioners of varying therapeutic approaches can orient or rewrite their practice, or within which practitioners can draw from techniques offered by multiple schools of therapy, integrating these within a coherent theoretical and ethical framework (Neimeyer 1988).

Therapists using a constructivist approach help clients to identify the individual dimensions or constructions that they use to make sense of their life experiences. With the client, the therapist explores the possibilities offered by these constructions, as well as the limitations, contradictions, and dilemmas that these constructions entail. The therapist also helps the client to generate predictions based on these constructions and to devise behavioral experiments to test these predictions (e.g., if I do this, then that will occur). The therapist helps the client to evaluate the outcome of these experiments and, when needed, helps the client to formulate alternate constructions that might offer more preferable outcomes. A particularly distinctive feature of constructivist therapy is creating new meanings or identifying new ways of organizing existing meanings through hypothetical or playful experiments within or outside of the therapy room, such as through role plays, alternative reframing of symptoms, or enactment of fictional roles. Distinct from the more rational approach of cognitive therapies, the assumption of constructivist therapy is that generation of more elaborate alternatives allows the client to change, even in the absence of explicitly disputing current constructions. Thus, constructivist approaches emphasize the creation of new meaning and new possibilities, rather than focusing on the past or on disputing and disproving current constructions (Kelly 1955, 1958; Harter 1988; Mahoney 1988a, 1988b).

21.3.2 OVERVIEW OF NARRATIVE THERAPY

Over the past 20 years, constructivist therapy has increasingly taken a narrative turn, moving from Kelly's (1955) metaphor of "personal scientist" to a metaphor of "personal storyteller" (Mair 1988, 1989; Harter 1995, 2004; Neimeyer 2000) as a designation for the meaning making and change process. At the same time, other descriptions of narrative meaning processes have developed within feminist, social constructionist, and postmodern communities (White and Epston 1990; White 2007), and there has been increasing dialogue and convergence in work across these communities. Although there are also other uses of narrative in psychotherapy, this chapter focuses on narrative therapy as described within these constructivist/constructionist communities. (For an overview of the uses of narrative across therapy schools and contributions of narrative methods to psychotherapy research, see McLeod 1997.)

Narrative therapy suggests that people are storytellers and historians. However, the narrative process is not an individual endeavor but is constructed through social discourse that may include internal dialogue. Thus, both storytelling and conversation are often used as metaphors for the meaning making and change process. Mair (1988, 127) suggested that we are born into the stories of our family and culture, and that we "live in" and "live by" these stories. This idea emphasizes the extent to which dominant narratives within families and cultures may be taken for granted as aspects of reality, rather than considered as one of many possible ways to understand or "story" an experience. Personal meanings do not occur in a vacuum but are constructed from what is available and what is familiar based on life experiences within meaning dimensions, metaphors, or stories offered within the family, other social systems, and the surrounding culture (White and Epston 1990; White 2007).

In generating responses to questions or in making choices in response to problems in living, people use the alternatives that are available. Sometimes, available meanings offer choices that work well for the person. Other times, however, people struggle to understand the meaning of an event or to reconcile available alternatives with other valued aspects of their identity. Particularly in the aftermath of traumatic experiences, people may have difficulty finding a way to meaningfully narrate or make meaning of the event that will allow them to integrate the experience into their life story and into their relationships with others (Harter 2004; Neimeyer 2000). Even within the same culture or family, people have differing roles that influence their stories of shared events. People and communities also differ in the extent to which their versions of experience are seen as credible within the family or social conversation. Marginalized persons and communities may have difficulty accessing stories of those who have shared similar experiences, or their versions of experience may be stigmatized (White and Epston 1990; Brown 2000; Paris and Epting 2004; Paris 2008).

Narrative therapists foster a wider collaboration and a more open and inclusive dialogue, to allow clients and others in their support networks to enrich their collection of experiences and the available meanings of those experiences. This collaboration also allows them to create stories for aspects of their own experience that have been "unstoried" due to the lack of available language to speak of the experience. As Kelly (1969, 335) states, "... people are usually ashamed of seeing what they are not supposed to see, so these are the stories that never get told." Through collaboration, people are able to move away from what they know and believe and to become aware of what they have the potential to know and adopt (White 2007). Considering alternatives does not require a person to adopt these alternative views permanently or completely. Acknowledging alternative views is enough, because recognizing alternative views increases the breadth of knowledge available to make future meaning.

21.4 APPLICATION OF RESEARCH: ENHANCING TREATMENT WITH EATING DISORDER CLIENTS USING CONSTRUCTIVIST AND NARRATIVE APPROACHES IN THERAPY

21.4.1 DIAGNOSING THE EATING DISORDER

Constructivist and narrative approaches to therapy place little emphasis on categorical diagnostic systems, such as the classification system in the *Diagnostic and Statistical Manual of Mental Disorders (DSM-IV-TR;* American Psychiatric Association 2000). However, these systems may be used for research purposes to identify similar patterns of construing or similar responses to therapy across symptom presentations or across people who have similar problems. Using a categorical diagnostic system in this way might provide some guidance for therapists when working with clients. Therapists also might discuss diagnoses within therapy, particularly when clients arrive with a diagnosis that they have received from past providers, or when they have derived diagnoses for themselves from reading, media, or conversations with others. For some clients, receiving a diagnosis can serve as a self-fulfilling prophecy, as they allow themselves to internalize it as a core aspect of their identity, sometimes adopting a healthcare provider's pre-emptive construing of their illness as defining them. Some clients may feel stigmatized or labeled by the diagnosis, even if they have readily adopted it as an aspect of their identity. Other clients find diagnoses helpful, especially when they are described from a collaborative stance that respects the person as much more than her experience of the illness and related symptoms. From such a stance, a diagnosis may provide an explanation for some problems that clients are experiencing in a way that situates them within shared experiences of other clients, therapists, and healthcare researchers. Diagnoses can provide some clients a sense of relief and a hope that others have had similar experiences, as well as confidence that the healthcare provider understands their problems and assurance that help is available. From a collaborative stance, therapists describe criteria in lay language and allow clients to provide examples of ways in which these criteria fit or do not fit their own experiences. Collaborative discussion also helps the therapist to avoid the danger of reifying the diagnosis, categorizing clients and their symptoms, and overgeneralizing from past experiences with other persons with similar diagnoses. Although it is often helpful to clients to recognize commonalities with others' experiences, each client's experience should also be regarded as personal and unique.

In assessing a client, constructivist and narrative approaches are interested in how symptoms of the disorder developed, in their family and wider cultural contexts, and in their meanings for the client, rather than just the presence of the symptoms themselves and their correspondence to diagnostic criteria. Although a diagnosis may offer one viewpoint for the client's problems, it is important to remember that it is not the only explanation or important story to be told. The relevance of medical diagnoses within the client's culture and the client's past experience within medical and related therapy systems may also influence the usefulness of diagnostic explanations for the client's symptoms and related treatment strategies.

21.4.2 RECOGNIZING AND EXPLORING CHOICES

Constructivist approaches emphasize the importance of choice and the way in which choices affect people's lives. "We must and do choose, even when we struggle to avoid choosing. Not choosing is a choice. We have no choice but to be always in the process of choosing" (Mahoney 2006, 19). Kelly (1955) described basic meaning processes as consisting of bipolar, contrasting constructs that define some events as similar to each other but different from other events. Our choices of construct dimensions to use in construing an event, or in constructing our identity, determine the availability and meaning of the alternatives available to us. In considering our own and others' choices, it is important to recognize the contrast or alternative to the existing choice and the meaning of the alternatives within the larger meaning system. Behavior that appears self-defeating or irrational becomes understandable in the context of available alternatives (Kelly 1955).

Although everyone has choices, all people have different choices and different views of their choices. One perception is that eating disorders develop in two ways: some people "choose" to develop eating disorders and other people "slip into" the "lifestyle." For instance, a parent might think that his or her daughter chose to develop anorexia nervosa, instead of thinking that she chose to diet to lose weight but her dieting reached a point of extreme restriction until managing a healthy diet seemed to be out of her control. Most people do not consciously choose to develop an eating disorder, but many do choose to engage in dieting or exercise behaviors in order to change some aspect of their physical appearance. Thus, the therapist should work with the client to challenge the idea that she is to blame for developing the eating disorder and instead talk about the current choices she is making to maintain the disorder.

Although a person may not consciously choose to develop a clinical eating disorder, she might have more control over the choices she makes to maintain the disorder. For example, a young woman might consciously choose to continue restricting her food intake or might choose to engage in inappropriate compensatory behaviors, such as self-induced vomiting, after beginning treatment for the disorder. She might believe that her only alternative is to gain weight and become fat, and she cannot imagine anything worse than gaining weight. When a young woman successfully changes her appearance and other people praise these changes, she might develop a different construct associated with her physical self. For example, she might think that, because her new body is now "acceptable," "desirable," or "attractive," her old body must not have been. Therefore, gaining weight and returning to her former appearance might mean losing this new acceptance, desirability, and attractiveness. As a therapist or someone trying to support a person with an eating disorder, it is important to be aware of her restricted range of choices and of related constructions circulating within the family, other social groups, and the culture in which she lives.

21.4.3 EXPLORING CONSTRUCTIONS USING THE ROLE CONSTRUCT REPERTORY GRID AND LADDERING TECHNIQUES

Personal construct psychology has provided a number of methods to assess personal meaning systems that are useful in working with eating-disordered clients. Many of these methods are versions or elaborations of Kelly's (1955) Role Construct Repertory Grid (RepGrid). The RepGrid is a form of structured interview, and the client is asked to describe dimensions along which some elements are similar and different from others. Originally, the elements of the grid were people in the person's social world, usually including parents, intimate partners, the self, and other persons with whom the client had important positive and negative experiences. Grids also often include the element "ideal self," representing the hypothetical person whom the client would ideally like to be. These elements are compared in triads (or, in some versions, in pairs), and the client is asked to describe a way in which two of them are similar and different from the third (or a way in which the two are similar or different). After this emergent construct pole is described, the client is asked to describe its contrast or opposite. Elicitation of the construct dimensions continues using different groups of elements until a representative number of construct dimensions has been elicited (often ten or twelve construct dimensions). Together, the emergent and contrasting poles represent bipolar dimensions along which the client then describes all of the elements, such as people being described in the grid, often using a Likert-type scale. These ratings result in a matrix of ratings that can be used to compute similarities between elements on grid. Common scores include average distances between ratings of the self and the ideal self (self-negativity), average distances between the self and other people described on the grid (self-isolation), and average distances between the ideal self and other people described on the grid (other negativity).

Principal components or correspondence analysis is often conducted on the RepGrid to estimate the amount of variance explained by the first common factor, which is used as an estimate of the degree to which the client's construing is unidimensional (i.e., high amount of variance explained by the first factor) or multidimensional (i.e., lower amount of variance explained by any one factor). Content analysis of the construct dimensions and their correlations with principal components also gives important information regarding dimensions the client uses in construing other people, or other domains of elements used on the grid. A number of authors have provided contemporary descriptions of the RepGrid (e.g., Fransella et al. 2003; Feixas and Alvarez 2010), and software programs are available to analyze grid data. One of these is available for free use on the internet (Shaw and Gaines 2010).

A number of researchers have adapted the RepGrid to explore interpersonal and self-constructions of persons with problems related to eating. For example, Mottram (1985) found that women diagnosed with anorexia nervosa differed from matched, nonclinical volunteers in construing themselves more negatively and as more different from others. Using cluster analysis, they found that participants with anorexia nervosa reported rigid, unidimensional social constructions. In contrast, the nonclinical volunteers construed similarities and differences between people in a more multidimensional manner. Results of this study suggested that, for women with anorexia nervosa, the obsession with thinness and physical appearance consumes one's thoughts and personal value is based heavily on physical attributes. Women who do not have eating disorders, however, are able to see value in themselves and in other people in various aspects of their lives.

Rather than using different people as elements to be construed, Neimeyer and Khouzam (1985) used the self in a variety of different eating situations (e.g., "when I've eaten a well-balanced meal, when I've over-eaten, when I've broken my diet, when I imagine my ideal weight") in a RepGrid study of restrained eating (i.e., chronic dieting, food deprivation, and binging-purging cycles) in college women. Women with highly restrained eating, in contrast to those with low restraint, had more negative and more unidimensional, simplistic constructions of themselves in relation to food.

Borkenhagen et al. (2008, 64) further adapted the RepGrid by using individual body parts and two body concepts, "real body" and "ideal body," as elements. This approach allows therapists to assess body acceptance and integration, and dissociation within the body image. Using this grid, they found negative constructions of the body for women with anorexia nervosa or bulimia nervosa. Analyzing the content of constructs that women used to describe their bodies, they found that those with anorexia nervosa or bulimia nervosa primarily described their bodies as objects or mechanisms, using constructs referring to external appearance and ability to function. These women used few constructs referring to feelings, such as emotions, sensuality, eroticism, and sexuality, and they used even fewer constructs referring to the body as a center of subjective experience.

These examples of RepGrid research offer potential ways to explore constructions of people, relationships, the self, and the body in clients with eating problems. They highlight the need to elaborate constructions of the embodied self, emotional meanings, and relationships to others in clients with eating disorders, rather than solely focusing on control of eating and binge–purge cycles. Focusing only on eating practices may further objectify the person, her body, and her relationships (Epston et al. 1995; Brown et al. 2008). Adaptations of the RepGrid offer a wealth of quantitative and qualitative data that can be used to identify possible pathways for change and obstacles to change in therapy. The RepGrid can also be used to create individualized indices of change. In addition to being a useful assessment technique, the experience of completing a RepGrid with a client may provide a relatively nonthreatening way to explore interpersonal or self-constructions. It also provides the client experience in generating multiple dimensions along which people, or the self, can be construed. As such, it may encourage multidimensional construing.

Using constructs identified from the RepGrid or constructs identified during therapy conversations, therapists may also use other personal construct methods to further explore relationships between constructs and their implications for behavior and for higher order core values. Simply considering the contrast to a construct pole for a client may clarify the meaning of the client's construct. This may be explored further using *laddering* (Hinkle 1965; cited in Fransella 2003), a technique in which the client is asked his or her preference between construct poles, and then the reason for that preference is used to ladder up to relatively superordinate or core constructions or to ladder down to explore the behavioral characteristics that are associated with a more subordinate construction.

A therapist might use laddering to understand the construction of attractiveness for a client with an eating disorder. The therapist might begin the exercise by asking the client what it means to be attractive. The client would then list qualities that she believes make a person attractive. For example, a woman with an eating disorder might suggest that being skinny and pretty makes a person attractive. The therapist would then ask the client to state the opposite of both qualities, such as fat and ugly. The therapist then encourages the client to think about other qualities of skinny, pretty, attractive people. If the client has difficulty generating additional qualities, the therapist could ask the question in a different way, such as asking her to list other characteristics for people who are "fat and ugly" or to list characteristics for people who are *not* "skinny and pretty." The client would then provide the opposite of each of these characteristics, which would reflect her ideas about what it means to be skinny, pretty, and attractive. The following is an example of the use of laddering for the construction of attractiveness.

What does it mean to be attractive?	What is the opposite of this?
Skinny ←	→ Fat
Pretty ←	→ Ugly
What else does it mean if someone is skinny and attractive?	What else does it mean if someone is *not* skinny and attractive?
Desirable ←	→ Disgusting
Good ←	→ Bad
Strong-willed ←	→ Weak
Hardworking ←	→ Lazy
Well-liked ←	→ Disliked
Popular ←	→ Unpopular
Pleasing ←	→ Disappointing
Happy ←	→ Unhappy
Healthy ←	→ Unhealthy
Proud ←	→ Ashamed
Pure ←	→ Tainted
In control ←	→ Out of control

The use of laddering in this example suggests that the client believes that people who are skinny are attractive, sexually desirable, good, strong-willed, hardworking, well-liked, popular, pleasing, happy, healthy, proud, pure, and in control of their lives. Those who are not skinny are fat, unattractive, disgusting, bad, weak, lazy, disliked, unpopular, disappointing, unhappy, unhealthy, ashamed, tainted, and do not have control over their lives. This hypothetical client has constructed a strong necessity to be skinny, because not being skinny automatically means being fat, ugly, lazy, and so on. The therapist can help "deconstruct" or break down this hierarchy of constructs by asking the client to challenge these beliefs. For example, the therapist might ask the client to think of all the attractive people she knows and determine if they all fit her entire perception of "attractive." Specifically, the therapist could ask, "Are all attractive people popular? Do you know any who are unpopular? Are all attractive people healthy? Can you think of any who are unhealthy? Are all 'fat' people unhappy? Do you know of any who are happy?"

Because of the restricted or chaotic relationship with food in those with eating disorders, it may be beneficial to explore the constructs the client has developed regarding food. The following is a hypothetical interaction with a client who binges and purges.

T: When is it okay to eat?
C: Only when I eat good food.
T: Good food? How do you define "good" food? Food that tastes good? Food that you like?

C: No, food that is safe to eat.

T: Safe to eat? What does it mean when food is "safe to eat"?

From here, the construct of "good food" and "bad food" can be explored.

Good food ←	→ Bad food
Consume in moderation ←	→ Off-limits
Nutritious ←	→ Empty
< 3 g of fat ←	→ > 3 g of fat
Low sugar ←	→ High sugar

Using these constructs, the client's idea of "good food" may include foods like bread, some cereals, pasta (without any type of sauce), rice cakes, most fruits and vegetables, and some "diet foods." Although "bad foods" might include foods that are not typically considered nutritious (e.g., candy, cake, and ice cream), nutritional foods, such as cheese, milk, meat, and nuts, may also be considered "off-limits" because of their fat content. Additionally, foods in the "good list" (e.g., rice cakes) may have very little nutritional value. A goal of the therapist or nutritional counselor might be to help the client "deconstruct" or dismantle this hierarchy, recognizing that some fat is necessary for proper development and health. Also, awareness that moderate amounts of "forbidden" foods can alleviate the urge to binge might be helpful in reframing her construction of good food and bad food.

Exploring other constructs might be effective as well. Sometimes, people with eating disorders have a difficult time separating themselves from the disorder, so an exploration of one's "identity" with and without the disorder may be helpful (Button 1985, 1992, 1993). Other examples might include exploring what it means to be "safe," what it means to be "in control," what it means to be "healthy," and what it means to be "happy." Button (1993) uses a version of the RepGrid that includes a number of hypothetical self elements, such as "me nowadays," "me when younger," "me a year ago," "me in the near future," "me in the far future," and "me as I would ideally like to be." This Self RepGrid also includes actual persons chosen for their relation to the person's self-constructions, such as "the person I'm closest to," "the person I am least like," "the person I am most like," and the person's mother and father. This approach may foster construction of the self as changing over time, rather than as static and unitary, opening space to experiment with change in therapy.

Damani et al. (2001) developed a semi-structured interview for use in exploring a client's image of the ideal woman and image of the ideal woman's body, and how these constructions relate to her own body image. Using this interview in conjunction with RepGrid techniques, they found that women with and without eating disorders emphasize the importance of slimness and physical appearance. However, for women with eating disorders, these constructs were more pervasive, core aspects of their self-construction. Almost all of the clients with eating disorders saw being thin or being slim as "the major issue in defining the kind of woman they wanted to be" (Damani et al. 2001, 177). In contrast, women in the nonclinical comparison group saw career as the most important issue and also emphasized family and interpersonal qualities. Both groups of women were aware of pressure to be thin and the media's influence in this regard, but nonclinical participants were less focused on this issue, also expressing concern about the many other competing demands upon women.

21.4.4 CONNECTING MIND, BODY, AND SPIRIT

Mahoney (2006) suggested that problems are discrepancies between reality and what is considered ideal, so solutions are reached by either changing the way things are (reality) or changing the expectation of how things should be (ideal). For a woman who develops an eating disorder, the belief that she should look like a supermodel might conflict with the composition of her body. Instead of changing her personal expectations, she might attempt to conquer biology and achieve unattainable standards by developing unhealthy behaviors, such as food restriction, self-induced vomiting, and compulsive exercise. When the mind, body, and spirit oppose one another, as illustrated in this example, chaos can be the result. Through self-care, self-soothing, and self-awareness, people can become more conscious of thought, more mindful of their bodies, and therefore more connected to their inner being.

Self-care is often a skill that clients lack. Sometimes, a lack of self-care can result in feeling "stuck" or feeling "out of control" and motivates the person to pursue professional help. A narrative study of clients diagnosed with anorexia nervosa found that many of these clients described their initial symptoms as misplaced self-care. They viewed taking control over food as a way to counter unhappiness, loss, lack of control, and dissatisfaction with themselves and their bodies. Sometimes, they developed overcontrolled, restrictive eating patterns in response to abuse, bullying, bereavement, or perceived failure to meet their parents' expectations or their own high expectations. As eating disorders and related physical debilitation progressed, the threat of chaotic loss of control increased as unsuccessful attempts to maintain control through eating practices increased (Dignon et al. 2006). That study indicates that clients with eating disorders can benefit from learning techniques that focus on relaxation, centering, and mindfulness. Although these techniques are useful to practice in the therapeutic setting, they can also be "tools that help teach ... living skills" (Mahoney 2006, 58), implying that clients can learn to live more efficient and fulfilling lives by increasing awareness of the self and their personal needs.

People often enter into therapy after losing their balance or after attempting to escape from "destructive or dysfunctional patterns" (Mahoney 2006, 57). Centering techniques are used to help clients find or return to "a sense of center and safety, and to experience from that sense ... and to help recover a sense of meaningful order" (Mahoney 2006, 69). Although most people know how to relax, it can be challenging to regularly apply this knowledge of relaxation, particularly when pressured or challenged (Mahoney 2006).

Teaching relaxation to someone struggling with an eating disorder can be beneficial, as stress may exacerbate symptoms of the disorder. Learning to breathe deeply can aid in relaxation and assist in gaining recognition of the body and increasing self-awareness. One possible technique is to explore varying levels of control in breathing, alternating between "tightening" control over breathing and "loosening" this control. Mahoney's (2006) method of pause breathing, exhaling to the count of one one thousand, two one thousand, three one thousand, four one thousand, pausing for a few seconds, then inhaling slowly and repeating the cycle can be used through several cycles as an exploration of controlled deep breathing. The client can be asked to alternate observing oneself using this controlled breathing for several repetitions, followed by breathing as naturally as possible. This exploration of control and release can then be generalized to life experience, reflecting the importance of finding balance between effort and surrender (Mahoney 2006).

For a client experiencing an extreme need for rigid control, as is often present among those who severely restrict their food intake, practicing this exercise in a therapeutic setting can offer an opportunity to practice letting go of the need or desire for excessive control. For clients desiring more consistency in experiences related to being in control, as may be true for a client experiencing cycles of binge eating and purging, this exercise can serve as a method of understanding varying levels of control and when it may be appropriate to "loosen" and "tighten" control. A similar approach is to experiment with control over breathing while engaging in varying levels of activity, as is used in some disciplines of yoga and martial arts, to further one's recognition of self-awareness and varying levels of control. Such practices might also help the client to view self-control as a process of experience rather than viewing oneself as an object to be manipulated.

21.4.5 Mirror Work

"I can fool most of the people a lot of the time, but I can't fool him (meaning himself)" (Mahoney 2006, 155, citing an unnamed colleague). For people with eating disorders, deceit, manipulation, and secrecy can accompany the illness to the point that others, even those close to the individual, are unaware of the personal struggle occurring. Thus, the eating disorder becomes a secret identity shared with no one or only those with similar difficulties with food. The person's relationship with her own body is often disrupted and dishonest (Damani et al. 2001; Borkenhagen et al. 2008). Use of the mirror can be helpful in re-establishing a relationship with the self, if the client is taught a new approach to the mirror and to the body. The therapist can guide the client in brief, graduated experiencing of the mirror image, alternating with closing the eyes, to process the experience in a more internal way (Mahoney 2006).

Like most process-level work, mirror time requires creativity and courage to examine oneself in the present moment (Mahoney 2006). Mirror work can be very difficult for people with eating disorders because they often do not experience viewing themselves in a positive way. For example, it may be very difficult for a woman who has just binged to look in the mirror and view herself as a worthy human being. Alternately, it may be less difficult for a woman who has just weighed herself and has achieved a number that she has deemed "acceptable" to look in the mirror and be affirming and appreciative. Because the intention of mirror work is to experience oneself as a human being, not an image, reflection, or object, mirror work may be especially difficult for a person who often evaluates the self and the image seen in the mirror harshly (Mahoney 2006). It may take time and practice to relate to oneself in the mirror without being evaluative and judgmental. In a therapy demonstration, Mahoney focused on eye contact with oneself and the experience of that eye contact, later expanding to larger facial expressions and then to body postures, to foster awareness of internal experience and dialogues, rather than self-criticism of physical attributes. For clients who become very anxious when asked to look at their images, the therapist can use gradual exposure by lowering the lights or covering the mirror with sheer material.

Although using mirror techniques might be challenging when working with clients with eating disorders, this technique also seems to have the potential to improve the experience of oneself as a person. "When a person really begins to experience herself, not only as the image in the mirror but also as the human being looking into that mirror, this can create a whole new realm of experiencing and communicating" (Mahoney 2006, 157). Indeed, this technique could be a powerful and important experience for a person who for a long time has not been able to view herself as a worthy, proud, beautiful human being.

21.4.6　Identifying the Problem

The purpose of problem solving in constructivist therapy is not merely to solve a current problem. Instead, the purpose is to develop ways of thinking analytically about the problem, experimenting with alternative approaches, and developing skills and ways of thinking that can be generalized to other current or future problems. However, identifying the problem can be a large part of the solution (Mahoney 2006). Not only can identifying the problem increase awareness within an individual, this insight might also allow a person to reframe her thoughts about the problem.

Simply observing and recording one's experience can be helpful. For clients with eating disorders, this can be achieved through food journaling (e.g., recording foods consumed and her associated feelings). Journaling can also include recording compulsive behaviors (e.g., weighing oneself, exercising, purging) and associated feelings. In this context, it may be important to expand the client's focus from self-vigilance of food intake and related rituals to the surrounding social contexts, self-talk, and emotional meanings. Although it can be helpful to increase awareness of food consumption during a binge, or lack of food consumption during a period of restriction, identifying "the problem" or behaviors associated with "the problem" are not always helpful. For a person who has just binged, it can be difficult and embarrassing to recall and admit to food indulgence and to identify the emotions that she experienced before and after the episode of binge eating and purging. Because of the shame often associated with binge eating, clients may be unable or unwilling to comply with this component of treatment. For clients who restrict their food consumption, journaling may serve as reinforcement, allowing the client to actually see how little she has consumed, and she might construe her food restriction positively. Additionally, because of the manipulation, secrecy, and resistance to change that is often present in clients with eating disorders, the potential to lie about food consumption or to be noncompliant in other ways provides additional challenges.

On the other hand, identifying problematic food behaviors can also be beneficial. Increasing awareness of problem behavior can help the client recognize patterns in that behavior and common triggers for maladaptive behaviors. Delay between action and consequence can be a source of struggle for self-control (Mahoney 2006), and poor habits or dysfunctional patterns or cycles may be the result of this struggle. Some bad habits might have positive, immediate effects but detrimental, long-term consequences. For example, self-induced vomiting after an episode of binge eating may provide immediate relief but may eventually result in rotten teeth or a damaged esophagus. Conversely, behaviors involving short-term pain may be construed as involving long-term benefits. For example, self-induced vomiting might allow a person to eat whatever she wants and remain thin, or severe food restriction might result in achieving the "ultimate goal" of being thin.

Exploring both the advantages and disadvantages of both continuing and changing eating-disordered behaviors may provide some understanding of apparent resistance to change and obstacles that will need to be overcome. For instance, a client may see abandoning restrictive patterns as having the possible advantage of preserving her life, but the disadvantage of becoming a disgusting failure. Changing these patterns may have the advantages of better health and increased energy, but the disadvantages of losing friends and being alone. The therapist and client may work together to test beliefs that normal eating will result in being fat, being disgusting to others, and losing friends. In addition, they might explore alternative ways to become close to others and valued by others (and oneself) that do not depend on thinness.

When working with clients with eating disorders, attempting to break cycles of both thought and action can be helpful. For example, for clients who binge and purge, it can be beneficial to attempt to break the binge and purge cycle. Although people who binge eat often report that they would like to stop binge eating, abstaining from this behavior is often difficult, as binge eating might be associated with emotional factors that have not been identified or resolved. One strategy is to focus on the aspect of the cycle that the client may have more control over, the purge. The therapist can acknowledge that binges may continue to occur but suggest that not "allowing" oneself to purge will eventually break the cycle, as the likelihood of binge eating may decrease if the client knows she will not be able to "relieve" herself (i.e., purge) after binge eating. The act of purging can be replaced with journaling, deep breathing, relaxation techniques, or another creative approach suggested by the client or therapist. This alternative to purging might give clients an opportunity to explore emotions associated with binge eating and purging and develop a better understanding of the cycle and associated problems. This approach should be used with caution, as the goal should not be to make the person comfortable with binge eating but to break the cycle and assist the client in identifying healthier alternatives to this behavior.

As is true with all therapeutic interventions, problem solving will not always be effective. This may be especially true when the problem that was focused upon and "solved" was not really the problem. For example, if an adolescent has anorexia nervosa, the problem may not be that she stopped eating. The problem may be that she is afraid to grow up and is afraid of displeasing her parents. By focusing only on helping her regain weight without exploring the associated emotions, her body size might increase but her fear of growing up and displeasing her parents will remain. Misidentifying the problem can create other problems or intensify difficulty (Mahoney 2006). For example, although an adolescent with anorexia begins eating and gains weight, she might be uncomfortable with her weight gain and might begin to engage in cycles of binge eating, purging, and food restriction. Also, problems can improve then return. For example, the problem with binge eating and purging could subside for an adolescent during high school but resurface after beginning college. Additionally, some clients are unsure how to exist without the problem. For instance, being "anorexic" or "bulimic" can become such a large part of one's identity that being without the disorder can result in feelings of loneliness, emptiness, and uncertainty. Therefore, the client and the therapist must work together to anticipate difficulties in the change process. It may be particularly important to work with the client in elaborating self-constructions that are independent of the eating disorder. When eating disorder symptoms are construed as a core part of the client's identity, change becomes very difficult (Button 1985, 1992, 1993).

21.4.7 EXTERNALIZING THE PROBLEM

Rather than describing anorexia, bulimia, and other disordered eating practices as illnesses within individual persons, narrative approaches view them as emerging and being sustained within dominant social forces related to gender, consumerism, the ideal female shape, and acceptable, marketable female and male identities (Gremillion 2003; Little and Hoskins 2004). These social forces may trap people into adopting a set of intense, limiting beliefs and related fears that maintain extreme self-vigilance and severely restricted or chaotic eating. Thus, anorexia and bulimia may be conceived as disempowering cultural practices that are similar to racism, homophobia, and classism (Maisel et al. 2004). For instance, Epston and Maisel (2009, 210) describe anorexia and bulimia as expressions of a "distinctly heinous morality of personhood ... that is remarkably successful in exploiting many dominant contemporary cultural values (e.g., thinness, self-discipline, self-control, individual achievement) in order to appeal to people's vulnerabilities and aspirations." The illusion of control offered by restricting eating behavior may allow adolescents, young adults, and others in identity transitions a temporary sense of self within multiple, conflicting family and cultural expectations. However, the demands of eating disorders eventually exclude other identities and relationships. Therapists must also be cautious not to reproduce ways of relating that encourage eating-disordered practices, such as coercion, adversarial relationships, and vigilant evaluation of bodies (Maisel et al. 2004).

Narrative therapists work with clients to create narratives that counter the version of the self prescribed by eating disorders and also work with clients to build communities of counterpractices. An initial step in this process is often externalizing the problem. The therapist consistently uses language that locates the problem within practices beyond the person and in the person's relationship to those practices. Thus, the eating disorder becomes a problem facing the person, not a defining aspect of the person (White 2007). As a first step in this regard, the problem is given a name in collaboration with the client. Then, the problem is spoken of as outside the person, often as a personalized force with strategies and intentions of its own. Relative influence questions are used to explore the effect of the problem in the lives of the client and the family, including ways that anorexia, for example, has disrupted relationships, dominated lives, and discouraged persons. Questions also explore ways the person or family has been able to stand up to the anorexia, times they have been able to resist its influence, and aspects of their identity that they have been able to protect or recover from anorexia, either individually or together as a family.

Separating the person from the problem opens space to consider other possible versions of the client's identity as well as alternative experiences and knowledge that can be drawn on to resist the eating disorder. It allows the client and family to work together against the problem by avoiding blame of individual persons. It also allows for forming a collaborative therapeutic alliance, as the therapist identifies herself or himself as opposing the eating disorder and promoting, rather than opposing, the client. For instance, when the therapist must act directively in life-threatening situations, this necessity can be presented as "not allowing anorexia to murder the client," and thus as valuing and furthering the relationship with the client, rather than as controlling the client. The therapist continues to validate the worth and experience of the client, even when it is necessary to take steps to ensure the safety to allow change to occur (Epston et al. 1995; Madigan and Goldner 1998; Epston and Maisel 2009).

The life story of a client with an eating disorder may initially appear saturated by the problem. For instance, bulimia may be so embedded in a person's past or current life that it seems impossible not to include it at the center of that person's narrative. For example, consider a woman who desires contentment and control but is unable to escape the unhealthy, self-defeating, destructive cycles of binge eating and self-induced vomiting. What would her narrative be and how could she *not* define herself within the context of this struggle? However, separating herself from bulimia may make it possible to see acts of resistance and wisdom that stand out as turning points in the struggle or that maintain her ability to resist. In this way, the woman herself becomes first author of her narrative, restricting bulimia to a more minor role.

Using a different example, consider the malnourished woman who fears weight gain and has spent the last 7 years of her life avoiding food and social interactions where food was present. Certainly, this constant battle is an important context of her narrative of the last 7 years. But what of foreclosed identities that have been submerged by this battle? What of potential allies, past or future, who could come to her aid? What of the person she is becoming and the person she will be in the future? What of people who have or could value her unique, individual voice and presence in the world, apart from her appearance or other achievements? What does her ability to live through 7 years of self-starvation say of her strength as a person? Although anorexia can become such a dominating reality that little else can be imagined, there are always other stories that could be told. The therapist's role is to create a space for their telling.

Healthcare providers and clients are vulnerable to social practices that locate disorders within persons. People may come to define themselves or others by their mental illness (e.g., "I am anorexic.") Even statements such as "I have anorexia" can locate it as a disorder within the person and potentially a part of her identity. Some people with eating disorders consciously *choose* to continue living with the illness. For example, consider members of "pro-ana" and "pro-mia" societies, where people view anorexia and bulimia as "alternative lifestyles" and support one another's decisions to maintain their eating disorders. These people who are "choosing" to be "anorexic" may be very aware that anorexia nervosa is a disorder. However, they may have poor insight regarding the harm they are doing to themselves by engaging in extreme food restriction. Some, however, may be fully aware of the dangers associated with anorexia nervosa but believe that excessive thinness is worth risking one's health, or even one's life, because engaging in intentional self-starvation can provide a sense of pride or purity. Each person's reasoning for choosing to remain "anorexic" or "bulimic" varies. In some instances, separating the person from the illness and attempting to reframe her thoughts will be quite challenging. Therapists need to be aware of their clients' involvement in communities supporting anorexic or bulimic identities, such as "pro-ana" or "pro-mia" websites, to identify the ways that these communities contribute to one's narrative and to discuss the advantages and disadvantages of participating in these communities (Lock et al. 2005).

While separating oneself from the illness and attempting to reframe thoughts about the disorder could be challenging for some clients, other clients might experience little difficulty viewing the problem as external, but nonetheless see it as benign. For example, a client might refer to her illness as "Annie," both giving the disorder life and offering herself the opportunity to "befriend" "Annie," or to experience "Annie" as befriending her. In such cases, narrative therapists might encourage the client to give "Annie" a "friendship test," exploring the costs of that friendship. Even after gaining insight about the destructive nature of "Annie," being without "Annie" may still seem terrifying. Externalizing eating disorders may give clients the opportunity to reclaim their agency, to take responsibility for their relationship to the problem, and to resist its demands. However, therapists should not minimize the difficulty of change and the associated anguish. This is a gradual process, with inevitable relapses, as the client struggles to construct new identities and practices outside of the disorder.

Although externalizing the problem is a frequent practice within narrative communities, there are some who are uncomfortable with this practice, seeing a potential for clients to experience themselves as victims of the problem and reducing, rather than enhancing, their ability to experience authorship of their life stories (Gremillion 2003). Constructivist and narrative practices offer the client and the therapist alternative languages within which to limit the implications of the problem for the client's life story. For instance, identity is considered multi-storied. The person may be seen as constructing a "community of selves," rather than as being or as having an essential, true self (Mair 1977; Button 1993). Thus, the "anorexic self" may be only one of a larger number of possible selves. Other "selves" might be asked what the "anorexic self" is trying to communicate through her eating disorder symptoms and if there are other ways to express these concerns.

21.4.8 PERFORMING AND THICKENING NEW STORIES

"Persons know life through their storing of lived experience" (Madigan and Goldner 1998, 381), and the stories that we construct about our lives are inherently social. They tell about relationships, and telling is a process of relating to others. Stories of identity are not only told but are performed with others. This performance gives them weight as a lived history or identity. Stories of anorexia, bulimia, and other eating disorders are entrenched in cultural practices and the media images that dominate our daily experiences. They have also often become entrenched in the client's way of being in the world and the client's way of relating to others, becoming a pervasive part of her interactions. The process of becoming disentangled from these eating disorder-saturated stories of identity and relationships requires developing and elaborating alternative stories so that their telling can be heard (White and Epston 1990; White 2007). The therapist assists the client in "re-storying" past, present, and future experience so that these alternative versions of identity become more sub- stantial parts of the self and of social conversations. This often requires recalling and telling about relationships and experiences that have remained relatively unstoried or neglected because they were inconsistent with the dominant problem-saturated story.

It is important to identify or recruit audiences for these new tellings. These audiences often include friends and family members. It can also be valuable for the therapist to provide alternative stories of recovery that offer the client possible pathways for change. As the client progresses in her struggle, new identities may also be strengthened by creating such stories for future audiences and by validat- ing the client by providing an opportunity to share what she has learned in the process. Clients may donate such stories to the therapist's archives to be shared with future clients. Additionally, anti- eating disorder communities, including therapists, allies, and former clients who have overcome eating disorders, can use the archives of material on successful resistance against eating disorders to participate in social activism and to provide support to other therapists and clients who are trying to overcome eating disorders (see Maisel et al. 2004 and www.narrativeapproaches.com).

21.5 CONCLUSION

The topics presented in this chapter provide a small sample of strategies that may be used within constructivist and narrative treatment approaches for eating disorders. They are intended as an introduction to approaches that emphasize the client's meaning making processes, and they view problems of meaning as located within the client's relationship to larger family and cultural stories or conversations. Each therapeutic interaction provides an opportunity to expand upon the strate- gies presented, as our lives are continually enriched by conversations and interactions with others.

To understand others, including clients with problems in their relationship with food, we must understand the personal construction determining their behavior, not only their externally observ- able behavior (Kelly 1958; Button 1993). As therapists, we must also be aware of how we make meaning and what we find meaningful to avoid imposing our own biases on clients. Although it is impossible to completely step outside of our own experience and cultural roles, therapists must attempt to understand clients from within the client's meaning system, created within experiences in the family and larger social and cultural communities. Gaining understanding often includes acknowledging culturally constructed power imbalances, such as gender, race, ethnicity, education, class, income, and sexual orientation, and their potential influence in the therapeutic relationship. The therapist works to validate the client as a maker of meanings and to empower the client as the primary author of her experience. New stories are created within the therapeutic relationship and are further elaborated outside the therapy room through new or revised partnerships with others. The client's active participation in these ongoing conversations is vital to elaborating a preferred identity outside of anorexia, bulimia, or other problems related to food. Meaning making is a personal and social process of continual dialogue and growth, not limited to the adoption of any specific beliefs or static view of reality.

As potential models for their clients, therapists must be aware of their own individual limits, develop their own creative self-care strategies, and reserve time for continued personal and professional development. This is particularly true when working with clients struggling with issues that permeate our culture, because these issues pervade the lives of clients and therapists and make it difficult for clients and therapists to work together therapeutically. Cultural stories of identity, gender, beauty, power, and personal worth are related to the food practices that are associated with eating disorders. Therapists and clients work together to create a space in which they can consider a new relationship to these stories and new roles within them that do not require the client to engage in eating-disordered practices.

REFERENCES

American Psychiatric Association. 2000. *Diagnostic and statistical manual of mental disorders* (4th ed, text revision). Washington, DC: American Psychiatric Association.

Berkman, N. D., K. N. Lohr, and C. M. Bulik. 2007. Outcomes of eating disorders: A systematic review of the literature. *Int J Eat Disord* 40: 293–309.

Borkenhagen, A., B. F. Klapp, E. Brähler, and F. Schoeneich. 2008. Differences in the psychic representation of the body in bulimic and anorexic patients: A study with the body grid. *J Constructivist Psychol* 21: 60–81.

Brown, C. G., S. Weber, and S. Ali. 2008. Women's body talk: A feminist narrative approach. *J Syst Ther* 27: 92–104.

Brown, L. S. 2000. Discomforts of the powerless: Feminist constructions of distress. In *Constructions of disorder: Meaning-making frameworks for psychotherapy*, eds. R. A. Neimeyer and J. D. Raskin, 287–308. Washington, DC: American Psychological Association.

Brownley, K. A., N. D. Berkman, J. A. Sedway, K. N. Lohr, and C. M. Bulik. 2007. Binge eating disorder treatment: A systematic review of randomized controlled trials. *Int J Eat Disord* 40: 337–348.

Bulik, C. M., N. D. Berkman, K. A. Brownley, J. A. Sedway, and K. N. Lohr. 2007. Anorexia nervosa treatment: A systematic review of randomized controlled trials. *Int J Eat Disord* 40: 310–320.

Button, E. 1985. Eating disorders and personal constructs. In *Advances in personal construct psychology, volume 2*, eds. R. A. Neimeyer and G. J. Neimeyer, 3–38. Greenwich, CN: JAI Press.

Button, E. 1992. Eating disorders: A quest for control. In *Personal construct theory and mental health: Theory, research, and practice*, ed. E. Button, 153–168. Cambridge, MA: Brookline Books.

Button, E. 1993. *Eating disorders: Personal construct therapy and change*. New York: Wiley.

Clausen, L. 2004. Review of studies evaluating psychotherapy in bulimia nervosa: The influence of research methods. *Scand J Psychol* 45: 247–252.

Damani, S., E. J. Button, and C. H. Reveley. 2001. The body image structured interview: A new method for the exploration of body image in women with eating disorders. *Eur Eat Disord Rev* 9: 167–181.

Dignon, A., A. Beardsmore, S. Spain, and A. Kuan. 2006. Why I won't eat: Patient testimony from 15 anorexics concerning the causes of their disorder. *J Health Psychol* 11: 942–956.

Epston, D., and R. Maisel. 2009. Anti-anorexia/bulimia: A polemics of life and death. In *Critical feminist approaches to eating disorders*, eds. H. Malson and M. Burns, 209–220. New York: Routledge.

Epston, D., F. Morris, and R. Maisel. 1995. A narrative approach to so-called anorexia/bulimia. In *Cultural resistance: Challenging beliefs about men, women, and therapy*, ed. K. Weingarten, 69–96. Binghamton, NY: Haworth Press.

Fairburn, C. G., and K. Bohn. 2005. Eating disorder NOS (EDNOS): An example of troublesome 'not otherwise specified' (NOS) category in DSM-IV. *Behav Res Ther* 43: 691–701.

Fairburn, C. G., Z. Cooper, and K. Bohn. 2007. The severity and status of eating disorder NOS: Implications for DSM-V. *Behav Res Ther* 45: 1705–1715.

Feixas, G., and J. M. Cornejo Alvarez. 2010. A manual for the repertory grid: Using the Gridcor programme (version 4.0). Accessed June 4, 2011 from http://www.terapiacognitiva.net/record/gridcor.htm.

Fransella, F., ed. 2003. *International handbook of personal construct psychology*. Chichester, England: Wiley.

Fransella, F., R. Bell, and D. Bannister. 2003. *A manual for the repertory grid technique, 2nd edition*. Chichester, England: Wiley.

Freedman, J., and G. Combs. 1996. *Narrative therapy: The social construction of preferred realities*. New York: Norton.

Gremillion, H. 2003. *Feeding anorexia: Gender and power at a treatment center*. Durham, NC: Duke University Press.

Harker, T. 1997. Therapy with male sexual abuse survivors: Contesting oppressive life stories. In *Narrative therapy in practice: The archaeology of hope*, eds. G. Monk, J. Winslade, K. Cricket, and D. Epston, 193–214. San Francisco, CA: Jossey-Bass.

Harter, S. L. 1988. Psychotherapy as a reconstructive process: Implications of integrative theories for outcome research. *Int J Pers Construct Psychol* 1: 349–367.

Harter, S. L. 1995. Construing on the edge: Clinical mythology in working with borderline processes. In *Constructivism in psychotherapy*, eds. R. A. Neimeyer and M. J. Mahoney, 371–383. Washington, DC: American Psychological Association.

Harter, S. L. 2004. Making meaning of child abuse: Personal, social, and narrative processes. In *Studies in meaning 2: Bridging the personal and social in constructivist psychology*, eds. J. D. Rasking and S. K. Bridges, 115–135. New York: Pace University Press.

Harter, S. L. 2007. Visual art making for therapist growth and self care. *J Constructivist Psychol* 20: 167–182.

Hinkle, D. 1965. *The change of personal constructs from the viewpoint of a theory of construct implications*. Doctoral dissertation, Ohio State Univ.

Kelly, G. A. 1955/1991. *The psychology of personal constructs, Volumes 1 and 2*. New York: Routledge.

Kelly, G. A. 1958/1969. Personal construct theory and the psychotherapeutic interview. In *Clinical psychology and personality: The selected papers of George Kelly*, ed. B. Maher, 147–162. New York: Wiley.

Kelly, G. A. 1969. Epilogue: Don Juan. In *Clinical psychology and personality: The selected papers of George Kelly*, ed. B. Maher, 333–351. New York: Wiley.

Little, J. N., and M. L. Hoskins. 2004. "It's an acceptable identity": Constructing "girl" at the intersections of health, media, and meaning-making. *Child Youth Serv* 26: 75–93.

Lock, A., D. Epston, R. Maisel, and N. de Faria. 2005. Resisting anorexia/bulimia: Foucauldian perspectives in narrative therapy. *Br J Guid Counc* 33: 315–332.

Lundgren, J. D., D. Danoff-Burg, and D. A. Anderson. 2004. Cognitive-Behavioral therapy for Bulimia-Nervosa: An empirical analysis of clinical significance. *Int J Eat Disord* 35: 262–274.

Madigan, S. P., and E. M. Goldner. 1998. A narrative approach to anorexia: Discourse, reflexivity, and questions. In *The handbook of constructive therapies: Innovative approaches from leading practitioners*, ed. M. F. Hoyt, 380–400. San Francisco, CA: Jossey-Bass.

Mahoney, M. J. 1988a. Constructive metatheory, I: Basic features and historical foundations. *Int J Pers Construct Psychol* 1: 1–35.

Mahoney, M. J. 1988b. Constructive metatheory, II: Implications for psychotherapy. *Int J Pers Construct Psychol* 1: 299–315.

Mahoney, M. J. 1991. *Human change processes: The scientific foundations of psychotherapy*. New York: Basic Books.

Mahoney, M. J. 2006. *Constructive psychotherapy*. New York: Guilford Press.

Mair, J. M. M. 1977. The community of self. In *New perspectives in personal construct theory*, ed. D. Bannister, 125–149. London, UK: Academic Press.

Mair, J. M. M. 1988. Psychology as storytelling. *Int J Pers Construct Psychol* 1:125–137.

Mair, J. M. M. 1989. *Between psychology and psychotherapy: A poetics of experience*. New York: Routledge.

Maisel, R., D. Epston, and A. Borden. 2004. *Biting the hand that starves you: Inspiring resistance to anorexia/bulimia*. New York: Norton.

Malowe, M. 2007. Mirror, mirror. *The Bulletin*. Accessed October 17, 2007 from the World Wide Web: http://www.apa.org/.

McLeod, J. 1997. *Narrative and psychotherapy*. London, UK: SAGE.

Mottram, M. A. 1985. Personal constructs in anorexia. *J Psychiatr Res* 19: 291–295.

Neimeyer, G. J., and N. Khouzam. 1985. A repertory grid study of restrained eaters. *Br J Med Psychol* 58: 365–367.

Neimeyer, R. A. 1988. Integrative directions in personal construct therapy. *Int J Pers Construct Psychol* 1: 283–297.

Neimeyer, R. A. 2000. Narrative disruptions in the constructions of the self. In *Constructions of disorder: Meaning-making frameworks for psychotherapy*, eds. R. A. Neimeyer and J. D. Raskin, 207–242. Washington, DC: American Psychological Association.

Neimeyer, R. A., and M. J. Mahoney, eds. 1995. *Constructivism in psychotherapy*. Washington, DC: American Psychological Association.

Paris, M. E. 2008. Looking for the context: Therapy as social critique. In *Studies in meaning 3: Constructivist psychotherapy in the real world*, eds. J. D. Raskin and S. K. Bridges, 329–359. New York: Pace University.

Paris, M. E., and F. Epting. 2004. Social and personal construction: Two sides of the same coin. In *Studies in meaning 2: Bridging the personal and social in constructivist psychology,* eds. J. D. Raskin and S. K. Bridges, 3–35. New York: Pace University Press.

Raskin, J. D., and A. M. Lewandowski. 2000. The construction of disorder as human enterprise. In *Constructions of disorder: Meaning-making frameworks for psychotherapy*, eds. R. A. Neimeyer and J. D. Raskin, 15–40. Washington, DC: American Psychological Association.

Shapiro, J. R., B. D. Berkman, K. A. Brownley, J. A. Sedway, K. N. Lohr, and C. M. Bulik. 2007. Bulimia Nervosa treatment: A systematic review of randomized controlled trials. *Int J Eat Disord* 40: 321–336.

Shaw, M., and Gaines, B. 2010. *WebGrid V*. Accessed April 16, 2010 from http://tiger.cpsc.ucalgary.ca/.

Smith, C., and D. Nylund. (eds). 1997. *Narrative therapies with children and adolescents*. New York: Guilford.

Vanderlinden, J. 2008. Many roads lead to Rome: Why does cognitive behavioural therapy remain unsuccessful for many eating disorder pations? *Eur Eat Disord Rev* 16: 329–333.

White, M. 2007. *Maps of narrative practice*. New York: Norton.

White, M., and D. F. Epston. 1990. *Narrative means to therapeutic ends*. New York: Norton.

22 Pharmaceutical Approaches for Treating Eating Disorders

Marta L. Hoes and Brigitte Curtis

CONTENTS

22.1 LEARNING OBJECTIVES

After completing this chapter, you should be able to

- Identify and explain the medications most commonly used to treat anorexia nervosa, bulimia nervosa, and binge eating disorders
- Identify the types of medications used to treat individuals with eating disorders who have other comorbid disorders

- Explain the limitations and side effects of medications for eating disorders
- Describe the importance of the interaction between physicians and mental health professionals in the treatment of individuals with eating disorders

22.2 BACKGROUND AND SIGNIFICANCE

The effects of eating disorders on the human body are always serious, often extremely deleterious, and sometimes even fatal. In fact, eating disorders are associated with the highest mortality rate of all mental illnesses. For patients with anorexia nervosa (AN) alone, the mortality rate can be as high as twelve times that of their unaffected peers (Sullivan 1995). The gravity of eating disorders is intensified by the expanding frequency of individuals meeting the criteria for eating disorder diagnoses, which has reached almost epidemic proportions and appears to be on the rise (Hudson et al. 2007).

In order to treat eating disorders, combat negative physical effects, and prevent the death of patients, a comprehensive plan must be developed to incorporate the healing of both the body and the mind. One method often employed for the treatment of eating disorders is the use of medication. Patients who are treated with both pharmaceutical and psychotherapeutic means exhibit fewer symptoms and are less likely to relapse than patients who only receive one of the two types of treatment (Jimerson et al. 1996; Mitchell and Selders 2005).

Existing research provides evidence that, while medication may not offer a true cure for eating disorders, it may be very beneficial in improving these disorders. Only a few patients improve from pharmacological treatment alone, but when combined with psychological therapy, medical treatment can be a powerful tool. There may not be a miracle drug to cure eating disorders, but there is reason to believe that medication will play an increasing role in the treatment of eating disorders by helping patients stabilize their weight, cope with stress, combat associated mental illnesses, and reduce the symptoms of eating disorders. Table 22.1 lists examples of common medications used in treating eating disorders and other mental disorders that often are associated with them.

The pharmaceutical treatment of eating disorders necessitates the expansion of the treatment team. In addition to psychotherapists and family counselors, physicians can play a large role in the diagnosis and treatment of eating disorders.

TABLE 22.1
Examples of the Types of Psychiatric Medications Used to Treat Eating Disorders and Other Mental Disorders Associated with Them

Types	Generic Names	Trade (Brand) Names
Antipsychotic	Chlorpromazine	Thorazine
	Olanzapine	Zyprexa, Zydis, Relprevv
Tricyclic antidepressants	Amitriptyline	Elavil
MAOIs	Tranylcypromine	Parnate
	Selegiline	Emsam
SSRIs	Fluoxetine	Prozac
	Sertraline	Zoloft
	Fluvoxamine	Luvox
Other antidepressants	Mirtazapine	Remeron
Anticonvulsants	Topiramate	Topamax

Note: MAOIs = monoamine oxidase inhibitors; SSRIs = selective serotonin reuptake inhibitors.

22.2.1 PHYSICAL PROBLEMS ASSOCIATED WITH EATING DISORDERS

Eating disorders produce a wide variety of effects on the human body, affecting almost every system of the body. The digestive system is not the only part of the body to suffer the effects of eating disorders; the cardiovascular, pulmonary, musculoskeletal, dermatological, endocrine, reproductive, and nervous systems are also affected. The main detrimental effects of AN on the human body come as a result of the lack of nutrients available to the body. In addition to the minor and often reversible side effects, such as dry skin and low body temperature, AN can produce serious or even deadly effects, including seizures or sudden cardiac arrest. Patients with bulimia nervosa (BN) or AN who engage in irregular eating patterns and purging behavior add a whole new dimension to the destructive nature of an eating disorder. Self-induced vomiting and laxative abuse are both extremely harmful to the body. The effects of binge eating disorder (BED) may overlap with symptoms of BN, but are almost entirely opposite of the effects of AN. Specifically, many patients with binge eating disorder are obese, and they often face problems, such as high blood pressure and an increased risk of contracting diabetes.

Medical treatment is especially necessary in extreme cases to stabilize a patient with an eating disorder. Doctors may introduce intravenous supplements of necessary chemicals to counteract deficiencies (e.g., potassium deficiency). In the majority of cases, however, normalizing eating patterns is typically the best way to restore health. Healthy eating is often the best medicine for replenishing the body and reversing the effects of eating disorders. The majority of medications prescribed for patients with eating disorders focus more on the neurological elements of the disorder.

22.2.2 THE NEUROLOGY OF EATING DISORDERS

Throughout the past century, a great deal has been discovered about the neurological background of many mental illnesses. Technology now allows us to take images of the brain, track its activity, and measure the levels of chemicals circulating through it. These technological advances have changed modern medicine by giving researchers a greater understanding of the physiological functioning behind mental illness and a clearer idea of pharmaceutical targets in treatment.

Originally, research on the neurology of eating disorders looked at the hypothalamus, which is the hunger and satiety center of the brain. The lateral hypothalamus initiates eating by creating the sensation of hunger, and the ventromedial hypothalamus gives the body a signal of satiety. Studies using test animals showed that alterations to these important regions of the brain could decrease or increase eating behavior (Leibowitz 1970). For example, destruction of the ventromedial hypothalamus in a rat would lead it to eat continuously until it became extremely obese.

As the field of neurology developed over the following decades, researchers began to observe that the brain mechanisms in eating disorders worked in a much more complicated manner than simple alterations to the hypothalamus. Entire nerve tracts are involved in the hunger and satiety responses of the body, and changes in these tracts could affect the function of the hypothalamus. The focus shifted to the role of neurotransmitters, particularly dopamine, norepinephrine, serotonin, and the endogenous opioids. The levels of these neurotransmitters were found to affect appetite, mood, cognition, and other factors related to eating disorders (Ferguson and Pigott 2000).

The discovery of the importance of neurotransmitters in the perpetuation of eating disorders paved the way for the introduction of medication to control the levels of neurotransmitters available in the brain. However, the relationship between neurotransmitter abnormalities and eating disorders is complicated by the fact that abnormal eating patterns have an effect on the availability of certain neurotransmitters in the brain. This makes it very difficult to determine whether neurotransmitter abnormalities are related to the disorder itself, the effects of disordered eating behaviors such as starvation and binge eating, or both.

Even though neurochemical abnormalities may exist, it is important to keep in mind the roles of environmental and emotional factors on young women and children. Genetics may predispose certain individuals, but the cause of eating disorders is actually a complicated sum of biological, sociological, and psychological factors. As such, treatment is never a simple matter of just taking the correct medication.

22.2.3 COMORBIDITY

Much existing research on eating disorders focuses on the relationship of AN, BN, and BED to other mental disorders. It is clear that some relationship exists between eating disorders and other mental health problems, including depression, anxiety disorders, bipolar disorder, and substance abuse, although the nature of the relationships remains somewhat unclear (Herzog et al. 1996). Medical treatment of comorbid disorders may improve patients' overall condition, and even lead to progress in treatment of the eating disorder.

22.2.3.1 Depression

Major depression is a common disorder among women with AN, BN, and BED. Depression is most often treated with the use of antidepressants, a class of drugs that includes tricyclic antidepressants, monoamine oxidase inhibitors, selective serotonin reuptake inhibitors, and serotonin and norepinephrine reuptake inhibitors. These medications are known for their ability to reduce symptoms of depression and improve mood.

The first antidepressants to be developed were the tricyclic antidepressants (TCAs). The antidepressant effect of these drugs was discovered somewhat accidentally in the 1950s, and TCAs have played a major role in the treatment of depression and other mental disorders ever since. In neurotransmission, the presynaptic cell releases neurotransmitters into the space between cells, called the synapse. From this space, neurotransmitters may pass on to the postsynaptic cell receptor, or they may be reabsorbed by the presynaptic cell. TCAs function as reuptake inhibitors to prevent the presynaptic cell from reabsorbing neurotransmitters, causing neurotransmitters to stay in the extracellular space or move on to the postsynaptic receptor. TCAs limit the reuptake of several neurotransmitters, including serotonin, norepinephrine, and dopamine. Although TCAs are still considered highly effective in the treatment of depression, their use has declined somewhat due to their possible side effects. Most of the side effects are mild and often go away over time, but in high doses, TCAs can be toxic to the heart and brain, resulting in overdose and possibly death. Despite this risk, the controlled use of TCAs is generally safe and effective.

Monoamine oxidase inhibitors (MAOIs) work, as their name implies, by inhibiting monoamine oxidase, an enzyme that breaks down several neurotransmitters including serotonin, norepinephrine, and dopamine. MAOIs are often effective in treating depression, even when other types of antidepressants have failed. However, MAOIs are often seen as the last alternative when prescribing an antidepressant because of the side effects associated with the drugs. As MAOIs pass through the body, they may react with other chemicals, producing negative and sometimes even lethal results. The diet of patients taking MAOIs must be carefully controlled, excluding foods containing tyramine, such as certain cheeses and wines. When combined with some other medications, including other types of antidepressants, some over-the-counter medications, and even some herbal supplements, MAOIs may react with these other chemicals to increase blood pressure and even cause a stroke. Due to the diet restrictions associated with MAOIs and the uncontrolled eating behaviors associated with eating disorders, MAOIs are generally not the best fit for patients with eating disorders. However, they may be used in cases when patients do not respond to TCAs or other antidepressants. The latest generation of MAOIs is available in patch form, which allows the drug to enter the bloodstream directly, without first passing through the digestive tract. Emsam is a skin patch that supplies the MAOI selegiline, which is more specific in its action than other MAOIs, which inhibit both MAO-A and MAO-B. Selegiline primarily inhibits MAO-B in the brain and has little effect on MAO-A in the digestive tract, so that there are fewer diet risks with its use. When administered in low doses, other MAOIs also do not have dangerous diet risks (Rosack 2006).

The newest and most common classes of antidepressants are selective serotonin reuptake inhibitors (SSRIs) and serotonin-norepinephrine reuptake inhibitors (SNRIs). These drugs work in the same way as TCAs, only with more specificity. SNRIs increase the neurotransmission of both serotonin and norepinephrine, whereas SSRIs work more selectively than TCAs on serotonin alone. Due largely to their specificity, SSRIs and SNRIs are the safest of all known antidepressants. They produce fewer and milder side effects, and have a much higher toxic dose, making overdose far less likely.

One major limitation to the use of antidepressants is the risk of side effects. The list of possible side effects related to antidepressants is extensive, and patients should be informed about them before they start taking antidepressants (Holmes 1997, 268; Nemeroff and Schatzberg 2007). These possible side effects include insomnia, drowsiness, nervousness, dryness of the mouth, blurred vision, difficulty with urination, weight gain, problems with digestion (nausea, constipation, or diarrhea), and sexual problems (diminished interest in sex or difficulty having orgasms). The severity of unpleasant side effects is usually directly related to the dosage of the antidepressants, so the side effects can be limited if the smallest effective dose of the medication is used. Fortunately, the side effects of antidepressants often become less of a problem as the person's body adjusts to the medication or the person learns to cope effectively with those side effects (Holmes 1997, 268).

Another major limitation to treating patients with antidepressants is the so-called black box warning applied by the Food and Drug Administration (FDA) of the United States government. This warning reflects research findings that adolescents who take antidepressants have an increased risk of suicidal thoughts or even suicide attempts (Bridge et al. 2007). Because individuals with eating disorders are at risk for attempting suicide, it is highly important to use caution when prescribing antidepressants to patients with eating disorders, especially if they are under the age of 25.

22.2.3.2 Anxiety Disorders

Anxiety disorders, such as generalized anxiety disorder (GAD), obsessive-compulsive disorder (OCD), and posttraumatic stress disorder (PTSD), are also very common among women and children with eating disorders. The relationship between anxiety disorders and eating disorders is especially marked for women with AN. In fact, there is even some overlap in the diagnostic criteria for AN and OCD, including a fixation on certain ideas and fears.

Anxiety disorders, such as GAD, OCD, and PTSD, are similar in their neurological response, and are generally treated with similar medications. Many patients with anxiety disorders may be treated with antidepressant medication. SSRIs, SNRIs, TCAs, and MAOIs are all commonly used in the treatment of anxiety disorders. Antidepressants are generally the safest way to treat anxiety disorders, especially in the long term. However, antidepressants often take a while to become effective. In some cases of anxiety disorders, antidepressants may be too slow to act and therefore may be ineffective. In these cases, a class of drugs known as benzodiazepines may be prescribed. Unlike antidepressants, benzodiazepines actually work by decreasing communication between neurons in the brain rather than increasing it. Benzodiazepines work by increasing the action of gamma-aminobutyric acid (GABA), which blocks receptors in the central nervous system, limiting the ability of neurons to become excited, and thus producing a sedative effect. In the short term, benzodiazepines are generally a safe and effective treatment for anxiety disorders. However, the cognitive and muscular sedative effects of benzodiazepines can be harmful if used for extended periods of time (a year or longer), and patients may become at risk for dependence (King 1992). Although toxicity is rare when benzodiazepines are taken alone, the potential for overdose increases when combined with other depressants, such as alcohol.

In addition to antidepressants and benzodiazepines, beta blockers are sometimes used in the treatment of anxiety disorders. Beta blockers block receptors of the sympathetic nervous system, limiting the "fight-or-flight" response of the body. For people with anxiety disorders, beta blockers prevent the increased heart rate, faster breathing, sweating, and tension associated with panic or other extreme levels of anxiety.

22.2.3.3 Bipolar Disorder

In addition to depression and anxiety disorders, patients with eating disorders are also more likely than their unaffected peers to have bipolar disorder (Lunde et al. 2009). The treatment of bipolar disorder is somewhat unique, as patients with bipolar disorder typically experience both manic and depressive episodes. If the correct balance is not achieved, medication may actually worsen manic or depressive behavior.

Bipolar disorder is typically treated with mood stabilizers, the oldest and most common of which is lithium. It remains unclear exactly how lithium works (Stahl 2000). The effectiveness of lithium is probably due to an alteration in neurotransmission in those brain areas that are responsible for a person's moods and where norepinephrine and serotonin are important neurotransmitters. One hypothesis is that lithium works by making those two neurotransmitters less available; another hypothesis is that lithium alters neurotransmission indirectly by stabilizing electrolyte balances (Carson et al. 1988, 572). Lithium is effective in treating bipolar disorder, mainly by preventing manic episodes. Lithium also reduces the risk of suicide in patients with bipolar disorder (Tondo and Baldessarini 2000). The benefits of lithium typically outweigh the side effects in patients with bipolar disorder, although the side effect of weight gain should be noted in the treatment of patients with eating disorders. One of the biggest drawbacks to the use of lithium is the slowness of its action. In some cases, an entire month may pass before the effects of lithium become apparent.

Because lithium works primarily to prevent manic episodes, patients with bipolar disorder may have antidepressants prescribed to decrease their depressive episodes. Patients with bipolar disorder should not be given antidepressants without mood stabilizers, as antidepressants taken alone may induce manic episodes or rapid cycling (Thase and Sachs 2000).

Although their use is less common, antipsychotics may also be prescribed for the treatment of bipolar disorder. Like lithium, the exact mechanism by which antipsychotics help individuals with bipolar disorder is unknown, but they seem to reduce manic episodes by blocking dopamine receptors in the central nervous system. The first generation of antipsychotic medications was marked by severe side effects, including seizures and tardive dyskinesia, a condition that causes involuntary jerking behavior. More recent antipsychotics, sometimes referred to as atypical antipsychotics, produce the same benefits as the first-generation antipsychotics with a lower instance of side effects. However, the drugs are relatively new, and side effects such as tardive dyskinesia may not appear for decades. Only with time will researchers know how much safer the newer generations of antipsychotic medication really are.

22.2.3.4 Substance Abuse

Patients with eating disorders are also more likely than their unaffected peers to abuse drugs and alcohol, and research shows that individuals who binge and purge are more likely to abuse substances than individuals who just severely restrict their food intake (Holderness et al. 1994). The use of medication in the treatment of substance abuse can be very effective in decreasing symptoms of withdrawal, inhibiting cravings, and preventing relapse. For the treatment of alcohol abuse, the FDA has approved three drugs: naltrexone, acamprosate, and disulfiram. The use of medication in the abuse of substances other than alcohol is more complicated and varies greatly for different types of drugs and for different patients.

For women and children with eating disorders, treating comorbid disorders can lead to significant progress in the treatment of the eating disorder itself. Although this method is indirect, treating depression, anxiety disorders, bipolar disorder, substance abuse, or any other mental illness can give the patient a surge of confidence, more energy to devote towards treatment of the eating disorder, and a more positive outlook.

Research on medications for depression, anxiety disorders, and bipolar disorder laid the foundation for research on the pharmaceutical treatment of eating disorders. The majority of medications used to treat eating disorders are the very same medications used to treat other mental disorders.

22.3 CURRENT FINDINGS

Compared to other mental disorders, less is known about the pharmaceutical treatment of eating disorders. The amount of research on medications to treat eating disorders is extensive, but largely unfocused. Many of the studies that exist are inconclusive, only focus on short-term effects, or have relatively small numbers of participants because many individuals with eating disorders discontinue participation before the study has been completed. In some ways, studies on eating disorder pharmacology seem to have brought more questions to the forefront than answers. However, despite the scarcity of conclusive results, existing studies have given researchers more tangible targets and have opened up new possibilities for future research. Researchers with backgrounds in psychology and medicine have an ever-increasing pool of information, as well as a growing hope for treatment in promising new drugs.

22.3.1 ANOREXIA NERVOSA

Among eating disorders, the least is known about the pharmacological treatment of AN. Although AN has the highest mortality rate of all known psychiatric disorders, there is no medication approved by the FDA for the treatment of AN. This is definitely not for lack of effort, as an unusually diverse body of research exists in this area, covering about ten different classes of drugs (Crow et al. 2009). Several factors may play a part in the lack of success of previous research, including participants' lack of willingness to comply, poor choices of pharmacologic targets, participants' nutritional states, the lack of availability of animal test subjects, and the complexity of interaction between physical and mental health. In spite of these factors, recent research indicates a renewed interest in finding an effective drug.

Although no medication is currently known to treat AN directly, psychiatrists and primary care physicians often use pharmacology to treat patients with AN in less direct ways. Medication may be useful in helping patients reach weight goals, treating comorbid disorders, and treating other symptoms of AN. By working indirectly, these drugs can help patients devote more energy towards psychotherapy, see the effects of the disorder more clearly, and achieve goals more quickly.

22.3.1.1 Weight Stabilization

When a patient has AN, the key to effective treatment is for her to reach a stable weight. Until a patient reaches a weight that is less than 15% below the target weight, with at least 10% body fat, weight restoration remains the treatment priority (Schlundt and Johnson 1990, 239). Until weight is restored, pharmacological treatment may have few if any positive results for patients with AN (Zerbe 2008, 38), but once a stable weight has been restored and a sense of trust has been established, pharmaceutical treatment may be a useful way to help the patient achieve her treatment goals. Depending on the patient's weight and condition, the treatment team may find hospitalization and monitored nutritional intake helpful or even necessary to restore a patient to a stable weight. Alternative methods of weight restoration are sometimes employed. Appetite stimulants, including zinc and cisapride, are sometimes used to increase weight, although studies of these supplements have produced inconclusive results (Zerbe 2008, 77).

In extreme cases, the use of a nasogastric feeding tube may be recommended to bring a patient to a stable weight. Using a nasogastric feeding tube allows the patient to receive nutrients while avoiding the act of eating itself. Existing research suggests that the use of a nasogastric feeding tube can be helpful in restoring weight stability, which may serve as a turning point in treatment. After the use of a feeding tube, some participants in a research study began not only to gain weight, but also to resume regular eating and drinking (Neiderman et al. 1999). Despite its effectiveness, the use of a nasogastric feeding tube raises several ethical and legal issues. Its purpose of restoring weight, by nature, goes against the wishes of a patient with AN. This is often a source of conflict between patients and treatment administrators and can lead to breaches in trust or even sabotage of treatment. Although this method is generally effective, it should be considered an option only if other means of improving nutrition become impossible (Neiderman et al. 1999).

22.3.1.2 Antipsychotic Medication

Some of the first drugs to be studied for the treatment of AN were antipsychotic medications, also referred to as neuroleptics or the major tranquilizers. This class of medication is traditionally intended for the treatment of psychotic disorders, such as schizophrenia. Antipsychotics were first investigated for the treatment of AN as a way to reduce the extremely unrealistic ideas associated with the disorder. Many patients with AN have psychotic-like symptoms, including an unrealistic belief system that can interfere with psychological treatment (Court et al. 2008).

Several different antipsychotic medications have been studied, including pimozide, sulpiride, amisulpride, olanzapine, and chlorpromazine. Antipsychotics work by affecting the levels of dopamine, norepinephrine, and serotonin available in the brain. Some of these studies, particularly of chlorpromazine, have concluded that antipsychotics have the ability to decrease psychotic symptoms of AN, including anxiety towards weight gain. In most of these studies, however, there was no significant difference in weight gain between women who were treated with psychotherapy alone and women who received drug therapy in addition to psychotherapy. Additionally, the first generation of antipsychotic medications came with the risk of severe side effects such as seizures and tardive dyskinesia. However, some evidence of a positive response has been noted among the second generation of antipsychotic medications, atypical antipsychotics, which do not have the same serious side effects (Pederson et al. 2003). The second generation antipsychotic olanzapine, for instance, may be useful in restoring weight and preventing relapse for patients with AN.

Antipsychotic medications seem to show promise for helping people with AN eliminate some of the anxiety associated with gaining weight, decrease their impulsive behaviors, and help them in decision making. Currently, not enough research exists to support or refute the use of antipsychotic medication for the treatment of AN. The continued use of antipsychotics in the treatment of AN is based largely on clinical experience and individual treatment procedures rather than a supporting body of research. Future research should include larger sample sizes, greater doses of medication, and more long-term follow-up of patients.

22.3.1.3 Antidepressants

Just as researchers hoped that antipsychotic medication could reduce the psychotic symptoms of AN, they looked to antidepressants to treat the depressive symptoms. Antidepressants are generally viewed as the first line of treatment for several disorders related to AN, such as depression, OCD, and BN, so it follows that antidepressants have been tested for the treatment of AN (Grilo and Mitchell 2010, 176). In fact, antidepressants have been prescribed for women with AN more than any other type of medication (Hsu 1990). Antidepressants work by changing the levels of neurotransmitters available in the brain through different mechanisms, including increased production, increased reception, decreased degradation, and decreased reabsorption. Because of the relationship between AN and altered levels of serotonin, norepinephrine, and dopamine, it follows that researchers attempted to treat AN with antidepressants that made more of these important neurotransmitters available in the brain.

Three different types of antidepressants have been studied for the treatment of AN: MAOIs, TCAs, and SSRIs. While some studies have shown positive results, the majority have found no difference between groups given antidepressants and control groups (Bulik et al. 2007). As with antipsychotics, the research on antidepressants has yet to produce any positive, conclusive results. Another possible direction for future research is to examine the combined effects of antipsychotics and antidepressants. A case study looking at olanzapine and mirtazapine used concurrently, for instance, showed positive results, although more studies are necessary to generalize results (Wang et al. 2006).

22.3.1.4 Hormone Therapy

Anorexia nervosa is associated with abnormal levels of several chemicals in the body. In addition to neurotransmitters, patients with AN often have abnormal levels of hormones. Researchers have attempted to use testosterone, growth hormones, estrogen, and progesterone in treating AN. While hormone therapy is associated with some positive outcomes, such as decreased depressed mood from testosterone supplementation, hormones do not appear to have an effect on the symptoms of AN itself (Bulik et al. 2007).

22.3.1.4.1 Menstrual and Reproductive Problems

A disturbance in one system of the body often creates disruption in another. Menstrual abnormality brought on by disordered eating behavior is an example of this relationship. Dietary inconsistency restricts the body's access to certain neurotransmitters and hormones, which can in turn stop production of the chemicals that induce the different phases of the menstrual cycle, particularly luteinizing hormone and follicle stimulating hormone.

A common occurrence in women with eating disorders is amenorrhea, the cessation of menstrual periods. Amenorrhea and other menstrual disturbances affect almost half of women suffering from BN, and are so common among women with AN that amenorrhea is a *DSM-IV* diagnostic criterion for the disorder (American Psychiatric Association 1994, 545; Zerbe 2008, 165). Because of the high frequency of occurrence, amenorrhea and other menstrual irregularities can be useful indicators of eating disorders to health professionals. Some women with eating disorders seek help from gynecologists to restore menstrual periods and increase fertility, often without informing the physician of the presence of other symptoms of an eating disorder. The administration of fertility treatments to women with eating disorders is strongly discouraged by the American Psychological Association, due to the physical and psychological burdens that accompany pregnancy (Zerbe 2008, 181). Additionally, doctors may not wish to induce menstrual periods in women with eating disorders because amenorrhea can serve as an indication that the disorder exists, even if other symptoms are hidden, and can also help in the determination of a healthy body weight for the specific individual (Garfinkel and Garner 1993, 165).

Menstrual irregularity and hormonal imbalances can produce serious detrimental effects on the female reproductive system. Not only is pregnancy itself more complicated for women with or recovering from eating disorders, but it can also be difficult or even impossible for them to become pregnant in the first place. Despite amenorrhea and other menstrual disturbances, disordered eating behavior is by no means a sure way of preventing pregnancy. While the likelihood of conceiving and carrying a child to term diminishes for women with AN, BN, or compulsive overeating, women with these disorders are often able to have children. However, health professionals must show extreme caution when working with pregnant women with AN and BN, as their symptoms often increase with pregnancy. Women with eating disorders who become pregnant often gain very little weight with pregnancy, and often deliver their children prematurely. Naturally, the mothers' health problems can have serious consequences on the health of their children. Babies born to mothers with eating disorders often have developmental problems resulting from inadequate nutrition in utero. Perinatal mortality, psychosocial deprivation, and growth retardation are more common for the children of women with eating disorders, as is a higher risk of failure to thrive in the first year of life. During pregnancy, women with eating disorders often report concerns about weight gain and loss of control of one's body, and may report either fear about infant malnutrition or the conflicting fear of bearing an overweight child (Zerbe 2008).

22.3.1.4.2 Osteoporosis

The effects of eating disorders on the body are often reversible with treatment, especially when the patient begins to consume necessary amounts of vital nutrients on a regular basis. However, some tissue loss is difficult to reverse, as the body does not continue to produce certain tissues at the rate at which they were destroyed. Bone loss is a frequently occurring problem among patients with AN, and begins to occur in the early stages of the disorder, even in younger patients (Audi et al. 2002; Bachrach et al. 1990). After only 6 to 12 months with AN, patients have an increased risk of significant bone mineral loss (Wong et al. 2001). Patients with osteoporosis have an increased likelihood of skeletal injury.

In postmenopausal women, hormone therapy is an effective and commonly used way to treat osteoporosis by minimizing its effects, such as decreased bone density. However, studies of the use of hormone therapy, including estrogen supplements and oral contraceptives, indicate that the same positive effects are not prevalent in women with AN (Mehler and Mackenzie 2009). One focus of current research is on the use of bisphosphonates, which may be more effective than estrogen supplements in restoring bone mineral density to women with AN.

22.3.2 Bulimia Nervosa

Compared to AN, the research background for BN is both more extensive and more optimistic. More studies have been conducted, some with positive results. While no drug is considered the cure for BN, several drugs seem to be effective in reducing symptoms and preventing relapse.

As with AN, patients with low body weight must achieve stability before medication can be fully effective. Normalization of nutritional intake should be the treatment priority, regardless of the patient's weight. After a regular, normal pattern of eating nutritious food has been established, pharmacological treatment is both safer and more effective.

22.3.2.1 Antidepressants

Antidepressants have been researched and prescribed in the treatment of BN more than any other type of drug (Pederson et al. 2003). All three major classes of antidepressants—TCAs, MAOIs, and SSRIs—seem to have positive effects on patients with BN (Bacaltchuk et al. 2000). Not only can antidepressants reduce the depressive symptoms that accompany BN, but they also improve mood and reduce the likelihood of relapse in recovered patients. Antidepressants may also be useful for patients who do not respond initially to cognitive behavioral therapies (Grilo and Mitchell 2010, 397).

Tricyclic antidepressants have been shown to reduce binge eating, lower preoccupation with food, and improve overall functioning. In addition to the benefits common to antidepressants, SSRIs have been linked to a reduction in binge eating, and a cessation of purging behavior. Perhaps the most extensive research in the field of eating disorder pharmacology has been that of the use of fluoxetine in the treatment of BN. Several studies supported the use of fluoxetine before it was accepted by the FDA, and it remains the only medication approved by the FDA for the treatment of BN (Ferguson and Pigott 2000, 248). Since its acceptance, further studies and clinical experience have supported its use, and it is currently considered to be the "gold standard" for the pharmacological treatment of BN (Grilo and Mitchell 2010, 390). The efficacy of fluoxetine extends beyond the specialty of psychiatry; the prescription of fluoxetine by primary care physicians may be a useful intervention for the treatment of BN (Walsh et al. 2004).

MAOIs have not been studied as extensively as TCAs and SSRIs in the treatment of BN. One major limitation of MAOI studies is the strict diet that must be maintained to prevent side effects of the medication. This is often difficult for patients with BN, a disorder marked by uncontrolled eating behavior. Results of several studies with MAOIs indicate a reduction in binge eating, but the diet restrictions associated with MAOIs pay prevent doctors from prescribing them to patients with BN (Zerbe 2008, 79).

Antidepressants seem to work in a variety of ways to treat BN. Not only do they reduce the depressive symptoms associated with the disorder, but they also help to decrease hunger and increase feelings of satiety, decrease the effects of stress, and even seem to reduce the core symptoms of BN (binge eating and compensatory behaviors, such as self-induced vomiting).

22.3.2.2 Anticonvulsants

The study of anticonvulsants in the treatment of BN stems from the view of a binge eating episode as a seizure-like behavior. Anticonvulsants were originally developed to treat epileptic seizures, but after their success in the treatment of bipolar disorder, studies were conducted to determine their effects on BN. These studies have produced some promising results, particularly from the relationship between anticonvulsant medication and reduced bingeing behavior. The anticonvulsant topiramate, for example, although not yet approved by the FDA, is associated with a reduced number of bingeing episodes as well as weight loss (Arbaizar et al. 2008).

22.3.2.3 Dental Problems

In addition to the other systems of the body, eating disorders can take a great toll on teeth. Behaviors such as self-induced vomiting and bingeing on foods high in sugar and other carbohydrates expose the teeth to an unhealthy amount of acid. Contact with acids can cause a number of dental complications, including enamel erosion, enlargement of salivary glands, increased sensitivity to hot or cold temperatures, and dryness of mouth, throat, palate, and lips. Damage to the teeth and gums is largely a cosmetic problem, but can also lead to increased susceptibility to infection, pain, difficulty eating, and even loss of teeth.

The dental problems associated with eating disorders introduce a new professional into the treatment of patients: the dentist. In addition to family members, physicians, psychotherapists, and other individuals involved in the recovery of patients with eating disorders, dentists often need to join the treatment team in combating these disorders and improving their patients' health. Cosmetic dentists play an additional role in treatment, as their work may help increase self-esteem and improve body image, which may help improve the patient's mental and emotional well-being. Dentists may also be able to provide helpful information in the early diagnosis of BN, as the effects of BN on the mouth provide a fairly reliable means of identifying the disorder. While no single symptoms stands alone as an indication of BN, the sum of several factors, such as swelling beneath the tongue, erosion of tooth enamel, and cracked lips, may help the dentist identify the disorder and encourage the patient to seek treatment (Kaplan and Garfinkel 1993, 101–112).

22.3.3 Binge Eating Disorder

Binge eating disorder was not identified as a potential disorder to be investigated and considered for inclusion in the next edition of the DSM until decades after AN and BN were firmly established as eating disorders (American Psychiatric Association 1994, 729–731). As a relatively new eating disorder, the pool of research on the pharmacological treatment of BED is fairly small but surprisingly promising (Brownley et al. 2007). Medical treatment for this disorder often overlaps with treatment for BN, as medication for both disorders attempts to focus on reduction of bingeing behavior.

22.3.3.1 Antidepressants

Antidepressants are the primary medication used in the treatment of BED, as well as other unspecified eating disorders. Comorbidity of depression in women with BED is common, and may make treatment of the eating disorder more complicated (Linde et al. 2004), which may explain the efficacy of antidepressants in women with BED. SSRIs are the most commonly prescribed medication, although other classes of antidepressants, such as TCAs, have also been studied.

Antidepressants—fluoxetine and fluvoxamine in particular—are associated with reduced frequency of binge eating, fewer symptoms of depression, and a reduction in obsessions and compulsions related to BED (Arnold et el. 2002; Brownley et al. 2007). Surprisingly, SSRIs are also associated with weight loss in patients with BED, although SSRIs can have a side effect of weight gain (Zerbe 2008, 80).

22.3.3.2 Anticonvulsants

Antidepressants are not the only medication to have met some success in the treatment of BED. Due to the seizure-like nature of bingeing episodes and promising results in studies of patients with BN, researchers have experimented with anticonvulsant medications in the treatment of BED.

Anticonvulsants, such as topiramate, are associated with a reduction in binge eating episodes over time, as well as fewer obsessions and compulsions related to binge eating disorder. However, anticonvulsants do not appear to have the same capacity for increasing weight loss or decreasing depressive symptoms as seen with antidepressants.

22.3.3.3 Anti-Obesity Medications

Although some patients with BED fall into a healthy weight category, a strong connection exists between BED and obesity. This connection has led researchers to the area of anti-obesity medication in the search for an effective treatment for BED. Anti-obesity medication is a broad term, encompassing appetite suppressants and medications intended to speed up caloric intake. Unfortunately, many anti-obesity medications have dangerous side effects, such as increasing blood pressure and risk of heart disease (Kolanowski 1999). In some cases, the costs of medication outweigh the benefits. While anti-obesity medications appear to be effective in reducing weight in patients with BED, further research is needed to evaluate the risks involved.

As with research on AN and BN, the sample size of many studies on BED medication has been small, and several studies have reported a high dropout rate (Brownley et al. 2007). Additionally, the relatively recent identification of the disorder means that most existing research has only taken place in the last few decades. Further studies should attempt to incorporate more participants, retain high enrollment in studies, and look at the effects of medication, including weight loss, over a longer period of time than in previous studies.

22.3.4 The Treatment Team

The medical problems resulting from eating disorders mandate the involvement of several different professionals in the treatment process. Not only must psychotherapists and family counselors be involved, but also primary care physicians, psychiatrists, dietitians, and dentists. Integrating the ideas of several professionals from different disciplines can complicate treatment. Without communication and agreement between the different professionals, the patient may receive different and even conflicting opinions about the direction of treatment, creating another roadblock on the path to wellness.

22.3.4.1 Legal Issues

Due to the strict code of privacy involved in the practice of psychology and medicine, communication between professionals can be difficult. Physicians and therapists must be very careful in sharing a patient's information with each other. Having the patient sign a release for information to be shared among a psychotherapist, a primary care physician, a psychiatrist, and a dietitian provides a way to ease the process and remind the patient of the teamwork involved in the treatment of eating disorders. With a release in place, each party involved in treatment is free to initiate communication with another without fear of legal difficulties. However, to prevent a breach of the patient's trust, it is still best to explain to the patient exactly what information will be shared.

22.3.4.2 Primary Care Physicians and Early Diagnosis

One important role physicians may be able to play in the battle against eating disorders is becoming more involved in early diagnosis. An earlier diagnosis, along with earlier intervention, is related to better outcomes in patients with eating disorders (Bryant-Waugh et al. 1988). Alternatively, failure to diagnose and to begin treatment of early-onset AN decreases the likelihood of a positive outcome (Pritts and Susman 2003). By observing certain symptoms more closely, primary care physicians may be able to identify the early warning signs and to refer the patient to a therapist earlier in the onset of an eating disorder.

Some indicators of AN may include low body weight, amenorrhea, intolerance to cold, growth of fine lanugo hair, fainting, fatigue, dry skin, and the loss of muscle mass, fat, or hair. Patients suffering from BN may report abdominal pain or sore throat and may have calluses on their knuckles, often referred to as Russell's sign. Patients with BED may be more difficult to identify, although obesity may be an indication of the disorder. Studies show that the very nature of the office visits of individual patients may be helpful in the early diagnosis of eating disorders (Lask et al. 2005; Ogg et al. 1997). Even one consultation about a patient's concern about her weight or shape may be a predictor of the early onset of an eating disorder. An unusually high number of psychological, gynecologic, and gastrointestinal consultations may also be an indicator of eating disorders in adults. Due to the higher frequency of certain mental health problems and obvious physical characteristics, primary care physicians may determine that certain patients are at a higher risk for developing eating disorders, and as such, should be screened during regular visits.

Simply being more educated about eating disorders is associated with a greater degree of eating disorder detection among primary care physicians (Hoek 1991). Physicians with a greater knowledge of eating disorders are more likely to suggest follow-up appointments to patients with symptoms of eating disorders (Currin et al. 2009). In addition to helping to catch early warning signs, the education of health professionals may help improve their attitudes towards patients with eating disorders, which are often negative (Fleming and Szmukler 1992; Hay et al. 2005). In fact, health professionals and medical students ranked AN low in status compared to other illnesses (Album and Westin 2008). Increasing health professionals' education in the field of eating disorders could lead to higher standards of treatment for patients in the future.

22.4 SUMMARY AND CONCLUSIONS

The medical treatment of eating disorders is complicated. Without a direct form of pharmaceutical intervention, doctors must focus on the symptoms and related disorders associated with AN, BN, and BED. Professionals involved in the treatment of eating disorders should be conscious of the harmful effects eating disorders have on many different parts of the body, and should be prepared to make patients aware of the risks.

The medical treatment of individuals with disordered eating behavior requires cooperation between physicians, psychologists, and other health professionals. All parties involved must keep the patient's interest as the main concern and come to an agreement about overall goals in treatment. By working together as a team, specialists in mental health and bodily health can contribute to the improvement of patients with eating disorders.

Despite current limitations, pharmaceutical intervention to treat eating disorders may help reduce symptoms, combat the effects of comorbid disorders, prevent relapse, or even serve as an important turning point in the treatment of a patient with AN, BN, or BED.

REFERENCES

Album, D., and S. Westin. 2008. Do diseases have a prestige hierarchy? A survey among physicians and medical students. *Soc Sci Med* 66: 182–188.

American Psychiatric Association. 1994. *Diagnostic and statistical manual of mental disorders* (4th ed.). Washington, DC: APA.

Arbaizar, B., I. Gomez-Acebo, and J. Llorca. 2008. Efficacy of topiramate in bulimia nervosa and binge-eating disorder: A systematic review. *Gen Hosp Psychiatry* 30: 471–475.

Arnold, L. M., S. L. McElroy, J. I. Hudson, J. A. Welge, A. J. Bennett, and P. E. Keck. 2002. A placebo-controlled, randomized trial of fluoxetine in the treatment of binge-eating disorder. *J Clin Psychiatry* 63: 1028–1033.

Audi, L., D. M. Vargas, M. Gussinye, D. Yeste, G. Marti, and A. Carrascosa. 2002. Clinical and biochemical determinants of bone metabolism and bone mass in adolescent female patients with anorexia nervosa. *Pediatr Red* 51: 497–504.

Bacaltchuk, J., P. Hay, and J. Mari. 2000. Antidepressant versus placebo for the treatment of bulimia nervosa: A systematic review. *Aust N Z J Psychiatry* 34: 310–317.

Bachrach, L. K., D. Guido, D. Katman, I. F. Litt, and R. Marus. 1990. Decreased bone density in adolescent girls with anorexia nervosa. *Pediatrics* 86: 440–447.

Bridge, J. A., S. Iyengar, C. B. Salary, R. P. Barbe, B. Birmaher, H. A. Pincus, L. Ren, and D. A. Brent. 2007. Clinical response and risk for reported suicidal ideation and suicide attempts in pediatric antidepressant treatment, a meta-analysis of randomized controlled trials. *JAMA* 297: 1683–1696.

Brownley, K. A., N. D. Berkman, J. A. Sedway, K. N. Lohr, and C. M. Bulik. 2007. Binge eating disorder treatment: A systematic review of randomized controlled trials. *Int J Eat Disord* 40: 337–348.

Bryant-Waugh, R., J. Knibbs, A. Fosson, Z. Kaminski, and B. Lask. 1988. Long term follow up of patients with early onset anorexia nervosa. *Arch Dis Child* 63: 5–9.

Bulik, C. M., N. D. Berkman, K. A. Brownley, J. A. Sedway, and K. N. Lohr. 2007. Anorexia nervosa treatment: A systematic review of randomized controlled trials. *Int J Eat Disord* 40: 310–320.

Carson, R. C., J. N. Butcher, and J. C. Coleman. 1988. *Abnormal psychology and modern life* (8th ed.). Glenview, IL: Scott, Foresman and Company.

Court, A., C. Mulder, S. E. Hetrick, R. Purcell, and P. D. McGorry. 2008. What is the scientific evidence for the use of antipsychotic medication in anorexia nervosa? *Eat Disord* 16: 217–223.

Crow, S. J., J. E. Mitchell, J. D. Roerig, and K. Steffen. 2009. What potential role is there for medication treatment in anorexia nervosa? *Int J Eat Disord* 42: 1–8.

Currin, L., G. Waller, and U. Schmidt. 2009. Primary care physicians' knowledge of and attitudes toward the eating disorders: Do they affect clinical actions? *Int J Eat Disord* 42: 453–458.

Ferguson, C. P., and T. A. Pigott. 2000. Anorexia and bulimia nervosa: Neurobiology and pharmacotherapy. *Behav Ther* 31: 237–263.

Fleming, J., and G. I. Szmukler. 1992. Attitudes of medical professionals towards patients with eating disorders. *Aust N Z J Psychiatry* 26: 436–443.

Garfinkel, P. E., and D. M. Garner. 1993. *The role of drug treatments for eating disorders*. New York: Brunner/Mazel.

Grilo, C. M., and J. E. Mitchell. 2010. *The treatment of eating disorders: A clinical handbook*. New York: Guilford Press.

Hay, P. J., C. de Angelis, H. Millar, and J. Mond. 2005. Bulimia nervosa mental health literacy of general practitioners. *Prim Care Community Psychiatr* 10: 103–108.

Herzog, D. B., K. M. Nussbaum, and A. K. Marmor. 1996. Co-morbidity and outcome in eating disorders. *Psychiatr Clin North Am* 19: 843–859.

Hoek, H. W. 1991. The incidence and prevalence of anorexia nervosa and bulimia nervosa in primary care. *Psychol Med* 21: 455–460.

Holderness, C. C., J. Brooks-Gunn, and M. P. Warren. 1994. Co-morbidity of eating disorders and substance abuse: review of the literature. *Int J Eat Disord* 16: 1–34.

Holmes, D. S. 1997. *Abnormal psychology* (3rd ed.). New York: Longman.

Hudson, J. I., E. Hiripi, H. G. Pope Jr., and R. C. Kessler. 2007. The prevalence and correlates of eating disorders in the National Comorbidity Survey Replication. *Biol Psychiatry* 61: 348–358.

Hsu, L. K. G. 1990. *Eating disorders*. New York: Guilford Press.

Jimerson, D. C., B. E. Wolfe, A. W. Brotman, and E. D. Metzger. 1996. Medications in the treatment of eating disorders. *Psychiatr Clin North Am* 19: 739–754.

Kaplan, A. S., and P. E. Garfinkel, eds. 1993. *Medical issues and the eating disorders: The interface*. New York: Brunner/Mazel.

King, M. B. 1992. Is there still a role for benzodiazepines in general practice? *Br J Gen Pract* 42: 202–205.

Kolanowski, J. 1999. A risk–benefit assessment of anti-obesity drugs. *Drug Saf* 20: 119–131.

Lask, B., R. Bryant-Waugh, F. Wright, M. Campbell, K. Willoughby, and G. Waller. 2005. Family physician consultation patterns indicate high risk for early-onset anorexia nervosa. *Int J Eat Disord* 38: 269–272.

Leibowitz, S. F. 1970. Reciprocal hunger-regulating circuits involving alpha- and beta-adrenergic receptors located, respectively, in the ventromedial and lateral hypothalamus. *Proc Natl Acad Sci* 67: 1063–1070.

Linde, J. A., R. W. Jeffery, R. L. Levy, N. E. Sherwood, J. Utter, N. P. Pronk, and R. G. Boyle. 2004. Binge eating disorder, weight control self-efficacy, and depression in overweight men and women. *Int J Obes* 28: 418–425.

Lunde, A. V., O. B. Fasmer, K. K. Akiskal, H. S. Akiskal, and K. J. Oedegaard. 2009. The relationship of bulimia and anorexia nervosa with bipolar disorder and its temperamental foundations. *J Affect Disord* 115: 309–314.

Mehler, P. S., and T. D. MacKenzie. 2009. Treatment of osteopenia and osteoporosis in anorexia nervosa: A systematic review of the literature. *Int J Eat Disord* 42: 195–201.

Mitchell, J. E., and A. Selders. 2005. Recent treatment research in bulimia nervosa. *Eat Disord Rev* 16: 1–3.

Neiderman, M., M. Zarody, M. Tattersall, and B. Lask. 1999. Enteric feeding in severe adolescent anorexia nervosa: A report of four cases. *Int J Eat Disord* 28: 470–475.

Nemeroff, C. B., and A. F. Schatzberg. 2007. Pharmacological treatments for unipolar depression. In *A guide to treatments that work*, ed. P. E. Nathan and J. M. Gorman, 217–288. New York: Oxford Univ. Press.

Ogg, E., H. Millar, E. Pusztai, and A. Thorn. 1997. General practice consultation patterns preceding diagnosis of eating disorders. *Int J Eat Disord* 22: 89–93.

Pederson, K. J., J. L. Roerig, and J. E. Mitchell. 2003. Towards the pharmacotherapy of eating disorders. *Expert Opin Pharmacother* 4: 1659–1678.

Pritts, S. D., and J. Susman. 2003. Diagnosis of eating disorders in primary care. *Am Fam Physician* 67: 297–304.

Rosack, J. 2006. MAOI skin patch wins FDA approval for depression. *Psychiatr News* 41: 31.

Schlundt, D. G., and W. G. Johnson 1990. *Eating disorders: Assessment and treatment.* Boston: Allyn and Bacon.

Stahl, S. M. 2000. *Essential psychopharmacology: Neuroscientific basis and practical applications* (2nd ed.). Cambridge, UK: Cambridge Univ. Press.

Sullivan, P. F. 1995. Mortality in anorexia nervosa. *Am J Psychiatry* 152: 1073–1074.

Thase, M. E, and G. S. Sachs. 2000. Bipolar depression: Pharmacotherapy and related therapeutic strategies. *Biol Psychiatry* 48: 558–572.

Tondo, L., and R. J. Baldessarini. 2000. Reduced suicide risk during lithium maintenance treatment. *J Clin Psychiatry* 61 Suppl 9: 97–104.

Walsh, B. T., C. G. Fairburn, D. Mickley, R. Sysko, and M. K. Parides. 2004. Treatment of bulimia nervosa in a primary care setting. *Am J Psychiatry* 161: 556–561.

Wang, T., C. Yuan-Hwa, and I. Shiah. 2006. Combined treatment of olanzapine and mirtazapine in anorexia nervosa associated with major depression. *Prog in Neuropsychopharmacol Biol Psychiatry* 30: 306–309.

Wong, J. C., P. Lewindon, R. Mortimer, and R. Shepherd. 2001. Bone mineral density in adolescent females with recently diagnosed anorexia nervosa. *Int J Eat Disord* 29: 11–16.

Zerbe, K. J. 2008. *Integrated treatment of eating disorders: Beyond the body betrayed.* New York: Norton.

Index

Note: Page numbers followed by "*f*" and "*t*" denote figures and tables, respectively.